ENVIRONMENTAL IMPACT DATA BOOK

ENVIRONMENTAL IMPACT DATA BOOK

by

JACK GOLDEN
Head, Environmental Assessment & Planning Department
MITRE Corporation, McLean, Virginia

ROBERT P. OUELLETTE
Associate Technical Director
Energy, Resources & Environment
MITRE Corporation, McLean, Virginia

SHARON SAARI
Technical Staff
MITRE Corporation, McLean, Virginia

PAUL N. CHEREMISINOFF
Consulting Engineer
Closter, New Jersey

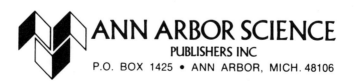

ANN ARBOR SCIENCE
PUBLISHERS INC
P.O. BOX 1425 • ANN ARBOR, MICH. 48106

This book will serve as a data reference, to supplement other sources used regularly in the preparation of environmental impact assessments and statements (EIS). It assumes the user is already involved in the environmental impact process and knows the format and data required by law. The intent of the book is to provide needed data from one composite source. Information is presented, usually in tabular format, to aid in quantification of impacts. Far too many EISs quantify only descriptive data for the existing environmental setting. When the impact chapter is written, words such as minimal, moderate or significant begin to creep into the text. It is our intent to provide quantifiable data to predict these impacts.

Another goal is to provide summary data that are used almost daily in environmental impact statement preparation. The data book is a compilation of other regularly used sources, from the *Federal Register*, to environmental law books, technical papers, textbooks and government publications. Since the authors are all involved professionally in EIS preparation, we have gathered the most often used data into shortened tables for ready reference. This allows the user to turn quickly to one source, rather than to hundreds of papers, to find needed information. The time and shelf space saved is intended to help shorten the normal 31-month time frame for EIS preparation. Data are provided on a national and statewide scope. No data are used which would be useful only on a site-specific case study.

This book, by its content and structure, addresses the environmental scientist or analyst rapidly drowning in the data made available to him through the marvel of technology. While this is a data book, it is not a "cook-book"; it does not provide ready-made, easy answers to complex and difficult problems. Chapters in the book represent the major technical aspects of an environmental assessment. This is not a book to be read but a book to be used.

The authors have exercised their best efforts to obtain the large volume of technical data contained in this book from reliable sources; but to avoid some errors that may have occurred in tables and text, it is recommended that users of this work evaluate carefully the data, facts and figures prior to their use. Figures and tables are referenced as to origin, unless specifically prepared for this book. Hopefully, only primary references or citations are used; if a secondary citation is used, please accept our apologies.

Jack Golden

Robert Ouellette

Sharon Saari

Paul Cheremisinoff

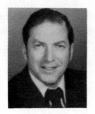
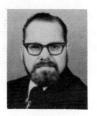
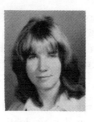
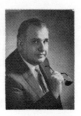

| Golden | Ouellette | Saari | Cheremisinoff |

Jack Golden is head of the Environmental Assessment and Planning Department of the MITRE Corporation, McLean, Virginia, where he has directed the preparation of numerous environmental impact assessments and environmental impact statements on a variety of subjects, including water-related construction projects, nuclear projects, new energy technology projects, energy fuel cycle studies, rate increase projects, and multiple–use potential studies dealing with large land sites. Mr. Golden graduated from City College of New York and earned master's degrees from New York University in meteorology and in environmental health science. He was a member of the New York University faculty as a research scientist. During the past ten years, he has authored articles on air pollution monitoring and environmental legislation.

Robert P. Ouellette is Associate Technical Director of Energy, Resources and the Environment for METREK, a division of the MITRE Corporation. Dr. Ouellette has been associated with MITRE in varying capacities since 1969 and has been associate technical director since 1974. Earlier, he was with TRW Systems, Hazelton Labs, Inc. and Massachusetts General Hospital. He graduated from the University of Montreal and received his PhD from the University of Ottawa. A member of the American Statistical Association, Biometrics Society, Atomic Industrial Forum and the NSF Technical Advisory Panel on Hazardous Substances, Dr. Ouellette has published numerous technical papers and books on energy and the environment. He edited the comprehensive survey, *Electrotechnology* (Ann Arbor Science, 1977).

Sharon Saari has been evaluating environmental problems since 1970, with both private and public agencies. She has worked on environmental impact statements from the Virgin Islands to Alaska and on assessment of projects in 42 states. Her experience includes impacts of energy development, highways, airports, dredging and filling, offshore oil facilities, dams, and housing and recreation developments, as well as federal government programs that affect natural resources. Ms. Saari received a baccalaureate degree in agricultural science from the University of Illinois in 1966. Her master's degree is from the School of Forest Resources of the University of Georgia. Her first job was with Georgia's Institute of Ecology, interpreting ecological issues for the public. A professional conservation representative and consultant on environmental issues from 1970 to 1972, Ms. Saari has written popular environmental articles and co-authored numerous environmental impact statements.

Paul N. Cheremisinoff, P.E., is Associate Professor of Environmental Engineering at New Jersey Institute of Technology and is a consulting engineer. He has almost thirty years of practical hands-on design, development and manufacturing engineering experience as well as being an authority in pollution control. A registered Professional Engineer, he is the author of many publications, including several Ann Arbor Science Handbooks (*Pollution Engineering Practice Handbook, Industrial Odor Technology Assessment, Industrial Noise Control Handbook, Environmental Assessment and Impact Statement Handbook*), associate editor of *Water & Sewage Works*, and editor-in-chief of *Reuse/Recycle* and *Environmental Impact News*.

CONTENTS

1. INTRODUCTION 1
2. TECHNIQUES FOR AIDING IN THE ASSESSMENT PROCESS . 23
3. DATA BASES 73
4. MODELS 147
5. LEGAL FRAMEWORK 241
6. AIR QUALITY 277
7. WATER RESOURCES 431
8. NOISE 505
9. PHYSICAL RESOURCES 549
10. ECOSYSTEMS 601
11. ECOSYSTEMS–EXAMPLES 665
12. TOXIC CHEMICALS 699
13. CULTURAL 731
14. ENERGY 767
15. TRANSPORTATION 811

INDEX 859

LIST OF TABLES

Table   Page

1-1   Summary of Environmental Impact Statements Filed with the CEQ 2

1-2   Agency NEPA Procedures (The Seventh General Report of the CEQ) 5

1-3   Environmental Impact Analysis Areas 18

2-1   Classification of Assessment Techniques 27

3-1   Summarized List of Environmental Data Services 74

3-2   Data Handling and Information Systems at the Federal Level. ... 79

3-3   Federal Data Retrieval and Information Systems—Air. 81

3-4   Federal Data Retrieval and Information Systems—Water 84

3-5   Federal Data Retrieval and Information Systems—Solid Waste .. 88

3-6   Federal Data Retrieval and Information Systems—Noise 88

3-7   Federal Data Retrieval and Information Systems—Toxicological Substances 89

3-8   Federal Data Retrieval Systems—Total Environment 92

3-9   EPA's Environmental Radiation Ambient Monitoring System Current Status 95

3-10   FEA Energy Program Summary 96

3-11   Energy Data Systems 97

3-12   State Energy Information Systems Matrix 99

3-13   Data System Scoring 104

3-14   Data Systems Applicable to Substance Identification 115

3-15   Data Systems Applicable to Production 118

3-16   Data Systems Applicable to Marketing. 119

3-17   Data Systems Applicable to Exposure 120

3-18   Data Systems Applicable to Epidemiology 121

3-19   Data Systems Applicable to Biological Effects. 123

3-20   Data Systems Applicable to Environmental Effects 124

3-21   Data Systems Applicable to Standards and Regulations. 125

3-22   Source of Data and the Proprietary Status of the Primary Systems. 126

3-23 Collections Identified in NESB Survey Classified According
       to Type of Collection.   130
3-24 Collections Identified in NESB Survey Classified According
       to Component of Interest in Specimens.   130
3-25 Collections Identified in NESB Survey Classified According
       to Use of Collection.   131
3-26 Collections Identified in NESB Survey Classified According
       to Collection Contents   132
3-27 Bibliographic Computerized Systems.   133
4-1   Sound Level Weighting Function for Overall Impact Analysis. . .   156
4-2   Weighting Function for Loss of Hearing/Severe Health Effects. .   158
4-3   Sample Standard Grid Analysis Printout   160
4-4   Summary of Cooling Tower Plume Models.   162
4-5   Comparison of Air Quality Models   174
4-6   Comparison of Water Quality Models   192
4-7   Methods and Models for Predicting Flow Changes in Estuaries . .   196
4-8   Methods and Models for Predicting Effects of Flow Changes
       on Water Quality in Estuaries—Literature Matrix.   197
4-9   Low-Resolution Models for Water Quality in Estuaries   198
4-10 Low-Resolution Models for Water Quality in Rivers   200
4-11 Summary of Certain Stream and Estuary Models.   202
4-12 Different Water Models.   208
4-13 Summary of the Characteristics of the Jet Models   218
4-14 Summary of the Characteristics of the Far-Field Models   220
4-15 Summary of the Characteristics of the Complete-Field Models. .   222
5-1   Federal Laws/Regulations Relating to Environmental Controls. .   243
5-2   Federal Laws/Regulations Pertaining to Wetlands of the U.S.. . .   250
5-3   Federal Noise-Related Regulations   253
5-4   Major EPA Regulations Under Consideration   258
5-5   State Statutory Provisions for Boundary-Delineation Techniques
       on Coast   267
5-6   Summary of State Codes and Attitudes Regarding Dredged
       Material.   268
5-7   State Coastal and Wetland Laws.   270
5-8   State Environmental and Water Laws   271
5-9   Data Update Regulations   275
6-1   National Ambient Air Quality Standards   278
6-2   List of Sources for which Emission Factors are Available   278
6-3   Emissions from Anthracite Coal Combustion Without Control
       Equipment—Emission Factor Rating B   280
6-4   Emission Factors for Heavy-Duty Construction Equipment. . . .   281
6-5   Emission Factors for Refuse Incinerators Without Controls—
       Emission Factor Rating A.   282
6-6   Average Emission Factors for Highway Vehicles—Emission
       Factor Rating B   283

6-7   Average Emission Factors for Highway Vehicles Based on
        Nationwide Statistics 284
6-8   Emission Factors for Motorcycles—Emission Factor Rating B . . 285
6-9   Emission Factors per Aircraft Landing-Takeoff Cycle—
        Emission Factor Rating B 286
6-10   Average Emission Factors for Inboard Pleasure Craft—
        Emission Factor Rating D 287
6-11   Emission Factors for Snowmobiles—Emission Factor Rating B. . 288
6-12   Emission Factors for Wheeled Farm Tractors and Nontractor
        Agricultural Equipment—Emission Factor Rating C 289
6-13   Organic Compound Evaporative Emission Factors for
        Petroleum, Transportation and Marketing Sources—
        Emission Factor Rating A 290
6-14   Emission Factors and Fuel Loading Factors for Open Burning
        of Agricultural Materials—Emission Factor Rating B. 291
6-15   Classification of Air Quality Control Regions 294
6-16   Pollutant Values for Determining Air Quality Control
        Region Classifications. 308
6-17   Standards of Performance 309
  A   National Emissions Report, U.S. Environmental
        Protection Agency 317
7-1   Water Quality Data from STORET Computer Printout of EPA. . 432
7-2   State STORET Codes. 433
7-3   Background Data Sources on Water Resources 434
7-4   Data and Methods for Stream Analysis 436
7-5   A Summary of Methods to Assess Fishery and Stream Habitat
        Flow Requirements 438
7-6   Annual Yield of Pollutants from Urban Runoff and
        Municipal Waste 442
7-7   Contributions of Various Sources to Oil in the Oceans 445
7-8   EPA Numerical Water Quality Criteria for Public Water
        Supply Intake. 445
7-9   EPA Numerical Water Quality Criteria for Marine Aquatic Life . 446
7-10   EPA Numerical Water Quality Criteria for Freshwater
        Aquatic Life. 447
7-11   Summary of Specific Quality Characteristics of Surface Waters
        That Have Been Used as Sources for Industrial Water Supplies . . 448
7-12   Ranges of Promulgated Standards for Raw Water Sources
        of Domestic Water Supply. 450
7-13   Summary of Categories for which Effluent Guidelines and
        Federal Standards Have Been Promulgated 451
7-14   State Numerical Water Quality Standards. 462
7-15   Recommended Maximum Concentrations of Biocides in Whole
        Unfiltered Water in Coastal Waters 481
7-16   Hazardous and Minimal Risk Concentrations of Selected
        Inorganic Chemicals (Including Heavy Metals) Which Should Be
        Considered for Protection of Marine Biota 482

7-17   Estimated Effects of Underwater Explosion Tests on Marine
       Life in the Patuxent River and Chesapeake Bay   483
7-18   Effects of Underwater Explosions on Aquatic Organisms   484
7-19   Maximum Range of Noise Audibility Generated by Different
       Charges of Underwater Explosions   487
7-20   Force in Pounds per Square Inch Expected at Different
       Distances as a Result of Detonating Different Charges of
       Explosives   488
7-21   Spawning Requirements of Fish   489
7-22   Low Flow Evaluation Matrix   494
7-23   Water Requirements for Domestic Service, Public Buildings,
       Schools and Camps   495
7-24   Consumption of Water in Condenser Cooling of 1000-MW
       Electric Power Plants   496
7-25   Estimated Cooling Pond Area and Water Consumption for
       1000-MWe Power Plants   497
7-26   Unit Water Requirements for Producing Energy   498
7-27   Measurement of Aesthetics of Rivers   499
8-1   Typical Noise Level   506
8-2   Typical Noise Levels During Construction   507
8-3   Noise Sources   507
8-4   Effects of Noise on Man   510
8-5   Human Effects for Outdoor Day-Night Average Sound Level . . .   512
8-6   Criteria for Outdoor Sound Levels for Analysis of Environ-
       mental Noise Impact for Various Land Uses   513
8-7   Summary of Preparation of a Noise Impact Analysis   515
8-8   Effects of Noise on Fish and Wildlife   516
8-9   Aircraft Disturbance to Wildlife   517
8-10   State Recreational and Off-Road Vehicle Noise Regulations . . .   520
8-11   State Noise Restrictions   522
8-12   Municipal Noise Ordinances   524
9-1   U.S. Geological Maps: Topographical   550
9-2   USDA—Soil Conservation Service—Soil Capability Classes   555
9-3   Typical Data Available from Soil Surveys   557
9-4   Soil Properties Comparisons of Three Classification Systems . . .   559
9-5   Types of Soils and Their Design Properties for Foundations   560
9-6   Typical Soils Data and K Values for Site-Specific Analysis   565
9-7   Indications of the General Magnitude of the Soil-Erodibility
       Factor K   566
9-8   Factor P Values for Components of Erosion and Sediment
       Control Systems   566
9-9   Maximum Permissible C Values for Indicated Gradient and
       Slope Length with Straight and Contoured Rows   567
9-10   Average Factor C Values for Various Surface Stabilizing
       Treatments   567
9-11   Matrix of Information on State Surface-Mined Area
       Reclamation Programs   569

9-12 BLM State Fire Code and Fire Numbers. 579
9-13 BLM Guide for Resource Damage Estimates from Fires 581
9-14 Length and Amount of Displacement Related to Earthquakes . . 588
9-15 State Mineral Production 592
9-16 Mineral Resource Maps of the United States. 594
9-17 U.S. Minerals Supply-Demand and World Production 596
9-18 Minerals Produced in the United States 598
10-1 Plant and Animal Food Chains on Uplands. 604
10-2 Plant and Animal Food Chains in Wetlands. 605
10-3 World Productivity for Land Areas. 606
10-4 Typical Wildlife Densities 609
10-5 U.S. Productivity for Agriculture 611
10-6 Agriculture Animal Units by State 612
10-7 Aquatic Ecosystems Annual Productivity Rates. 614
10-8 Standing Crops of Fish. 616
10-9 Endangered, Threatened and Rare Species of the U.S. 619
10-10 Status of State Endangered Species Programs 633
10-11 Rare, Threatened or Endangered Plants and Animals 636
12-1 Legislative Responsibilities of Agencies in the Control of
       Chemicals 700
12-2 Major Indicators 701
12-3 Common Degradation Reactions 704
12-4 Toxicity of Acids to Aquatic Biota. 710
12-5 Summary of the Acute and Chronic Toxicity of Inorganic and
       Organic Pollutants to Freshwater Fish. 713
12-6 Phytotoxic Effects Exerted by Lead on Plants of Economic
       Importance in Illinois. 715
12-7 Comparison of Carcinogenicity, Mutagenicity and Teratogenicity 716
12-8 Effects of Toxic Chemicals 717
12-9 Sources of Information. 719
13-1 Estimated Work Force Requirements for Various Energy
       Technologies 732
13-2 Multipliers 734
13-3 Environmental Loadings from Community Expansion 737
13-4 Area Required for Community Development 739
13-5 Community Cost Analysis. 739
13-6 Service Factors for Expanding Populations. 740
13-7 Factors for Expanding Populations. 740
13-8 Typical Parkland and Recreation Area Needs 741
13-9 Recreation Activities Needs. 741
13-10 Measurements of Aesthetics on Rivers. 742
13-11 Illustration of Variety Class Breakdown of a Steep Mountain
       Slope Subtype 756
13-12 Guidelines for the Visual Management of Lands under
       Consideration. 760

14-1   Earth Characteristics   768
14-2   Glossary of Resource Terms   776
14-3   Estimate of U.S. Coal Resources.   777
14-4   Reserve Base of Western States by Sulfur Content   779
14-5   Reserve Base of Eastern States by Sulfur Content   780
14-6A   Proven and Indicated Reserves of Crude Oil and Production
        by State.   781
14-6B   Distribution of Proved Reserves of Natural Gas and
        Production by State.   787
14-7   Oil Shale Resources of the U.S.   788
14-8   U.S. Uranium Resources by Forward Cost Category.   788
14-9   U.S. Geothermal Resource Base and Estimated Recoverable
        Heat by Resource Type   789
14-10   Shipment of Bituminous Coal from the Mine, 1960-1974   791
14-11   Petroleum Transportation, 1938-1974.   792
14-12   Crude Oil and Natural Gas Worldwide Proved Reserves.   793
14-13   Middle East Proved Reserves of Crude Oil and Natural Gas   793
14-14   Centrally Planned Economies Proved Reserves of Crude Oil
        and Natural Gas   794
14-15   North American, Caribbean American and Other American
        Proved Reserves of Crude Oil and Natural Gas.   794
14-16   Western European Proved Reserves of Crude Oil and
        Natural Gas   795
14-17   Africa, Far East and Oceania Proved Reserves of Crude Oil
        and Natural Gas   796
14-18   Worldwide Oil Production and Refining.   797
14-19   Worldwide Energy Consumption, 1950-1973   798
14-20   U.S. Coal Production Under Selected Scenarios (1985).   801
14-21   U.S. Natural Gas Production Under Selected Scenarios (1985). .   802
14-22   U.S. Crude Oil Production Under Selected Scenarios (1985) . . .   803
14-23   U.S. Nuclear Generation of Electricity Under Selected
        Scenarios (1985).   805
15-1   Comparison of Passenger Transportation Modes in the
        United States   814
15-2   Comparison of Major Freight Transportation Modes in
        the United States.   815
15-3   Cars and Population.   819
15-4   U.S. Estimated Freight Bill   825
15-5   Estimated Truck Travel Data for the United States   827
15-6   Comparative Statistics: Bus, Rail, Auto   828
15-7   Atmospheric Pollutants from U.S. Transportation   831
15-8   Water Pollutant Characteristics of Storm Runoff
        (Highways, Urban and Industrial Areas).   833
15-9   Typical Widths for Highway Rights-of-Way Transportation   833
15-10   Motor Vehicle Accidents, Deaths and Injuries According
        to Urban and Rural Places.   834

15-11 Age of Drives—Total Number and Number in Accidents 835
15-12 Report of Traffic Fatalities Based on Early Reports 836
15-13 Animals Killed per Mile of Highway 838
15-14 U.S. Transportation Energy 846
15-15 Automobile Usage and Efficiency—by Trip Purpose 848
15-16 Urban Passenger Ground Transportation Energy Consumption . . 850
15-17 Urban Passenger Ground Transportation Energy
      Consumption Rates 851
15-18 Summary Table of Social Impact Analysis 855

LIST OF FIGURES

Figure   **Page**

2-1 Model Elements   24
2-2 Battelle Hierarchical System   39
2-3 Commonwealth Environmental Analysis System   40
2-4 Portions of Circular 645 Matrix   45
2-5 Typical Impact Value Function   54
3-1 Standard Metropolitan Statistical Areas   144
4-1 Sound Level Weighting Function for Overall Impact Analysis. . .   157
4-2 Example of Computer Plot   158
4-3 Maximum Visible Distance of Plume for Pasquill Classes
      C, E and F   167
4-4 Maximum Visible Distance of Plume for Pasquill Classes B and D.   168
4-5 Coordinate System Showing Gaussian Distributions in the
      Horizontal and Vertical   183
4-6 Flowchart of the Possible Model Building Pathways   190
4-7 Pollutant Material Balance for Water and Sediment Phases
      of a Stream   212
5-1 Hierarchy of Laws and Regulations of the Federal and State
      Governments   242
6-1 Isopleths of Mean Annual Morning Mixing Heights   315
6-2 Isopleths of Mean Annual Afternoon Mixing Heights   316
7-1 Land Use vs Mean Total Phosphorus and Mean Orthophosphorus
      Stream Concentrations   443
7-2 Land Use vs Mean Total Nitrogen and Mean Inorganic
      Nitrogen Stream Concentrations   444
7-3 Typical U.S. Surface Water Temperature Isotherms   491
7-4 Relationship Between Pressure and Distance from Explosion
      for Two Charge Weights   492

7-5	Seasons of Lowest Stream Flow	493
7-6	Water Consumption in Energy Conversion and Refining	502
7-7	Wild and Scenic Rivers of the U.S.	503
8-1	Speech Interference Levels	511
8-2	Average Mean Subjective Rating as a Function of Maximum Noise Level	514
8-3	Noise Limits (Approach) and Aircraft Noise Levels	518
8-4	Noise Limits (Takeoff) and Aircraft Noise Levels.	519
9-1	Physical Divisions of the U.S..	551
9-2	Soil Orders of the U.S.	552
9-3	A Comparison of Grain-Size Limits in the Three Classification Systems.	558
9-4	Rainfall-Erosion Losses from Eastern U.S.	562
9-5	Rainfall-Erosion Losses from the Midwest	563
9-6	Slope-Effect Chart	564
9-7	Percentages of Fires Caused by Lightning.	583
9-8	Potential Earthquake Risk (Velocities)	584
9-9	Potential Earthquake Risk (Accelerations).	585
9-10	Probable Levels of Earthquake Shaking Hazards	586
9-11	Prediction: Seismic Risk Map.	587
9-12	Energy Release on the Richter Scale for Earthquakes.	589
9-13	Physical Criteria for Site Selection and Evaluation	590
9-14	Volcanoes of the U.S..	591
10-1	Biomes of the United States	602
10-2	Standing Crops of Fish per Acre by Species	617
10-3	Distribution of Endangered Species that are Geographically Isolated	632
11-1	Beach and Primary Dune (Severely Disturbed)	665
11-2	Primary Dune, Trough and Secondary Dune (Drifting)	666
11-3	Beach; Primary Dune and Trough (Impacted by Off-Road Vehicles); and Backdune and Bayshore	666
11-4	Beach Colonization	667
11-5	Primary Dune Building.	667
11-6	Dune Stabilization.	668
11-7	Beach Trough.	668
11-8	Secondary Dune	669
11-9	Backdune.	669
11-10	Northern Spruce Forest Fire (Alaska)	670
11-11	First Seral Stage After Fire—High Brush Regrowth.	671
11-12	Second Seral Stage After Fire—Hardwood (Birch)	671
11-13	Spruce/Hardwood Ecotone	672
11-14	Black Spruce Forest.	672
11-15	Tundra Biome; Black Spruce/Muskeg (Alaska)	673
11-16	Tundra Biome (Alaska); Moist Tundra.	673
11-17	Wetland Type: Coastal Salt Meadow (*Spartina*).	674
11-18	Wetland Type: Inland Fresh Meadow (Everglades).	675

11-19 Wetland Type: Coastal Open Brackish (Eelgrass Floating) 675
11-20 Wetland Type: Coastal Shallow Fresh Marsh (Emergent). 676
11-21 Wetland Type and Tropical Biome: Mangrove Swamp. 676
11-22 Wetland Type: Inland Shallow Fresh Marsh (Cattail) 677
11-23 Wetland Type: Inland Open Fresh Water 677
11-24 Tropical Biome (Caribbean); Cleared Hardwood Forest. 678
11-25 Tropical Biome (Caribbean); Early Seral Stage of Hardwood
      Forest. 679
11-26 Tropical Biome (Caribbean); Hardwood Forest Climax. 679
11-27 Tropical Biome (Caribbean); Cactus/Agave Shrub 680
11-28 Tropical Biome; Everglades Hammock. 680
11-29 Tropical Biome; Hardwood Forest (Mature Stage) 681
11-30 Tropical Biome; Mangrove Forest. 681
11-31 Southern Mixed Forest Biome; Southern Floodplain Forest/
      Swamp (Mature). 682
11-32 Southern Mixed Forest Biome; Palmetto Prairie 683
11-33 Southern Mixed Forest Biome; Sand Pine Scrub 683
11-34 Southern Mixed Forest Biome; Cypress Swamp
      (Immature Stage) 684
11-35 Southern Mixed Forest Biome; Southeastern Pine Forest
      (Immature Stage) 684
11-36 Deciduous Forest Biome; Old Field Prairie/Red Cedar
      (First Seral Stage) 685
11-37 Deciduous Forest Biome; Immature Hardwood Brush (Early
      Seral Stage) 685
11-38 Deciduous Forest Biome; Mixed Mesophytic Forest
      (Immature Stage) 686
11-39 Deciduous Forest Biome; Oak/Hickory/Maple (Immature Stage) 687
11-40 Northern Coniferous Biome: Northeastern Spruce/Fir 687
11-41 Northern Coniferous Forest Biome; Great Lakes Spruce/Fir
      (Mature Stage) 688
11-42 Grassland Biome; Shortgrass (Wheatgrass/Grama)/Prairie
      (Mature Stage) 689
11-43 Grassland Biome; Tallgrass (Bluestem) Prairie (Mature Stage). . . 689
11-44 Deciduous Forest Ecotone with Grassland Biome; Bluestem
      (Tallgrass) Prairie (Mature Stage) 690
11-45 Grassland Biome; Eastern Ponderosa Forest and Northern
      Badlands 690
11-46 Grassland Biome; Southern Badlands (South Dakota). 691
11-47 Grassland Biome; Live Oak Savanna 691
11-48 Grassland Biome; Juniper Oak Savanna 692
11-49 Western Coniferous Forest Biome; Aspen (Intermediate Seral
      Stage). 692
11-50 Western Coniferous Biome; Western Spruce/Fir Forest
      (Aspen in Foreground). 693
11-51 Western Coniferous Forest Biome; Douglas Fir/Ponderosa Pine
      (Mature Stage) 693

11-52   Western Coniferous Forest; Petran Subalpine Forest (Mature
       Stage).   694
11-53   Western Coniferous Forest; Alpine (Above Treeline)   694
11-54   Western Coniferous Forest Biome; Spruce/Cedar/Hemlock
       Forest (Immature Stage).   695
11-55   Western Coniferous Forest Biome; Redwood Forest
       (Immature Stage)   695
11-56   Sagebrush Biome; Sagebrush Steppe   696
11-57   Steppe Biome; Coastal Sagebrush and Rocky Coast   696
11-58   Desert Scrub Pine (Mature Stage)   697
11-59   Western Coniferous Biome; California Mixed Evergreen   697
12-1   Movement of Chemicals   703
12-2   The Linear Regression Between the Logarithms of the Partition
       Coefficient and the Bioconcentration of Various Chemicals
       in Trout Muscle.   707
12-3   Dose Response Relationship   708
13-1   Relationship Between System Elements.   755
14-1   Energy Rates—Some Comparisons   769
14-2   Energy Flow Patterns in the U.S.   770
14-3   U.S. Economic Growth and Energy Use.   771
14-4   U.S. Gross Consumption of Mineral Energy Resources and
       Electricity from Hydropower and Nuclear Power, 1947-1985 . .   772
14-5   U.S. Consumption of Coal by Consuming Sector, 1950-1985. . .   773
14-6   U.S. Consumption of Petroleum by Type of Customer,
       1950-1975.   774
14-7   Classification of Mineral Resources   775
14-8   U.S. Coal Supply Regions Used by FEA-PIES Model   778
14-9   Middle East Proved Reserves of Crude Oil and Natural Gas   782
14-10   Centrally Planned Economics Proved Reserves of Crude Oil
       and Natural Gas   783
14-11   North American, Caribbean American and Other American
       Nations Proved Reserves of Crude Oil and Natural Gas   784
14-12   Western European Proved Reserves of Crude Oil and Natural Gas.   785
14-13   Africa, Far East and Oceania Proved Reserves of Crude Oil
       and Natural Gas   786
14-14   Potential of Solar Energy   790
14-15   World Oil Reserves.   799
14-16   World Oil Production and Consumption.   799
14-17   Coal Reserves of the World   800
14-18   Free World Reserves of Uranium   804
14-19   World Reserves of Lithium   804
14-20   Total Energy Consumption in Ford Foundation Scenarios.   806
14-21   Total Energy Consumption in ERDA Scenarios.   807
14-22   U.S. Energy Supply Curves for SRI "Nominal Scenario".   807
14-23   Oil Import Prices (SRI Scenarios)   808
15-1   Transportation Contribution to GNP.   812

15-2   Trends of Transportation Expenditures and Revenues
        (1962-1972).. 813
15-3   Average Number of Full-Time and Part-Time Employees by
        Transportation Section (1962-1972)..................... 816
15-4   Average Annual Earnings per Full-Time Employee by
        Transportation Sector (1962-1972)...................... 816
15-5   Personal Consumption Expenditures, by Type of Product
        (1962-1972).. 817
15-6   Personal Consumption Expenditures by Transportation Sectors
        (1962-1972).. 818
15-7   Current Use of Automobile.............................. 820
15-8   Auto Ownership vs Transit Patronage (1930-1973)........ 820
15-9   U.S. Urban/Rural Population (1900-2000)................ 821
15-10   Fifteen-Year Growth in Airline Capacity and Utilization....... 822
15-11   Airline Passenger and Ton Mile Load Factors (1959-1974).... 823
15-12   Fifteen-Year Growth of Airline Revenues................ 823
15-13   Cost Trends in Airline Lift (1959-1974)................ 824
15-14   1972 Domestic Air Travel Market........................ 825
15-15   Freight Handled by Mode................................ 826
15-16   Relative Distribution of Freight Revenues (1947-1972) and
        1972 Revenues of Regulated Carriers 826
15-17   Travel by Public Carrier 827
15-18   Relative Growth of Intercity Passenger Service 829
15-19   Atmospheric Pollutants on a Weight Basis in the U.S........ 830
15-20   Emissions for Various Transportation Modes at Cruise Speed... 832
15-21   Number of Train Accidents and Percentage Caused by
        Maintenance of Way Deficiencies 837
15-22   U.S. Total Energy Budget by Sector and Energy Resource..... 838
15-23   U.S. Transportation Energy Distribution by Mode........ 839
15-24   U.S. Transportation Energy Consumption by Mode 840
15-25   Distribution of Transportation Energy by Mode 841
15-26   Distribution of Transportation Energy by Purpose....... 841
15-27   Automobile Ownership by U.S. Households 842
15-28   Energy Consumption and Vehicle Weight—Vehicle-Mile Basis... 843
15-29   Energy Consumption and Vehicle Weight—Passenger-Mile Basis . 844
15-30   Composite Energy Consumption Rates 844
15-31   Automobile Energy Intensiveness—by Trip Purpose 849
15-32   Modal Comparison of Fuel Economy 852
15-33   Causal Path Flow Diagram of the Direct and Significant
        Impacts on Individuals................................. 853
15-34   Theoretical Motor Vehicle Fuel Savings................. 854

CHAPTER 1

INTRODUCTION

With the introduction of the National Environmental Policy Act of 1969, which required each federal agency to prepare a detailed environmental impact statement (EIS) for each major action that significantly affected the quality of the human environment, more than 8,000 statements have been prepared and submitted to the Council on Environmental Quality (Table 1). Undoubtedly, thousands more environmental assessments and related studies have been performed.

When the nature of the proposed project and its impact are such that the need for the preparation of an EIS is not obvious, an initial evaluation takes the form of an environmental assessment, which evaluates the anticipated effects of the proposed action. On the basis of data developed during the assessment, a conclusion can be drawn as to whether the proposed action, if implemented, will significantly affect the quality of the human environment, and, therefore, require the preparation of an EIS. If the determination is made that an EIS is not warranted because there will be no significant impact on the environment, then the assessment normally serves as the basis for a "negative determination."

In accordance with NEPA, the Council on Environmental Quality (CEQ) issued guidelines to federal departments and agencies for preparing environmental statements (38FR147, August 1973). Based on these, federal agencies issue guidelines for internal agency use. These policies and procedures [CEQ Guidelines (10 CFR 11)] typically provide guidance for:

1. identifying the agency's environmental appraisal process, those actions requiring environmental assessments and statements, and the appropriate time prior to agency decision for requisite federal, state, local and public consultation **and review;**
2. obtaining information to allow the potential environmental impact of budget decisions and proposed policy determinations, procedures,

1

Table 1-1. Summary of Environmental Impact Statements Filed with the CEQ
Through May 31, 1977 (by agency)[a]

Agency	Draft 102s for Actions on Which no Final 102s have yet been Received	Final 102s on Legislation and Actions	Supplements	Total Actions on Which Draft or Final Statements have been Received
Agriculture, Department of	188	810	7	1005
Appalachian Regional Commission	1	0	0	1
Architect of the Capitol	0	144	0	186
Atomic Energy Commission	42	144	0	186
Canal Zone Government	0	1	0	1
Civil Aeronautics Board	0	2	0	2
Commerce, Department of	24	74	3	101
Consumer Product Safety Commission	0	1	0	1
Defense, Department of	10	8	1	19
Air Force	11	27	2	40
Army	4	29	2	35
Army Corps of Engineers	557	1132	32	1721
Navy	14	43	2	59
Delaware River Basin Commission	2	8	0	10
Energy Policy Office	0	1	0	1
Energy Research & Development Administration	9	9	0	18
Environmental Protection Agency	52	110	2	164
Federal Energy Administ Administration	10	9	2	21
Federal Maritime Commission	3	0	0	3
Federal Power Commission	81	68	5	154
Federal Trade Commission	1	0	0	1
General Services Administration	19	108	3	130
Health, Education and Welfare, Department of	3	18	0	21
Housing and Urban Development, Department of	84	264	4	352
Interior, Department of	156	396	6	558
International Boundary and Water Commission—U.S. and Mexico	0	10	0	10

Table 1-1. Continued

Agency	Draft 102s for Actions on Which no Final 102s have yet been Received	Final 102s on Legislation and Actions	Supplements	Total Actions on Which Draft or Final Statements have been Received
Interstate Commerce Commission	9	15	0	24
Justice, Department of	2	3	0	5
Labor, Department of	5	5	0	10
National Aeronautics and Space Administration	11	25	3	39
National Capitol Planning Commission	5	8	0	13
National Science Foundation	0	7	0	7
New England River Basins Commission	3	0	0	3
Nuclear Regulatory Commission	8	42	9	59
Office of Science and Technology	0	1	0	1
Ohio River Basin Commission	0	1	0	1
Pacific Northwest River Basins Commission	3	0	0	3
Pennsylvania Avenue Development Corporation	0	1	0	1
Scuris-Red-Rainy River Basins Commission	1	0	0	1
State Department	3	6	0	9
Tennessee Valley Authority	9	29	0	38
Transportation, Department of	1023	2309	24	3356
Treasury, Department of	4	7	0	11
Upper Mississippi River Basin Commission	1	0	0	1
U.S. Postal Service	3	4	0	7
U.S. Water Resource Council	7	9	0	16
Veterans Administration	4	9	0	13
TOTAL	2372	5754	107	8233

[a]Source: *102 Monitor* 7(5) (June 1977).

regulations and legislation to receive full consideration in the agency decision-making process;

3. obtaining information and internal review required for the preparation of environmental assessments and statements; and

4. designating the officials who are to be responsible for preparation, review and approval of environmental assessments and statements.

A list of agency procedures is provided in Table 1-2. These agencies do not, as a rule, give guidance in the techniques to be used in preparing their analysis. Rather, broad statements such as defining air and water quality, noise impact, social impact, etc., are outlined. It is often left to the individual analyst to translate the broad regulations into the more practical day-by-day analytical tools.

NEPA STATUTORY REQUIREMENTS

According to Section 102(2) (c) of NEPA, for every recommendation or report on proposals for legislation and other major federal actions significantly affecting the quality of the human environment, a detailed statement is to be prepared, which describes:

1. the environmental impact of the proposed action,

2. any adverse environmental effects which cannot be avoided should the proposal be implemented,

3. alternatives to the proposed action,

4. the relationship between local short-term uses of man's environment and the maintenance and enhancement of long-term productivity, and

5. any irreversible and irretrievable commitments of resources which would be involved in the proposed action should it be implemented.

Despite the statutory requirement that environmental impact statements be prepared for "major Federal actions significantly affecting the quality of the human environment," NEPA does not provide criteria, procedures or guidelines for interpreting these major and significant requirements or for identifying specific actions that require the preparation of an environmental impact statement. The CEQ Guidelines on Preparation of Environmental Impact Statements (40CFR1500) address this subject on a general level and specify that "the identification of those actions that require an environmental impact statement is the responsibility of each Federal agency, to be carried out against the backdrop of its own particular operations."

For a NEPA environmental impact statement to be required for a proposed action, the action must: be a "federal" action, be a "major" action, be "significant" and affect the quality of the human environment.

Table 1-2. Agency NEPA Procedures as of March 1, 1976
(The Seventh General Report of the Council on Environmental Quality, September 1976)

U.S. Agency	Current Procedures		Amendments		Revision	
	Date	Citation[a]	Date	Citation	Date	Citation[a]
Agriculture						
Departmental	5/29/74	39 Fed. Reg. 18678				
Agricultural Stabilization and Conservation Service	5/29/74	39 Fed. Reg. 18678	12/20/74	39 Fed. Reg. 43993		
Animal and Plant Health Inspection Service	1/29/74[b]	39 Fed. Reg. 3696[b]				
Farmers Home Administration	8/29/72	37 Fed. Reg. 17459				
Forest Service	5/3/73	38 Fed. Reg. 20919	10/30/74	39 Fed. Reg. 3244		
Rural Electrification Administration	5/20/74	39 Fed. Reg. 23240				
Soil Conservation Service	6/3/74	7 C.F.R. Part 650 39 Fed. Reg. 19646				
Appalachian Regional Commission	6/7/71	36 Fed. Reg. 23676				
(Atomic Energy Commission)						
Nuclear Regulatory Commission (regulatory)	7/18/74	10 C.F.R. Part 51 39 Fed. Reg. 26279				
Energy Research and Development Administration (nonregulatory)	2/14/74	10 C.F.R. Part 11 39 Fed. Reg. 5620				
Canal Zone Government	10/20/72	37 Fed. Reg. 22669				
Central Intelligence Agency	1/28/74	39 Fed. Reg. 3579				

Table 1-2, Continued

U.S. Agency	Current Procedures		Amendments		Revision	
	Date	Citation[a]	Date	Citation	Date	Citation[a]
Civil Aeronautics Board	7/1/71	14 C.F.R. §399.110 36 Fed. Reg. 12513	8/25/75 12/19/75	40 Fed. Reg. 37182 14 C.F.R. 312 40 Fed. Reg. 59925		
Department of Commerce National Oceanic and Atmospheric Administration, Coastal Zone Management	10/23/71 8/21/74	36 Fed. Reg. 21368 36 Fed. Reg. 30153	2/4/75	40 Fed. Reg. 5175	2/28/75	40 Fed. Reg. 8546
Economic Development Administration	11/13/74	39 Fed. Reg. 40122				
Department of Defense	4/26/74	32 C.F.R. Part 214 39 Fed. Reg. 14699				
Army Corps of Engineers	4/8/74	33 C.F.R. §209.410 39 Fed. Reg. 12737				
Delaware River Basin Commission	7/11/74 7/11/74	18 C.F.R. Part 401 39 Fed. Reg. 25473				
Environmental Protection Agency	4/14/75	40 Fed. Reg. 16813				
Export-Import Bank (no regulations)						
Federal Communications Commission	12/19/74	39 Fed. Reg. 43884	11/18/75	40 Fed. Reg. 53391		
Federal Energy Administration	1/30/76	41 Fed. Reg. 4722 10 C.F.R. 208				
Federal Power Commission	12/18/72	Commission Order No. 415-C 37 Fed. Reg. 28412	6/7/73	Commission Order No. 485 guidelines to applicants		

Federal Trade Commission	11/19/71	16 C.F.R. §1.81-1.85	36 Fed. Reg. 22814
General Services Administration			
Departmental	4/4/75	40 Fed. Reg. 15131	
Property Management and Disposal Service	12/30/71	PMD Order 1095.1A	36 Fed. Reg. 23704
Public Buildings Service	3/2/73	PBS Order 1095.1B	
Telecommunications Service	6/30/71	TCS 1095.1	7/1/75 40 Fed. Reg. 27733
Health, Education and Welfare			
Departmental	10/17/73	HEW General Administration Manual, Chapters 30-10 through 30-16	
Food and Drug Administration	3/15/73	21 C.F.R. Parts 6, 601	4/16/74 39 Fed. Reg. 13741
		38 Fed. Reg. 7001	
Consumer Product Safety Commission (no regulations)			
Department of Housing and Urban Development			
Community Development Block Grants	7/16/75	40 Fed. Reg. 29992	2/19/76 41 Fed. Reg. 7515
Other programs	7/18/73	38 Fed. Reg. 19182	11/4/75 39 Fed. Reg. 38922
Interior			
Departmental	9/27/71	36 Fed. Reg. 19343	
Bonneville Power Administration	1/19/72	37 Fed. Reg. 815	
Bureau of Indian Affairs	1/21/74	Bureau Transmittal Memo	
Bureau of Land Management	5/4/72	Bureau Manual Release	
Bureau of Mines	2/9/72	37 Fed. Reg. 2895	
Bureau of Outdoor Recreation	3/24/72	37 Fed. Reg. 6501	
Bureau of Reclamation	11/23/72	37 Fed. Reg. 24910	
Fish and Wildlife Service	11/8/74	Bureau Transmittal Memo	

Table 1-2, Continued

U.S. Agency	Current Procedures		Amendments		Revision	
	Date	Citation[a]	Date	Citation	Date	Citation[a]
U.S. Geological Survey	3/11/72	37 Fed. Reg. 5263				
National Park Service	7/29/74	Bureau Manual Release				
Interstate Commerce Commission	3/28/72	49 C.F.R. §1100.250				
Department of Justice	2/6/74	28 C.F.R. Part 19				
Law Enforcement Assistance Administration		39 Fed. Reg. 4736				
Department of Labor	3/15/74	29 C.F.R. Part 1999				
		39 Fed. Reg. 9959				
National Aeronautics and Space Administration	4/10/74	14 C.F.R. §1204.11				
		39 Fed. Reg. 12999				
National Capital Planning Commission	8/72[b]	37 Fed. Reg. 16039				
National Science Foundation	1/28/74	45 C.F.R. Part 640				
		39 Fed. Reg. 3544				
Small Business Administration	10/20/72	37 Fed. Reg. 22697				
State						
Departmental	8/31/72	37 Fed. Reg. 19167				
Agency for International Development	8/1/75	Policy Determination 63 (supersedes 39 Fed. Reg. 22686-7 of 10/20/72)				
International Boundary and Water Commission	3/14/74	39 Fed. Reg. 9868				
Tennessee Valley Authority	2/14/74	39 Fed. Reg. 5671				

Transportation				
Departmental	9/30/74	39 Fed. Reg. 35232		
Federal Aviation Adminis-tration	6/19/73	FAA Order 1050.1A		
Airport Development Act	12/7/70	FAA Order 5050.2A:		
Federal Highway Administration	12/2/74	36 Fed. Reg. 7724 39 Fed. Reg. 41804		
U.S. Coast Guard	10/22/75	33 C.F.R. 771 40 Fed. Reg. 49383		
Urban Mass Transportation Administration	2/1/72	DOT Order 5610.1		
National Highway Traffic Safety Administration	11/10/75	37 Fed. Reg. 22692 40 Fed. Reg. 52395 49 C.F.R. 520		
Saint Lawrence Seaway Development Corporation	11/71	Procedure SLS 2-5610.1A	4/24/75	40 Fed. Reg. 18026
Treasury				
Departmental	4/26/74	39 Fed. Reg. 14796		
Internal Revenue Service	8/12/71	36 Fed. Reg. 15061		
Veterans Administration	6/17/74	39 Fed. Reg. 21016	8/25/75	40 Fed. Reg. 37126
Water Resources Council	2/10/71	36 Fed. Reg. 23711		
U.S. Postal Service	7/6/72	37 Fed. Reg. 13322		

[a] For procedures that have been published in the *Federal Register* or have otherwise been formally issued.
[b] Issued in proposed form and currently followed on an interim basis.

Federal Action

The NEPA requirement for environmental impact statements applies only to federal actions; NEPA environmental statements are not required for nonfederal actions. For an action to be construed under NEPA as federal, it must be one that is either undertaken directly by a federal agency, one that involves a federal lease, permit, etc., or one that is supported, in whole or part, through federal assistance. This assistance may be in the form of funding, facilities or personnel.

In the case of federal assistance, there must be "sufficient" federal control and responsibility over the action for it to be covered by NEPA [CEQ Guidelines (40CFR1500)]. The term "sufficient" is not defined in the CEQ Guidelines, but is intended to imply a threshold of federal control and responsibility. For example, when federal funds are distributed in the form of general revenue sharing for use by state and local governments, there is no federal agency control over the subsequent use of the funds. Consequently, actions resulting from the use of the revenue sharing funds would not be federal actions under NEPA and would not require a NEPA environmental statement; however, state and local laws may require that some sort of environmental statement be prepared. On the other hand, federal funding assistance, for which the funds must be used for a specified purpose, such as in highway construction or for specific research and development programs, does constitute sufficient federal control and responsibility so that the action is covered by NEPA. In general, as long as a federal agency makes a decision that permits some party, either private or governmental, to take a specific action, the action is construed as a federal action under NEPA, however, any action taken by the agency is ultimately subject to judicial review.

Major Action

Interpretation of the term major is interwoven with interpretation of the term significant. Normally, if an action is major it is significant, and vice versa. Most agencies rely on the definition of significant to define major.

The terms major and significant are intended to imply thresholds of importance and impact that must be met by the federal action before an environmental statement is required. Actions that exceed these thresholds require environmental impact statements; actions that do not exceed them do not require environmental impact statements. The evidence that the action does not meet the criteria for an EIS is termed a "Negative Declaration" or "Negative Determination." While NEPA does not provide any guidance for determining whether an action is major and significant, CEQ Guidelines and various court decisions have addressed this issue.

CEQ Guidelines state that the identification of major and significant actions affecting the quality of the human environment is the responsibility of each federal agency. The Guidelines suggest that the terms major and significant be "construed by Federal agencies with a view to the overall cumulative impact of the action proposed, related Federal actions and projects in the area, and further actions comtemplated." The Guidelines further state that while "such actions may be localized in their impact, if there is a potential that the environment may be significantly affected, the statement is to be prepared . . . an environmental statement should be prepared if it is reasonable to anticipate a cumulatively significant impact on the environment from Federal actions." These guidelines imply that the significance of the action is the overriding criterion in determining whether an environmental impact statement is required.

Various court decisions have provided further guidance on the interpretation of the term significant and on the ability of each federal agency to make its own determination of what constitutes a significant action under NEPA. For example, the opinion of the court in *First National Bank v. Richardson* states that:

> "In discussing the proper interpretation of the term "significant," the court (in Hanly II, 471, F.2d at 830) noted a complete lack of Congressional or administrative guidelines and stated that: Congress apparently was willing to depend principally upon the agency's good faith determination as to what conduct would be sufficiently serious from an ecological standpoint to require use of the full-scale (environmental impact statement) procedure. The majority opinion then concluded that: in deciding whether Federal action will significantly affect the quality of the human environment, the agency in charge, although vested with broad discretion, should normally be required to review the proposed action in the light of at least two relevant factors:
>
> 1. the extent to which the action will cause adverse environmental effects in excess of those created by existing uses in the area affected by it; and
>
> 2. the absolute quantitative adverse environmental effects of the action itself, including the cumulative harm that results from its contribution to existing adverse conditions or uses in the affected area.*

The first factor is a measure of the action's relative effect on a site area, *i.e.,* how its impacts compare to existing impacts. The second factor is a measure of the cumulative impact of the action and all other activities in any affected area. Both of these effects should be considered in determining the significance of a proposed action.

First National Bank v. *Richardson, Environment Reporter—Cases,* 5 ERC 1833, The Bureau of National Affairs, Washington, D.C. (1974).

Quality of the Human Environment

For a major federal action to require a NEPA environmental statement, it must "significantly affect the quality of the human environment."

The CEQ Guidelines state that the quality of the human environment may be affected either by impacts directly affecting humans or by impacts indirectly affecting humans through adverse effects on the environment. Adverse significant effects include those that degrade the quality of the environment, curtail the range of beneficial uses of the environment and serve short-term uses to the disadvantage of long-term environmental goals. The CEQ Guidelines further provide that "significant" effects can also include actions that may have both beneficial and detrimental effects, even if the agency believes that the overall effect will be beneficial.

ENVIRONMENT IMPACT ASSESSMENT

There are three basic steps to determine whether a proposed major federal action requires an environmental impact statement. These steps are:

1. definition of the purpose and scope of the proposed action;
2. preparation of an initial environmental assessment; and
3. evaluation of whether there could be significant impacts from the proposed action.

Definition of Purpose and Scope

The first step in determining whether a proposed action requires an environmental impact statement is to define the purpose and scope of the proposed action. This involves identifying why the proposed action is to be undertaken as well as determining what it involves and where it will occur. The following questions should be considered:

1. Is the proposed action an independent action or is it part of some larger project?
2. If the proposed action is not part of a larger project, are there any other actions proposed for the same site?
   If there are other actions proposed for the same area and either one or more of the actions would have a potential for cumulative significant impact, an EIS may be necessary.
3. Is the proposed action similar to any other proposed actions in other areas.
   If it is, then it should be determined whether a study is necessary to cover impacts of all individual actions as part of the overall program.

4. If the proposed action is part of a larger decision, has a programmatic statement been prepared for the overall project?

   If a programmatic statement has been prepared which evaluates the site-specific impacts of the proposed action, an additional site statement may not be required for the proposed action.

5. If the proposed action is part of a larger project, is the proposed action separately authorized and funded?

   If the proposed individual action is not separately funded and authorized, the individual action cannot be evaluated separately to determine whether an environmental impact statement is required. The entire authorized and funded project must be the subject of the environmental assessment and any subsequent environmental impact statement.*

   If the actions will all occur at the same site, consideration should be given to the preparation of a site statement for the entire action. If the actions will occur at diverse sites, consideration should be given to the preparation of a programmatic statement for the entire action.

6. If the proposed action is part of a larger project, is it a necessary prior step to other contemplated future action?

   If it is a necessary prior step, consideration should be given to the preparation of a site statement or programmatic statement.

If all components of the overall project do not occur at the same site, then it may be necessary to prepare both a site statement for the individual action (or for all actions at that site) and a programmatic statement for the overall project.

A programmatic statement should be prepared for all major technological research and development programs that are likely to have a significant environmental impact. The opinion in *Scientists' Institute v. The Atomic Energy Commission* addressed the point of whether the AEC's liquid metal fast breeder reactor (LMFBR) program required an environmental impact statement while the program was still in the research and development stage and no specific implementing action yet taken that would significantly affect the environment. The court found that NEPA required an EIS for the program early in the development because of the potential future effects of the program. The opinion states that "we thus tread firm ground in holding that NEPA requires impact statements for major Federal research programs, such as the AEC's LMFBR program, aimed at development of new technologies which, when applied, will significantly affect the quality of the human environment." The opinion also states that "development of the technology serves as much to affect the environment as does an AEC decision granting a construction permit

---

Save Crystal Beach Association v. *Callaway, Environmental Reporter Decisions No. 19,* No. 45, 8 ERC 1645, The Bureau of National Affairs, Washington, D.C. (March 5, 1976).

(to a utility company which will permit it to take action affecting the environment by building LMFBR power plants) . . . development of the technology is a necessary precondition of construction of any plants."* Thus, the actual determination that must be made for a major technological research and development program is not whether environmental impact statements should be prepared, but when is the preparation of a programmatic statement appropriate.

For most major federal actions, it is not possible to determine automatically whether the action could cause significant environmental impacts. Rather, it is first necessary to assess the environmental impacts associated with the action and then to evaluate these impacts to determine whether the action could cause significant environmental effects.

An environmental assessment is an environmental report prepared expressly to determine whether a proposed action requires the preparation of an environmental impact statement. The environmental assessment may be based on procedures such as checklists, matrices, networks, overlays and specific studies. The environmental assessment should:

1. describe the proposed action,†
2. describe the environment to be affected,†
3. identify all relevant environmental impact areas,‡
4. evaluate the potential environmental impacts,†**
5. identify adverse impacts that cannot be avoided should the action be implemented,†**
6. identify irreversible and irretrievable commitments of resources,**
7. discuss the relationship between local short-term uses of man's environment and long-term productivity,†**
8. identify conflicts with state, regional or local plans and programs**
9. evaluate alternatives to the proposed action**, and
10. discuss any existing controversy regarding the action††

---

*Scientists' Institute v. AEC, Environmental Report - Cases, 5 ERC 1423-1425, The Bureau of National Affairs, Washington, D.C. (1974).
†CEQ Guidelines, 10CFR711.
‡Hanley v. Mitchell, Environmental Reporter - Cases, 4 ERC 1152-1158, The Bureau of National Affairs, Washington, D.C. (1973); Maryland Planning Commission v. Postal Service, Environmental Reporter - Cases, 5 ERC 1725-1726, The Bureau of National Affairs, Washington, D.C. (1974).
**Save Crystal Beach Association v. Callaway, Environmental Reporter, Decisions No. 19, No. 45, The Bureau of National Affairs, Washington, D.C. (March 5, 1976).
††CEQ Guidelines for the implementation of NEPA state that whenever an action is controversial, an EIS is required. Although controversial can be defined many ways, in Rucker v. Wills it was ruled that controversy does not refer to opposition to the project, but to cases "when substantial dispute exists as to the size and nature of effect of the major Federal action."

If the environmental assessment indicates that there would not be any significant effects from the proposed action, an environmental impact statement is not required. (The assessment, if it is determined that an EIS is not required, is used as the basis of the negative determination.) Factors that tend to indicate that an environmental impact statement is necessary include: (1) significant controversy expected; (2) the proposed action is of a type for which environmental impact statements have been prepared in the past; and (3) the proposed action is "similar" to actions for which environmental statements have been prepared previously.

While it may be highly probable that an environmental impact statement is required in such cases, the preparation of the statement should not be initiated automatically. There may be some fundamental differences in the action or in the environment that will eliminate the significant impacts. Normally, such differences can be assessed very quickly. However, if the previous type of action had the potential for causing widespread significant impacts, it may be most practical to prepare an environmental statement without first preparing an environmental assessment.

Decisions not to prepare an EIS should never be made without first preparing an environmental assessment, even if the proposed action is identical to previous actions that did not require environmental impact statements. Any change in the site could result in a potential for significant impacts. For example, the proposed action may be located adjacent to a National Historic Landmark or in an ecologically important and fragile area such as a salt-water marsh, whereas the previous similar actions may have been located in less-sensitive environmental areas. The opinion for *Maryland Planning Commission* v. *Postal Service* stated that one criterion for use in judging whether a federal agency has supplied convincing reasons why potential impacts are insignificant is to determine whether "the agency took a hard look at the problem, as opposed to bold conclusions, unaided by preliminary investigations."*

Another type of environmental assessment is referred to as a generic assessment. The generic assessment discusses the various activities involved in a general type of action, the required inputs, the types of environmental residuals generated and the components of the environment likely to be affected. To the greatest extent possible, the generic assessment provides factors for quantifying the inputs and the environmental residuals. In addition, the generic assessment may identify analytical techniques for evaluating the environmental impacts resulting from a series of similar actions. It may present tables, monographs or other reference material to use in estimating the environmental impacts of these actions.

Maryland Planning Commission v. *Postal Service, Environmental Reporter - Cases,* 5 ERC 1725, The Bureau of National Affairs, Washington, D.C. (1974).

A generic assessment is valuable because it contains discussions, factors and reference material that could be incorporated directly into future environmental assessments, thereby decreasing the time required to prepare such assessments. However, preparation of such a generic assessment does not in itself satisfy legal requirements for preparation and filing of environmental statements.

The preparation of a generic assessment is best undertaken after several assessments have been prepared for the recurring type of action. This assures that sufficient information and expertise are available for preparing a comprehensive generic assessment. In evaluating whether the preparation of a generic assessment would be worthwhile, a consideration should be made on how many additional times in the future the action will recur and the degree of similarity between the numerous actions and their resulting residuals.

Scope of Environmental Assessment

The initial step in preparing an environmental assessment for a proposed action is to determine its scope, which requires identification of the activities involved in the proposed action, the conjunctive developments involved, the type of ecosystem likely to be affected and the time-frame over which the activity will occur.

Data Collection

The data requirements for an environmental assessment can normally be satisfied by a visit to the site and by obtaining data on the general characteristics of both the site area and the proposed action. Depending on the size of the site, the site visit typically would require from one day to two to three months (exclusive of "raw" data generation).

Selection of Analytical Techniques

This activity involves selecting the methods to be used to measure the impact of specific project actions. Selection of analytical techniques typically requires from one to three weeks. If a generic assessment is available for the proposed action, the generic assessment will contain some analytical techniques and little extra time will be required for this activity.

Preparation of Environmental Assessment

The preparation of the environmental assessment consists of analyzing the impacts associated with the proposed action. This involves quantifying those impacts that can be quantified and evaluating those impacts that cannot be quantified. The objective of NEPA is to build into the federal agency decision-making process, beginning at the earliest possible point, an appropriate and careful consideration of the environmental aspects of proposed actions so that decisions can meaningfully reflect national environmental concerns.

Timing of Environmental Assessments

There are two purposes behind the preparation of environmental impact assessments: (1) to determine whether a proposed action requires the preparation of an environmental impact statement, and (2) to ensure that environmental values are considered as early as possible in the decision-making process (even if these potential impacts are not "significant" but are, nevertheless, adverse). Each purpose affects the time at which an environmental assessment should be prepared.

With regard to the first purpose, the environmental assessment must be completed early enough to allow timely preparation of an environmental impact statement if one is deemed necessary by the assessment. Thus, in all instances, the environmental assessment must be completed prior to the date the environmental impact statement would be initiated, if one is deemed necessary. Review of the environmental assessment consists of determining the adequacy of the assessment. The review process and any necessary revisions can typically require at least double the time for the actual preparation.

There are no specific congressional or administrative guidelines as to the interpretation of "significance." Because the point at which an impact becomes significant will vary, based on the many factors, a precise definition of environmental significance that is valid in all contexts cannot be formulated.

Table 1-3 lists the types of potential impacts to be considered in determining the environmental significance of a proposed project. The impacts have been categorized according to the environmental area affected, i.e., physical, biological or human. This allows for considerable flexibility and ease in determining the overall impacts from diverse activities affecting the same environmental area.

In determining the significance of the proposed action, both adverse and beneficial effects are to be considered. Significant effects include both beneficial and adverse effects, and an environmental statement is required even if, on balance, the effect of the proposed action is believed to be beneficial. Significant adverse effects include those that degrade the quality of the environment, curtail the range of beneficial uses of

Table 1-3. Environmental Impact Analysis Areas

Potential Impacts to the Physical Environment	Ecological Relationships
Air	Ecological balance
Climate	Critical species in food chain
Air emissions	Productivity
Air quality	Diversity
Water	Potential Impacts to Human Environment
Water requirements	Socioeconomic Impacts
Water availability	Population and demographic changes
Water quality	Economic conditions
Physiography	Employment
Soils	Wages
Geology	Tax base
Topography	Social Conditions
Drainage modifications	Noise
Solid Wastes	Pressure on services such as police,
Quantity	fire, schools, and hospitals and on
Disposal	utilities and transportation
Mineral Resources	Changes in daily living patterns
Consumption	Land use
Depletion	Water use
Potential Impacts to the Biological Environment	Aesthetics
Flora	Special Interest Points
Terrestrial	Archaeological
Aquatic	Paleontological
Endangered species	Historical
Fauna	Recreational
Terrestrial	Human Health Effects
Aquatic	Air emissions
Endangered species	Water residuals
	Solid wastes

the environment and serve short-term benefits to the disadvantage of long-term environmental goals.

Furthermore, significant environmental effects encompass both primary (direct) and secondary (indirect) environmental effects. Primary effects may include direct destruction of animal habitat by construction activities, the generation of environmental residuals and the introduction of the operational population into the project area. Secondary effects may include effects from reduction of animal habitats, from impacts to water quality and from the additional population required to support the plant work force. Primary effects are not given greater consideration than secondary effects in determining significance.

Proposed actions, which are likely to be highly controversial, most probably will entail the preparation of an environmental impact statement. The term "controversial" refers to instances where a substantial dispute exists as to the size, nature, location or effect of the proposed action rather than to the existence of opposition to a use, the effect of which is relatively undisputed. The suggestion that "controversial" must be equated with neighborhood opposition has been rejected.

The court opinion in *Hanly* v. *Kleindienst** described two relevant factors to be considered in determining the significance of a proposed action. The first factor is:

> "the extent to which the action will cause adverse environmental effects in excess of those created by existing uses in the area affected by it."

This factor views the relative effect of the action. It considers the magnitude of the additional impacts caused by the proposed action in relation to those impacts already occurring in the area. Since the relative impact of the proposed action will vary with the environmental setting, an action that is significant in one area may not be significant in another. For example, construction of an additional power plant in a heavily industrialized area will usually have less of an adverse impact than if it were constructed in a low-density residential area.

The dissent to the majority opinion in *Morningside Renewal Council* v. *AEC* further stated:

> "it would (not) be inconsistent with, or stretching, this language to say that the true first test is the extent to which the action has the *potential of causing* adverse environmental effects . . . If the potential is substantial then the impact statement must be forthcoming; NEPA speaks of making an initial determination 'as to whether the proposal would have a significant effect,' not whether it 'does have' such an effect."†

Environmental Reporter - Cases, 4 ERC 1789, The Bureau of National Affairs, Washington, D.C. (1973).

†*Hanly* v. *Kleindienst, Environmental Reporter - Cases,* 4 ERC 1789, The Bureau of National Affairs, Washington, D.C. (1973).

The second relevant factor proposed by the *Hanly* v. *Kleindienst* court for evaluating significance is as follows:

> "the absolute quantitative adverse environmental effects of the action itself, including the cumulative harm that results from its contribution to existing adverse conditions or users in the area."*

This factor views the cumulative effect of the proposed action. Actions that do not have a relative significant effect may have an absolute significant effect due to their existing contribution to an existing adverse effect.

The opinion for *First National Bank* v. *Richardson,* illustrating this second factor, states:

> "while speaking in terms of normative conditions, we understand from the inclusion of this test that the standard for invoking the scrutiny of the full-scale procedure goes beyond protection and preservation of the environmental status-quo."†

For broad research and development programs, determination of the time at which environmental impact statements should be prepared is extremely subjective. There is no one specific time when the statement has to be prepared either to satisfy the requirements of NEPA or to avoid significant delays in the program development. In fact, the basic question to be resolved is not when the statement should be prepared, but rather when it becomes meaningful to prepare the statement to satisfy the intent of NEPA. Determination of when it is meaningful to prepare a programmatic statement requires reconciliation of two competing needs. There is the need to prepare the statement early enough in the program's decision process so that environmental concerns can be factored into the decision process; however, there is also the need to prepare the statement late enough in the program so that the statement can contain meaningful information.

In the early stages of a research and development program, little is known about the technologies to be developed through the program. Future applications of the technologies and the impacts from such applications are uncertain. Predictions of the possible effects from implementation of the technologies would necessarily have to be very general and would be based more on guesswork than on any real analysis. The value of a statement prepared at such a time would be very questionable. The

---

Hanly v. *Kleindienst, Environmental Reporter - Cases,* 4 ERC 1789, The Bureau of National Affairs, Washington, D.C. (1973).
†*First National Bank* v. *Richardson, Environmental Reporter - Cases,* 5 ERC 1833, The Bureau of National Affairs, Washington, D.C.

opinion rendered for *Scientist's Institute* v. *AEC** in deciding that a programmatic statement was then required for the liquid metal fast breeder reactor program stated that "NEPA requires predictions, but not prophecy."

On the other hand, in the late stages of the program, when commercial feasibility of the technologies has been demonstrated, detailed and valid data would be available for the preparation of an environmental impact statement. A statement prepared at such a late date would present a thorough and accurate description of the effects of the program. However, such a statement would be of little value in ensuring that pertinent environmental concerns are considered in the decision-making process. By that time the program would have reached such a stage of investment or commitment to future developments that future options would probably be precluded or restricted, regardless of their environmental desirability.

There will be no one instance when it is apparent that such a point has been reached. Rather, these competing requirements for timeliness of preparation and availability of meaningful information will continually have to be balanced against each other to determine an appropriate point at which to prepare a programmatic statement. Important factors to be considered in such a balancing include:

1. the magnitude of federal investment in the program and the extent to which such investment has slowed down the development of alternative technologies;
2. the extent to which continued investment in the program is likely to foreclose or restrict future alternatives;
3. the extent to which irretrievable commitments are being made and options precluded as the program progresses;
4. the likelihood that the technology will prove commercially possible and how soon this may occur;
5. the degree of environmental impact that could occur in the event the technologies involved in the program were widely applied;
6. the extent to which meaningful information is available to estimate the effects from the application of the technologies involved in the program; and
7. the extent to which meaingful information is available to estimate the effects from the application of alternative techologies.

Periodic evaluation of such factors is required to determine when it has become practical to prepare a programmatic statement. According to CEQ guidelines (40 CFR 1500), such an evaluation should be performed

---

**Environment Reporter - Cases,* 5 ERC 1427, The Bureau of National Affairs, Washington, D.C. (1974).

periodically for research and development programs, and when such a periodic evaluation procedure determines that a statement is still premature, the agency should briefly set forth the reasons for its determination that a statement is not yet necessary.

CHAPTER 2

TECHNIQUES FOR AIDING IN THE
ASSESSMENT PROCESS

INTRODUCTION

The environmental assessment process surfaces a large volume of unorganized raw data. One of the challenges facing the analyst is to create order out of this chaos. A number of procedures, aids, techniques and methods have been developed and tested with the multiple aims of:

1. organizing an heterogeneous mass of data;
2. summarizing these data;
3. aggregating the data into a smaller set with a minimum loss of information;
4. extracting saliant features; and
5. displaying the raw data and the derived information in a meaningful way

The proposed model of impact assessment is shown as Figure 2-1 in terms of its major elements, each one of which is described below.

I. Definition of Impact
    1. Definition of individuals and/or classes of events or changes that may impact on the environment.
    2. Categorizing the areas of activities in which such impact may occur.
    3. For a class of events, specifying the kind of action associated with it through which impact may occur.
    4. Through the application of explicit or implicit criteria, matching the classes of action (*e.g.*, building a nuclear power plant) to areas of human activity (*e.g.*, industrial production) to determine more specifically the potential impact associated with a given class of events.

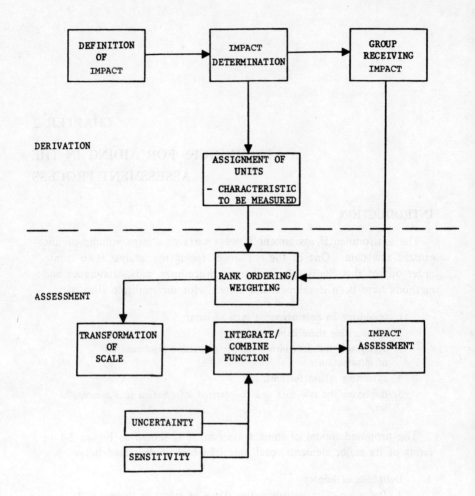

Figure 2-1. Model elements.

II.   Impact Determination

1. The translation of potential impact into a level of concreteness represented by specific advantageous and disadvantageous changes capable of observation by human senses or instrumentation.

2. Establishing the kind and level of impact which may be received by different segments of the population engaged in different activities.

3. Selection of a specific observable or sensible characteristic to be used as a measure of specific impact.

III. Impact Allocation

1. Segmentation of some general population into subsets (*e.g.,* government vs industry workers, or population at different distances from a site, etc.) which are affected differently.

2. Determination of how the impacts defined for a given class of events affect each segment of the population differently.

3. Assignment of a specific characteristic to be measured as an expression of the impact received by each segment of the population.

IV. Measurement of Impact

1. Determination of the units in which impact is to be measured (*e.g.,* pounds of SO_2, per capita income, etc.).

2. Methods or techniques for obtaining a measurement (*e.g.,* survey, expert judgment).

3. Means for actually securing the measurement (*e.g.,* subjective opinion can be obtained by interview or questionnaire).

V. Transformation of Scale

1. Determination of scale to be used (*e.g.,* ordinal, cardinal, interval, ratio).

2. Selection of a common basis for all parameters (*e.g.,* transformation to dollar value or 0-1 scale).

3. Actual transformation by the use of such techniques as cost or equivalents, imputed worth, etc.

VI. Rank Ordering/Weighing

1. Determining the relative rank of different impact (*e.g.,* health effect being more important than economic gain).

2. Determining relative weights to be attached to each input and for each population segment.

VII. Impact Integration

1. Determination of the dimensionality to be used (*e.g.,* each impact presented separately or as a summary).

2. Summary of the impact either by the use of statistics, indicators or graphical means.

VIII. Sensitivity/Validation

1. Testing the results predicted by the model for changes in the basic parameters.

2. Documentation of similar impact from an alternative source.

IX. Treating Uncertainty

1. Documentation by some statistical measures, of variation.

2. Treatment by sensitivity analysis.

Table 2-1 summarizes the applicability of each technique to be described below to one or more of the aims of environmental assessment.

- Definition of generic impact
- Determination of specific impact

- Allocation of impact to population groups
- Measurement of impact
- Rank ordering/weighting of kinds of impact
- Transformation of scale
- Aggregation of impact

Additionally, techniques are specified for dealing with uncertainty (Duckstein *et al.*, 1977) in regard to impact levels and for examining the results of the model for sensitivity to changes in the input data.

PRINCIPLES OF SELECTION

A few important principles should guide the analyst in selecting techniques to assist him in preparing an environmental assessment.

The Systems Approach

A systematic approach is the single most important attribute for the preparation of a useful environmental assessment.

Quantification

Quantification is a two-edged sword; but on the whole, greater insight into a problem is provided by some form of quantification, even if it is just forcing numerical value into subjective judgment.

A Predictive Process

It is essential to remember that an environmental assessment is essentially a predictive process. While necessary, a baseline case does not an assessment make.

Exogeneous Factors

Factors external to the actions or outside the control of the decision-maker should not be ignored. Their effect is sometimes decisive.

CRITERIA FOR SELECTING A METHODOLOGY

Listed below are some of the most important criteria for selecting a methodology.

1. *Comprehensiveness.* The methodology must embrace all significant alternatives, criteria aspects and major points of view. Without this approach, decisions are almost certain to be less than optimal and intellectually unacceptable.

Table 2-1. Classification of Assessment Techniques

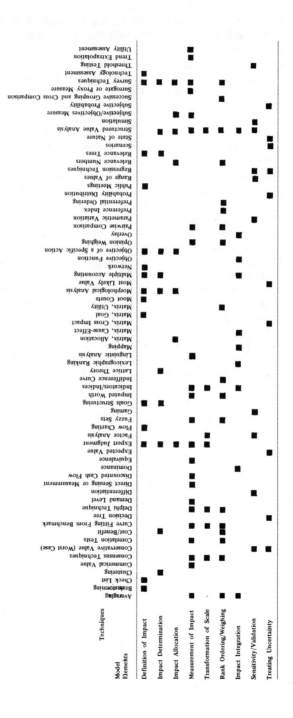

2. *Workability.* The methodology must be simple enough to be learned and applied by a small staff with limited knowledge on a small budget in a short time.

3. *Portrayability.* The conclusions derived must lend themselves to summarization and visual presentation so as to instill perspective, understanding, and confidence in the public and secure their participation.

4. *Expandability.* The methodology must permit initial screening of broad alternatives, and yet must be readily expandable to provide detailed focus on key aspects. Thus, the same methodology should permit either an overview analysis or a detailed examination.

5. *Explicitness of Criteria.* The methodology must include an explicit statement of all relevant criteria, systematically arrayed and weighed to reflect their relative importance.

6. *Holism.* The methodology must reflect an understanding of the environmental socioeconomic system as a whole and the major interrelationships among the various criteria.

7. *Separation of Effects.* The methodology must reflect the changes that would occur in moving from a "without the alternative" to a "with the alternative" future and must allow for measuring or sensing the "distance" between sets of alternatives.

8. *Commensurability.* Various criteria are conventionally measured in a wide variety of objective and subjective units (dollars, biomass, recreation days, good-bad, jobs, etc.). It is highly desirable to employ a means of translating these ratings into commensurate units as a tool to facilitate comparison.

9. *Data Input.* Difficulty of providing the required data input for a technique is a key criterion for the successful implementation of any model. Potentially excellent techniques may not be feasible because of the difficulty of data acquisition.

OVERVIEW

There have been several surveys of assessment methodologies published or presented at technical conferences. The papers of Andrews (1973) and Bishop (1972) are particularly well written and comprehensive. Schlesinger and Daetz (1973) provide a discussion of matrix methods, and Morrison *et al.* (1973) provide a survey of methodologies for siting power plants.

DESCRIPTION OF SPECIFIC TECHNIQUES

The techniques tabulated in Table 2-1 will be described in generic terms. Unless the technique is part of common knowledge or is very well known, a few references will be given to provide the theoretical foundations as well as applications and case studies.

AVERAGING

Averaging is a procedure based on the summation of all values in a set and then division by the number of values. It is a standard technique for summarizing a set of numerical data items into a single number representing the point of central tendency of the underlying distribution. It is the most commonly used summarization technique.

BRAINSTORMING

Brainstorming can be structured or unstructured. In both of its expressions it is a free-flowing generation of ideas among experts. A brainchild of the aerospace industry, it is some times a useful process for generating ideas and for simultaneously examining a phenomenon at many angles and optics. Brainstorming, whether carried-on individually or in groups, is based on the premise that among any large group of ideas a few should be good ones. Basic rules for brainstorming sessions have been identified as follows (Anderson, 1973):

1. State the problem in basic terms.
2. Do not stop to explore an idea or challenge it when it arises.
3. Reach for any idea even if on the surface its relevancy appears remote.
4. Provide the climate and support necessary to liberate participants from inhibiting attitudes.

Uninhibited atmosphere and expert knowledge are the essential ingredients for successful brainstorming.

CHECKLISTS

The use of checklists is one of the most common means for identifying and standardizing the activities to be included in subsequent analyses. It guarantees that topics of interest to a particular agency are considered, independent of the type of project or the interests of the reviewer. It also makes explicit which activities have been considered significant and those considered irrelevant or insignificant by the analyst. This can be very important as an aid to the agency or individuals reviewing the work. If done properly, it is also a means of ensuring exhaustive coverage of the issues involved. The main disadvantage is the tendency to rely on the checklist and to ignore items of special interest that may not be on the standard checklist.

A checklist for environmental threshold assessment was developed by The MITRE Corporation (Golden *et al.,* 1973) for the Interstate Commerce Commission as a simple means of determining whether an environmental impact statement was necessary. It also provided the reviewable record needed for a negative declaration in those cases in which an environmental impact statement is not required.

If the checklists are systematically developed and subjected to wide and thoughtful public exposure, they can be very useful in ensuring that all issues have been examined and that an explicit finding has been made that nothing of substantial relevance has been found that has not been made visible and analyzed in the evaluation (McHarg, 1969; Belknap and Furtado, 1967). The principal example of the checklist approach is the Water Resources Council method, defined in the Water Resources Council's (WRC) *Principles and Standards* (1971). Of all the methodologies considered herein, this one has received much public attention.

In addition to checklists, the need for other inputs in determining a comprehensive list of key factors is cited by Andrews (1973). Public meetings, personal contacts, multidisciplinary groups, listening sessions and opinion surveys are all used and will be described.

CLUSTERING

Clustering (Day and Heller, 1971) is the grouping of related elements in an organized manner, usually in the form of a hierarchy. A number of mathematical techniques based on similarity measures (distance, minimum intergroup variance, etc.) are available for manual and computerized handling of data on many scales. Graphic techniques (such as Dendrograms, tree diagrams) have been developed for displaying the results of clustering data analysis techniques.

COMMERCIAL VALUE

The evaluation of an economic product by the marketplace is one measure of its value. If the product is not bartered in a market, surrogate products that are may be substituted in an evaluation. This method is often used for quantifying impacts on a dollar scale (Howe, 1971; Schlaifer, 1969).

CONSENSUS TECHNIQUES

Consensus is an interactive communication technique used by a group until a group value is selected by common agreement (Jantsch, 1967).

This goal of achieving a consensus is found in most studies, and a number of methods are used from general meetings to brainstorming, to analytical techniques, to general citizen participation.

CONSERVATIVE VALUES

The selection of a less favorable outcome, which is highly likely to be exceeded, is often used as a lower bound of a distribution of outcome. This is a method used for sensitivity analysis as well as for evaluating uncertainty.

CORRELATION

Correlation is a statistical technique used to determine the strength of relationships between variables. The linear product moment correlation is most useful when dealing with quantitative data. Alternatively, a rank correlation technique is available for dealing with ordinal information.

Once a correlation matrix is developed, partial correlation coefficients or techniques for extracting latent structure from the correlation matrix (factor analysis, principal component analysis, Fischer discriminant function analysis, cannonical correlation analysis) are available and described in standard statistical texts for dealing with the complexity of multi-attributes analysis.

COST/BENEFIT ANALYSIS

Benefit/cost analysis is a technique that compares the impacts (benefits or disadvantages) of a program (usually spending public funds) with the costs of the program (Gsellman, 1977).

Cost-effectiveness and cost/benefit analyses have identical objectives, *i.e.,* to provide information to the decision-maker to improve the efficiency of decisions. However, cost-effectiveness analyses differ from cost/benefit analyses in two major respects. The cost-effectiveness analysis methodology is designed to handle programs in which all benefits cannot be conveniently or effectively measured in terms of dollars, and to consider alternative program levels as an integral part of the analysis.

Costs

The costs of the program are simply the discounted dollar expenditures over the life of the program. In theory, the costs should be equal to the benefits lost as a result of selecting the program over its next best alternative. In practice, applying this concept is difficult and expensive since it requires one to identify and evaluate the next best alternative. In a free market economy, resource prices reflect the value of the resource used in the next best alternative. Therefore, for all practical purposes, equating the cost of the program to its dollar cost is satisfactory.

Discounting is a very important part of performing cost/benefit studies. Both costs and benefits vary in magnitude over time. If discounting were not used, the cost and benefit stream for a program would be expressed as a function of time, $i.e.,$ $b(t)/c(t)$. Discounting permits the stream of costs and benefits to be presented as numbers which are not functions of time. This single number is referred to as the present value of the stream of costs or benefits. Economic literature is filled with discussions of the appropriate rate to use in discounting. In general, however, the discount rate to be used for cost/benefit studies of federal programs is specified by the Office of Management and Budget to be 10%/yr.

Benefits

Benefits (or disadvantages) are the impacts resulting from the implementation of the results of the program (Watson et $al.,$ 1974). Traditionally, cost/benefit analyses have concentrated on quantifying all benefits in terms of a single measure, $i.e.,$ dollars. From a practical standpoint, this is unfortunate. Many of the factors required to convert all quantitative measures of benefits to dollars generate significant amounts of debate which tend to detract from and, in some cases, destroy the usefulness of an analysis. In addition, converting all benefits to dollars tends to reduce the value of the study to the decision-maker. In light of the above, the most desirable approach is to develop a set of benefit indicators (with the traditional cost/benefit ratio being one of the indicators) and to use this set as a basis for performing the analysis and presenting the results. This approach, in effect, is a combination of part of the cost-effectiveness and cost/benefit analysis concepts.

The present state-of-the-art in performing cost/benefit analyses does not permit all the program benefits or values to be qualified. Further, many of those benefits which can be quantified cannot be converted to a common measure. These limitations, in conjunction with the inherent uncertainties associated with planning, reduce the potential value of cost/benefit in supporting planning.

The tools available for performing cost/benefit studies fall into three categories: (1) those used to estimate the benefits, (2) those used to combine benefits, and (3) those used to allocate resources.

Techniques to support resource allocation or project selection decisions range from formal analytical procedures such as dynamic programming and mathematical programming to informal ad hoc techniques using criteria defined to reflect the relative values of the various projects. Final selection of projects using this approach tends to rely heavily upon subjective judgment.

In the informal approach, the decision-maker identifies the advantages and disadvantages of each attribute and discusses a possible rationale for his choice with other members of the decision-making body. This method can be applied successfully when the number of attributes is small and good communications exist among members of the decision-making body.

The second group, formal quantitative methods, can be separated into a number of subgroups: (1) weighting schemes, and (2) economic.

CURVE FITTING FROM BENCHMARKS

A small number of key entries are selected because their worth is readily agreed on or can be defined in terms of objective criteria. A smooth curve is then fitted to these benchmarks either by eye or using mathematical techniques. The technique provides a means of converting different kinds of impact to a common utility scale (*e.g.,* from 0-1) for subsequent comparison (O'Connor, 1972; Rowe, 1970). For example, incremental economic increases expected to result in a depressed locality from a nuclear power station could be so plotted, using as a benchmark for lower threshold the amount required to bring the per capita income up to the poverty level; as an upper threshold the amount required to bring the per capita income to the top 5% level for the country as a whole, and as a midpoint the addition needed to match the average level of some larger geographic areas in which the locality exists.

DECISION TREES

Decision trees are used to portray alternative courses of action, and to relate them to alternative decisions showing all consequences of the decision. The tree represents alternative courses or series of actions related to a previous decision (Moskowitz, 1973; Rainer and White, 1969). Decision trees have been widely used as a discipline to organize information and ensure exhaustive coverage. Trees are basically hierarchical structures and allow for level to be given to each action or decision and following the logic of a progressive sequence.

DELPHI TECHNIQUE

The Delphi technique originated in Rand in 1964. Since then it has been time-tested and modified in many directions and dimensions. The main attribute of this technique is that it forces a group (typically an expert panel) to think in a structured fashion using explicit assumptions; to minimize the dominance of one or a few individuals by requiring consensus or convergence; and to maximize the utility of the procedure by identifying new alternatives or options not part of the starting set.

The Delphi technique (Turoff, 1972; Dalkey and Helmer, 1963; Wood and Campbell, 1970) is a systematic attempt to discipline the input of expert judgment for the purposes of assessing, evaluating and forecasting. It uses the opinion of knowledgeable experts and, through an iterative process, converges toward group consensus. The method can be both qualitative and quantitative. It can be done in a group meeting, by telephone, or by filling-in questionnaires or forms.

Perhaps currently the most popular means of acquiring a satisfactory consensus of subjective opinion is the Delphi technique, which involves iterative use of questions and answers. Quantitative responses to each question are statistically assessed to find the mean value and then are fed back to each participant, who is given an opportunity to change his estimate, if he so desires. Anonymity of the answers is preserved to prevent undue influence of any particular individuals whose views might be regarded as dominant, while each respondent personally weighs the strength of his own convictions against group estimates. Although time-consuming, this technique has been found effective, in a number of applications, both in reaching a reasonable consensus and in uncovering unsuspected factors that account for strongly divergent views.

While the Delphi technique is commonly employed with subject matter experts, it is occasionally combined with opinion surveys to get the public's attitudes. Some methodologies attempt to sample public opinion by means of mailed questionnaires or interviews conducted either in person or by telephone. These surveys are typically intended to provide estimates of the extent of potential support of or opposition to proposed action among the populace in a specific locality. But they may also seek attitudes about relevant social values and other particular environmental considerations and attempt to make explicit relative rankings or weights implicitly accorded to various criteria by the public. Assessment of public opinion is a relatively recent addition to the repertoire of impact assessment methodologies and reflects awareness by the industry and their contractors of the increasing public concern over the physical and social impacts of new developments (Martino, 1970a, b; Wright, 1972; Mandanis, 1969).

Techniques are available, although not in wide use, for measuring aspects of public reaction to projects which are particularly difficult to quantify while at the same time possibly critical. The Delphi technique has a strong basis in intuitive thinking, a more or less systematic use of expert speculations and much variation in the organized search for new ideas. It can be equated to a series of interactive brainstorming sessions.

Recently, Brockhaus (1975) has developed a methodology that can be used to gather, improve and refine judgments. The methodology is called POSTURE, meaning policy specification technique using realistic environments. A new judgmental method named *Shang* (Ford, 1975) has been proposed as an alternative to Delphi to avoid some of the problems of Delphi associated with its pressure to converge and the need for response commitment. An interesting quantification of the Delphi technique is to merge it with a Bayesian probability viewpoint (Sahal and Yee, 1975). The validity and reliability of the Delphi technique itself has also been reviewed (Hill and Fowles, 1975; Salancik, 1973).

DEMAND LEVEL

Borrowed from the economic field, demand level is a representation of expected impact in terms of a predicted demand curve. It has been used extensively in cost/benefit analyses (Cicchetti *et al.,* 1972; Green and Rao, 1970).

DIFFERENTIATION

The mathematical process of differentiation expresses the rate of change of one variable with respect to change in the value of another. This is a useful technique for sensitivity analysis. In many cases, the rate of change of a variable is equally, if not more, important than the amplitude of the effect.

DIRECT SENSING OR MEASUREMENT

The direct determination of value by examination, *e.g.,* accounting records, physical measurement, etc., is the first step in developing a data base for impact assessment (Rowe, 1972; Tarascio and Murphy, 1972). The whole spectrum of physical devices, platforms, media and techniques is used to collect raw data as input to the assessment process.

DISCOUNTED CASH FLOW

The use of an appropriate interest rate to discount all cash flows to the same point in time is an essential step in econometric analyses. These analyses are an essential part of the environmental assessment process since impact can no longer be measured, estimated or formulated without reference to an economic or another common denominator.

DOMINANCE

Dominance relationship is a means of assessing multidimensional representations (vectors) of the value of different alternatives by finding an alternative for which all (or a maximum number of) elements have values equaling or exceeding the value of any corresponding element. For example, the vector 8, 6, 4 dominates the vector 4, 3, 2 (Foldes, 1972). This technique has been used in the social sciences and is just now being applied to problems of environmental assessment.

EQUIVALENCE

Like dominance, equivalence is a concept used in social science studies. It consists of measuring the impact associated with an action, in terms of the value of something regarded as an equivalent or which could have been used as a substitute (Arrow, 1951; Rainer and White, 1969).

EXPECTED VALUE

The expected value of a variable is the evaluation of an uncertain numerical event by weighting all possible events by their probability of occurrence and averaging. This technique is often used as a best "guestimate" of value.

EXPERT JUDGMENT

The reliance on opinions of persons knowlegeable in an area for estimating possible futures, alternatives, impact type and intensity is an accepted technique. Experts are most useful in throwing light on a difficult problem. But like all specialized groups, they have their special biases and prejudices, and the analyst must recognize this deficiency and be ready to deal with it.

FACTOR ANALYSIS

Factor analysis is a structural technique for multidimensional analysis in which the statistical correlations among a set of measurements expressed as n-dimensional points are used to derive an orthogonal basis in m ($\leq$ n) dimensions. The new basis is taken to represent a set of m mutually independent "factors" accounting for the differences among the measurements. The measurements can then be equivalently expressed as points in m-dimensional space or linear combinations of the m factors, using a new scale.

Factor analysis is a powerful technique for reducing the dimensionality of the event space. Other techniques include principal component analysis, cannonical correlation, and discriminant function analysis.

FLOWCHARTING

Many impacts are not amenable to mathematical modeling, but rather are best determined on the basis of the insights and experience of environmental specialists. The difficulty with this type of intuitive approach is that it does require training in environmental sciences. Therefore, to implement it, this intuitive knowledge is crystallized by translating it into a flowchart where the major axis can be time or stage of development or steps in a cycle.

FUZZY SETS

The theory of fuzzy sets has been established by Zadeh (1973). Items that possess in varying degree an abstract quality (*e.g.*, "youth") can be considered as members of a qualitative or "fuzzy" set; the extent to which a given item is considered to exhibit the specific quality can then be expressed by a number representing on a common scale the degree of membership in that set. For example, a newborn infant might have 100% membership in the fuzzy set comprising "youth," whereas a centenarian approaches 0 membership, age 30 may represent a midpoint (50%), etc. (Saaty, 1972).

GAMING

This technique usually uses models and sophisticated computers to explore the implications and consequences of assumptions, decisions and choices. Several gaming techniques have been attempted that profit by group interactions and the feedback of cause-effect displays. Armstrong and Hobson (1970) describe a NEXUS procedure designed to elicit key factors and conflicting assumptions about potential impacts. Kane *et al.,* (1973) have a sophisticated simulation language, KSIM, feeding back impacts as an aid to identifying important activities. Other important source documents in game theory are Milnor (1954), Hurwicz (1953) and Luce and Raiffa (1957).

Games originated in the military and have been used in the industry for 10-15 years for staff training (Warneryd, 1975). They are seen as a means for education, as a research method and as a planning instrument. Their main advantage is that they promote a holistic or total approach they foster interprofessional cooperation, they are a form of education that allows the finding of new problems, they generate new data and are a most useful planning and forecasting tool (Duke, 1968).

Apex is a typical simulation of a metropolitan area containing data on population, employment, land utilization, municipal services and meteorological conditions.

GOALS STRUCTURING

Goals structuring is any systematic procedure for extending goals to one or more levels of greater detail and concreteness as a result of which specific impact can be ultimately defined (Sayeki and Vesper, 1973).

Goals themselves are defined as a statement from an authoritative or official source defining the goals or aims of any specific action or ongoing activity or of the policy to be pursued toward end-results thereof (Beckerhoff, 1970; Davenport, 1972; Awerbuch and Wallace, 1977).

IMPUTED WORTH

Imputed worth is the estimation of the value on item by equating costs of protection from an uncertain event and the probability of recurrence. Examples of the use of this concept are presented by Mohring (1965) and Strayk (1970).

INDICES AND INDICATORS

Indices representing an integrated measure of the status of the environment are often used to compare different regions, different time periods or the impact of different scenarios (Bisselle, 1973, 1977; Sanderson, 1977; Munn, 1977).

Also, when comparing different sites, techniques may be employed to represent in terms of some reference value the final rating scores of each

site. One such is the Impact Quotient (IQ) used in a methodology by
Dames and Moore. The IQ expresses the algebraic difference between the
calculated environmental state at a given location with and without the
projected action or facility. The procedure represents both a normaliza-
tion of the rating for each potential site and a measure of whether the
impact of locating a plant or other action will be beneficial (positive IQ)
or adverse (negative IQ).

A matrix structure in which siting criteria or elements of potential
impact appear as terms in a vector is used both as a specialized checklist
format to ensure inclusiveness of considerations and as a graphic device
to facilitate visual analysis. The vectors themselves are typically either
alternative locations or aspects of a proposed plant at a particular location.
In the second situation, each location (or each plant configuration at a
single location) is characterized numerically be an entire matrix, resulting
in greater comprehensiveness of detail but also in the need to compare
matrices for assessing alternatives.

The Battelle Environmental Evaluation System uses a hierarchical arrange-
ment to aggregate the individual impacts into a total environmental impact
rating (Figure 2-2). The initial level includes Ecology, Environmental

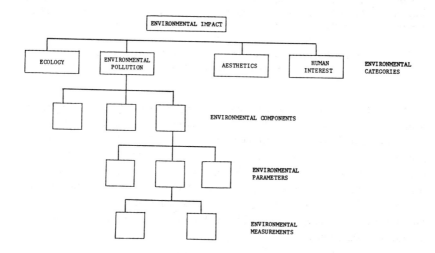

Figure 2-2. Battelle hierarchical system (Bennington *et al.*, 1974).

Pollution, Aesthetics and Human Interest. To calculate the total impact rating, the system works from the bottom level to the top. At level four, each impact measurement is transformed into a standardized environmental quality value (EQ) on a continuing scale from zero to one. The relative importance of each of the 78 parameters at level four is expressed in Parameter Importance Units (PIU), and a value for each parameter is is calculated in terms of environmental impact units (EIU), which are calculated by the formula EIU = (PIU) (EQ). These EIU values are then cumulated up through the levels to compute category scores at level one and finally a total environmental impact score.

Another hierarchical system, the Environmental Analysis System, has been developed for Northern States Power Company by Commonwealth Associates. The categories for the first two levels of the five levels employed are shown in Figure 2-3.

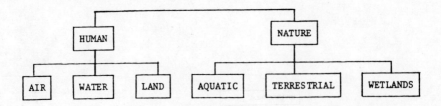

Figure 2-3. Commonwealth environmental analysis system (Bennington *et al.*, 1974).

At the bottom level, a magnitude and importance are derived independent of all other impacts. These are measured on a zero to ten scale. The upward addition of the impacts leads to the total environmental impact number. An external weighting scheme is applied at every level to combine the different types of information. It is stressed that these external weights must be consistent for all alternatives if the method is to be useful. Two dimensional spatial plots of differential cost vs impact number are then provided to highlight dominated alternatives and assist in trade-off decisions.

INDIFFERENCE CURVES

Indifference curves are functional relationships of value expressed as equivalent quantities of an alternative which are identical in value (Keeney, 1972).

LATTICE THEORY

Lattice Theory is a branch of set theory in which sets are partially ordered in terms of commonality of members and which is applied in the present context to order impact clusters or groups of interrelated impact in terms of degrees of uniqueness and commonality among the clusters (Gulliksen, 1961).

LEXICOGRAPHIC RANKING

Lexicographic ranking is the ordering of vectors or sets of elements or discrete numerical values in a fashion analogous to alphabetical indexing. It is based on priority assigned to each element of the vector so that all vectors with maximum value in the element of highest priority are ranked first; within those having the same value for highest priority element, sub-ordering is by value of the element of second priority, and so on. For example, if the positioning of elements in the following vectors corresponds to their priority for lexicographic ranking, then 10, 7, 1, 2 ranks ahead of both 10, 6, 10, 10 and 2, 8, 9, 7. It is useful in assessing impact vectors or multiple scoring of noncomparable impact if the relative significance of the different impact can be determined on an ordinal but not an interval or ratio scale (Thuesen, 1971).

LINGUISTIC ANALYSIS

Linguistic analysis is the conversion of qualitative characteristics or judgments from an expression in words into a numerical representation based on precise values or mathematical conversion functions assigned to each term. It is especially suitable for combination with the use of fuzzy sets by evaluating the qualitative terms numerically in terms of their degree of membership in a fuzzy set (Yu, 1973).

MAPPING

Maps constitute one of the quickest and most easily understood means of presenting environmental data. Most data are already available for the mapping of spatial data using computer techniques. Typically, maps have been used to describe *status quo* conditions. These include topography, soil type, vegetation, resource distribution, land use, etc. Maps are often based on extensive ground surveys and aerial photography, with some use of satellite imagery. Sometimes it is possible to identify unique combinations of historical and natural resources by using a set of overlay maps (McHarg, 1969).

Maps have the great virtue of literally giving the viewer a total picture; and development or future plans can be seen in relation to existing features, natural or man-made.

MATRICES

Of all the methods for impact evaluation, matrices are the most popular. In general, alternative plans (measures, projects, sites, actions or designs) are listed as column headings. The rows are the criteria that should dictate the choice. A conclusion is recorded, in each cell within the body of the matrix, that the indicated alternative will impact favorably or adversely on the indicated criterion. In most systems, a range of numbers is used to allow evaluators the opportunity to record shades of intensity. Some methodologies show how the evaluator might use a combination of objective indicators, expert opinions and impressions to score each cell. Most, however, emphasize the inescapability of the need for impressionistic ratings because: (1) many criteria do not lend themselves to numerical or other forms of objective analysis; (2) even where numerical data or indices are readily available, they are often relevent to only a part of the particular rating; and (3) the very large number of cells usually required precludes extensive data acquisition and analysis for each cell, any one of which might be expandable into a complex study of its own.

In some applications of the matrix method, the relative importance of the individual criteria is reflected in numerical ratings which are then normalized to 1.000 or 100%. Sometimes the weighting is done by an individual, sometimes by a team. In all weighting schemes, it is fully recognized that these weights are solely value judgments. It is also stressed, however, that it is realistically impossible to decide any issue with multiple criteria without such judgments. In this methodology the judgments are explicitly defined in commensurable units. To the extent desired, many people can make these judgments, and the final conclusion (selection of the best overall alternative) can be tested for sensitivity over the full range of value weights suggested.

A few methodologies multiply the severity rating (within each cell) by the importance rating of each criterion (row), and add up the totals to get an overall single-number index, which summarizes each alternative.

Most of the reviewed matrix methodologies have the following drawbacks:

1. They concentrate primarily on environmental parameters, ignoring the existence of economic and social criteria.
2. None provides adequate systematic guidance to the evaluator as to how he should consistently approach the rating in each cell.
3. Most concentrate almost entirely on adverse effects under the undefended assumptions that beneficial effects will be minor.
4. Some matrices are very difficult to portray. The Leopold method, for example, would use a master sheet with 8,700 cells for each alternative.

The checklists are often used as an input to a cause-effect matrix to identify the possible impacts of the project activities. The U.S. Geological Survey's Circular 645 (Leopold *et al.,* 1971) is an example of such a system. A portion of the matrix is shown in Figure 2-4. The entire matrix consists of 100 columns representing examples of causative actions and 88 rows representing environmental components and characteristics. Although the list of actions is not intended to be exhaustive, it is comprehensive enough to indicate the general type of actions to consider and to stimulate further discussion. The first step in this procedure is to check each column corresponding to an action associated with a particular project. For each column that is marked, the boxes coresponding to the impacts are examined. For each box, a magnitude and importance are specified on a scale of 1 to 10. These two numbers are placed in the box and separated by a slash. Each project would have a separate matrix, and the basis for assessing the activities and the values associated with the project were to be based on the professional judgment of the planners.

The Bechtel Environmental Assessment Matrix (Schlesinger and Hughes, 1972) is adapted from the U.S.G.S. system for site selection studies and incorporates a time-shared computer program and an automated sensitivity analysis. Battelle's Environmental Evaluation System (Dee *et al.,* 1973) and the Optimum Pathway Matrix Technique of the University of Georgia (1971) also use checklists as part of these procedures, which will be discussed below.

Another approach that combines the previous ideas is Sorenson's (1971) stepped matrix procedure that was developed for analyzing coastal zone resource utilization. Sorenson's procedure starts with a matrix relating various uses (residential development, crop farms, etc.) to causal effects. A network is then defined to trace out the possible effects. For example, the causal effect of "dredging an enclosed basin into an estuary shoreline"

INSTRUCTIONS

1. IDENTIFY ALL ACTIONS (LOCATED ACROSS THE TOP OF THE MATRIX) THAT ARE PART OF THE PROPOSED PROJECT.
2. UNDER EACH OF THE PROPOSED ACTIONS, PLACE A SLASH AT THE INTERSECTION WITH EACH ITEM ON THE SIDE OF THE MATRIX IF AN IMPACT IS POSSIBLE.
3. HAVING COMPLETED THE MATRIX, IN THE UPPER LEFT-HAND CORNER OF EACH BOX WITH A SLASH, PLACE A NUMBER FROM 1 TO 10 WHICH INDICATES THE MAGNITUDE OF THE POSSIBLE IMPACT: 10 REPRESENTS THE GREATEST MAGNITUDE OF IMPACT AND 1 THE LEAST (NO ZEROES). BEFORE EACH NUMBER PLACE + IF THE IMPACT WOULD BE BENEFICIAL. IN THE LOWER RIGHT-HAND CORNER OF THE BOX PLACE A NUMBER FROM 1 TO 10 WHICH INDICATES THE IMPORTANCE OF THE POSSIBLE IMPACT (e.g. REGIONAL vs. LOCAL): 10 REPRESENTS THE GREATEST IMPORTANCE AND 1, THE LEAST (NO ZEROES).
4. THE TEXT WHICH ACCOMPANIES THE MATRIX SHOULD BE A DISCUSSION OF THE SIGNIFICANT IMPACTS, THOSE COLUMNS AND ROWS WITH LARGE NUMBERS OF BOXES MARKED AND INDIVIDUAL BOXES WITH THE LARGER NUMBERS.

SAMPLE MATRIX

	a	b	c	d	e
a		2/1	8/8	3/1	8/5
b		7/2			9/7

PROPOSED ACTIONS

A. MODIFICATION OF REGIME
a. EXOTIC FLORA OR FAUNA INTRODUCTION
b. BIOLOGICAL CONTROLS
c. MODIFICATION OF HABITAT
d. ALTERATION OF GROUND COVER
e. ALTERATION OF GROUND WATER HYDROLOGY
f. ALTERATION OF DRAINAGE
g. RIVER CONTROL AND FLOW MODIFICATION
h. CANALIZATION
i. IRRIGATION
j. WEATHER MODIFICATION
k. BURNING
l. SURFACE OR PAVING
m. NOISE AND VIBRATION

B. LAND TRANSFORMATION AND CONSTRUCTION
a. URBANIZATION
b. INDUSTRIAL SITES AND BUILDINGS
c. AIRPORTS
d. HIGHWAYS AND BRIDGES
e. ROADS AND TRAILS
f. RAILROADS
g. CABLES AND LIFTS
h. TRANSMISSION LINES, PIPELINES AND CORRIDORS
i. BARRIERS INCLUDING FENCING
j. CHANNEL DREDGING AND STRAIGHTENING
k. CHANNEL REVETMENTS
l. CANALS
m. DAMS AND IMPOUNDMENTS
n. PIERS, SEAWALLS, MARINAS AND SEA TERMINALS
o. OFFSHORE STRUCTURES
p. RECREATIONAL STRUCTURES
q. BLASTING AND DRILLING
r. CUT AND FILL
s. TUNNELS AND UNDERGROUND STRUCTURES

C. RESOURCE EXTRACTION
a. BLASTING AND DRILLING
b. SURFACE EXCAVATION
c. SUBSURFACE EXCAVATION AND RETORTING
d. WELL DRILLING AND FLUID REMOVAL
e. DREDGING
f. CLEAR CUTTING AND OTHER LUMBERING
g. COMMERCIAL FISHING AND HUNTING
a. FARMING
b. RANCHING

EARTH
a. MINERAL RESOURCES
b. CONSTRUCTION MATERIAL
c. SOILS
d. LAND FORM

A. PHYSICAL AND CHEMICAL CHARACTERISTIC	2 WATE	d. QUALITY
		e. TEMPERATURE
		f. RECHARGE
		g. SNOW, ICE AND PERMAFROST
	3 AT-MOSPHERE	a. QUALITY (GASES, PARTICULATES)
		b. CLIMATE (MICRO, MACRO)
		c. TEMPERATURE
	4 PROCESSES	a. FLOODS
		b. EROSION
		c. DEPOSITION (SEDIMENTATION, PRECIPITATION)
		d. SOLUTION
		e. SORPTION (ION EXCHANGE, COMPLEXING)
		f. COMPACTION AND SETTLING
		g. STABILITY (SLIDES, SLUMPS)
		h. STRESS-STRAIN (EARTHQUAKE)
		i. AIR MOVEMENTS
B. BIOLOGICAL CONDITIONS	1 FLORA	a. TREES
		b. SHRUBS
		c. GRASS
		d. CROPS
		e. MICROFLORA
		f. AQUATIC PLANTS
		g. ENDANGERED SPECIES
		h. BARRIERS
		i. CORRIDORS
	FAUNA	a. BIRDS
		b. LAND ANIMALS INCLUDING REPTILES
		c. FISH AND SHELLFISH
		d. BENTHIC ORGANISMS
		e. INSECTS
		f. MICROFAUNA

Figure 2-4. Portions of circular 645 matrix (Leopold, 1971).

leads to four principal categories. Each category has several levels of subcategories. One of the categories is given below:

101: Estuary Surface Area Increase
    101:1   Creation of New Water Areas Isolated from General Circulation Patterns of Estuary
    101:2   Possible Salinization or Other Contamination of Underlying Freshwater Aquifer by Puncturing Aquatard
    101:3   Increase Shoreline Perimeter

There are two more levels of subcategories as well as references to corrective actions, control mechanisms and references to a publication index. The network is a tree structure that shows multiple impacts resulting from an action but does not show cross effects or cumulative effects.

Once the possible impacts have been identified, the next step in impact assessment is forecasting effects or predicting impacts. If soil erosion is a potential impact, how much erosion will there be and over what time period?

The procedures vary from intuitive predictions sometimes utilizing Delphi procedures to the use of computer simulations. The U.S.G.S. proposal in Circular 645 suggests and encourages the use of expert judgment.

The U.S.G.S. Circular 645 matrix method includes an importance value of each impact in addition to the magnitude value. The importance value is intended to include the subjective evaluation of this impact; however, no guidance is provided on how to combine these two numbers or accumulate the effects.

The U.S.G.S. procedure is carried one step further by the Bechtel Environmental Assessment Matrix. A single environmental weighting scale is used for each plan and a total environmental score is computed. A sensitivity analysis is also performed by varying the environmental impact weights.

The University of Georgia Optimum Pathway Matrix Analysis uses a similar weighting scheme except that the short and long-term impacts are determined to measure the duration of the impact. These two effects are then combined by multiplying the long-term factors by 10. The cost of the project is included in the score with a weight of 25. This is one of the few approaches to directly combine cost and environmental impacts. In addition, a sophisticated sensitivity analysis is included to provide a 95% confidence limit on the credibility of the results.

Another method for determining an environmental quality value was used in 1974 by Commonwealth Associates in a corridor selection study in upstate New York. A suitability factor for each area grid cell to be considered for a proposed corridor is determined from an activity vs objec tive function matrix. The cells and associated data are available from a land use and natural resources data base (LUNR) maintained by the state government. For each activity, a suitability graph is determined by an interdisciplinary group of professionals. This graph relates the level of activity to a uniform scale of zero to ten. For example, routing a transmission line through a cell with two dairy farms would receive a score of seven with respect to the objection of minimizing conflict with existing land uses while a cell containing an existing transmission line might receive a score of one. Other objectives in the study are to: (1) minimize damage to natural systems; (2) minimize conflict with proposed land uses; (3) minimize conflict with culturally significant features; and (4) maximize potential for right-of-way sharing. If more than one activity affects the objective for a cell, an average suitability is determined. The resultant scores are then weighted relative to each other and averaged according to weight to form an objective score. The objective scores for the several objectives are then plotted by computer and transmission line routes selected.

Generally speaking, in terms of impact assessment, we recognize five broad classes of matrices (Pinkel, 1969; Gordon and Hayward, 1968; Gordon and Becker, 1972; Cetron, 1972).

Matrix Allocation

Matrix allocation is a procedure for estimating the distribution of impact, in which the numerical entry at the intersection of the ith row with the jth column expresses as the product of the respective row and column weights the relative share of the ith impact received by the jth population segment. Typically, both row and column weights are normalized so that the set of values for each sums to unity.

Cross Impact Matrix

Cross impact matrix is a device for expressing numerically the relationships between contingent events and anticipated future conditions. In the matrix, the intersection of the ith row with the jth column expresses a measure of the impact which the ith contingency will have on the jth condition. In a specific documented application, the "conditions" represented technological advances whereas the "contingencies" represented possible future events which would affect the technological achievements.

Goal Matrix

Goal matrix is the representation of progress toward multiple goals under each alternative action by elements of a vector. At a minimum, the direction of progress is determined.

Utility Matrix

Utility matrix is a matrix in which the numerical entry at the intersection of the ith row with the jth column measures as the product of the respective row and column weights the utility which the ith variable had for the jth purpose. In a documented application, the row variables represented kinds of information developed from a specific model whereas the purposes were uses expected to be made of the information classes. By considering rows as impact areas and columns as population segments, the technique coincides with matrix allocation of impact.

Cause-Effect Matrix

Cause-effect matrices are difficult to derive if we abide by the formal determinism of causation. In a weaker context, a matrix relating the general causing agent to the expected effect can be derived.

MOOT COURTS

This is a variation on gaming. It allows for utilizing the time-tested court hearing process to derive a better understanding of the implications associated with a proposed action.

MORPHOLOGICAL ANALYSIS

Morphological analysis is a technique of exhaustive search. It is based on the systematic asking of questions about the state of technological development. It was formulated first by Zwicky in 1957. Another important source is Bridgewater, 1968.

In morphological analysis, a problem is divided into subproblems. All the logical ways to solving the problems are sought. Then all combinations of solutions to the subproblems are studied. Morphological research has been defined as just "an orderly way of looking at things," and in so doing, achieving a "systematic perspective over all possible solutions of a given large-scale problem" (Jantsch, 1967).

MOST LIKELY VALUE

The assignment of the value with the highest probability of occurrance to a stochastic process in contemplating alternative actions is called the most likely value. This assignment can be made by numerical methods or by intuitive judgment or expert knowledge.

MULTIPLE ACCOUNTING

Multiple accounting is the evaluation of progress towards multiple goals by alternative data.

NETWORKS

A methodology, originally developed by Travelers Research Corporation (later CEM) (1969) and greatly expanded by Sorenson (1971), uses the sequential relationship, causal factor → environmental impact → effect. For each of four major uses of the California coastal zone (residential - commercial - agricultural, recreational, extractive, and industrial - transportation) Sorenson suggests certain causal factors (*e.g.*, protection of species, fences, slips and berths). Each causal factor, in turn, produces a possible adverse impact. Each of these possibly adverse initial conditions, in turn, produces consequent "conditions" or "effects." More than any other method thus far, it responds to a holistic criterion. Rather severe problems of workability, portrayability, separation of effects and commensurability would probably be encountered by using this method to compare a number of competing alternatives simply and systematically.

In another study, Nathan Associates' Deepwater Port Study (1972) developed a network-based system to aid in determining the secondary activities and potential impacts of major projects. The Deepwater Port Study starts with the problem of offloading petroleum and proceeds to redefine it into alternative delivery systems, disaggregating the systems into their components such as dredging, processing, etc. In addition, a set of environmental components are defined, *e.g.*, shoreline uses, increases in turbidity, etc. A network of interrelations is then defined to show primary and secondary effects of the various alternatives.

OBJECTIVE FUNCTION

A specified mathematical relationship between a dependent variable (*e.g.*, overall measure of impact) and a set of independent variables (*e.g.*, individual impact measures and their relative weights) is an objective function. In choosing among alternatives, the decision-maker typically seeks to maximize the (dependent variable of the) objective function (Smith, 1956).

OBJECTIVES OF SPECIFIC ACTION/ACTIVITY

The defined aims (either in qualitative or numeric terms) of a planned action or an activity undertaken with the expectation of specified results is an objective. Typically, the objectives are defined in an official or quasilegal manner by persons authorized to plan or undertake the action. In this context, "specific objectives" are narrower and more precise than "official goals."

OPINION WEIGHING

Any procedure for combining the results obtained from diverse sources by giving to the opinions expressed by the different sources, weights which are not proportional to the numerical strength of each source is an opinion-weighing scheme. For example, opinions of a group of quasi-experts might be weighted according to the degree of expertise each member of the group is believed to have; in a sampling survey of impact expected from a specific action, opinions from different groups might be given weights proportional to some estimate of the degree to which each group is affected by the action.

OVERLAY TECHNIQUE

Overlay technique is a form of mapping, starting with a basic map and using the same scale, translucent overlays may be used to display distribution of species or effects. When they are stacked on top of each other, a vivid display of impact is provided.

These techniques, emphasized principally by McHarg (1969), select explicit mappable parameters and illustrate their combined effects by stacking overlays. They are most useful when all the selection criteria can be systematically defined, weighed, and mapped. They are strongest in using absolutely limiting criteria to screen out disallowed alternative locations. Therefore, they are often employed in narrowing the search for (say) all potential nuclear power sites. Their weakness lies in the fact that few criteria are "absolutely limiting."

PAIRWISE COMPARISON

A procedure for ranking n different items through conditions of each one of the total $1/2(n)$ $(n-1)$ pairs, x_i, x_j and indicating that x_i is either preferred to, not preferred to, or equivalent to x_j (Green and Rao, 1971; Pardee, 1969).

PARAMETRIC VARIATION

This is a technique for sensitivity analysis of any given model by systematically varying the values of parameters which are input to the model's calculation to observe how such variation affects the model's output (especially ranking of alternatives) (Sawicki, 1972).

PREFERENCE INDEX

This technique converts pairwise comparison on n different items into numerical ranking (interval or ratio scale) in terms of the number of preferences expressed for each item.   In one documented application, the preference index of item x_i was the ratio "number of times x_i was preferred/number of pairwise comparisons involving x_i."   Details of application of this method can be found in Luce and Suppes, 1965; Koo and Hasenkamp, 1972; Keeney, 1971; and Dbreu, 1954.

PREFERENTIAL ORDERING

This refers to the ranking of alternative outcomes in order of preference without any evaluation of degree of preference (Herstein and Milnar, 1953).

PROBABILITY DISTRIBUTION

The representation of a repeatable stochastic process by a function satisfying the axiom of probability theory (Shubik and Brewer, 1972).

PUBLIC MEETINGS

Successful environmental assessments have taken into account the view of polarized pressure groups as well as the often ill-defined feelings of the public at large.   Public meetings are a double-edged sword, when well conducted they serve to enlighten many issues by providing a common-sense view of the world and a very narrow view of the people directly affected by the proposed action.

People affected by a project are usually eager to participate in the evaluation and decision-making process. This tendency needs to be disciplined and should not be a limiting factor in the orderly process; but well-channelled, public participation is to the advantage of all involved.

An experiment has recently been conducted with great benefits using *Plato* (Lamont, 1975) as an interactive computer language for citizen participation in decision-making.

RANGE OF VALUE

This means evaluation of an uncertain outcome by estimation of maxima and minima for the event. The range is defined as the distance between the maximum and the minimum number in a set.

REGRESSION TECHNIQUES

These are the methods by which statistical relationships between random variables are determined. This is a standard statistical technique for partitioning the variance and is fully described in all statistics texts.

RELEVANCE NUMBERS

This is numerical representation of the extent to which one variable impacts on another and typically is associated with relevance areas to quantify the contributions of elements at a lower level of abstraction (*e.g.,* specific objectives) to an element at a broader level (*e.g.,* general impact) (Martin and Sharp, 1973). Examples of practical applications can be found in the literature (Esch, 1968; Sheppard, 1970).

RELEVANCE TREES

Relevance trees, like decision trees, is a technique allowing the development of the full set of all possible options or alternatives for a technology or an action (Fischer, 1970).

SCENARIOS

Scenarios are alternative descriptions of the future. They also allow the implications associated with different views of the future to derive. Originally used in social sciences, it is now used extensively to deal with energy and environmental issues when the future is uncertain. It is wise to postulate a few alternative futures (the scenarios) and to analyze the implications and impact of these cases. A good practice is to use scenarios to bound the future possibilities by having a largest (or lowest) scenario and a midpoint among the continuous spectrum of future possibilities.

SIMULATION

Simulation is the application of mathematical techniques for describing the behavior of a conceptual or physical model of the phenomena under study.

A new mathematical language (KSIM) (Kane, 1973), has been developed and designed for interactive team use. Many features of KSIM make it particularly appropriate in formulating environmental policy: (1) it is easily grasped by the nonmathematical specialist and can communicate the workings of complex, nonlinear feedback systems to such people; (2) it allows for ready entry of such 'soft' subjective variables as environmental quality and national sovereighnty; (3) it emphasizes the significance of structural relations rather than numerical prediction; and (4) it is flexible and easily generalized.

Input output models have been used to depict environmental impacts associated with time-dependent technological changes (Herzog, 1973).

Some of the major world models such as Forester's *Dynamo* and *World* are beyond the scope of most environmental assessment. Even large but more modest models such as EPA/ERDA's *SEAS* (strategic environmental assessment studies) can be applied only at gargantuous expenses of money and computer time. Still, similar models have found use and will find increasing applications as integral parts of the environmental assessment process.

STATE OF NATURE

This is a concept from Decision Theory. In decision-making under uncertainty, the outcomes (numerical results) associated with each available alternative are considered to be predictable as a set of n discrete values depending on conditions beyond the decision-maker's control and for which he has no useful estimates of their respective probabilities. The n sets of conditions under which each one of the outcomes is expected are termed States of Nature, and are considered potentially applicable in the present context to a situation in which the level of one or more impacts would be estimated as a set of discrete values with no means of estimating the probabilities governing the occurrence of the particular values.

STRUCTURED VALUE ANALYSIS

Structured Value Analysis is a method of determining the impacts or values of projects in terms of an abstract set of value criteria. The basic comparison is straightforward and merely relates project parameters or characteristics to a measure of value specified by the decision-makers. These relationships provide the basis for obtaining a numerical value for the project.

The analysis uses value judgments of experts, either individually or by consensus, to provide information and data where hard data are unavailable. As such, much of the information going into the model is subjective, but the results can be of high utility.

Four principles were considered central in developing the SVA technique. It should: (1) be adaptive; (2) be as simple to use as possible; (3) yield repeatable conclusive results; and (4) give a complete measure of the project, using expert value judgments as part of the evaluation process (Rowe, 1970).

Essentially, Structured Value Analysis is a procedure which separates a complex decision process into a set of relatively simple, but inter-related, decisions. Each of these simple decisions is quantified and then combined, according to rules established by the decision-maker, to arrive at a single measure of project value. The steps for performing a structured value analysis are to identify the parameters, to establish measurement scales for parameters, to establish value functions, to establish weights, to calculate structural value and perform sensitivity analysis.

The weighting schemes essentially are all the same. The measurements of the impacts are converted to some magnitude (Figure 2-5). The magnitude is then scaled by an importance weight, and, finally, the impacts are combined into an overall project impact by another weighting. This form of a weighting scheme has been used by MITRE (1973) and others (Mottley and Newton, 1959), and is not a new procedure for multiobjective decision-making.

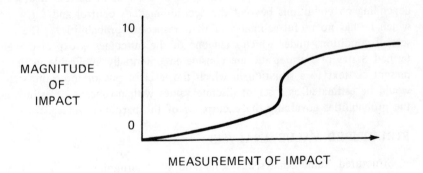

Figure 2-5. Typical impact value function.

SUBJECTIVE-OBJECTIVE MEASURED

This refers to the relationship of subjective measures of value to related objective characteristics. An example is the Leopold use of matrices (1969) described previously.

SUBJECTIVE PROBABILITY

This is the assignment of subjective weights to possible outcomes of an uncertain event in which weights assigned satisfy axioms of probability theory (Peterson and Seo, 1972; Raiffa and Schlaifer, 1961).

SUCCESSIVE GROUPINGS AND CROSS COMPARISON

In this technique for converting subjective preference into a numeric measure, subsets of the items to be ranked are formed and judgment is made as to whether pairs of subset are equivalent or, if not, which is preferred. By observing the influence individual items have in con-tributing to a preference subset, ranking on an interval scale may be achieved according to some chosen method of scoring (Churchman and Ackoff, 1959).

SURROGATE OR PROXY MEASURES

This is the use of a related quantity as a proxy for an unknown or difficult-to-measure value. The relationship may be established by arm-chair analysis, correlation techniques, scientific studies, etc. This is done quite often even if the analyst is sometimes unaware that he is using a surrogate or proxy measure. The choice of measure is often dictated by technical ease or economics of data acquisition.

SURVEY TECHNIQUES

These techniques apply to any procedure for obtaining by oral or written interrogation, or both, the views of any portion of the affected population as to benefit levels expected, their utility and/or relative im-portance. Typically, scientific sampling procedures would be used to maximize (for a given level of effort) the accuracy and precision of the results obtained. It borrowed from market research the full set of techniques for securing information in the form of opinions, judgments or quantitative appraisal from diverse groups affected by the proposed action, and includes interview, polling and citizen participation (Carroll, 1971; Pool, 1973; Leonard, 1971; Syncon, 1973; Sheridan, 1973; Scoville, 1973; Corwin, 1969; Tribus, 1969; Howard, 1972).

TECHNOLOGY ASSESSMENT

This comprehensive technique for evaluating impacts follows the following steps (Coates, 1972, 1975; Jones, 1973; Jones *et al.*, 1971; Hetman, 1973; Sahal, 1977; Arnstein, 1977; Cetron, 1972; Cetron and Bartocha, 1972): (1) examines problem statements; (2) specifies systems alternatives; (3) identifies possible impacts; (4) evaluates impacts; (5) identifies the decision apparatus; (6) identifies action options for decision apparatus; (7) identifies parties at interest; (8) identifies macro system alternatives (other routes to goal); (9) identifies exogenous variables or events possibly having an effect on 1-8; and (10) makes conclusions (and recommendations).

Technology assessment incorporates a description of the technology to be assessed, a description of the context or the setting in which technology is to be introduced, an identification of anticipated consequences and an evaluation of each of the consequences in terms of their impact, timing, severity, etc. (Roessner and Frey, 1974).

THRESHOLD TESTING

This is a technique for sensitivity analysis. By holding constant the values of other parameters, the threshold can be determined at which a change in relative ranking of alternatives occurs as the value of one or more parameters is varied.

TREND EXTRAPOLATION/PROJECTION

A trend is defined as an influence on human affairs that increases or decreases in a noticeable function over time. This trend must extend from past to present and is assumed to continue into the foreseeable future. Trend identification can be done intuitively, using graphical or mathematical means. After the trend has been identified, the most important question still remains—where will such a trend take us?

Trends and tendencies in the absence of any theory are at best a naïve procedure limited to assuming that the future will be much like the past. One of the many techniques for predicting the future, it starts with historical information and provides a judgmental view of the future. Under the terms Technological Forecasting, a large body of theoretical and empirical knowledge about the systematic identification of future scenarios, options and alternatives has been assembled and tested (Ayres, 1969; Martino, 1972; Jantsch, 1966).

UTILITY ASSESSMENT

This is a process for obtaining and estimating subjective human values for the outcomes of decision and is part of the group of behavioral decision theory aimed at improving the quality of decision.

Johnson (1977) describes the utility assessment methodology as follows:

"The usual utility assessment process has the following steps.

1) Identify the perspective from which utility is to be assessed, *i.e.,* "utility to whom," which individual or organizational unit.

2) Determine the scope of the problem and identify the objectives, purposes, or uses of the objects or events whose utilities are to assessed.

3) Identify the set of alternatives to be evaluated.

4) Determine the relvant attributes or factors on which each of the alternatives are to be assessed.

5) Develop operational measures for each attribute or factor.

6) Choose an appropriate technique for assessing the utility of each attribute or factor, *i.e.,* for converting the physical measure into a utility or value measure.

7) Assess the utility or value of each alternative on each attribute or factor.

8) Choose an assessment model.

9) Evaluate each alternative using this model.

10) Select the "best" alternative."

Multiattributes utility measurement, Monte Carlo simulation and conditional probabilities have all been used for utility assessment.

Several authors (Edwards, 1977; Gardiner, 1977; Pearl, 1977; Swalm, 1966; Pollak, 1971; Friedman and Savage, 1952; Fishburn, 1970; Turnban, 1971; Keeney, 1972; Marschak, 1950; Bryon, 1970; Azardiadis, 1972; Stimson, 1969; Breit and Culbertson, 1970; Hausner, 1954) have recently expanded the theoretical foundation and the range of applications of utility assessment.

REFERENCES

Anderson, G. "Methods in Future Studies: A View from the Theory of Science," *Technol. Forecast. Social Change* 5:303-317 (1973).

Andrews, R. N. L. "Approaches to Impact Assessment: Comparison and Critique," presented at Short Courses on Impact Assessment in Water Resource Planning, Amherst, Massachusetts, May/June 1973.

Armstrong, R. H., and Hobson. "The Use of Gaming/Simulation Techniques in the Decision Making Process," United Nations Paper No. ESA/PA/ MMTS/21, (August 31, 1970).

Arnstein, S. R. "Technology Assessment: Opportunities and Obstacles," *IEEE Trans. SMC* 7(8):571-582 (1977).

Arrow, K. J. "Alternative Approaches to the Theory of Choice in Risk-Taking Structure Situations," *Econometrica* 19:404-437 (1951).

Awerbuch, S., and W. A. Wallace. "A Goal-Setting and Evaluation Model for Community Development," *IEEE Trans. SMC* 7(8):589-597 (1977).

Ayres, U. "Technological Forecasting and Long-Range Planning" (New York: McGraw-Hill Book Co., 1969).

Azardiadis, C., *et al.* "Partial Utility Approach to the Theory of the Firm," *So. Econ. J.* 38:485-494 (1972).

Beckerhoff, D. "Goal Systems for R&D Planning," *Technol. Forcasting* 1:363-369 (1970).

Belknap, R. K., and J. G. Furtado. *Three Approaches to Environmental Resource Analysis,* Landscape Architecture Research Office, Graduate School of Design, Harvard Universty (Washington, D.C.: The Conservation Foundation, 1967).

Bennington, G., *et al. Resources and Land Investigations (RALI) Program: Methodologies for Environmental Analysis,* MTR-6740, Vol. 1 (McLean, Virginia: The MITRE Corporation, 1974).

Bishop, B. "An Approach to Evaluating Environmental, Social and Economic Factors in Water Resources Planning," *Water Resources Bull.* 8(4):724-736 (August 1972).

Bisselle, C. *Strategic Environmental Assessment System Radiation Residuals,"* MTR-6511 (McLean, Virginia: The MITRE Corporation, 1973).

Bisselle, C. *Strategic Environmental Assessment System: Air and Water Pollution Indicators,* MTR-6565 (McLean, Virginia: The MITRE Corporation, 1977).

Breit, W., and W. P. Culbertson, Jr. "Distributional Equality and Aggregate Utility: Comment," *Am. Econ. Rev.* 60:435-443 (1970).

Bridgewater, A. V. "Morphological Methods—Principles and Practice," in *Technol. Forecasting,* R. V. Arnfield, Ed., (Edinburgh: University Press, 1968).

Brockhaus, W. L. "A Quantitative Analytical Methodology for Judgmental and Policy Decisions," *Technol. Forecast. Social Change* 7:3127-3137 (1975).

Bryon, R. P. "Simple Method for Estimating Demand Systems Under Separate Utility Assumptions," *R. Econ. Stud.* 37:261-274 (1970).

Carroll, J. D. "Participatory Technology," *Science* (February 1971), pp. 647-653.

Cetron, M. J., and B. Bartocha, Eds. *The Methodology of Technology Assessment* (New York: Gordon and Breach Science Publishers, 1972).

Cetron, M. J. "The Trimatrix—An Integration Technique for Technology Assessment," in *The Methodology of Technology Assessment,* M. J. Cetron and B. Bartucha, Eds. (New York: Gordon and Breach Science Publishers, 1972), pp. 137-162.

Chase, G. H. "Matrix Techniques in the Evaluation of Environmental Impacts," *Environmental Impact Assessment,* M. Blissett, Ed., Engineering Foundation (1975).

Churchman, C. W., and R. L. Ackoff. "An Approximate Measure of Value," *J. Oper. Soc. Am.* 2:172-189 (1959).

Cicchetti, C. J., *et al.* "Recreation Benefit Estimation and Forecasting: Implications of the Identification Problem," *Water Resources Res.* 8(4): pp. 840-850 (1972).

Coates, J. F. "Some Methods and Techniques for Comprehensive Impact Assessment," *Environmental Impact Assessment,* M. Blissett, Ed., Engineering Foundation (1975).

Coates, V. T. "Technology and Public Policy: The Process of Technology Assessment in the Federal Government," Program of Policy Studies in Science and Technology, The George Washington University, Washington D.C. (July 1972).

Corwin, E. J. Technological Data. Citizens Response, 200 Central Park South, New York, New York 10019.

Dalkey, N., and O. Helmer. "An Experimental Application of the Delphi Method to the Use of Experts," *Managemt. Sci.* 9:362-374 (1963).

Davenport, S., Ed. "Planning and Evaluation of Multiple Purpose Water Resources Projects in a Multiobjective Environment: An Overview and Post-Audit Analysis," INTASA, Menlo Park, California.

Dawes, M. Comprehensive Models as a Guide to Preference *IEEE Trans. SMC* 7(5):355-357 (1977).

Day, G. S., and R. M. Heller. "Using Cluster Analysis to Improve Marketing Experiments," *J. Marketing Res.* 8:304-347 (1971).

Debreu, G. "Representation of a Preference Ordering by a Numerical Function," in *Decision Process,* R. N. Thrall, C. H. Coombs and R. L. Savis, Eds. (New York: John Willey & Sons, Inc., 1954).

Dee, N., *et al.* "Environmental Evaluation System for Water Resource Planning," Report to Bureau of Reclamation, U.S. Department of the Interior, Battelle Columbus Laboratories (1972).

Duckstein, L., *et al.* "Practical Use of Decision Theory to Assess Uncertainties About Actions Affecting the Environment," PB-269-011, Office of Water Research and Technology (February 1977).

Duke, R. "*Apex,* A Gaming Simulation for Air Pollution Experience in a Simulated Metropolitan Environment," Environmental Simulation Laboratory, The University of Michigan, Ann Arobr (1968).

Edwards, W. "How to Use Multiattribute Utility Measurement for Social Decision Making," *IEEE Trans. SMC* 7(5):326-340 (1977).

Esch, M. E. "Planning Assistance through Technical Evaluation of Relevance Numbers," in *Technol. Forecasting,* F. V. Arnfield, Ed. (Edinburgh: University Press, 1968).

Fischer, M. "Toward a Mathematical Theory of Relevance Tress," *Technol. Forecasting* 1:381-389 (1970).

Fishburn, P. C. *Utility Theory for Decision Making* (New York: John Wiley & Sons, Inc., 1970).

Foldes, L. "Expected Utility and Continuity," *R. Econ. Stud.* 39(40):7-21 (1972).

Ford, D. A. "SHANG Inquiry as an Alternative to Delphi: Some Environmental Findings," *Technol. Forecast. Social Change* 7:139-164 (1975).

Friedman, M., and L. J. Savage. "The Expected−Utility Hypothesis and the Measurability of Utility," *J. Pol. Econ.* 60(6):436-474 (1952).

Golden, J., *et al. Environmental Threshold Assessment as Applied to Proposed Railroad Abandonment Authorizations,* MTR-6581, Vol. I and II (McLean, Virginia: The MITRE Corporation, 1973).

Gordon, T. J., and H. Hayward. "Initial Experiments with the Cross Impact Matrix Method of Forecasting," *Futures* 1(2):100-116 (1968).

Gordon, T. J., and H. A. Becker. "The Use of Cross-Impact Matrix Approaches in Technology Assessment," in *The Methodology of Technology Assessment,* M. J. Cetron and B. Bartucha, Eds. (New York: Gordon and Breach Science Publishers, 1972), pp. 127-136.

Gardiner, P. C. "Decision Spaces," *IEEE Trans. SMC* 7(5):341-349 (1977).

Green, P. E., and V. R. Rao. "Rating Scales and Information Recovery− How Many Scales and Response Categories to Use?" *J. Marketing* 34: 33-39 (1970).

Gsellman, L. R. *Cost/Benefit Analysis and R&D Planning,* M77-12 (McLean, Birginia: The MITRE Corporation, 1977).

Gulliksen, H. "Linear and Multidimensional Scaling," *Psychometrika* 26:9-25 (1961).

Hausner, M. "Multidimensional Utilities," in *Decision Processes,* R. M. Thrall, C. H. Coombs and R. L. Davis, Eds. (New York: John Wiley & Sons, Inc., 1954).

Herstein, I. N., and J. Milnor. "An Axiomatic Approach to Measurable Utility," *Econometrica* 23:291-297 (1953).

Herzog, H. W. "An Environmental Assessment of Future Production-Related Technological Change: 1970-2000 (An Input-Output Approach)," *Technol. Forecast. Social Change* 5:75-90 (1973).

Hetman, F. "Society and the Assessment of Technology," Organization for Economic Co-Operation and Development, Paris (1973).

Hill, K., and J. Fowles. "The Methodological Worth of the Delphi Forecasting Technique," *Technol. Forecast. Social Change* 7:179-192 (1975).

Howard, R. A., J. E. Matheson and D. W. North. "Decision to Seed Hurricanes," *Science* 196:1191-1201 (June 16, 1972).

Howe, C. W. "Benefit-Cost Analysis for Water System Planning," *Water Resources Monograph 2* (Washington, D.C.: American Geophysical Union, 1971).

Hurwicz, L. "What Has Happened to the Theory of Games?" *Am. Econ. Rev.* 43(2):398-405 (1953).

Jantsch, E. *Technological Forecasting in Perspective* (Washington, D.C.: Organization for Economic Co-Operation and Development, 1966).

Jantsch, E. *Technological Forecasting in Perspective* (Washington, D.C.: Organization for Economic Co-Operation and Development, 1967).

Johnson, M. "The Technology of Utility Assessment," *IEEE Trans. SMC* 7(5):311-325 (1977).

Jones, M. V. "A Comparative, State-of-the-Art Review of Selected U.S. Technology Assessment Studies," (Washington, D.C.: National Science Foundation, 1973).

Jones, M. V., et al. *Technology Assessment, 1) Some Basic Propositions; 2) Automotive Emissions; 3)Computers-Communications; 4) Enzymes (Industrial); 5) Mariculture (Sea Farming); 6) Water Pollution: Domestic Wastes* (McLean, Virginia: The MITRE Corporation, 1971).

Kane, J., I. Vertinsky and W. Thomson. "KSIM: A Methodology for Interactive Resource Policy Simulation," *Water Resources Res.* 9(1):65-79 (1973).

Keeney, R. L. "Illustrated Procedure for Assessing Multiattributed Utility Functions," *Sloan Mgtmt R.* 14:37-50 (1972).

Keeney, R. L. "Utility Functions for Multiattributed Consequences," *Managemt. Sci.* 18:276-287 (1972).

Keeney, R. L. "Utility Independence and Preferences for Multiattributed Consequences," *Oper. Res.* 19:875-893 (1971).

Koo, A. Y. C., and G. Hasenkamp. "Structure of Revealed Preference: Some Preliminary Evidence," *J. Pol. Econ.* 80(4):724-744 (1972).

Lamont, V. C. "New Directions for the Teaching Computer: Citizen Participation in Community Planning," *Technol. Forecast. Social Change* 5:145-162 (1975).

Leonard, E., A. Etzioni, H. A. Hornstein, P. Abrams, T. Stephens and N. Ticky. "MINERVA: A Participatory Technolgoy System," *Bull. Atomic Scientists* (November 1971), pp. 4-12.

Leopold, L. B. *Quantitative Comparison of Some Aesthetic Factors Among Rivers* U.S. Geological Survey Circular 620 (Washington, D.C.: U.S. Geological Survey, 1969).

Leopold, L.B., E. Clarke, B. B. Hanshaw and J. B. Balsley. *A Procedure for Evaluating Environmental Impact,* U.S. Geological Survey Circular 645 (Washington, D.C.: U.S. Geological Survey, 1971).

Luce, R. D., and H. Raiffa. *Games and Decisions: Introduction and Critical Survey* (New York: John Wiley & Sons, Inc., 1957).

Luce, R. D., and P. Suppes. "Preference, Utility, and Subjective Psychology," in *Handbook of Mathematical Psychology,* Vol. III, R. D. Luce, R. P. Bush and K. Calanter, Eds. (New York: John Wiley & Sons, Inc., 1965).

Mandanis, G. P. "The Future of the Delphi Technique," *Technology Forecasting,* R. V. Arnfield, Ed. (Edinburgh: University Press, 1968). pp. 159-169.

Marschak, J. "Rational Behavior, Uncertainty Prospects, and Measurable Utility," *Econometrica* 18:111-141 (1950).

Martin, W. T., and J. M. Sharp. "Reverse Factor Analysis: A Modification of Relevance Tree Techniques," *Technol. Forecast. Social Change* 4:355-373 (1973).

Martino, J. "The Lognormality of Delphi Estimates," *Technol. Forecasting* 1:355-358 (1970a).

Martino, J. P. "The Precision of Delphi Estimates," *Technol. Forecasting* 1:293-299 (1970b).

Martino, J. P. *Technological Forecasting for Decision Making* (New York: American Elsevier Publishing Co., Inc., 1972).

McHarg, L. *Decision with Nature* (Garden City, New York: The Natural History Press, 1969).

Milnor, C. J. "Games Against Nature," in *Decision Processes*, R. M. Thrall, C. H. Coombs and R. L. Davis, Eds. (New York: John Wiley & Sons, Inc., 1954), pp. 49-59.

MITRE Corporation. "Use of Structured Value Analysis in Resource Allocation Models," M72-5 (January 1972); "Tropical Storn Agnes: Long-Range Flood Recovery," MTR-6429 (August 1973).

Mohring, H. "Urban Highway Investments," in *Measuring Benefits of Government Investments*, R. Dorfman, Ed. (Washington, D.C.: Brookings Institute, 1965), pp. 231-291.

Morrison, D. L., J. T. McGinnis and R. A. Mayer. "General Environmental Siting Criteria for Power Plants," presented at the American Nuclear Society Winter Meeting, San Francisco, California, November 11-16, 1973.

Moskowitz, H. "An Experimental Investigation of Decision Making in a Simulated R&D Environment," *Managemt. Sci.* 19(6):676-687 (1973).

Mottley, C. M., and R. D. Newton. The Selection of Projects for Industrial Research, *Oper. Res.* 7(6):740-751 (November/December 1959).

Munn, R. E., M. L. Phillips and H. P. Sanderson. "Environmental Effects of Air Pollution: Implications for Air Quality Criteria, Air Quality Standards, and Emission Standards," *Sci. Total. Environ.* 8:53-67 (1977).

O'Connor, M. F. "The Application of Multiattribute Scaling Procedures to the Development of Indices of Value," Department of Psychology, University of Michigan, Ann Arobr, Michigan (1972).

"Optimum Pathway Matrix Analysis Approach to the Environmental Decision Making Process—Testcase: Relative Impact of Proposed Highway Alternatives," Institute of Ecology, University of Georgia (1971).

Pardee, F. S., *et al.* "Measurement and Effectiveness of Transportation System Effectiveness," (1969).

Pearl, J. "A Framework for Processing Value Judgments," *IEEE Trans. SMC* 7(5):349-354 (1977).

Peterson, R. E. and K. K. Seo. "Public Administration Planning in Developing Countries, A Bayesian Decision Theory Approach," *Policy Sci.* 3:371-378 (1972).

Pinkel, B. "On the Decision Matrix and the Judgment Process: A Developmental Decision Example," The Rand Corp., Santa Monica, California (1969).

Pollak, R. A. "Additive Utility Functions and Linear Engal Curves," *R. Econ. Stud.* 38:401-414 (1971a).

Pollak, R. A. "Conditional Demand Functions and the Implications of Separable Utility," *So. Econ. J.* 37:423-433 (1971b).

Pool, I. de S., Ed. *Talking Back: Citizen Feedback and Cable Technology* (Cambridge: The MIT Press, 1973).

Raiffa, H., and R. Schlaifer. *Applied Statistical Decision Theory* (Cambridge, Massachusetts: Harvard University Press, 1961).

Rainer, R. P., and C. R. White. "Identification and Interrelationships of Secondary Benefits in Waterways Development," Water Resources Research Institute, Auburn University, Georgia (1969).

Roessner, J. D., and J. Frey. "Methodology from Technology Assessment," *Technol. Forecast. Social Change,* 6:167-169 (1974).

Rouse, W. B., and T. M. Sheridan. "Computer-aided Group Decision Making: Theory and Practice," *Technol. Forecast. Social Change* 7:113-126 (1975).

Rowe, W. D. *The Application of Structure Value Analysis to Models Using Value Judgments as a Data Source,* M70-14 (McLean, Virginia: The MITRE Corporation, 1970).

Rowe, W. D. *The Environment: A Systems Approach with Emphasis on Monitoring* (McLean, Virginia: The MITRE Corporation, 1972).

Saaty, T. L. "Operations Research: Some Contributions to Mathematics," *Science* 178:1061-1070 (1972).

Sahal, D., and K. Yee. "Delphi: An Investigation from a Bavesian Viewpoint," *Technol. Forecast. Social Change* 7:165-118 (1975).

Sahal, D. "Structural Models of Technology Assessment," *IEEE Trans. SMC* 7(8):582-589 (1977).

Salancik, J. R. "Assimilation of Aggregated Inputs into Delphi Forecasts: A Regression Analysis," *Technol. Forecast. Social Change* 5:243-247 (1973).

Sanderson, H. P. "Observations on Local and National Air Quality Indices," *Sci. Total Environ.* 8:39-51 (1977).

Sawicki, D. S. *Break-even Benefit-Cost Analysis of Alternative Express Transit Systems* (Washington, D.C.: Urban Mass Transit Administration Department of Transportation, 1972).

Sayeki, Y., and K. H. Vesper. "Allocation of Importance in a Hierarchial Goal Structure," *Managemt. Sci.* 19:667-675 (1973).

Schlaifer, R. *Analysis of Decisions Under Uncertainty* (New York: McGraw-Hill Book Co., 1969).

Schlesinger, B., and D. Daetz. "A Conceptual Framework for Applying Environmental Assessment Matrix Techniques," *J. of Environ. Sci.* 16(4):11-16 (1973).

Schlesinger, B., and R. A. Hughes. *Environmental Assessment of Alternate Shipbuilding Sites* (San Francisco: Bechtel Corporation, 1972).

Scoville, A. "Citizen Participation in State Government," Report for NSF, The Citizen Participation Project, The Environmental Planning Information Center, Montpelier, Vermont (1973).

Shepphard, W. J. "Relevance Analysis in Research Planning," *Technol. Forecasting* 1:371-379 (1970).

Sheridan, T. "Progress Report of the MIT Community Dialogue Project " (July 1973).

Shubik, M., and G. D. Brewer. "Models, Simulations and Games—A Survey," Report R-1060-ARPA/RC, Rand, Santa Monica, California (1972).

Smith, J. W. "A Plan to Allocate and Procure Electronic Sets by the Use of Linear Programming Techniques and Analytical Methods of Assigning Values to Qualitative Factors," *Naval Res. Logistic Quart.* (1956).

Sorenson, J. C. "A Framework for Identification and Control of Resource Degradation and Conflict in Multiple Use of the Coastal Zone," Department of Landscape Architecture, University of California at Berkeley, 1971.

Stimson, D. H. "Utility Measurement in Public Health Decision Making," *Managemt. Sci.* 16:1317-1330 (1969).

Strayk, R. J. "Agricultural Flood Control Benefits and Land Values," Corps of Engineers, Institute for Water Resources, Ft. Belvoir, Virginia (1970).

Swalm, R. O. "Utility Theory: Insights into Risk Taking," *Harvard Bus. Rev.* 44(6):123-136 (1966).

"SYNCON: A technique developed by the Committee for the Future, Inc.," International Headquarters and New Worlds Training and Education Center, 2325 Porter Street, N.W., Washington, D.C. 20008.

Tarascio, V. J., and J. L. Murphy. "Uncertainty, Learning and Dynamic Utility Theory," *Quart. Rev. Econ. Bus.* 12:19-33 (1972).

Thuesen, G. J. *A Study of Public Attitudes and Multiple Objective Decision Criteria for Water Pollution Control Project* (Atlanta, Georgia: Institute of Technology, School of Industrial and Systems Engineering, 1971).

Travelers Research Corporation (later CEM). "The Development of a Procedure and Knowledge Requirements for Marine Resource Planning," prepared for the Marine Resources Council of the Nassau-Suffolk Regional Planning Board, Hartford, Connecticut (1969).

Tribus, M. *Rational Descriptions Decisions and Designs,* Pergamon Unified Engineering Series: Engineering Design Section (Elmsford, New York: Pergamon Press, 1969).

Turban, E., and M. L. Metersky. "Utility Theory Applied to Multivariate System Effectiveness Evaluation." *Managemt. Sci.* 17:13817-13828 (1971).

Turoff, M. "Delphi Conferencing: Computer-Based Conferencing with Anonymity," *Technol. Forecast. Social Change* 3:159-204 (1972).

U.S. Deepwater Port Study, Vol. IV. The Environmental and Ecological Aspects of Deepwater Ports, IWR Report 72-8, R. R. Nathan Associates (1972).

Warneryd, O. "Games for Urban and Regional Planning: A Pedagogical Tool," *Technol. Forecast. Social Change* 7:397-412 (1975).

Water Resources Council. "Proposed Principles and Standards for Planning Water and Related Land Resources," *Federal Register* 36(245) (December 21, 1971).

Watson, J., R. Kuehnel and J. Golden. "A Preliminary Study of a Concept for Categorizing Benefits," MTR-6569, The MITRE Corporation (January 1974).

Wood, W. D., and H. F. Campbell. "Cost-Benefit Analysis and the Economics of Investment in Human Resources: An Annotated Bibliography," Industrial Relations Centre, Queen's University, Kingston, Ontario (1970).

Wright, J. P. "Delphi—Systematic Opinion-Gathering," *GAO Rev.* (Spring 1972), pp. 20-27.

Yu, P. L. "A Class of Solutions for Group Decision Problems," *Managemt. Sci.* 19:926-946 (1973).

Zadeh, L. A. "Outline of a New Approach to the Analysis of Complex Systems and Decision Processes," *IEEE Trans. SMC,* 3(1):28-44 (1973).

Zwicky, F. *Morphological Astronomy* (New York: Springer-Verlag, 1957).

SELECTED REFERENCES

Ackoff, R. L., Ed. *Progress in Operations Research,* Vol. 1 (Publications in Operations Research No. 5) (New York: John Wiley & Sons, Inc., 1961).

Alberts, D. S. *A Plan for Measuring the Performance of Social Programs: The Applications of Operations Research Methodology.* (New York: Praeger, 1970).

Alexander, E. K. "Choice in a Changing World," *Policy Sci.* 1:325-328 (1970).

American Institutes for Research. *Evaluative Research: Strategies and Methods.* Pittsburgh, Pennsylvania (1970).

Andrews, R. N. L. "Committee on An Environmental Evaluation System for Water Resource Planning," *Water Resources Res.* 10(2):376-378 (1974).

Asmi, S. K. "Benefit-Cost Ratio of Projects: Its Most General Form and a New Graphical Method for Its Evaluation," *Inst. Civil Eng. Proc.* 50:161-168 (1970).

Atomic Energy Commission. "Preparation of Environmental Reports for Nuclear Power Plants," Regulatory Guide 4.2, Directorate of Regulatory Standards (March 1973).

Bates, J. "A Model for the Science of Decision," *Phil. Sci.* 21:326-339 (1954).

Battelle's Columbus and Pacific Northwest Laboratories. "Methodology for Ranking Energy Systems, Appendix B of Environmental Considerations in Future Energy Growth, Volume I, Fuel/Energy Systems: Technical Summaries and Associated Environmental Borders," report to EPA Office of Research and Development (April 1973).

Bliss, C. A. "Absolutism in the Realm of Uncertainty," *Calif. Managemt. Rev.* 11:35-42 (1969).

Bishop, B. "An Approach to Evaluating Environmental, Social and Economic Factors in Water Resources Planning," *Water Resources Bull.* 8(4):724-734 (August 1972).

Bromley, D. W., N. L. Meyer, J. Stoltzenberg and M. Warner. "Water Resource Projects and Environmental Imapct: Towards a Conceptual Model," (Madison, Wisconsin: Water Resources Center, University of Wisconsin, 1972).

Bross, I. D. J. *Design for Decision* (New York: MacMillan Co., 1953).

"Bureau of the Budget," Circular 81 (January 1958).

Cambell, A. B. "Impact of Energy Demands," *Physics Today* 23:1137-1140 (1970).

Carresse, L. M. and C. G. Baker. "The Convergence Technique: A Method for the Planning and Programming of Research Efforts," *Managemt. Sci.* 13(8):420-438 (1967).

Cartwright, D., and L. Festinger. "A Quantitative Theory of Decision," *Psych. Rev.* 50:595-621 (1943).

Christian, J. J. "Social Subordination, Population Density, and Mammalian Evolution," *Science* 168:84-90 (1970).

Cicchetti, C. J., R. K. Davis, S. H. Hawke and R. H. Haveman. "Evaluating Federal Water Projects: A Critique of Proposed Standards," *Science* 181:723-728 (August 24, 1973).

Commonwealth Associates, Inc., Landplan Systems Division, "Ontario 500 KV Transmission Line Right of Way Lennox-Oshawa Technical Report, Corridor Selection Methodology," Jackson, Michigan (1973).

Commonwealth Associates, Inc., Jackson, Michigan. "Environmental Analysis Systems," prepared for Northern States Power Company, report R-1447 (Appendix B under separate cover) (September 1972).

Conrath, D. "From Statistical Decision Theory to Practice," *Managemt. Sci.* 19(8):873-883 (1973).

Cross, F. L., Jr. "Assessing Environmental Impact," *Poll. Eng.* 5:34-35 (1973).

Crum, L. W. "Value Engineering—A Challenge to Management," *Aero. J.* 74:608-613 (1970).

Davidson, D., et al. *Decision-Making: An Experimental Approach* (Los Angeles: Stanford University Press, 1957).

Deal, R. E., and M. H. Halbert. "The Application of Value Theory to Water Resources Planning and Management," Institute for the Study of Inquiring Systems, Philadelphia, Pennsylvania (1971).

Dean, B. V., and M. J. Nishry. "Scoring and Profitability Models for Evaluating and Selecting Engineering Projects," *Oper. Res.* 13(4):550-369 (1965).

Dickens, P. "Some Aspects of the Decision Making Behavior of Business Organizations," *Econ. Geog.* 47:426-437 (1971).

Didis, S. K. "Value Analysis of Information Systems." *J. Systems Managemt.* 20:9-11 (1969).

Dyer, J. S. "A Time Sharing Computer Program for Solution of the Multiple Criteria Problem," *Managemt. Sci.* 19(12) (1973).

Eckenrode, R. T. "Weighing Multiple Criteria," *Managemt. Sci.* 12(3): 180-192 (1965).

Edwards, W. "The Theory of Decision Making," *Psych. Rev.* 51(4):380-417 (1954).

Eishel, L. M., and J. J. Gaudette. "Comments on An Environmental Evaluation System for Water Resource Planning," *Water Resources Res.* 10(2):379-380 (1974).

English, J. M., Ed. *Cost-Effectiveness—The Economic Evaluation of Engineered Systems* (New York: John Wiley & Sons, Inc., 1968).

Environmental Aspects of Nuclear Power Stations (Vienna: International Atomic Energy Agency, 1971).

Ference, T. P. "Induced Strategies in Sequential Decision-Making," *Human Relations* 25(5):377-389 (1972).

Festinger, L., and D. Katz, Eds. *Research Methods in the Behavioral Sciences* (New York: Dryden Press, 1953).

Fifield, I. "Value of Value Analysis as an Administrative Tool," *Personnel* 49:27-33 (1972).

Fishbein, M, Ed. *Readings in Attitude Theory and Measurement* (New York: John Wiley & Sons, Inc., 1967).

Frederiksen, H. "Feedbacks in Economic and Demographic Transition," *Science* 166:347-848 (1969).

Frei, M. D. "Administrative and Socio-Psychological Constrains of the Business Decision-Making Process," *Managemt. Int. Rev.* 11(2-3):67-81 (1971).

Friedman, M., and L. J. Savage. "The Expected—Utility Hypothesis and the Measurability of Utility," *J. Pol. Econ.* 60(6):436-474 (1952).

Gilpin, R. "Technological Strategies and National Purpose," *Science* 169: 441-448 (1970).

Goldman, T. A., Ed. *Cost-Effectiveness Analysis* (New York: Praeger, 1967).

Grauhan, R., and W. Strubelt. "Politcal Rationality Reconsidered: Notes on the Integrated Evaluative Scheme for Policy Choices." *Policy Sci.* 2:249-270 (1971).

Green, P. E., and V. R. Rao. "Rating Scales and Information Recovery—How Many Scales and Response Categories to Use?" *J. Marketing* 34:33-39 (1970).

Green, P. E., and V. R. Rao. "Multidimensional Scaling and Individual Differences," *J. Marketing Res.* 8:71-77 (1971).

Green, P. E., and V. R. Rao. "Configuration Synthesis in Multidimensional Scaling," *J. Marketing Res.* 9:65-68 (1972).

Green, P. E., Y. Wind and A. K. Jain. "Benefit Bundle Analysis," *J. Advert. Res.* 12(4):31-36 (1972).

Hadar, J., and W. R. Russell. "Rules for Ordering Uncertain Prospects," *Am. Econ. Rev.* 59:25-34 (1970).

Hakansson, N. H. "Friedman-Savage Utility Functions Consistent with Risk Aversion," *Quart. J. Econ.* 84(3):472-487 (1970).

Hart, A. G. *Anticipation, Uncertainty, and Dynamic Planning* (New York: Augustus M. Kelley, 1951).

Hartman, R. S. *The Structure of Value* (Southern Illinois University Press, 1967).

Heath, J. "What is Value?" *Fin. Exec.* 39:13-15 (1971).

Helmer, O., and P. Oppenheim. "A Syntactical Definition of Probability and of Degree of Confirmation," *J. Symbolic Logic* 10:25-60 (1945).

Hertz, D. B., and J. Melise, Eds. *Proc. Fourth Int. Conf. Oper. Res.* (New York: Wiley-Interscience, 1966).

Hill, M. "A Goal-Achievement Matrix for Evaluating Alternative Plans." *Am. Inst. Planners J.* 34:19-29 (1968).

Holmes, T. H., and R. H. Rahe. "The Social Readjustment Rating Scale," *J. Psychosomatic Res.* 11:213 (1967).

Holt, C. C. "System of Information Centers for Research and Decision Making (with discussion)," *Am. Econ. Rev. Papers Proc.* 60:149-168 (1970).

Howard, R. "Bayesian Decision Models for System Engineering," *IEEE Trans. Syst. Sci. Cybern.* SSC-1(1) (1965).

Howard, R. "Value of Information Lotteries," *IEEE Trans. Syst. Sci. Cybern.* SSC-3(1):54-60 (1967).

Howard, R. "The Foundations of Decision Analysis," *IEEE Trans. Syst. Sci. Cybern.* SSC-4(3):211-219 (1968).

Hurwicz, L. "The Theory of Economic Behavior," *Am. Econ. Rev.* 34:908-925 (1945).

Jacoby, J., and M. S. Matell. "Three-Point Likert Scales are Good Enough," *J. Marketing Res.* 8:495-500 (1971).

Jantsch, E. "Toward a Methodology for Systematic Forecasting," *Techol. Forecasting* 1:409-419 (1970).

Jeffrey, R. C. *The Logic of Decision* (New York: McGraw-Hill Book Co., 1965).

Joskow, J. "Cost-Benefit Analysis for Environmental Impact Statement," *Pub. Util. Fortnightly* 91(2):21-25 (1973).

Kadish, M. R. "Toward a Theory of Decision," Ph.D. Thesis, Columbia University (1971).

Kamier, M. I., and N. L. Schwartz. "Direct Approach to Choice Under Uncertainty," *Managemt. Sci.* 18:470-477 (1972).

Klarh, D. "Decision Making in a Complex Environment: The Use of Similarity Judgments to Predict Preferences," *Managemt. Sci.* 15(11): 595-618 (1969).

Krupp, S. R., Ed. *The Structure of Economic Science: Essays on Methodology* (Englewood Cliffs, New Jersey: Prentice Hall, 1966).

Kruskal, J. B. "Analysis of Factorial Experiments by Estimating Monotone Transformations of the Data," *J. Roy. Stat. Soc. Series B* 27:251-263 (1965).

Leclercq, R. "The Use of Generalized Logic in Forecasting," *Technol. Forecast. Social Change* 2:189-194 (1970).

Lord, W. B. and M. L. Warner, "Aggregates and Externalities: Information Needs for Public Natural Resource Decision-Making," *Nat. Resources J.* 13(1):106-117 (January 1973).

Lowi, T. "Decision Making vs. Policy Making: Toward an Antidote for Technocracy," *Pub. Admin. Rev.* 30:314-325 (1970).

McCullough, J. D. "Cost Analysis for Planning-Programming-Budgeting Cost-Benefit Studies," The RAND Corp., Santa Monica, California (1966).

Machol, R., Ed. *Information and Decision Processes* (New York: McGraw-Hill Book Co., 1960).

Mack, R. P. *Planning on Uncertainty* (New York: Wiley-Interscience, 1971).

Miller, J. *Professional Decision Making* (New York: Praeger, 1970).

Mitroff, I. I., L. V. Blankenship. "On the Methodology of the Holistic Experiment: An Approach to the Conceptualization of Large-Scale Social Experiments," *Technol. Forecast. Social Change* 4:339-353 (1973).

Montana Power Co., Puget Sound Power and Light Co., Portland General Electric Co., The Washington Water Power Co., and Pacific Power and Light Co. "Colstrip Generation and Transmission Project: Applicants Environmental Analysis" (November 1973).

Muir, A. H., *et al.,* "Cost-Effectiveness Analysis of On-the-Job and Institutional Training Courses," Planning Research Corp., Los Angeles (1967).

National Academcy of Engineering, Ed. *Perspectives on Benefit-Risk Decision Making,* Colloquium by the Committee on Public Engineering Policy, Washington, D.C. (April 26-27, 1971).

Ng, Y. K. "Value Judgements and Economists' Role in Policy Recommendation," *Econ. J.* 82:1014-1018 (1972).

Oberlin, T. L., and R. L. Kashyap. "Bayes Decision Rules Based on Objective Priors," *IEEE Trans. Sys. Man. Cybern.* SMC-3:59-64 (1973).

O'Connor, M. F. "The Application of Multi-Attribute Scaling Procedures to the Development of Indices of Value," Engineering Psychology Laboratory, The University of Michigan, Ann Arbor, Michigan (June 1, 1972).

Ortolano, L., and W. Hill. "An Analysis of Environmental Statements for Corps of Engineers' Water Projects," U.S. Army Engineer Institute for Water Resources, Alexandria, Virginia, IWR Report 72-3 (AD 747-374) (June 1972).

Ortolano, L. "Impact Assessment in the Water Resources," paper presented at the Short Course on Impact Assessment in Water Resources Planning, Amherst, Massachusetts; Ann Arbor, Michigan, and East Sound, Washington, May/June, 1973.

Otway, H. J., Ed. *Risk vs. Benefit: Solution or Dream,* Informal Report LA-4860-MS, Los Alamos, New Mexico (1972).

Paykel, E. S. "Dimensions of Social Adjustment in Depressed Women," *J. Nervous Mental Dis.* 152:158-172 (1971).

Prest, A. R., and R. Turvey. "Cost-Benefit Analysis: A Survey," *Econ. J.* 75(12):683-735 (1965).

Rader, T. "Resource Allocation with Increasing Returns to Scale," *Am. Econ. Rev.* 60:814-825 (1970).

Rao, V. R., and R. Katz. "Alternative Multidimensional Scaling Methods for Large Stimulus Sets," *J. Marketing Res.* 8:488-494 (1971).

Reutlinger, S. "Techniques for Project Appraisal Under Uncertainty," World Bank Staff Occasional Papers No. 10. (Baltimore, Maryland: Johns Hopkins Press, 1970).

Rivard, J. B. "Risk Minimization by Optimum Allocation of Resources Available for Risk Reduction," *Nucl. Safety* 12(4):305-309 (1971).

Rochester Gas and Electric, Naigara Mohawk Power Corporation. "Application to the State of New York Public Service Commission for Certificate of Environmental Compatibility and Public Need (Technical Appendix B, under separate cover) (January 1974).

Samuelson, P. A. *The Collected Scientific Papers,* Vol. 1. (Cambridge, Massachusetts: MIT Press, 1966).

Savage, L. J. "The Theory of Statistical Decision," *J. Am. Stat. Assoc.* 46(3):55-67 (1951).

Shelly, M. W., and G. L. Bryan, Eds. *Human Judgments and Optimality* (New York: John Wiley & Sons, Inc., 1964).

Shubik, M. "A Note on Decision Making and Replacing Sure Prospects with Uncertain Prospects," *Managemt. Sci.* 19(2):711-712 (1973).

Simon, J. L. "Toward Formal Valuation of Scientific Research Projects: A Case Study in Population Control," *Policy Sci.* 3:177-181 (1972).

Smith, D. V. "Decision Rules in Chance—Constrained Programming," *Managemt. Sci.* 19(6):688-702 (1973).

Smith, H. L., and W. L. Heilman. "Numerical Rating of Environmental Impacts for Power Planting Siting," presented at the American Nuclear Society Symposium, Portland, Oregon, August, 1974.

Smith, N. M., Jr., *et al.* "The Theory of Value and the Science of Decision—A Summary," *J. Oper. Res. Soc. Am.* 1(3):103-113 (1953).

Sowby, F. D. "Radiation and Other Risks," *Health Physics* 11:879-887 (1965).

Stanley, J. "Environmental Factors Related to Land Use Planning and Industrial Development," paper no. 73-51, presented at the 65th Annual Meeting of the Air Pollution Control Association, Miami Beach, Florida, June 18-22, 1972.

Stretchberry, D. M. "General Methodology: Costing, Budgeting, and Techniques for Benefit-Cost and Cost-Effectiveness Analysis," NASA, Washington, D.C. (1972).

Swager, W. L. "Summary of Technological Forecasting Seminar, Battelle Seattle Research Center, No. 5-7, 1969," *Technol. Forecasting* 1:359-361 (1970).

Swalm, R. O. "Utility Theory: Insights into Risk Taking," *Harvard Bus. Rev.* 44(6):123-136 (1966).

Trinkl, F. H. "Allocations among Programs Having Counteractive Outcomes," *Policy Sci.* 3(2):163-176 (1972).

Tucson Gas and Electric Co., Tucson, Arizona. "Applicants Environmental Analysis: 345 KV Transmission Line from Westwind Substation to Vail Substation."

Tucson Gas and Electric Co., Tucson, Arizona. "Applicants Environmental Analysis: 345 KV Transmission Line from Vail Substation to San Juan Power Plant" (September 1971).

Upchurch, S. B., and D. C. N. Robb. "Mathematical Models: Planning Tools for the Great Lakes," *Water Resources Bull.* 8(2):338-348 (April 1972).

Wald, A. *Statistical Decision Functions.* (New York: John Wiley & Sons, Inc., 1954).

Weisbrod, B. A. "Costs and Benefits of Medical Research: A Case Study of Poliomyelitis," *J. Pol. Econ.* 19(3):527-544 (1971).

White, D. J. *Decision Theory* (Chicago: Aldine Publishing Co., 1969).

Wilson, A. G. "Forecasting 'Planning,'" *Urban Studies* 6:347-367 (1969).

Wold, H. "Ordinal Preferences of Cardinal Utility," *Econometrica* 20:661-664 (1952).

Young, F. W., and W. S. Torgenson. "TORSCA, a FORTRAN IV Program for Shepard-Kruskal Multidimensional Scaling Analysis," *Behavioral Sci.* 12:498 (1967).

CHAPTER 3

DATA BASES

INTRODUCTION

Data bases and data banks exist in every size and form. They have been much maligned for being expensive to build, difficult to use, over-crowded with useless information and usually out-of-date on becoming operational. Despite these difficulties, the collection of raw and/or pro-cessed information is an essential tool for the conduct of environmental assessments.

We will differentiate between scientific literature indexing and abstract-ing services and the collection of observational data items. Most of the relevant information useful to the assessment process is not in organized, computerized, maintained data systems. It is indeed diffusely distributed, varigated, uncertified, conflicting, difficult to assess and not summarized. Still, the quantity which is organized is not trivial and provides, as a minimum, a point of departure for the analyst.

DIRECTORIES OF DIRECTORIES

A number of directories of computerized information resources have been compiled (Green, 1976; Olson, 1977; Barrett, 1976; A. D. Little, 1974). Green (1976) made a summary of useful computerized systems, which is reproduced as Table 3-1.

The Regional and Urban Studies Information Center (RUSTIC) is a part of the Oak Ridge Computerized Hierarchical Information System (ORCHIS). It contains a large number of data bases from diversed sources available for on-line retrieval using the ORLOOK Program (Olson, et al., 1977). Associated software packages, display and plotting routines facilitate the preparation of statistical summaries and displays.

For additional sources a number of directories of directories should be consulted (Kruzas, 1974; Christian, 1975; Brown et al., 1975; NTIS, 1974).

Table 3-1. Summarized List of Environmental Data Services (Green et al., 1976)

FUNCTIONS AND SERVICES	Literature Searches — Computer	Literature Searches — Manual	Publications of Bibliographies	Microform Services	Publications	Abstracting and Indexing — Computer	Abstracting and Indexing — Manual	Referral/Reference	Selective Dissemination of Information	Copying	Data Collection/Storage and Retrieval	Data Analysis	Advisory/Consulting	State-of-the-Art Compilation	Interlibrary Loan	Bibliographic Research and Compilation	Translation	Computer Tapes	Available only to Government Contractors	Data Base	Information Center	Computer Program	Computer System	Data Bank
1. American Agricultural Economics Documentation Center (USDA)	X		X	X	X													X			X			
2. CAIN System (Cataloging and Indexing), 1970–present			X																	X				
3. Center for Air Environment Studies; The Pennsylvania State University		X	X	X	X		X			X	X										X			
4. Air Pollution Technical Information Center (APTIC) (EPA)		X	X	X	X		X		X	X	X	X				X		X		X	X			
5. National Air Data Branch, Air Pollution Office (EPA)										X	X	X								X	X			
6. Air Quality Implementation Planning Program, Computer Program Tape																						X		
7. Projection Algorithm for Vehicular Emissions (PAVE-I)																						X		
8. Hazardous Air Pollutants Enforcement Management System (HAPEMS)																								X
9. Central Abstracting and Indexing Service, American Petroleum Institute	X			X		X		X	X	X	X	X	X	X				X			X			
10. Franklin Institute Research Laboratories	X	X				X					X	X	X	X				X			X			
11. General Electric Company, Space and RESD Divisions	X	X						X	X		X	X	X	X		X					X			
12. Center for Urban Regionalism; Kent State University				X	X		X				X	X	X	X	X						X			
13. Textile Research Center; Illinois Institute of Technology	X	X			X		X		X		X	X	X		X				X		X			
14. Freshwater Institute Numeric Database (FIND)											X								X	X				
15. Environmental Information Retrieval On-Line (EPA)	X										X						X			X				
16. Tatsch Associates	X	X											X	X										
17. Eric Clearinghouse for Science, Mathematics, and Environmental Education; U.S. National Institute of Education								X	X	X	X		X		X			X			X			
18. Computerized Products and Services; Data Courier, Inc.	X	X	X	X	X	X			X	X	X	X	X					X			X			
19. Waterways Experiment Station; U.S. Army Corps of Engineers	X	X	X	X	X	X	X		X	X	X	X	X		X		X	X			X			
20. NASA Regional Center; Los Angeles					X														X					
21. American Society of Civil Engineers				X	X		X		X															
22. Smithsonian Science Information Exchange; Smithsonian Institution	X			X		X		X		X	X	X	X					X			X			
23. Center for Short-Lived Phenomena; Smithsonian Institution				X			X		X		X	X	X					X			X			
24. Conservation Library Center; Denver Public Library	X	X	X		X		X	X			X			X							X			
25. Ronald J. Scheidelman and Associates; Searchline	X	X		X				X		X	X	X	X								X			
26. Scientists' Institute for Public Information	X	X			X		X	X	X	X	X										X			
27. Ecology Forum, Inc.; Environmental Information Center	X	X		X	X	X	X	X	X	X	X	X	X		X	X	X	X			X			

28. Biosciences Information Services of Biological Abstracts
29. Environmental Mutagen Information Center
30. Biological Information Service
31. Geographic Information Systems; Geographic Applications Program (USGS)
32. Bibliography and Index to the Literature in the NBS Alloy Data Center
33. Mineral Supply; U.S. Bureau of Mines
34. Soil Data Storage and Retrieval Unit; Soil Conservation Service (USDA)
35. Rock Mechanic Information Retrieval System; University of London
36. ENDEX/OASIS NOAA Environmental Data Key
37. Overview of the Water Quality Control Information System (STORET)
38. Matrix of Environmental Residuals for Energy Systems (MERES)
39. Institute for Scientific Information
40. National Weather Service River Forecast System
41. The Defense Documentation Center
42. RECON (ERDA)
43. Land Base–1973
44. Oil Shale Project, 1969 to Present
45. Battelle Energy Information Center (BEIC)
46. Natural Resources Library; U.S. Department of the Interior
47. Federal Aid in Fish and Wildlife; Denver Public Library
48. Environmental Technical Information Center; Institute for Paper Chemistry
49. Transportation Noise Research Information Service; National Academy of Sciences
50. Noise Information Retrieval System; Office of Noise Abatement and Control
51. Toxicology Information Program; U.S. National Library of Medicine
52. Analysis and Evaluation of Sources, Transport, Fate and Effects of Nuclear and Nonnuclear Contamination in the Biosphere
53. Oil and Hazardous Materials; Battelle Memorial Institute
54. Poison Control Toxicological Inquiry, 1956-1973
55. Pesticides Data Bank (EPA)
56. Pesticides Information Center
57. Office of Pesticide Programs (EPA)
58. Analytical Methodology Information Center; Battelle Memorial Institute
59. Mathematical Model for Outfall Plume
60. National Center for Resource Recovery, Inc.
61. Simulation of the Time-Dependent Performance of the Activated Sludge Process Using the Digital Computer
62. A Generalized Computer Model for Steady-State Performance of the Activated Sludge Process

Table 3-1, continued

FUNCTIONS AND SERVICES	Literature Searches: Computer	Literature Searches: Manual	Publications of Bibliographies	Microform Services	Publications	Abstracting and Indexing: Computer	Abstracting and Indexing: Manual	Referral/Reference	Selective Dissemination of Information	Copying	Data Collection/Storage and Retrieval	Data Analysis	Advisory/Consulting	State-of-the-Art Compilation	Interlibrary Loan	Bibliographic Research and Compilation	Translation	Computer Tapes Available only to Government Contractors	Data Base	Information Center	Computer Program	Computer System	Data Bank
62. A Generalized Computer Model for Steady-State Performance of the Activated Sludge Process												X	X									X	
63. National Water Data System (USGS)			X						X			X	X						X			X	X
64. State of Washington Water Research Center; Washington State University			X					X													X		
65. Hydrological Information Storage and Retrieval System; Water Resources Research Institute						X					X	X	X	X		X							
66. Water Resources Scientific Information Center Network; U.S. Department of the Interior						X		X	X			X	X	X				X			X		
67. Environmental Systems Applications Center; Indiana University		X								X			X				X	X			X		
68. Main I: A System of Computerized Models for Calculating and Evaluating Municipal Water Requirements		X								X											X		
69. Main C: Computerized Methodology for Evaluation of Municipal Water Conservation Research Programs												X										X	
70. Forecasting Municipal Water Requirements												X										X	
71. Mathematical Simulation of Ammonia Stripping Towers for Wastewater Treatment												X										X	
72. Dam 2, Fortran IV Computer Program												X										X	
73. Project Formulation—Hydrology, Fortran IV Computer Program												X										X	
74. Computer Program for Preliminary Design of Wastewater Treatment Systems												X										X	
75. Preliminary Design and Simulation of Conventional Wastewater Renovation Systems Using the Digital Computer												X										X	
76. Wastewater Treatment Plant Cost Estimating Program												X										X	
77. Watershed Conservation and Development Master File, 1973												X											X
78. Water Surface Profile Program												X										X	
79. Mathematical Model of Natural Draft, Wet Cooling Towers																						X	

#	Source	1	2	3	4	5	6	7	8	9	10	11	12
80.	Data Bases: Solid Earth and Solar-Terrestrial Environmental Data					X	X	X			X	X	
81.	Data Bases: Oceanography			X			X	X				X	
82.	Analyses of Natural Gases						X						X
83.	Data Bases: Climatology			X		X	X				X	X	
84.	Energy and Environmental Systems Division (ALC)						X		X		X	X	
85.	NUS Corporation Technical Library	X	X			X						X	
86.	SDC/POLLUTION	X			X		X				X		
87.	SDC/COMPENDEX	X			X		X				X		
88.	American Geological Institute			X	X		X				X		
89.	National Technical Information Service (NTIS)	X		X	X		X				X	X	
90.	Chemical Abstracts Service, Division of American Chemical Society		X	X	X		X				X	X	
91.	Nuclear Science Abstracts (ERDA)			X	X					X			

ENVIRONMENTAL DATA BASES

Data bases of historical information are kept by a variety of groups—government agencies, trade associations, industries, foundations—in the discharge of their functions (research, monitoring, enforcement administration). These data bases are either bibliographic, *i.e.*, they are a compilation of technical journal citations or references to books and reports or are substantive and contain raw or processed data and information on the study of the environment. This information is most useful for establishing an environmental baseline, for characterizing an area or for establishing trends in parameters of interest.

The following tables and references provide an orientation to the data bases in existence, the major characteristics and availability. Table 3-2 identifies the major data handling systems in the fields of air pollution, water pollution, solid waste, toxic substances, noise and integrated assessment as they are sponsored and/or maintained by federal government agencies or specialized groups. Tables 3-2 to 3-8 describe in detail each of the data systems identified in Table 3-2.

ENVIRONMENTAL RADIATION AMBIENT MONITORING SYSTEM AND DATA BASES

Continuing surveillance of radioactivity levels is maintained through EPA's Environmental Radiation Ambient Monitoring System (ERAMS). This system was formed in July 1973 from the consolidation and redirection of separate monitoring networks formerly operated by the U.S. Public Health Service prior to EPA's formation. These previous monitoring networks had been oriented primarily to measurement of fallout levels. They were modified by changing collection and analysis frequencies and sampling locations and by increasing the analyses for specific radionuclides. The emphasis of the current system is toward identifying trends in the accumulation of long-lived radionuclides in the environment.

Table 3-9 is a summary of the current status and historical perspective of ERAMS. The system involves over 7,000 individual analyses per year on samples of air, water, milk and bone from approximately 150 locations throughout the continental United States, Alaska, Hawaii and the U.S. territories. Samples are collected by state and local health agencies and forwarded to the Eastern Environmental Radiation Facility in Montgomery, AL for analysis. From 1960 until December 1974, the ERAMS results were published in *Radiation Data and Reports* and its predecessors, *Radiological Health Data and Reports* (1966-1971) and *Radiological Health Data* (1960-1965). This monthly publication was suspended in 1974 and will

Table 3-2. Data Handling and Information Systems at the Federal Level (Fennelly *et al.*, 1976)

Sponsor	Air	Water	Solid Waste	Toxic Substances	Noise	Comprehensive Environmental Data
U.S. Environmental Protection Agency	AEROS - Aerometric and Emissions Reporting Systems NEDS - National Emissions Data System SAROAD - Storage and Retrieval of Aerometric Data QAMIS - Quality of Aerometric Data SOTDAT - Source Test Data Storage HATREMS - Hazardous and Trace Substance Inventory System SIP - State Implementation Plan EDS - Energy Data System FPC-67 - Cumulative FPC Form 67 Data System APTIC - Air Pollution Technical Information Center UNAMAP - Users Network for Applied Modeling of Air Pollution	STORET - Storage and Retrieval of Water Quality Data ENVIRON - Environmental Information Retrieval On-Line GPSF - General Point Source File NEI - National Estuarine Inventory Water Quality Standards	SWIRS - Solid Waste Information Retrieval System		NOISE - Noise Information Retrieval System	NERC - National Environmental Research Center PRES - Program Review and Evaluation Environmental Impact Statement System
U.S. National Oceanic and Atmospheric Administration		ENDEX - Environmental Data Index EDS - Environmental Data Service				EDBD - Environmental Data Base Directory ESIC - Environmental Science Information Center
U.S. Geological Survey, Water Resources Division		OWDC - Office of Water Data Coordination NWDS - National Water Data System				

Table 3-2, continued

Sponsor	Air	Water	Solid Waste	Toxic Substances	Noise	Comprehensive Environmental Data
U.S. Department of the Interior	WRSIC	Water Resources Scientific Information Center Network				
Oak Ridge National Laboratory				EISO - Environmental Information System Office		
				TMIC - Toxic Materials Information Center		
				EMIC - Environmental Mutagen Information Center		
				TIRC - Toxicology Information Response Center		
				ESIC - Ecological Sciences Information Center		
U.S. Public Health Service				NIOSH - National Institute of Occupational Safety and Health, Technical Information Services Branch		
				NIEHS - National Institute of Environmental Health Sciences - Information Services		
				CHEMLINE - Chemical Dictionary On-Line		
				TOXLINE - Toxicology Information Program (TIP)		
Battelle Memorial Institute				EIAC - Environmental Information Analysis Center		
Council on Environmental Quality (CEQ)				EIC - Energy Information Center		
				MERES - Matrix of Environmental Residuals for Energy Systems		
The Center for Short-Lived Phenomena, Cambridge, MA				United Nations Environment Program		
Ecology Forum, Inc.				EIC - Environmental Information Center		
Pollution Abstracts, Inc.				Pollution Abstracts		

Table 3-3. Federal Data Retrieval and Information Systems—Air (Fennelly, _et al._, 1976)

Name of System and Sponsor	Brief Description	Scope	Input Data Sources	Access to System	Users Guide Manual Available	Form of Data Output	Use Restrictions
U.S. Environmental Protection Agency Air Pollution Office National Air Data Branch (NADB) NEDS SAROAD	Collection, analysis, and publication of emission and ambient air data by way of two computer systems: 1. NEDS - National Emissions Data System 2. SAROAD - Storage and Retrieval of Aerometric Data. SAROAD contains national ambient air quality data, statistically analyzed and reduced from nationwide ambient monitoring systems. NEDS is comprised of emissions data from individual point and area sources.	Air pollution, air quality and emissions data. NEDS - 75,000 point sources 3,500 area sources. SAROAD - 3,000 air monitoring stations, 27 million entries to data base since 1958.	Data generated by EPA and its contractors, and collected from state and local agencies.	TSO and batch access systems are available in all 10 EPA regional offices, linked to central computer at Research Triangle Park, North Carolina.	NEDS: APTD-1135, "Guide for Compiling a Comprehensive Emission Inventory" Volume II of the AEROS manual. SAROAD: A complete directory of SAROAD site data published annually. Also refer to Volume III of the AEROS manual.	NEDS: Point and area source data can be arranged in multiple ways. The more common outputs are emissions according to pollutant, geographic area, source category, type ownership; specific fuel usage; control equipment; compliance status of sources. SAROAD: The following are common data reports: yearly data inventory by site, by pollutant; yearly or quarterly frequency distribution; composite listing; yearly report by quarters; air standards reports; parameter/ sampling method/unit listing; raw data listing for 1 hr or 24 hrs.	Services are available within EPA without restrictions, exchange agreements are available for other organizations with some restrictions on data available.
U.S. Environmental Protection Agency Users Network for Applied Modeling of Air Pollution (UNAMAP)	UNAMAP provides access to a network of air pollution models and associated meteorological and emissions data bases in order to determine effectiveness of controls and administer charges as required.	A variety of models pertaining to air pollution models made available to states, regions and other qualified users.	A series of mathematical models for determining effects on air quality of various air pollution control actions.	Access available to regions, states, and other qualified users via a remote terminal network.	An inventory of models and capabilities will be made available so users can select appropriate models.	Once on-line with the network, the user can select any model, data base, and test desired control strategies.	The system is available to EPA personnel and a variety of other eligible users.
U.S. Environmental Protection Agency Aerometric and Emissions Reporting System (AEROS)	AEROS is comprised of input forms, procedures, programs, files and reports established by the EPA to collect, maintain and report information describing air quality and emissions sources. *AEROS was formed by merging NEDS and SAROAD. NEDS and SAROAD forms provide the primary input to AEROS. AEROS now encompasses other information systems such as OAMIS, SOTDAT, HATREMS, SIPS, EDS and RAPS as described below.	AEROS allows for: 1. Evaluation of state implementation plans 2. Evaluation of emissions and control equipment for developing new source performance standards 3. Support of enforcement of EPA regulations and inspection/monitoring 4. Determination of status and trends in air pollution for reports and progress evaluation 5. Studies of fuels, usage and availability 6. Research on monitoring of sources and ambient air for modeling	Punch cards and tape generated from NEDS and SAROAD forms. Forms are submitted to EPA by the states on a quarterly and semiannual basis.	All AEROS reports can now be obtained directly from the National Air Data Branch. The objective is to provide full interactive and remote batch use of AEROS by all regional offices.	the AEROS manual	According to user requirements, various mathematical techniques can be used for data reduction and output of summaries, listings raw data listings and published reports.	Similar to that described above

Table 3.3, continued

Name of System and Sponsor	Brief Description	Scope	Input Data Sources	Access to System	Users Guide Manual Available	Form of Data Output	Use Restrictions
U.S. Environmental Protection Agency Quality of Aerometric Data (QAMIS) (see AEROS)	QAMIS is an interim system for evaluating the quality control activities of groups that collect ambient air data, analyze the data, convert the data, and, finally, submit the data into SAROAD. There are no plans to update QAMIS as it will either be re-designed or superseded.	QAMIS consists of three files: agency, laboratory and site. In general, each file contains the results of general questionnaires solicited by EPA from representatives of each of the three quality control points for each monitoring system. There is the capability to "grade" the performance of agencies based on the data contained in QAMIS.	Questionnaires completed by agencies and laboratories responsible for acquiring data for input to SAROAD. The system analyzes quality control activities of these groups.	N/A	N/A	The following information is available on a nationwide or state basis: 1. Site information 2. Site-pollutant information 3. Agency information	This system is used mainly by EPA personnel for the improvement of the SAROAD data base.
U.S. Environmental Protection Agency Source Test Data Storage (SOTDAT)	The system is designed to store and retrieve relevant technical data acquired during the performance of point source pollutant emission tests.	Data are included from source tests of stationary combustion facilities, chemical processes, mineral products industries, food and agriculture production, etc. Approximately 500 source tests were input to SOTDAT as of February, 1975. Annual increase is expected to be 300-500 source tests from EPA and other organizations.	Data is obtained from the EPA Emission Measurement Branch test reports, state and local air pollution control agencies, control equipment, manufacturers, consultants, and installations identified through information retrieved from the NEDS point source file.	System not yet operational	Source Test Data System (SOTDAT) National Air Data Branch - Monitoring and Data Analysis Division August, 1973 by J. H. Sutherland W. M. Vatavuk of E. J. Dale & J. B. Turner, System Sciences, Inc.	Data can be output according to specific pollutant; SCC codes; or by name and address of source.	Available on a time-sharing basis to OAQPS and EPA personnel.
U.S. Environmental Protection Agency Hazardous and Trace Substance Inventory System (HATREMS)	The system is being designed to store operating parameters and annual emissions of sources of noncriteria pollutants. HATREMS is included in the NEDS file. The HATREMS source identification hierarchy is plant, point source, process, and pollutant.	HATREMS is comprised of two basic data files: point and area sources. A great deal of data included is derived from the NEDS file. The system is in the final stages of file maintenance and program design.	Emission factors from AP-42 and EPA 450/2-73-001, Emission Factors for Trace Substances will be used to develop the initial data base.	System not yet operational	Currently under development	Similar to NEDS	When system is developed access will be on a basis similar to NEDS.
U.S. Environmental Protection Agency State Implementation Plans (SIP)	The system stores the full text of all state implementation plan regulations and subsequent revisions	The file contains 5000 state regulations, with expected addition of maximum of 200 pages of revised or new regulations per year.	The complete text of all State Implementation Plans for the purpose of air pollution abatement.	Access is available through NADB		Two outputs are available: 1. Full text retrieval of each regulation as it applies to one of approximately 160 identifying codes e.g. source surveillance record keeping or SO_x control regulations for steam electric power plants. 2. Total number of regulations that meet the retrieval specifications.	

System	Description	Content	Input	Access	Reference	Output	Restrictions
U.S. Environmental Protection Agency Energy Data System (EDS)	EDS is currently under design and is intended to integrate all energy-related air quality data banks presently in EPA's data banks (see above).	EDS will contain fuel use summaries by geographical region and fuel consumption category; emissions and control equipment at large fuel burning sources; regulations applicable to fuel burning sources; compliance schedules; modeling results; and ambient air quality data in vicinity of large power plants.	All energy-related data available in other EPA data banks.	System not yet operational		Output will be in a form similar to NEDS	
U.S. Environmental Protection Agency and Federal Power Commission Cumulative FPC-Form 67 Data System	The FPC collects data yearly from each power plant of greater than 25 MW capacity and incorporates them into the Form 67 data system. Each boiler within each plant is assigned applicable NEDS plant and point identification codes and SCC codes. The FPC-67 system is completely compatible with NEDS and is accessible by a number of NEDS retrieval packages.	Information includes monthly and annual fuel use by boiler with associated sulfur and ash content; and detailed breakdowns of environmental control systems and costs. Form 67 includes 400 subject items and is completed by approximately 800 plants.	FPC form 67 questionnaire as completed by power plants of greater than 25-MW capacity. EPA receives coded data on magnetic tapes.	Access is available through NADB, which maintains a file of FPC-67 data on microfiche or on the original FPC questionnaires. A cross reference table between NEDS ID and FPC plant ID allows for use of NEDS retrieval codes.	The AEROS manual Volume III - Summary and Retrieval Manual Contract No. 68-02-1376, September, 1975	The complete FPC-67 information for all years for a given power plant can be retrieved. Selection can be made by geographic area, NEDS plant I.D., NEDS point I.D., SCC code, or fuel type.	Use restrictions are similar to NEDS
U.S. Environmental Protection Agency Air Pollution Technical Information Center (APTIC)	Collects and disseminates all domestic and foreign technical literature pertaining to air pollution. Services include: a. Monthly abstracts b. Literature searches c. Response to inquiries concerning the dissemination of federally produced air pollution-related documents d. Preparation of air pollution bibliographies.	Air pollution effects, atmospheric interactions, measurement, and control. 50,000 technical documents, hard copy and microfilm.	Domestic and foreign serials, patents, preprints, technical society papers, proceedings, and U.S. Government reports.	Accessible by telephone to the Air Pollution Technical Information Center, Research Triangle Park, North Carolina (919-549-8411)	Unknown	Technical documents in hard cover on microform Air Pollution Abstracts available monthly from the Superintendent of Documents, U.S. Government Printing Office, Washington, D.C. 20402	Free services primarily intended for EPA only; some services also free to qualified requesters.

Table 3-4. Federal Data Retrieval and Information Systems—Water (Fennelly *et al.*, 1976)

Name of System and Sponsor	Brief Description	Scope	Input Data Sources	Access to System	Users Guide Manual Available	Form of Data Output	Use Restrictions
U.S. Environmental Protection Agency Storage and Retrieval of Water Quality Data (STORET)	Storage and retrieval system for environmental data related to the discharge of pollutants to waterways. STORET provides information on water quality standards, waste discharges, abatement needs, construction costs, implementation schedules and manpower needs. STORET is intended to aid in determining cause and effect relationships of water pollution.	Nationwide data base with data on 20,000 pollutant discharges and 20 million monitoring observations from over 150,000 locations and 20 million monitors data on ambient conditions in the nations waterways.	Data gathered through permits issued for waste water discharge, monitoring data collected by a variety of agencies at the federal, state and local levels, stored as the result of various laboratory analyses of water samples.	Access by remote users via telephone terminals in 350 locations including 10 EPA regional offices and offices in 40 state capitals.	The STORET Handbook	Data base available as tape, punched cards, and computer printout.	Direct usage limited to primary pollution control authorities on the federal state and local levels.
U.S. Environmental Protection Agency Environmental Information Retrieval On-Line (ENVIRON)	EPA-wide, on-line, full text data storage and retrieval system utilizing the Computer Network (COMNET) in Washington, D.C. The primary input in environmental literature and data received from various environmental monitoring and surveillance networks.	Data collection and literature searching in multiple fields of environmental concern.	Input from active and proposed R&D project descriptions, published literature, and various environmental quality surveillance networks.	EPA users by telephone throughout the U.S. The user needs keyboard terminals with EBCDIC correspondence or ASCII codes for on-line access to data.			Commercial access available on contract basis through Informatics, Inc., Rockville, MD.
U.S. Environmental Protection Agency General Point Source File (GPSF)	GPSF collects and analyzes data describing unique point sources of water pollution discharge, and institutes data quality control procedures.	Enables user to specify report information and format. User can select discharges according to discharge data conditions, select parameters for retrieval, retrieve various levels of the data, and design a specific output format.	Input data is derived from other computerized systems such as STORET after appropriate validation and editing.			User can design his own output format.	
U.S. Environmental Protection Agency National Estuarine Inventory (NEI)	NEI compiles information on the coastal zones of the U.S. to identify present and potential users, and the extent of pollution damage.	NEI serves as a repository for all estuarine data without regard for its individual characteristics, volumes, or special processing needs. Complete flexibility in data processing. The data base consists of 200 million items.	New information cataloged, validation criteria are determined for each data element, update characteristics are determined and a standard print format is designed.			A standard print format is output. NEI is designed to have complete flexibility in data processing.	

U.S. Environmental Protection Agency Water Quality Standards	System provides EPA headquarters and regions with the various individual state water quality standards on microfiche for analyses and reference.	Water quality standards including numerical and narrative criteria applied to specify stream use classifications; and an antidegradation statement.	Water quality standards are established by the states and reviewed for approval by the EPA regional office. Upon acceptance, they are relayed to headquarters for formatting and microfiching.		One copy of final microfilm is sent to each EPA region.
National Water Data System (NWDS) U.S. Geological Survey Water Resources Division	The NWDS was established to assess the quality of U.S. water resources. NWDS provides statistical data and summary reports to planners, developers and managers. In future, NWDS will identify and make available to all users all water data acquired in the U.S. by government and private interests.	Surface water stage and discharge; chemical quality parameters; radiochemistry; sediment; pesticide and certain biological concentrations in water, groundwater and surface water levels; geologic data on ground water; flood frequency and inundation mapping.	Measurements and observations collected by U.S. Geological Survey, states, counties and local interest groups. 9,000 streamflow gauging stations; 4,000 water quality measuring stations; 30,000 groundwater observation wells. Data back to 1890.	Catalog of information on water data. Memorex 1600 computer output on microfilm system; publication data available on magnetic tape or cards; and 9-channel 800 BPI tapes are available.	Services are available without restrictions; users are required to pay the computer costs involved in the selection and duplication of data.
Water Resources Scientific Information Center (WRSIC) Network U.S. Department of the Interior	Organized to disseminate information to the water resources community via state-of-the-art reviews and computer-aided retrieval of pertinent literature, WRSIC consists of 3 information processing centers located at University of Wisconsin, Cornell University, and North Carolina State University, which are linked to computer facilities at the University of Oklahoma Research Institute and Oklahoma State University, which acts as coordination and evaluation of network activities. The 3 centers provide technical consultation, reference service and library services to each of 3 multistate regions.	Water resources supply conservation, management, protection, law, engineering, planning and pollution; an interdisciplinary coverage of the natural, physical and social sciences related to water resources.	Literature, research in progress, patents, conference proceedings, final reports, and abstracting and indexing services. Primary input sources include WRSIC supported "centers of competence," the 51 water resources research institutes, and grantees and contractors of Office of Water Resources Research and other federal water agencies.	Computer literature searching available but no magnetic tapes are presently available.	Abstract journal, annual catalog, computer searches periodic bibliographies, and state-of-the-art reviews available for purchase without restrictions.

Table 3-4, continued

Name of System and Sponsor	Brief Description	Scope	Input Data Sources	Access to System	Users Guide Manual Available	Form of Data Output	Use Restrictions
U.S. NOAA (National Oceanic and Atmospheric Agency) Environmental Data Index (ENDEX)	The ultimate goal of the system is to maintain files of available marine environmental data for all United States coastal waters. The file descriptions give the types of records and data held by federal, state and local government agencies, industry and universities. The system is essentially a reference library of available information.	The files pertain to a wide variety of pollution-related coastal water characteristics. Information regarding when a particular program was started, what parameters are monitored, where analysis is performed, etc., is contained in the files.		By request, along with stipulation of type and range of information required.	Available on request from any EDS (see below) center or library.		No restrictions. Services provided on a reimbursable fee basis.
U.S. NOAA Environmental Data Service (EDS) National Oceanographic Data Center (NODC)	NODC acquires, processes, exchanges, stores and retrieves globally oriented physical, chemical and biological data related to oceanography. NODC provides data compilations along with evaluations of data accuracy. Services include: abstracting and indexing; data collection and analysis; literature searching; consulting; microreproduction; and research into ENDEX (see above).	Data from all oceans, seas and estuaries.	Data submitted by foreign and domestic corporations, national data centers, and the World Data Center system.		User's guide for NODC data processing system.	Data tapes are available in various formats and combinations.	Requests should contain: 1. Definition of required data 2. Geographic area 3. Other pertinent information Small amounts of data free of charge, otherwise cost estimates made and receipt of funds required.
Office of Water Data Coordination (OWDC)	The purpose of OWDC is to coordinate the acquisition of water data by federal agencies, design a national water data network, and establish a catalog of information on water data acquisition activities (see NWOS below). Other services include preparation of indexes giving acquisition activities, responses to requests for information, and assistance to users in obtaining data on acquisition activities.	All water data acquisition activities, including data collection, processing, storage, retrieval and dissemination; also included are the identification of standardized procedures for acquiring and handling water data and quality control techniques.	All input from federal and nonfederal organizations acquiring and or using water data. Covers: 24,000 surface water stage stations; 18,000 water quality stations; 29,000 groundwater observation wells; 1,800 aerial investigations.		Catalog of information on water data; 21 volumes corresponding to U.S. water resource regions.		Services are available without restriction.

U.S. National Oceanic and Atmospheric Administration, National Ocean Survey, Lake Survey Center	Lake Survey Center studies the Great Lakes and their outflow rivers, Lake Champlain, New York State Barge Canal, and the Minnesota-Ontario Border Lakes. It compiles and publishes charts and related material, collects data related to the Great Lakes and issues these data in the form of summaries and technical reports.	Hydrographic surveys, charts and cartography, water levels motion and river flow, water characteristics and hydrology, and limnologic systems.	Field observations, survey drawings, aerial photographs, notebooks, computations, soundings, published literature, data from vessels and field parties, paper and magnetic tape, punch cards and printouts.	The Center uses a Xerox Data Systems Sigma 3 Computer.	A list of technical publications and charts, and a guide to ordering publications are available through the Superintendent of Documents, U.S. Government Printing Office, Washington, D.C. or from the Distribution Office in Detroit, MI.	Annual Data Summaries, Field Activities Reports, and Indexes of Area Coverage Surveys are issued. Microform copies of computer holdings are available. Data listings and bibliographies generated by literature searching are also available.
						Services available to all without restriction.
University of California, Water Resources Center	WRC serves the State of California and the West by funding, coordinating and disseminating data concerning water resources. The Center makes referrals to other agencies and specialists in the water field. Two archives are maintained which are collections relating to all aspects of development and use of water in California and the West, and on water resources in general.	Engineering, economic, social and legal aspects of water; water as a natural resource and its use; irrigation and reclamation; flood control; municipal and industrial water uses and problems; water rights; water development projects; associated environmental problems and concerns.	Reports and information received from a variety of public and private sources.		Contact University of California, Water Resources Center, Davis, CA 95616	The Center issues research reports, pamphlets, conference reports, and bibliographies. On-site use of literature collections are available.
						Services available to all without restriction.
U.S. Environmental Protection Agency Region 5 –Chicago Power Plant Program Management Information System	System will maintain location and technical data on thermal pollution from power plants and the status of their permits. Monitoring process is designed to assist the enforcement procedure.	System will produce a sorted list of power plants along with identification of receiving waters, type, heat load, priority, dates of operation, and 7-year average flow.	Monitoring data from power plants located within Region 5.		Contact the Power Plant Program Management Information System, EPA Region 5, 230 South Dearborn, Chicago, IL 60604	User can ask the file for characteristics, give limits and extract data.
						Services are provided primarily for EPA use.

Table 3-5. Federal Data Retrieval and Information Systems—Solid Waste (Fennelly, et al., 1976)

Name of System and Sponsor	Brief Description	Scope	Input Data Sources	Access to System	Users Guide Manual Available	Form of Data Output	Use Restrictions
U.S. Environmental Protection Agency Office of Solid Wastes Management Programs Solid Wastes Information Retrieval System (SWIRS)	SWIRS maintains a file of abstracts of publications concerning solid waste management. SWIRS responds to technical inquiries, provides literature searches and compiles bibliographies on solid waste.	Solid waste management; water pollution; air pollution; urban, industrial and environmental health.	Books, patents, vendor's catalogs, and scientific periodicals.	Contact EPA, Office of Solid Wastes Management Programs, 1835 K. St., N.W., Washington, D.C. 20460	1. Information Retrieval Services of EPA's Office of Solid Waste Management Programs. 2. User's Guide to the Solid Waste Information Retrieval System Thesaurus. Both documents are available on request.	Solid Waste publications, abstracts and bibliographies.	SWIRS is open to outside users provided requests are channeled.

Table 3-6. Federal Data Retrieval and Information Systems—Noise (Fennelly et al., 1976)

Name of System and Sponsor	Brief Description	Scope	Input Data Sources	Access to System	Users Guide Manual Available	Form of Data Output	Use Restrictions
U.S. Environmental Protection Agency Office of Noise Abatement and Control Noise Information Retrieval System, NOISE	NOISE serves as an integrated, centralized information center that collects technical and non-technical data on noise and noise sources. NOISE supplies copies of any information abstract to interested individuals. NOISE is a part of the ENVIRON system.	All aspects of environmental noise, including: aircraft, truck, train, bus and auto-mobile noise; ultra and infra-sonic sounds; health and biological effects of noise; abatement and control of noise; measurement standards and methodology; and legal and enforcement experience. NOISE consists of ~15,000 articles, 1/5 of which have been computerized.	Journals, newspapers, professional and trade papers, government publications, EPA hearings, reports to Congress and witness statements. Special efforts have been made to acquire data from Western Europe, Japan and the USSR.	Part of the NOISE data base has been computerized and is accessible via a terminal linked to an IBM 360-65 computer system.	A thesaurus to be used with the NOISE data base can be provided upon request.	Output consists of either complete referencing to literature of interest or copies of publications.	Manual literature searching is available to all without charge.

Table 3-7. Federal Data Retrieval and Information Systems—Toxicological Substances (Fennelly *et al.*, 1976)

Name of System and Sponsor	Brief Description	Scope	Input Data Sources	Access to System	Users Guide Manual Available	Form of Data Output	Use Restrictions
Oak Ridge National Laboratory Environmental Information System Office—EISO, P.O. Box X, Oak Ridge, TN 37830	EISO is composed of topical, mission-oriented environmental information centers, various data base groups, scientific project teams, and a unit which provides response and referral services to the environmental research community. Component information centers include: the Toxicology Information Response Center (TIRC), Toxic Materials Information Center (TMIC), Environmental Mutagen Information Center (EMIC), Energy Information Center (EIC), Current Energy Research and Development, and Environmental Response and Referral Service (ERRS).	EISO provides abstracting and indexing input to all its information centers and data bases, consulting services in environmental, computer, and information system disciplines, and literature searches. The Office issues state-of-the-art reports on the topics of toxicology and pesticides. EISO provides coverage of environmental research including: ecological sciences, materials resources and recycling, environmental impact of electrical energy, and regional modeling.	EISO inputs a number of commercially available computerized files including CA Condensates, BA-Previews, Bioresearch Index, Nuclear Science Abstracts, Chemical and Biological Sections of CA (CABS), and Government Research Announcements (GRA).	Contact ORNL, Environmental Information System Office P.O. Box X, Oak Ridge, TN 37830 The Office uses IBM 360-75 and 360-91 computers.	The Environmental Directory; a computerized compilation of information centers, research projects and individual investigators.	EISO maintains a large number of data sets on magnetic tape and large data bases not formally established as information services are accessible through EISO. EISO has access to ORNL libraries; Information Division. Advisory and consulting services are also available.	Services are available to U.S. government agencies their contractors, research and educational institutions, and industry.
Toxic Materials Information Center (TMIC), Environmental Information System Office, Oak Ridge National Laboratory	The objective of the system is to establish a data base on environmental levels of toxic materials. TMIC answers inquiries, provides R & D information, provides literature searching and abstracting and indexing services, distributes publications and makes referrals to other information sources.	Two classes of materials are included in data base: toxic metals and synthetic and natural organic compounds. Types of data are: materials balances in and around mining, smelting, and power facilities; natural and induced levels toxic and potentially toxic materials in various areas of the country; and information on the levels of toxic substances in plants and animals inhabiting these areas.	Published literature, conference papers, and internally produced reports.	On-site use of collection is permitted.		Publication abstracts and bibliographies, and data listings. Portions of data base can be made available externally on magnetic tapes.	Services are available to those with a professional interest in the ecology and analysis of trace contaminants, both inside and outside ORNL.
Oak Ridge National Laboratory Environmental Mutagen Information Center (EMIC)	EMIC was established to accumulate, store and disseminate all information pertinent to the chemical compounds in the environment which have been tested for mutagenicity. The Center works with two other information centers sponsored by ORNL, the TMIC and TIRC, in areas of mutual interest to provide comprehensive coverage to users of the other centers.	Chemical mutagenesis, including genetic effects of drugs, food additives, cosmetics and industrial chemicals.	Journal articles, laboratory reports, symposium proceedings, abstracting publications, scientific newsletters and bulletins, and commercially available computerized data bases.	The EMIC uses an IBM 360 computer. Contact ORNL, Environmental Mutagen Information Center, P.O. Box Y, Bldg. 9224, Oak Ridge, TN 37830	EMIC issues annual indexed bibliographies of the chemical mutagenesis literature.	Publication abstracts and bibliographies generated from computer literature searches. State-of-the-art reviews on currently important subjects are also available.	Services are available without restriction to the scientific community.

Table 3-7, continued

Name of System and Sponsor	Brief Description	Scope	Input Data Sources	Access to System	Users Guide Manual Available	Form of Data Output	Use Restrictions
Oak Ridge National Laboratory Toxicology Information Response Center (TIRC)	TIRC was formed to serve as national and international center of toxicology information. One of TIRC's principal functions is to provide literature searches, answers to toxicological questions, production of annotated bibliographies, critical reviews and state-of-the-art reports.	Toxicology, including: pharmacology, adverse effects, untoward reactions, drug interactions, side effects, biotransformation, pesticides, food additives, metal, chemicals carcinogenicity, veterinary toxicology, industrial chemistry and environmental pollutants.	Center utilizes various computerized services such as MEDLINE and TOXLINE.	The Center uses the Environmental Information System Office equipment consisting of IBM 360-75 and 360-91 computers.	TIRC publication list is available on request.	Bibliographies generated from literature searches and state-of-the-art reports.	Services are available without restriction.
Oak Ridge National Laboratory Ecological Sciences Information Center (ESIC)	ESIC provides information support to the Environmental Sciences Division of the Oak Ridge National Laboratory. Services include identification collection, analysis, storage and retrieval of data relevant to the radioecology interests of sponsors.	Radioecology including radionuclide cycling in various ecosystems, radiation effects on ecosystems or their components basic ecology, and thermal effects and other aquatic impacts; special emphasis is given to the environmental aspects of plutonium and uranium.	Input data is selected from a complex of specialized libraries, current awareness services from automated sources (NSA, BA, CA, and GRA), and individual collections of material.	Computerized information files are available on-line through a working relationship with the Environmental Information System Office.		Publication abstracts and indexes, bibliographies compiled from literature searches, and data listings.	Services are available to all, with requests answered on the basis of availability of staff and resources.
U.S. Public Health Service National Institute of Occupational Health & Safety	The TISB disseminates scientific and technical information on occupational safety and health. TISB answers questions concerning industrial health and maintains an information storage and retrieval system for literature covering occupational safety and health.	TISB includes information on all aspects of occupational health including industrial hygiene, medicine, toxicology, pathology, engineering, nursing and chemistry. Approximately 20,000 documents are incorporated in the system.	Derived from current literature on occupational safety and health.	Contact NIOSH Division of Technical Services, Technical Information Services Branch, P.O. and Court House Building, Cincinnati, OH 45202	A list of publications is available from the Office of Technical Publications, NIOSH.	Computer literature searches, copies of solicited publications, etc.	Services are available to all, limited only by staff time and work load.
U.S. Public Health Service National Institute of Environmental Health Sciences, NIEHS Information Services	Information Services serves the information needs of the scientific staff and administrators of the NIEHS. The Institute maintains a library and provides bibliographic services through MEDLINE to outside requestors.	Mutagenesis; toxicology; pharmacology; teratology; veterinary science and technology; environmental pollutants; analytical methodology.	Derived from EPA publications, Edgewood Arsenal reports, NIOSH, and the EPA Pesticide Information Center.	NIEHS library and computer literature searching through MEDLINE.		The Institute maintains a library (4000 volumes and periodicals) and provides bibliographic services both manually and by outline terminal through MEDLINE.	Services intended for NIEHS personnel, others may use library during work hours.
CHEMLINE Chemical Dictionary On-Line	This system is sponsored by the Toxicology Information Program and the Chemical Abstracts Service.	Approximately 60,000 chemical substances identified by CAS Registry Numbers, molecular formulas, preferred chemical nomenclature, etc., can be searched on-line.					

U.S. National Library of Medicine Toxicology Information Program (TIP) TOXLINE	TIP was established to provide the scientific community with a toxicology information service. TOXLINE is a nationwide, on-line literature retrieval service.	TOXLINE covers human and animal toxicity studies, effects of environmental chemicals and pollutants, adverse drug reactions, and analytical methodology. The data base includes approximately 325,000 references.	TIP contains files from various private and government sources.	TOXLINE can be accessed by different types of terminal devices at many locations. Entry points to the computer are located throughout the U.S.	Whole text output of over 270,000 citations are available.	Services available to scientific community without restriction. Direct requests to Director, Toxicology Information Response Center, Oak Ridge National Laboratory, P.O. Box Y, Oak Ridge, TN 37830

Table 3-8. Federal Data Retrieval Systems—Total Environment (Fennelly *et al.*, 1976)

Name of System and Sponsor	Brief Description	Scope	Input Data Sources	Access to System	Users Guide Manuals Available	Form of Data Output	Use Restrictions
U.S. Environmental Protection Agency National Environmental Research Center (NERC) Information Center and Library	Information center and library of NERC is the scientific and technical information focal point for the EPA. Computer literature searches of 33 data bases with citations to 97 million documents. Book catalog made available for participating EPA libraries.	Air and water pollution (including standards and analysis); solid waste, noise, thermal pollution, radiation, pesticides and related ecological and environmental topics. Major emphasis is on water quality, with such peripheral subjects as chemistry, engineering, biomedicine and microbiology.	Input from U.S. National Technical Information Service, U.S. Government Printing Office, and states and universities. Periodicals, reports, proceedings, newspapers, and computerized data bases.	Data bases available through on-line or batch services at University of Georgia, Lehigh University Informatics, Inc.; Battelle Memorial Institute, University of Cincinnati, and Ohio State University.	Contact NERC, Information Center and Library, Cincinnati, OH 45268	Bibliographies, microreproduction of publications, full text copies, and library loan are available.	Computer searches are available to EPA staff, consultants and contractors; all other services are available to all cooperating libraries.
Ecology Forum, Inc. Environment Information Center (EIC) The Environmental Clearinghouse, Inc., Washington, D.C., is an affiliate and serves as its input agent for congressional and other government information.	EIC is a computer-assisted central data bank which gathers, indexes, abstracts analyzes and disseminates information on environmental matters. EIC monitors, abstracts and cross-references information in some 500 scientific publications. Ecology Forum, a nonprofit organization, attempts to fill information and communication-gaps, to facilitate access to environmental data and to increase the speed with which new information can be assimilated.	Environmental issues, including air, noise, land pollution; wildlife; geophysical change; energy; recreation; transportation; population control, and ecological imbalance.	Materials from primary and secondary source journals, research reports, conference proceedings, government and private documents, films, books and legislation.	Information available to subscribers in a biweekly publication or through computer searches and bibliography assemblies requested by mail or telephone order.		Abstracted items are available in microfiche or hard copy form on a single item or subscription basis.	Services are available to all. Retrieval services are for personal reference purposes only.
Pollution Abstracts, Inc. Pollution Abstracts	This periodical service indexes and abstracts journals on environmental pollution. It performs literature searches for outside users on a contract basis and provides a document retrieval service for subscribers to its journals.	This service covers 30,000 citations in all major areas of pollution. Pollution Abstracts subscribes to 750 periodicals.	Domestic and foreign journals, technical reports, books, symposia, and government documents.	Subscription to Pollution Abstracts Pollution Abstracts, Inc. P.O. Box 2369 La Jolla, CA 92037	N/A	Bimonthly periodical	Services and publications are available to subscribers only; manual literature services are offered on a contract basis.

Source	Description	Subject Coverage	Input	Access	Output	Availability
Battelle Memorial Institute-Columbus Laboratories Energy Information Center (EIC) 505 King Avenue Columbus, OH 43201 (614) 299-3151 x3711	The EIC was established as part of the Battelle Energy Program to provide energy information and data to users inside and outside Battelle who are involved in energy-related research. The EIC is intended to be the nation's major source of evaluation energy information and data.	Present coverage includes coal, oil, natural gas; nuclear, geothermal, solar, tidal, wind and hydro sources of energy. All aspects of energy systems are covered from resource extraction to final consumption.	Input is derived from 120 journals, technical reports, and other appropriate reference materials.	User needs an appropriate remote terminal and communication link.	Results of computer literature searching, and data listings	Services are available to all with interest in the nation's energy problems.
U.S. Environmental Protection Agency Environmental Impact Statement System	System will assist in monitoring environmental impact statements through the review process and by generating reports for publishing in *Federal Register.*	The system will identify impact statements which have been commented upon, statements under current review and number of statements per region, in order to monitor processing of statements.	Office of Federal Activities prepares input from Environmental Impact Statement logs which are received weekly from all EPA regions.		Four reports produced: 1. Biweekly register 2. Monthly frequency report 3. Quarterly statement 4. Listing of total file off-line.	
U.S. Environmental Protection Agency Program Review and Evaluation System (PRES)	PRES compiles in one location specific information on all monitoring-oriented programs operated throughout EPA. Central file used as starting point for all agency technical personnel to identify where and who is performing specific monitoring operations.	PRES will identify the following information for a particular monitoring program: 1. Who is performing the work 2. Where work is being done 3. Major results	File includes all fiscal year 1973 accomplishment plans for all monitoring operations performed at the National Environmental Research Centers by the EPA regions.			Use is intended primarily for EPA personnel.
Battelle Memorial Institute Environmental Information Analysis Center (EIAC)	Objective of the center is to provide a basis for information collected and used in support of various environmental research programs. The primary emphasis is devoted to environmental and health protection associated with nuclear facilities and activities. The center answers inquiries; provides consulting, reference, literature searching, abstracting and indexing services; provides R&D information; lends materials; permits on-site use of collection.	Power plant siting; nuclear reactor; thermal effluent effects; water quality management; radionuclide cycling in the environment; system ecology; solid waste management; environmental monitoring and analysis, combustion research; environmental impact assessments; environmental **aspects** of urban regional planning; mathematical modeling of ecosystems; environmental information management.	Not a computerized service. Holdings include periodicals, technical papers, research and development reports and other similar data.	Documents are manually accessible by an inverted coordinate index searchable by author, organization and key words.	Data are available on microfiche or hard copy, primarily in the form of abstracts.	Services are provided on a contract basis. Qualified users include government and industry.

Table 3-8, continued

Name of System and Sponsor	Brief Description	Scope	Input Data Sources	Access to System	Users Guide Manuals Available	Form of Data Output	Use Restrictions
The Center for Short-Lived Phenomena, Cambridge, Massachusetts United Nations Environment Program	The center has developed a major data base on existing, long-term pollution monitoring programs in 78 countries. It contains information on the purpose of each program, how the programs are administered and the pollutants monitored. Information is given on the physical medium monitored, geographical area covered, number of sites, sampling frequency, methods of sampling and data acquisition, measurement techniques, methods of sample analysis, precision of analysis, mode of data storage and the date the program began.	The data base includes information on 141 monitoring programs in the United States. The data base includes administrative, operational and technical data on each program. Programs covered include those monitoring SO_2, sulfates, POM, CO, CO_2, NO_x, oxidants, radioactive HC's; Hg, Pb, Cd, DDT, PCB's, asbestos, HC's, toxins of biological origin, nitrates, nitrites, ammonia, BOD, DO, pH, coliform bacteria, radionuclides, soluble salts of alkaline earth metals.	Information received from worldwide environmental monitoring programs.	Contact the Center for Short-Lived Phenomena 185 Alewife Brook Parkway, Cambridge, MA 02138 (617) 868-4793		A variety of outputs are available depending upon the specificity and detail required. For example, one can obtain a list of programs monitoring a specific pollutant in a given medium in a specific ocean area.	Fee charged for services, but available to all.
Matrix of Environmental Residuals for Energy Systems (MERES) Sponsored by the Council of Environmental Quality (CEQ)	MERES is a computerized data base specifying the water pollution, air pollution, solid waste, land use and occupational health effects of present and future energy systems. MERES also includes data on energy efficiencies and costs. A major reason for the development of MERES is to provide simplification of preparation and review of environmental impact statements, concerning energy-related projects. The complete system including the MERES data base, computer software, and computational models is termed the Energy Model Data Base (EMDB)	Data is included relating to the entire spectrum of energy supply systems and environmental impact. The following activities are considered: resource, extraction, transportation, processing, distribution, storage, conversion, electric generators and end uses. For each activity, MERES contains coefficients estimating environmental impact, efficiency, and capital and operating costs. Energy sources covered include those derived from coal, oil, natural gas, nuclear fission, and new technologies such as coal gasification and liquefaction, oil, shale, solvent-refined coal, and fluidized-bed coal combustion. Residuals specified in MERES include air, water and solid wastes. Air pollutants covered are NO_x, SO_x, HC's, CO and aldehydes. Water pollutants covered include acids, bases, dissolved solids, BOD, COD and heat. Land impacts such as area required, are also considered.	Most of original data contained in MERES came from "Environmental Impacts, Efficiency, and Cost of Energy Supply and End Use" prepared by Hittman Associates, Inc. Updating and refinement of the data is a continuous process carried out at Brookhaven.	MERES data are stored in a computer at the Brookhaven National Laboratory, Long Island, NY. The data and programs for performing computations are available from the Brookhaven computer via remote terminal or on the users own computer system.	Energy Model Data Base Users Manual, Brookhaven will provide copies of programs and data. Additional information concerning MERES and EMDB is available from the Energy/Environmental Data Group, Brookhaven National Laboratory, Upton, NY 11973.	Data is available on magnetic tape and in the two printed volumes, Environmental Impacts, Efficiency, and Cost of Energy Supply and End Use. Information is presented in a matrix format. Columns are environmental residuals, energy requirements, and costs; and the rows are activities and processes involved in a particular energy resource.	The system is available to all on a cost basis.

Table 3-9. EPA's Environmental Radiation Ambient Monitoring System Current Status

Component	Number of Sampling Sites	Sampling Frequency	Analyses Performed	Frequency of Analysis	Previous Network	Initially Established
Air Monitoring Program						
Gross Radioactivity and Deposition	20 Active, 54 Standby[a]	Semiweekly	Gross β[b], Gamma Scan[c]	Semiweekly	Radiation alert network	1956
Deposition	20 Active, 54 Standby[a]	As rain occurs	Gross β, Gamma Scan[d], Tritium, ^{238,239}Pu, ^{234,235}U	As rain occurs, As rain occurs, Monthly composite, March-May Composite	Radiation alert network	1956, 1967, 1974
Plutonium and Uranium in Air	20	Semiweekly	^{238,239}Pu, ^{234,235}U	Quarterly[e], Quarterly[e]	Plutonium in airborne Particulates	1965
^{85}Kr in Air	12	Semiannually	^{85}Kr	Semiannually	No network, but individual measurements for 1962	1973
Water Analysis and Sampling Program						
Surface Water	55	Quarterly	Tritium, Gamma Scan	Quarterly[e], Annually[e]	Tritium surveillance system	1964
Drinking Water	76	Quarterly	Tritium, Gross α, Gross β, Gamma Scan, ^{226}Ra, ^{90}Sr, ^{238,239}Pu, ^{234,235}U	Quarterly, Annually[e], Annually[e], Annually[e], Annually[f], Annually[g], Annually[e], Annually[e]		1970
Interstate Carrier System	658, ~220/year	Triannually	Gross α, Gross β, ^{90}Sr, ^{226}Ra	Triannually	Interstate Carrier Drinking Water Project	1960
Milk Analysis Program						
Pasteurized Milk	65	Monthly	Gamma Spectrometry[h], ^{89,90}Sr	Monthly	Pasteurized milk network	1960
Special Milk Analysis	9	Monthly	Tritium, ^{14}C	Annually[e]	^{14}C	1965
Human Organ Program						
Bone Analysis	Varies	Annually	Stable Calcium, ^{90}Sr	Annually, Annually	Human bone network	1961

[a] Activate if contaminating event occurs (e.g., atmospheric nuclear test in the Northern Hemisphere).
[b] Field estimate and subsequent laboratory determination.
[c] If gross beta is greater than 10 pCi/m^3
[d] If deposition exceeds gross beta of 15nCi/m^3.
[e] Composite sample analyzed.
[f] If gross alpha level exceeds 3 pCi/liter.
[g] If gross beta level exceeds 10 pCi/liter.
[h] For ^{131}I, ^{137}Cs, ^{140}Ba, and K.

be succeeded by annual topical reports and quarterly summaries of the ERAMS data. An annual summary of ERAMS data along with an evaluation of trends and their significance is presented in each year's publication of EPA's Radiological Quality of the Environment. ERAMS data are presently maintained by Environmental Protection Agency, Eastern Environmental Radiation Facility, P.O. Box 3009, Montgomery, AL 36109.

ENERGY DATA SYSTEMS

The FEA (1974) has published a comprehensive survey of existing energy data gathering programs and summarized each according to the format in Table 3-10. Additional energy information is available from Energy Information Act Hearings (1974). Table 3-11 is a compilation by FEA (1975) of the energy data banks maintained by a variety of government agencies. Table 3-12 is a compilation prepared by the National Governors' Conference on State Energy Information Systems (DeForest, 1975).

In spite of and maybe because of this mass of interrelated but poorly coordinated data gathering programs, the General Accounting Office (1976) called for improvements in energy data collection, analysis and reporting.

TOXIC CHEMICAL DATA BANKS

With the passage of the Toxic Substance Control Act of 1976, a massive effort has been initiated to define data requirements associated with the Act and to compile on a comparative basis all existing toxic

Table 3-10. FEA Energy Program Summary

Program Name
Contract
Objective
Date Available As
Use Made of Data by Parent Agency
Contribution of Data or Information
Collection Format
Verification Performed
How Often Updated
Mechanism for Exchange of Data
Products Resulting from Program
Survey Forms Used
Data in Existing Data Bases
Energy Cycles Covered
Date Last Updated

Table 3-11. Energy Data Systems (FEA, 1976)

Code	Agency	No. of Programs	Coal	Electricity	Energy-Related	Geothermal	Natural Gas	Nuclear	Oil Shale	Organic Waste	Petroleum Products	Petroleum	Solar	Tar Sands
ARC	Appalachian Regional Commission	4	X	X	X		X		X			X		
DOC BEA	Department of Commerce, Bureau of Economic Analysis	17	X	X	X		X	X			X	X		
DOC BDC	Department of Commerce, Bureau of Domestic Commerce	23	X	X	X	X	X	X	X	X	X	X	X	X
DOA	U.S. Department of Agriculture	19	X	X	X	X	X	X	X	X	X	X	X	X
CIA	Central Intelligence Agency	5	X	X	X		X	X	X		X	X		
CAB BAS	Civil Aeronautics Board, Bureau of Accounts and Statistics	9	X	X	X						X	X		
DOD DIA	Department of Defense, Defense Intelligence Agency	2	X	X	X		X	X			X	X		
DOD AF	Department of Defense, Air Force	19	X	X			X	X			X	X		
DOC DIB	Department of Commerce, Domestic and International Business Administration	3	X	X	X		X					X		
DOC IER	Department of Commerce, International Economic Policy and Research	3		X	X						X	X		
DOC MA	Department of Commerce, Maritime Administration	1	X	X			X				X	X		
DOC NOA	Department of Commerce, National Oceanic and Atmospheric Administration	6	X	X	X		X	X			X	X		
DOC NBS	Department of Commerce, National Bureau of Standards	2	X	X	X		X	X						
DOC PO	Department of Commerce, U.S. Patent Office	13	X	X	X		X	X						
DOC TS	Department of Commerce, U.S. Travel Service	8	X	X	X		X	X			X			
DOI GSC	Department of the Interior, Geological Survey Conservation Division	11	X	X	X		X	X			X	X		
DOI BOM	Department of the Interior, Bureau of Mines	6	X	X	X		X	X			X			
DOD OAS	Department of Defense, Office Assistant Secretary of Defense	30	X	X	X	X	X	X			X	X	X	
DOD NVY	Department of Defense, Navy	1	X	X	X		X	X			X	X		
DOD DSA	Department of Defense, Defense Supply Agency	2	X	X			X	X			X	X		
DOJ	U.S. Department of Justice	21	X	X			X				X	X		

Energy Sources Covered

Table 3-11, continued

Agency	No. of Programs	Coal	Electricity	Energy-Related	Geothermal	Natural Gas	Nuclear	Oil Shale	Organic Waste	Petroleum Products	Petroleum	Solar	Tar Sands
DOI GSG Department of the Interior, Geological Survey Geologic Division	5	X	X	X		X	X			X	X		
FPC BNG Federal Power Commission, Bureau of Natural Gas	3	X	X	X		X	X			X	X		
FEA U.S. Federal Energy Administration	1	X	X	X						X	X		
ERDA U.S. Energy Research and Development Administration	6	X	X	X		X	X			X	X		
EPA U.S. Environmental Protection Agency	1	X	X	X		X				X	X		
DOT U.S. Department of Transportation	2	X	X	X						X	X		
DOS U.S. Department of State	1	X	X			X				X	X		
DOL BLS Department of Labor, Bureau of Labor Statistics	1	X	X	X		X	X			X	X		
GSA PBS General Services Administration, Public Building Services	1	X	X	X		X				X	X		
GSA FSS General Services Administration, Federal Supply Service	1	X	X	X		X					X		
GSA FPA General Services Administration, Federal Preparedness Agency	2	X	X	X		X				X			
FTC U.S. Federal Trade Commission	2											X	
FPC OE Federal Power Commission, Office of Economics	4	X	X	X		X	X			X	X		
FPC OAF Federal Power Commission, Office of Accounting and Finance	1	X	X	X		X	X			X	X		
FPC BOP Federal Power Commission, Bureau of Power	5	X	X	X		X	X			X	X		
HUD U.S. Department of Housing and Urban Development	9	X	X			X	X				X		
ICC U.S. Interstate Commerce Commission	4	X	X			X	X		X	X	X		
NRC U.S. Nuclear Regulatory Commission	1				X							X	
NSF National Science Foundation	1	X	X						X	X			
SBA U.S. Small Business Administration	1	X	X			X				X	X		
SEC U.S. Securities and Exchange Commission	1	X	X	X		X				X	X		
DOC BOC Department of Commerce, Bureau of the Census	1	X	X			X	X				X		
TOTAL		34	29	29	3	35	25	3	2	32	31	4	1

Table 3-12. State Energy Information Systems Matrix (Energy Program, National Governor's Conference, 1975)

State	Energy Flow or Budget Document[a] Available Y	N	Institution	Users[c]	Planning Y	N	Operational Y	N	Energy Models[b] Institution	Planning Y	N	Institutional Process for Transferring Information to Policy-Makers	Overall Energy Management Coordination
Alabama	X		Energy Management Board	Energy Management Board			X			X		No formal mechanism	Energy Management Board
Alaska		X	Alaska Energy Office		X		X		Alaska Energy Office	X		No formal mechanism	Alaska Energy Office
Arizona	X		University of Arizona	Governor's Office and Legislature				X	Office of Economic Planning (Arizona Trade-Off Model)			Mechanism under development	Office of Economic Planning and Development
Arkansas	X				X		X					No formal mechanism	State Energy Office
California		X	Energy Resources Conservation and Development Commission			X		X	Rand Corporation, Stanford Research Institute, and others			Employment of researchers in state government as policy-makers	Energy Resources Conservation and Development Commission
Colorado	X		Colorado School of Mines	General Public			X		Colorado Energy Research Institute	X		No formal mechanism	Colorado Energy Research Institute (research only)
Connecticut	X		Department of Planning and Energy Policy				X		Department of Planning and Energy			Commissioner is policy advisor to Governor	Department of Planning and Energy
Delaware		X						X		X		No formal mechanism	Proposed energy plan under study
Florida	X		Florida Energy Office	State Government, utilities and universities			X		Florida Department of Commerce and universities			Formal structure under development	Department of Administration (State Energy Office)
Georgia	X		State Energy Office	State Government and universities			X		State Energy Office	X		Energy Office is in Office of the Governor	State Energy Office
Hawaii	X		Department of Planning and Economic Development	Department of Planning and Economic Development			X		Department of Planning and Economic Development			Director of Planning is State Energy Coordinator	Department of Planning and Economic Development
Idaho	X		Office of Energy (gasoline only)	Confidential use only				X				No formal mechanism	Independent state agency action
Illinois	X		University of Illinois	State government, universities, industry			X		Division of Energy	X		No formal mechanism	Division of Energy
Indiana		X					X			X		No formal mechanism	Indiana Energy Office

Table 3-12, continued

State	Energy Flow or Budget Document[a]					Energy Models[b]					Institutional Process for Transferring Information to Policy-Makers	Overall Energy Management Coordination
	Available Y	N	Institution	Users[c]	Planning Y / N	Operational Y / N	Institution	Planning Y / N				
Iowa	X		Energy Policy Council	State government and		X	State Geological Survey				Employment of researchers	Energy Policy Council
Kansas	X		Kansas Geological Survey	State and federal agencies, legislature		X	Kansas State University				Formal mechanism under development	(New) Energy Agency
Kentucky	X		Kentucky Energy Office	Kentucky Energy Office		X	University of Kentucky				Informal communications by Energy Office	Kentucky Energy Office
Louisiana	X		Private Contractor (Jack Faucett Assoc.)		X (plan)	X	Comprehensive Energy Management Program	X (plan)			No formal mechanism	Division of Natural Resources and Energy
Maine	X		Work with New England Regional Commission		X (plan)	X	Department of Commerce and Industry				New England Energy Management Information System Program (NEEMIS)	Not specified
Maryland	X		Governor's Science Advisory Council	General Public		X	Energy Policy Office				No formal mechanism	Not specified
Massachusetts	X		Private contractors (Arthur D. Little, and Intermetrics)	Energy Policy Office and state agencies		X	New England Regional Commission	X (plan)			Interaction between energy policy and executive offices. Also, in NEEMIS program	Energy Policy Office
Michigan	X		Public Service Commission		X (plan)	X	Public Service Commission and private contractor (Arthur Young & Co.)				No formal mechanism	Governor's Task Force on Energy
Minnesota	X		Minnesota Energy Agency	State government offices, universities and suppliers		X	Energy Agency and University of Minnesota				Director of Energy Agency receives reports and advises Governor	Minnesota Energy Agency
Mississippi	X		State Research and Development Center		X (plan)	X	State Research and Development Center				No formal mechanism	Not specified
Missouri	X		Department of Natural Resources	Various state agencies		X	Division of State Planning and University of Missouri				No formal mechanism	Missouri Energy Agency
Montana		X			X	X					No formal mechanism	Montana Energy Advisory Council
Nebraska	X		State Energy Office			X					No formal mechanism	State Energy Office

State		Organization	Disseminated to		Cooperating agency / source		Coordination with other agencies	Energy policy office
Nevada	X	Public Service Commission				X	No formal mechanism	Public Service Commission
New Hampshire	X	Private contractor (MITRE Corp.)	General public	X	New England Regional		No formal mechanism	Not specified
New Jersey	X	Governor's Task Force on Energy	Energy Office and universities			X	State Energy Office link with agencies and Governor	Cabinet Energy Committee
New Mexico	X	Energy Resources Board				X	Energy Resources Board	Energy Resources Board
New York	X	Emergency Fuel Office	State government, utilities and universities	X	Emergency Fuel Office and other institutions in the state		Fuel Office work submitted to Governor's Office and other agencies	Governor's Office and Emergency Fuel Office
North Carolina	X	Department of Military and Veterans Affairs (Energy Division)		X	Energy Division	X	Energy Policy Council	Energy Policy Council
North Dakota	X	Legislative Council				X	Natural Resources Council	Office of the Governor
Ohio	X	Private contractor (Mathematica)		X	Ohio Energy Emergency Commission		No formal mechanism	Formal cooperation among agencies
Oklahoma	X	Governor's Energy Advisory Council	General public	X	Energy Advisory Council	X	Energy Advisory Council	Energy Advisory Council
Oregon	X	Department of Energy	General public	X	Department of Energy	X	Formal mechanism under development	(New) Department of Energy
Pennsylvania	X	Governor's Energy Council		X	Energy Council	X	Council of agency heads, chaired by Lt. Governor	Energy Council
Rhode Island	X	Work with New England Regional Commission		X	New England Regional Commission		No formal mechanism	Not specified
South Carolina	X	Energy Management Office		X	Energy Management Office	X	Energy Office links to Governor and Regional Planning Districts	Energy Management Office
South Dakota	X	Office of Energy Policy		X	University of South Dakota	X	Energy Office inputs to various agencies	Office of Energy Policy
Tennessee	X			X	Energy Policy Office	X	No formal mechanism	Not specified
Texas	X	Houston Energy Institute	General public	X	Governor's Office and universities	X	Governor's Energy Advisory Council and Division of Planning Coordination	Governor's Energy Advisory Council
Utah	X	State Science Administration		X	Department of Natural Resources		No formal mechanism	Not specified
Vermont	X	Work with New England Regional Commission				X	Energy Office link to Governor and Legislature	State Energy Office

Table 3-12, continued

State	Energy Flow or Budget Document[a]			Energy Models[b]			Planning Y N	Institutional Process for Transferring Information to Policy-Makers	Overall Energy Management Coordination
	Available Y N	Institution	Users[c]	Planning Y N	Operational Y N	Institution			
Virginia	X	Virginia Energy Office		X	X		X	No formal mechanism	State Energy Office
Washington	X	University of Washington	General public		X	University of Washington		Formal mechanism under development	Office of the Governor
West Virginia	X			X	X	Appalachian Regional Commission (Resource Planning Associates)		No formal mechanism	Not specified
Wisconsin	X	Office of Emergency Energy Assistance		X	X	University of Wisconsin		Informal distribution of reports, testimony at hearings, and workshops	No overall coordination
Wyoming	X	Department of Economic Planning and Development		X	X	Private contractor		No formal mechanism	Office of the Governor
Puerto Rico	X	Office of Petroleum Fuels Affairs		X	X	Office of Petroleum Fuels Affairs		Technical presentations to Governor, legislature and the public	Office of the Governor

[a]This document is typically a report covering a recent "base year" and highlights energy Btu flows from primary sources through conversion processes by sector to final end-use.
[b]These models are usually computerized operations of varying sophistication regarding data quality and program design. They enable the user to run alternative scenarios for assessing the potential impact of policy options.
[c]Users in most cases include Fuel Allocation Offices.

substances data banks to decide whether legitimate requirements are met or could be met by existing data systems or if now one should be devised to satisfy current or anticipated needs (Bracken, *et al.*, 1977).

Two hundred and sixty data files are compiled in Table 3-13 in eight toxic substances categories. Each system is given a utility score as follows. The first element of the score denotes the importance of the information to toxic substances research and regulation. This importance varies from a high of "1" to a low of "4."

The second element of the score is a measure of the value of the data and is determined by the following criteria:

* the number of records contained in the system;
* the specificity of the information;
* the extent to which the data were evaluated;
* the ease in accessing the data by both system and subject; and
* the breadth of coverage by the information in the data system.

The "value factor" was scored from a high of "a" to a low of "d."

Two additional columns have been included in Table 3-14, which provide supplemental file characteristics. One shows whether the system is manual or automated, while the other indicates the data base ownership. These files are considered to be of primary importance and are designated by an asterisk in Table 3-13.

When selecting files for inclusion in an information system, it is necessary to compare those systems containing data in similar subject areas. Tables 3-14 through 3-21 contain descriptions of the selected data files by subject category. The primary systems designated on Table 3-13 by a "1a" or "1b" in a given data category are included on these category-specific tables. On these tables, the primary systems are scored for the presence of applicable information in a series of subcategories. A column is also included for comments.

In addition, the primary systems were examined to determine: (1) whether data were generated internally or **were** merely compiled from external sources of information; (2) whether they contain proprietary information; and (3) whether they are collected as a result of a mandatory solicitation. This information is included in Table 3-22.

Table 3-13. Data System Scoring (Bracken et al, 1977)

System	Acronym	Owner	I Substance Identification	II Production Aspects	III Marketing	IV Exposure	V Epidemiology	VI Biological Effects	VII Environmental Effects	VIII Standards and Regulations	Computerized (C) or Manual (M)
*Advisory Center on Toxicology		NAS/NRC	1b	—	3c	2b	1a	1a	1a	1a	M
*Aerometric and Emission Reporting System	AEROS	EPA	2b	1b	—	1a	—	—	—	—	C
*Agricultural On-Line Access	AGRICOLA	NAL/USDA	2b	2b	1a	1a	—	—	1a	—	C
Agricultural Research Service		ARS/USDA	—	2c	—	3c	—	—	—	—	C
*Air Pollution Technical Information Center	APTIC	EPA	2b	3b	—	2a	—	—	1a	1a	C
Air Quality Implementation Planning Program		EPA	3c	2b	—	2b	—	—	—	2b	C
American Statistical Index	ASI	Cong. Info. Serv.	2b	—	—	—	—	3c	—	—	C
Animal History Data System		FDA/HEW	3c	—	—	—	1a	—	—	—	M
*Annual Survey of Injuries and Illnesses		BLS/DOL	—	1b	—	—	—	—	—	—	C
APILIT		Amer. Pet. Inst.	3c	2b	2b	—	1a	—	—	—	M
Army Chemical Information and Data System		Army/DOD	2b	—	—	2b	—	—	—	—	C/M
*Astro-4 Drug Information System		FDA/HEW	1a	1b	2a	2c	1b	—	—	2a	C
*Atlas of Cancer Mortality		NCI/NIH/HEW	—	—	—	—	—	—	—	—	M
*Biological Data Storage and Retrieval System	BIO-STORET	EPA	2b	—	—	2a	1a	3c	1a	—	C
*Biological Sciences Information Service	BIOSIS	Biosciences Info. Servs.	2b	—	—	2a	1a	1a	1a	—	C
*Biomedical Studies Group		EPA	2b	1a	1a	1a	1a	1a	1a	—	M
Bird Toxicity & Repellency Data Base		FWS/DOI	2b	—	3c	—	3c	3c	—	—	C
Boston Collaborative Drug Surveillance Program		Boston Univ.	3c	—	—	2a	—	2b	—	—	C
Cancer Information On-Line	CANCERLINE	NCI/NIH/HEW	2a	2b	—	1a	1a	1a	—	—	C
CANCERLIT		NCI/NIH/HEW	2b	—	—	—	—	2b	—	—	C
Cancer Projects	CANCERPROJ	NIC/NIH/HEW	2b	—	—	—	—	1a	—	—	C
Carbon-13 Nuclear Magnetic Reasonance Spectral Search System	CNMR	NIH/EPA	1a	—	—	—	—	—	—	—	C

Data Base	Acronym	Source								
Carcinogen Use Registry		NIH/HEW	2b							C
*Carcinogenesis Bioassay Data System	CBDS	NCI/NIH/HEW	1a				1a			C
Catalog of Information on Water Data		USGS/DOI	3c			2c		2c		M
*Census Bureau Foreign Trade Statistics		Census/DOC	2b	1a						M
*Census of Manufacturers		Census/DOC	2b	1a						C
CG-388 Chemical Data Guide for Bulk Shipment by Water		USCG/DOT	2c			3c				M
Chemical Abstracts Condensates	CA-CON	Amer. Chem. Soc.	2b	2b			3c			C
*Chemical Abstracts Service Chemical Registry System		Amer. Chem. Soc.	1a							M
*Chemical Abstracts Service Information System		Amer. Chem. Soc.	1a	2a	2b				3b	C
Chemical-Biological Data Base for Herbicidal Information		Army/DOD	2a	2b			3c	2b		C
Chemical Data Center		Chem. Data Ctr.	1b	2b			3c			C
*Chemical Dictionary of the U.S. ITC		U.S. ITC	1b	1a	2b				1b	C
*Chemical Dictionary On-Line	CHEMLINE	NLM/NTH/HEW	1a							C
*Chemical Economics Handbook		SRI	2b	1a	1a					M
Chemical Hazard Response Information System	CHRIS	USCG/DOT	2b			3c	3c			C/M
Chemical Industry Notes	CIN	Predicasts/ Chem. Abs. Serv.	—		1a	3c				C
*Chemical Information & Data System	CIDS	Army/DOD	1a		1a					C
*Chemical Information System		NIH/EPA	1a			2b				C
*Chemical Monograph Referral Center	CHEMRIC	CPSC	1b				1c			C
*Chemical Names File		NCI/NIH/HEW	1b			2b	4c			C
Chemical Toxicological Data Retrieval System		FWS/DOI	4d				2b			M
*Chemical Transportation Emergency Center	CHEMTREC	Mfg. Chem. Assoc.	1b				2b	2b		C
Chemistry Data System		FDA/HEW	3c			2c				C
Chick Embryo System		FDA/HEW	3c				3b			C
*Clinical Toxicology of Commercial Products	CTCP	Univ. of Rochester	2b	2c			1b			C
Clintox Literature System		CDC/HEW	2c				2c	2c		C
Combination Chemotherapy Master File		NCI/NIH/HEW	3c				3c			C
Compendium of Toxicology		AFIP/DOD	2b	2a			2b			C
Compliance Data System		EPA	3c	3c		2c			2a	C
*Component Information for Chemical Consumer Products		CPSC	1a			3c	3b			C

Table 3-13, continued

System	Acronym	Owner	I Substance Identification	II Production Aspects	III Marketing	IV Exposure	V Epidemiology	VI Biological Effects	VII Environmental Effects	VIII Standards and Regulations	Computerized (C) or Manual (M)
Computerized Engineering Index	COMPENDEX	Eng. Index, Inc.		3b							C
Comprehensive Dissertation Index	CDI	Univ. Microfilm International	2b			2b	2b	2b	2b		C
Conformational Analysis of Molecules in Solution	CAMSEQ	NIH/EPA	1c								C
*Congressional Information Service Index	CIS Index	Cong. Info. Serv. Inc.								1a	C
*Congressional Record Abstracts	CRECORD	Capitol Services			2c					1a	C
Cosmetics Information System		FDA/HEW	2b	2c				2b		3b	C
Cosmetics, Toiletry and Fragrance Assoc. Ingredient Dictionary		CFTA	2a								M
*CPSC Chemical Abstracts		CPSC	1a	2c	2b			2b			C
*Current Employment Statistics		BLS/DOL		1b		1a					M
Current Energy Research Information Retrieval System	CERIRS	ANL/ERDA		1a						1b	C
*Data Base of U.S. International Trade Commission		US ITC	2b		1a				2a	2b	C
Data Bases for Energy Systems		ILL/ERDA	2a	2b	3c	2a	2a	2a	2a	2b	C
Data Extraction & Analysis		ORNL/NLM		2c	2a						C
*Defense Documentation Center	DDC	DLA/DOD	1a	1a					1b		C
Diagnostics Subsystem		FDA/HEW	3c								C
*Directory of Chemical Producers	DCP	SRI	2b			2c		3c			M
*Distribution Register of Organic Pollutants in Water		EPA	2c				2a	2a	1a		M
Document Reference System	WATERDROP	NCI/NIH/HEW	2b			2b	2a	2a		2b	C

Database	Acronym	Source									Type
Drug Distribution & Inventory System		NCI/NIH/HEW	2b	—	2a	2b	—	2b	2a	2b	C
Drug Efficacy Study Implementation		FDA/HEW	2b	—	—	2c	—	2c	—	—	C
Drug Experience Information System		FDA/HEW	2b	2b	—	2c	—	2b	—	—	C
Drug Experience Reports		FDA/HEW	3b	2b	—	3c	—	3c	—	—	C
*Drug Registration & Listing System		FDA/HEW	1a	—	—	—	—	1a	—	—	C
Drug Research & Development Biological Data		NCI/NIH/HEW	2b	—	—	3c	—	2b	3c	—	C
Drug Research & Development Chemical Information Bibliography File		NCI/NIH/HEW	2b	—	—	—	—	2b	—	—	C
*Drug Research & Developmental Chemical Information System		NCI/NIH/HEW	—	—	—	—	—	—	—	—	C
*Dun's Market Identifiers	DMI	Dun & Bradstreet	1a	—	2b	—	1b	1a	—	—	C
Effluent Data System	EDS	EPA	3c	1b	2b	2b	2b	3c	—	—	C
EIS Industrial Plants		Predicasts	2c	3c	1a	—	—	2c	—	—	C
Emissions Data System	EDS	EPA	3c	2b	2b	2b	2b	3c	2b	3c	C
Energy Data System		EPA	3d	—	3c	—	1a	—	—	—	C
Energy Information		ERDA	2a	—	—	—	2a	—	—	—	C
Energy Line		Env. Info. Ctr.	—	2b	—	2b	—	2b	—	—	C
Energy Research and Development Inventory		ORNL/ERDA	—	—	—	—	—	2c	—	—	C
Environmental Contaminant Evaluation Program		FWS/DOI	3b	—	2b	—	2c	—	1b	—	M
*Environmental Contaminant Monitoring Program		FWS/DOI	3b	—	2b	—	2c	—	—	—	M
Environmental Data Index	ENDEX	NOAA/DOC	2b	—	1a	—	1a	—	1a	—	C
Environmental Data System	EDS	NOAA/DOC	2b	—	2b	—	2b	—	2a	—	C
Environmental Information System	EIS	Swedish CEI	3b	2b	2b	2b	2b	2b	2b	—	C
*Environmental Mutagen Information Center	EMIC	NIEHS/NIH/HEW	1b	—	—	—	1a	1a	—	—	C
Environmental Pollution Effects on Aquatic Resources		NOAA/DOC	—	—	—	—	—	—	2a	2a	M
*Environmental Reports Summaries		EPA	2c	—	—	—	—	—	—	1b	C
Environmental Residual Information System		EPA	3c	2b	—	—	—	—	—	—	C
Environmental Resource Center		ORNL/ERDA	—	4c	2b	—	3b	3b	2b	—	C
Environmental Science Information Center	ESIC	NOAA/DOC	3b	—	2a	—	3c	3c	2b	—	C
*Environmental Teratology Information Center	ETIC	NIEHS/NIH/HEW	1c	—	—	—	1b	1a	1a	—	C
EPA Reports System		NTIS/DOC	2b	2a	1c	1a	2b	1a	1a	1a	C
Epidemiological Studies Program System		EPA	3c	—	—	2b	—	—	—	—	C
Establishment/Product Licensing System		FDA/HEW	2b	2b	—	—	—	3c	—	3b	C

Table 3-13, continued

System	Acronym	Owner	I Substance Identification	II Production Aspects	III Marketing	IV Exposure	V Epidemiology	VI Biological Effects	VII Environmental Effects	VIII Standards and Regulations	Computerized (C) or Manual (M)
Establishment Registration Support System	ERSS	EPA	2c	2a	–	–	–	3b	–	–	C
Excerpta Medica		Information Sys.	2b	–	–	2c	2c	2a	–	–	M
*Exposure Dictionary for National Occupational Hazards Survey	EDNOHS	NIOSH/HEW	1a	–	–	–	–	–	–	–	C
*Federal Inventory on Environmental and Safety Research		ERDA	2c	–	–	2b	2b	2a	1b	–	C
*Fish Control Laboratory–Data Base Information		FWS/DOI	2b	–	2c	–	–	2b	1a	–	M
*Fish-Pesticide Research		FWS/DOI	2b	–	–	2c	–	1b	1a	–	C
Food Information Storage and Retrieval		FDA/HEW	2b	–	–	–	–	2b	–	–	C
Foreign Trade of Member Countries of the OECD Data Base		ERS/DOC	3b	2b	2b	3b	3b	2b	3c	2b	M
Fuel Additive Registration		EPA	2b	2b	2c	–	–	2b	–	–	C
Funk & Scott (F&S) Indexes		Predicasts	3c	1b	1a	–	–	–	2b	–	C
Geophysical Monitoring for Climate Change		NOAA/DOC	–	–	–	–	–	–	2b	–	C
Graphical Interactive NMR Analysis Program		NIH/EPA	3c	–	–	–	–	2b	2a	–	C
Great Lakes Fishery Information		EPA	3c	–	–	1b	–	2b	2a	–	C
Hazardous and Trace Emissions System	HATREMS	EPA	2b	–	–	2b	2a	3c	–	1b	M
*Health Hazard Evaluations		PHS/CDC/HEW	4d	2a	2a	2c	–	2b	2b	–	M
Heavy Metals		TVA	3c	–	–	–	–	–	–	–	C
*Index Chemicals Registry System	ICRS	ISI	1a	–	–	1c	2b	3b	–	2a	C
Industrial Hygiene Automated Data System		TVA	2b	2b	3c	1b	1b	3b	–	2b	M
*Industrywide Studies		NIOSH/CDC/HEW	3b	3a	3a	–	–	–	–	–	M
*Information Bulletin of the Survey of Chemicals Being Tested for Carcinogenicity		WHO	1b	–	–	–	–	1b	–	–	M

Database	Abbrev.	Source										
Information Center for Energy Safety		ORNL/ERDA	2c	—	—	—	—	1b	—	—	2b	C
*Information Storage and Referral Section		NIEHS/NIH/HEW	—	1a	2b	2b	2b	—	1a	—	—	C
*Inorganic Chemical Computer Toxicology Parameter Data Base		EPA	3b	—	—	—	1b	—	1b	1a	—	C
INSPEC Science Abstracts		Inst. of Elec. Engineers, U.K.	2b	2b	—	—	—	—	—	—	—	C
*International Cancer Epidemiology Clearinghouse		ICRDB/IARC/CCR	2b	—	—	1a	—	1b	1b	—	—	C
International Classification of Diseases for Oncology	ICD-O	WHO	—	—	—	—	—	—	2b	2b	—	M
International Registry of Potentially Toxic Substances		UNEP	—	—	—	—	—	—	—	—	—	C
Investigational New Animal Drug Index		FDA/HEW	2b	2b	3c	2b	—	—	—	—	2b	C
Iowa Drug Information Service	IDIS	Univ. of Iowa	2b	—	—	—	—	—	2b	—	—	M
*IPC Chemical Data Base		IPC Industrial Press, U.K.	2b	1b	1a	—	—	—	—	—	—	C
Isotopic Label Incorporation Determination		NIH/EPA	3c	—	—	—	—	—	—	—	—	C
*Kirk-Othmer Encyclopedia of Chemical Technology		Interscience Publishers	2b	1a	1b	—	—	—	—	—	—	M
Laboratory Analysis Data Base		CPSC	2c	—	—	—	—	—	2b	2b	2b	C
*Laboratory Animal Data Base	LADB	NIH/HEW	2c	—	—	—	—	—	1a	1a	1b	C
Laboratory Management System		EPA	3c	—	3c	—	—	—	—	—	—	C
*Mammal Toxicity and Repellency Data Base		FWS/DOI	2c	—	3c	—	—	—	1b	1b	—	C
Marine Ecosystem Analysis Program	MESA	NOAA/DOC	2b	—	—	2b	—	—	1a	1a	1a	C
Mass Spectrometry Data Centre		Atomic Weapons Research Estab., U.K.	1a	—	—	—	—	—	—	—	—	C
Mass Spectrometry Bulletin Search		NIH/EPA	2a	—	—	—	—	—	—	—	—	C
Mass Spectral Identification		NIH/EPA	—	—	—	—	—	—	—	—	—	C
Mass Spectral Search System		NIH/EPA	1a	—	—	—	—	—	—	—	—	C
*Meat & Poultry Inspection Monitoring Program		APHIS/USDA	2b	1b	—	—	—	—	—	—	2b	M
*Medical Literature Analysis and Retrieval System On-Line	MEDLINE	NLM/NIH/HEW	2a	—	—	1a	1a	—	1a	—	—	C
Medical Subject Headings Vocabulary	MESH	NLM/NIH/HEW	1c	—	—	—	—	—	—	—	—	C
*Microconstituents in Fish and Fishery Products		NOAA/DOC	3c	2b	—	—	2b	—	—	3b	1a	C
*Military Entomology Information Service	MEIS	Army/DOD	2b	2a	—	—	2a	1a	1a	1a	—	C

Table 3-13, continued

System	Acronym	Owner	I Substance Identification	II Production Aspects	III Marketing	IV Exposure	V Epidemiology	VI Biological Effects	VII Environmental Effects	VIII Standards and Regulations	Computerized (C) or Manual (M)
*Mineral Commodity Survey System		BOM/DOI	1b	1b	1b	–	–	–	–	–	C
Multilateral Trade Negotiations Data Base	MTNDB	DOC	2c	1b	1b	–	–	–	–	–	C
*NASA Scientific and Technical Information System		NASA	1b	–	–	2b	–	2b	2b	–	C
National Air Surveillence Network	NASN	EPA	2b	–	–	1b	–	–	–	–	C
National Cancer Institute (NCI) Carcinogenesis Program File		NCI/NIH/HEW	3c	–	–	3c	–	2b	3c	–	C
*National Center for Health Statistics	NCHS	HEW	–	–	–	–	1a	–	–	–	C
*National Center for Toxicological Research (NCTR) Integrated Research Support System		FDA/NCTR	3c	–	–	–	–	1b	–	–	C
National Clearinghouse for Mental Health Information		NIMI/NIH/HEW	2b	–	–	–	–	2c	–	–	C
*National Electronic Injury Surveillance System	NEISS	CPSC	2b	–	–	1a	1a	–	–	2b	C
National Emissions Data	NEDS	EPA	2b	1b	2b	2a	–	–	–	–	C
National Fire Data Center		DOC	3c	–	–	–	–	3c	–	–	M
National Index of Energy and Environmental Related Data		ERDA	3d	–	–	3c	–	2b	3b	–	C
National Index of Energy and Environmental Related Models		ERDA	4d	–	–	3b	3b	3b	3b	–	C
*National Occupational Hazard Survey File	NOHS	NIOSH/CDC/HEW	2b	2b	1a	1a	–	–	–	–	C
National Park Service (NPS) Pest Control System		NPS/DOI	3c	3c	3b	4d	–	–	3c	–	C
National Pollutant Discharge Elimination System	NPDES	EPA	3c	2b	–	3c	–	–	–	2b	C
National Referral Center		Library of Cong.	3b	–	–	–	–	–	–	–	C

Database	Acronym	Agency										M/C
*National Technical Information Service	NTIS	DOC	2b	2a	1a	1a	1a	1a	1a	1a	1a	M
National Water Data Systems	NWDS	USGS/DOI	3c	–	2b	–	–	2c	–	2c	–	M
Navy Environmental Protection Support Services		Navy/DOD	2b	3c	–	2b	2b	–	2b	1b	–	C
Nevada Applied Ecology Information Center		ERDA	2b	2b	–	2a	–	–	–	–	–	C
New Animal Drug Applications		FDA/HEW	2b	3c	3c	2b	3c	3c	3c	2c	2b	C
New York Times Information Bank		New York Times	3c	3c	3c	3c	3c	1a	1a	4d	–	C
*NIOSH Technical Information Center	NIOSHTIC	NIOSH/HEW	3c	2b	3c	1a	2c	–	–	3c	2b	C
Occupational Safety and Health		OSHA/DOL	3c	2c	2b	2c	2b	2b	2c	1a	–	C
*Oceanic Abstracts		Data Courier, Inc.	2b	–	–	–	–	–	–	–	–	C
*Oceanic and Atmospheric Scientific Information Service	OASIS	NOAA/DOC	2c	–	2b	2b	2b	–	1b	1b	1b	C
*Office of Standard Reference Data Chemical Files		NBS/DOC	1b	4d	–	–	–	–	–	–	–	C
*Oil & Hazardous Materials Technical Data System	OHM-TADS	EPA	2a	2b	2b	2b	–	1b	1b	2a	1b	C
*Organic Chemical Producers Data Base		EPA	2c	1a	2c	2c	–	1b	1b	–	1b	C
PaperChem	Kwik Index	Inst. of Paper Chemistry	3c	2b	2b	–	–	–	–	–	–	C
Parklawn Health Library		PHS/HEW	3c	–	–	–	2b	2b	2b	–	2b	C
Pathology Data System		FDA/HEW	3c	–	–	2c	2c	2c	2c	–	2c	C
Permit Compliance System (Water)		EPA	3c	3c	2b	–	–	–	–	–	–	C
P/E News		Amer. Pet. Inst.	3c	2b	–	2c	2b	2b	2b	–	2b	M
*Pesticide and Industrial Chemicals		FDA/HEW	1b	–	2b	–	–	3c	3c	1b	3c	C
Pesticide Enforcement Management System	PEMS	EPA	2b	2b	–	–	2b	–	–	2b	–	C
Pesticide Import File Region X		EPA	2b	2b	2c	3b	2c	–	–	–	1b	C
Pesticide Registration Systems	now PARCS	EPA	2b	2c	–	–	2c	–	–	1a	2b	C
*Pesticide Reporting System		FDA/HEW	2d	2c	3c	2b	3c	–	–	2b	–	C
Pesticide Sampling Information System - Region X		EPA	2c	2c	2c	2b	2c	–	–	–	1a	C
*Pesticides Analysis Retrieval and Control System	PARCS	OPM/EPA	1a	1a	1b	1b	2b	–	–	2a	2b	C
Pharmaceutical News Index	PNI	Data Courier, Inc.	–	2b	2b	2b	–	–	–	2b	–	C
Pilot Data Base for Hazardous Substances		CPSC	2c	–	–	–	–	2b	2b	–	2a	C
*POISINDEX		Micromedex	1b	–	–	2c	–	1b	1b	–	2b	M
Poison Control Centres of Canada		Consumer & Corp. Affairs, Canadian Govt.	2a	–	3c	2a	–	2a	2a	–	–	C/M

Table 3-13, continued

System	Acronym	Owner	I Substance Identification	II Production Aspects	III Marketing	IV Exposure	V Epidemiology	VI Biological Effects	VII Environmental Effects	VIII Standards and Regulations	Computerized (C) or Manual (M)
*Poison Control On-Line Inquiry System		FDA/HEW	1b				1a	1b			C
*Pollution		Data Courier Inc.				2b			1a		C
*Population Studies System		EPA	2c			1a	1a	1b			C
Predicasts Domestic Statistics		Predicasts	3c	2b	1a						C
Predicasts Federal Index		Predicasts								2b	C
Predicasts International Statistics		Predicasts	3c	2b	1a						C
Predicasts Market Abstracts		Predicasts	3c	2a	1a						C
*Predicasts Marketing Systems		Predicasts		2a	2b					2b	C
Product Safety Indexed Document Collection		CPSC	2a	3b							C
Program for Toxicology of Combustion Products		NBS/DOC		2b		3b	3b	3b	2a		C
Proton Affinity Retrieval		NIH/EPA	1b					2c			C
Psychological Abstracts		Am. Psychological Assn.						3d			C
*Registry of Toxic Effects of Chemical Substances	RTECS	CDC/HEW	1a					1a			C
*Reporting of Economic Data for Negotiation of International Transportation Conventions	REDNITRAC	DOC	2b	1a	1a	4d			2b	1a	M
Research Materials Information Center		ORNL/ERDA	2a	1a	1a						C
*Research Program of Chemicals that Impact Man		NCI/NIH/HEW	1a			1b	1a	1a	1a		M
Retirement History Study		OPP/HEW				2c	2b	2c			C

Database	Acronym	Source									C/M
RINGDOC		Derwent Publ.	2b	—	—	—	—	2b	—	—	C
Science & Technical Division		Lib. of Cong.	2c	—	—	—	—	—	—	2b	C
Science Citation Search	SCISEARCH	ISI	2b	—	—	2b	2c	1b	—	—	C
Scientific Manuscript Bibliographic System		FDA/HEW	3c	—	—	4d	—	4d	2b	—	C
Scientific Reference Services Branch		CDC/HEW	4c	—	1b	—	—	2b	—	—	M
Selective Dissemination of Information On-Line	SDILINE	NLM/NIH/HEW	2b	—	—	—	1b	1b	1a	—	C
Single Drug Master File		NCI/NIH/HEW	3c	—	—	—	—	3b	1b	—	C
*Smithsonian Scientific Information Exchange	SSIE	SSIE	2b	—	—	1a	—	2b	—	—	M
*Solid Waste Information Retrieval System	SWIRS	EPA	2b	—	—	—	—	—	—	—	C
Special Reports—Grant-Supported Literature Index	GENIUS	NCI/NIH/HEW	2b	—	—	—	2a	2a	—	—	C
*Special Trade Representatives Centralized Data Bank	STRCDB	Off. of Spec. Representative for Trade Neg.	2b	1a	1b	—	—	—	—	—	C
*Standards Completion Program		NIOSH/CDC/HEW	4d	—	—	1b	1b	4d	—	1b	C
State Implementation Plans	SIPS	EPA	3c	—	—	2c	—	—	—	—	C
Statistical Center for the Tyler Texas Asbestos		NCI/NIH/HEW	4d	—	—	4d	4d	4d	2c	—	C
Strategic Environmental Assessment System	SEAS	EPA	4d	—	—	—	—	—	—	—	C
*Storage and Retrieval for Water Quality Data	STORET	EPA	2b	—	—	1a	—	—	—	2b	C
Storage and Retrieval of Aerometric Data	SAROAD	EPA	2b	—	—	2a	—	—	—	—	C
*Subject Content-Oriented Retriever for Processing Information On-Line	SCORPIO	Lib. of Cong.	2c	—	—	—	—	—	—	2b	C
Substructure Searching System		NIH/EPA	1b	—	—	1b	—	1a	—	—	C
*Supplementary Data System		BLS/DOL	2b	—	—	—	1a	1b	—	—	C
*Survey of Compounds which have been tested for Carcinogenic Activity		NCI/PHS/HEW	2b	—	—	—	—	—	—	—	M
*Technical Data Center	TDC	OSHA/DOL	1b	—	—	1a	1a	1a	—	1b	M
Technical Files		TVA	2b	3c	3c	2b	2a	2a	—	2b	M
Technical Library—TVA		TVA	—	3c	—	—	—	—	3c	—	M
Technical Library Information Office		Army/DOD	—	—	—	—	—	—	—	—	M
The Environment Information Retrieval System	TEIRS	Purdue Univ.	2b	—	—	—	—	—	—	—	M
*Thermophysical Properties Research Center		Purdue Univ.	1a	—	—	—	—	—	—	—	M
Toxic Materials Information Center		ERDA/NSF	2b	2b	3c	2a	2a	2a	2a	—	C

Table 13-13, continued

System	Acronym	Owner	I Substance Identification	II Production Aspects	III Marketing	IV Exposure	V Epidemiology	VI Biological Effects	VII Environmental Effects	VIII Standards and Regulations	Computerized (C) or Manual (M)
Toxicological Studies		NIOSH/CDC/HEW	2a	2c	2b	2b	–	2a	–	2b	M
*Toxicology Data Bank	TDB	NLM/NIH/HEW	1a	1a	2a	2a	1a	1a	2a	–	C
*Toxicology Information On-Line	TOXLINE	NLM/NIH/HEW	2b	2b	2b	1a	1a	1a	1a	–	C
Toxicology Information Response Center	TIRC	ERDA	2b	–	–	2b	2b	2b	2b	–	C
Toxicology Research Projects Directory		NLM/NIH/HEW	2b	–	–	1a	1a	1a	1a	–	M
*Toxicology Testing in Progress	TOX-TIPS	NLM/NIH/HEW	2a	2b	2b	2a	2a	1a	2b	–	C
TOXLINE Backfile	TOXBACK	NLM/NIH/HEW	2b	2c	2b	1a	1b	1a	1a	–	C
*Tradename Ingredient Clarification	TNIC	CDC/HEW	1a	–	–	1	–	–	–	–	C
USDA–ERS Use of Pesticides		ERS/USDA	3c	2c	2b	3c	–	2a	–	–	M
VIOLOG		EPA	3c	–	–	3c	–	–	2b	2b	C
Walter Reed Army Institute of Research, Biological Data System	WRAIR	Army/DOD	2b	–	–	–	–	2a	–	–	
Walter Reed Army Institute of Research, Chemical Inventory System	WRAIR	Army/DOD	2b	–	–	–	–	–	–	–	
Walter Reed Army Institute of Research, Chemical Structure System	WRAIR	Army/DOD	2a	–	–	–	–	–	–	–	
Walter Reed Army Institute of Research, Index File	WRAIR	Army/DOD	2a	–	–	–	–	–	–	–	
Water Quality Data Base		TVA	2b	–	–	2b	–	–	–	–	
Water Resources Scientific Information Center	WRSIC	DOI	2b	–	–	2a	–	2b	2b	2a	
Water Storage Data and Retrieval System	WATSTORE	USGS/DOI	2b	–	–	2b	–	–	–	–	
X-Ray Crystal Data Retrieval System		NIH/EPA	1a	–	–	–	–	–	–	–	
X-Ray Crystal Structure Retrieval System		NIH/EPA	1a	–	–	–	–	–	–	–	
X-Ray Powder Diffraction Retrieval System		NIH/EPA	1a	–	–	–	–	–	–	–	

Table 3-14. Data Systems Applicable to Substance Identification

System	Cas #	Nomenclature	Structure	Chemical/Physical Properties	Composition (Including Impurities)	Chemical Analysis a	Bibliographic (Totally)	Comments
Advisory Center on Toxicology	X	X		X	X		X	Manual card file
Astro-4 Drug Information System	X	X	b	X	X			Drug production and registration information
Carcinogenisis Bioassay Data System	X	X	b	X	X			Lab experiment data
Chemical Abstracts Service Chemical Registry System	X	X	X					
Chemical Abstracts Service Information System		X	X	X			X	
Chemical Dictionary of the U.S. ITC	X	X	b				X	Tariff information
Chemical Dictionary On-Line	X	X	X					
Chemical Information & Data System	X	X	b					CIDs registration system
Chemical Information System	X	X	c	X				Also X-ray CNMRs and Mass spec.
Chemical Monograph Referral Center		X		X				Referral system to monographs with these data
Chemical Names File	X	X	b					Compounds tested for carcinogenicity
Chemical Transportation Emergency Center		X		X				File used in case of accidental spill
Component Information for Chemical Consumer Products	X	X			X			Formulation of 15,000 products to 0.1% level
CPSC Chemical Abstracts	X	X						3,487 consumer products

Table 3-14, continued

System	Cas #	Nomenclature	Structure	Chemical/Physical Properties	Composition (Including Impurities)	Chemical Analysis	Bibliographic (Totally)	Comments
Defense Documentation Center	X	X		X	X		X	
Drug Registration and Listing System	X	X		X	X		X	
Drug Research & Development Chemical Information System	X	X	c	X				
Environmental Mutagen Information Center	X	X	b				X	May be expanded for data sources of mutagen information
Exposure Dictionary for NOHS	X	X						
Index Chemicals Registry System		X	b		X			12,000 chemical names
Information Bulletin of the Survey of Chemicals Being Tested for Carcinogenicity		X						
IPC Chemical Data Base		X						Imports/exports
Mineral Commodity Survey System		X			X			Survey of mineral industry
NASA Scientific and Technical Information Center		X		X			X	Environmental information
Office of Standard Reference Data Chemical Files		X		X				
Pesticides and Industrial Chemicals	X	X			X	X		Pesticide chemistry
Pesticides Analysis Retrieval and Control System		X			X			New system, use and formulation
Poison Control On-Line Inquiry System		X			X			Contains 10,000 household products and drugs

						Notes
POISINDEX						Contains 160,000 entries
Registry of Toxic Effects of Chemical Substances	X	X	b		X		Basic toxicology of 22,000 chemicals
Research Program of Chemicals that Impact Man	X	X			X		(1,500 chemicals by SRI)
Technical Data Center	X	X			X	X	Documentation on occupational safety and health
Thermophysical Properties Research Center			X	X			
Toxicology Data Bank	X	X	b		X	X	New system, on-line access to toxicology data
Trade Name Ingredient Clarification			X		X		

aNot on original questionnaire.
bWiswesser line notation.
cSubstructure searching.

Table 3-15. Data Systems Applicable to Production

	Manufacturer[a]	Production Quality	Plant Location	Production Process	By-products/ Impurities	Control Technology	
Aerometric and Emission Reporting System	X	X	X	X			NEDS
Annual Survey of Injuries	X	X	X				All establishments > 111 employees by SIC code
Astro-4 Drug Information System	X	X	X	X			Drug producers and amounts
Biomedical Studies Group	X	X	X	X	X	X	For 14 compounds
Census Bureau Foreign Trade Statistics		X	X				Imports/exports
Census of Manufacturers	X	X	X				By SIC code
Chemical Economics Handbook	X	X					
Data Base of the U.S. International Trade Commission	X	X					Manufacturers and Importers in summary form
Directory of Chemical Producers	X	X	X				Manual
Employment and Earnings	X	X					Size of work force
IPC Chemical Data Base	X	X	X				Imports/exports on 100 chemicals
Kirk-Othmer Encyclopedia of Chemical Technology	X	X	X	X	X	X	Manual
Mineral Commodity Survey System		X	X				200 mineral industries
Multilateral Trade Negotiations Data Base		X					Imports/exports
Organic Chemical Producers Data Base	X	X	X	X	X	X	400 chemicals
Pesticides Analysis Retrieval and Control System	X	X					Formulation information by producer
Predicasts Marketing Systems	X	X	X	X	X	X	F & S, EIS of Predicast
Reporting of Economic Data for Negotiation of International Transportation Conventions							Import/export
Research Program of Chemicals that Impact Man	X	X	X		X		On 1,500 chemicals SRI
Special Tarde Representatives Centralized Data Bank		X	X				Imports/exports
Toxicology Data Bank	X	X		X			1,000 chemicals (new system)
Inorganic Chemical Computer Toxicology Parameter Data Base			X	X	X	X	172 inorganics (new system)

[a]Not on original questionnaire.

Table 3-16. Data Systems Applicable to Marketing

System	Usage	Users	Substitutes	Economics	Place of Use	Bibliographic Only	Comments
Agricultural On-Line Access	X	X		X		X	Agricultural chemicals
Biomedical Studies Group	X	X	X	X	X		On 14 chemicals
Chemical Economics Handbook	X			X			Manual
Data Base of U.S. International Trade Commission	X			X			8,000 chemicals—some manufacturers, some imports
Dun's Market Identifiers				X			
IPC Chemical Data Base				X			Import/export on 100 chemicals
Kirk-Othmer Encyclopedia of Chemical Technology	X		X				
Mineral Commodity Survey System	X	X	X	X			Survey of 200 industries
National Occupational Hazard Survey	X				X		Workplace uses
National Technical Information Service	X	X	X	X	X	X	Government reports
Pesticide Analysis Retrieval and Control System	X		X				Pesticides
Predicasts Marketing Systems	X	X	X	X	X	X	All systems
Reporting of Economic Data for Negotiation of International Transportation Conventions				X			
Research Program of Chemicals that Impact Man	X	X	X	X	X		SRI file on 1,500 chemicals
Special Trade Representatives Centralized Data Bank				X			Import/export

Table 3-17. Data Systems Applicable to Exposure

System	Occupational	Consumer	Environmental	Monitoring[a]	Bibliographic Only	Air	Water	Comments
Aerometric and Emission Reporting System	X		X	X		X		Includes NEDS, SAROAD, HATREMS, EDS, 1
Agricultural On-Line Access		X	X			X	X	
Biomedical Studies Group	X	X	X		X	X	X	
Cancer Information On-Line	X		X		X	X	X	14 chemicals only
Current Employment Statistics	X							
Dun's Market Identifiers	X							
Industrywide Studies	X							100 occupational studies
Meat and Poultry Inspection Monitoring Program		X		X				Levels of pesticides, drugs, metals and residues
National Electronic Injury Surveillance System		X	X	X				Emergency room injuries associated with consumer products
National Occupational Hazard Survey	X			X				
National Technical Information Service	X	X	X	X	X	X	X	Government reports
Oceanic and Atmospheric Scientific Information Service			X	X		X	X	ENDEX
Population Studies Program				X				
Research Program of Chemicals that Impact Man	X	X	X			X	X	1,500 chemicals - SRI file
Smithsonian Scientific Information Exchange	X	X	X	X	X	X	X	Research in progress
Standards Completion Program	X		X					
Storage and Retrieval for Water Quality Data			X	X			X	400 chemicals - includes WATSTORE, ECMS, NPDES, LAM
Supplementary Data Center	X							
Technical Data Center	X				X			
Toxicology Information On-Line	X				X	X	X	5,000 chemicals Including TOXBACK

[a]Not included on original questionnaire.

Table 3-18. Data Systems Applicable to Epidemiology

System	Occupational	General	Bibliographic Only	Comments
Advisory Center on Toxicology	X	X		Manual (minimal added data)
Annual Survey of Injuries and Illnesses	X			BLS biannual survey
Atlas of Cancer Mortality		X		
Biomedical Studies Group	X	X		14 chemicals
Biological Sciences Information Service	X	X	X	
Cancer Information On-Line	X	X	X	
Industrywide Studies	X			100 studies performed by NIOSH
Information Storage and Referral Section	X		X	New system
International Cancer Epidemiology Clearinghouse	X	X		
Medical Literature Analysis and Retrieval System On-Line	X	X	X	Includes SOILINE
Military Entomology Information Service	X	X	X	
National Center for Health Statistics		X		Baseline information
National Electronic Injury Surveillance System		X		Consumer epidemiology
National Occupational Hazard Survey File	X			Plant profiles
National Technical Information Service	X	X	X	Government reports
NIOSH Technical Information Center	X	X	X	8,000 chemicals
Poison Control On-Line Inquiry System		X		Procuring incidence reports
Population Studies System	X			CHESS
Research Program of Chemicals that Impact Man	X	X		SRI
Standards Completion Program	X			Surveillance re. 400 chemicals with standards
Supplementary Data System	X			State Unemployment Insurance Records
Technical Data Center	X	X	X	OSHA data bank
Toxicology Data Bank	X	X	X	New system—now covers 1,000 chemicals and drugs
Toxicology Information On-Line	X	X	X	Including TOXBACK

Table 3-19. Data Systems Applicable to Biological Effects

System	Clinical Studies	Acute Toxicology	Carcinogenicity	Mutagenicity	Teratogenicity	Metabolism	Testing Methodology	Bibliographic Only	Comments
Advisory Center on Toxicology	X	X		X	X	X			Manual card index
Biomedical Studies Group	X	X	X	X	X	X			14 chemicals
Biological Sciences Information Service	X	X	X	X	X	X		X	
Cancer Information On-Line	X	X	X	X	X	X	X	X	Cancer proj.
Carcinogenesis Bioassay Data System	X	X	X			X	X		
Clinical Toxicology of Commercial Products	X	X							20,000 trade names with toxicity
Environmental Mutagen Information Center			X	X				X	
Environmental Teratology Information Center					X			X	
Fish Pesticide Research		X					X		
Information Bulletin of the Survey of Chemicals Being Tested for Carcinogenicity			X				X		
Information Storage and Referral Section	X		X	X	X	X		X	New system
International Cancer Epidemiology Clearinghouse			X			X			
Laboratory Animal Data Base		X	X				X		50,000 animals
Mammal Toxicity and Repellency Data Base		X	X						
Medical Literature Analysis and Retrieval System On-Line	X	X	X	X	X	X		X	
Inorganic Chemical Computer Toxicology Parameter Data Base		X							172 inorganics

Data Base									Notes
Military Entomology Information Service	X			X	X	X		X	
National Technical Information Service	X			X	X	X	X	X	Govt. reports
National Center for Toxicology Experiment Integrated Research Support System			X	X					
NIOSH Technical Information Center	X	X	X	X	X	X	X	X	MESA sub
Oceanic and Atmospheric Scientific Information Service			X	X	X	X			
Oil and Hazardous Materials			X	X	X	X			
Organic Chemical Producers Data Base			X	X	X				400 chemicals
POISINDEX			X	X					
Poison Control On-Line Inquiry System	X		X	X					10,000 products
Population Studies Program			X	X	X				
Registry of Toxic Effects of Chemical Substances	X		X	X	X	X		X	
Research Program of Chemicals that Impact Man	X		X	X	X	X		X	
Smithsonian Scientific Information Exchange	X		X	X	X	X	X	X	TRPD subset
Supplementary Data Base		X	X						Injuries, illness
Survey of Compounds That Have Been Tested for Carcinogenicity			X	X					
Technical Data Center	X		X			X		X	
Toxicology Data Bank	X		X	X	X	X		X	
Toxicology Information On-Line	X		X	X	X	X	X	X	Including TOXBACK
Toxicology Testing in Progress		X	X		X	X			

Table 3-20. Data Systems Applicable to Environmental Effects

System	Bioaccumulation	Ecological Effects	Physical Effects	Degradation	Monitoring and Analysis Technol.[a]	Bibliographic Only	Comments
Advisory Center on Toxicology	X	X					Manual file
Agricultural On-Line Access	X	X		X		X	
Air Pollution Technical Information Center		X	X	X	X	X	
Biomedical Studies Group	X	X	X	X	X		For 14 chemicals
Biological Sciences Information Service	X	X	X				
Biological Data Storage and Retrieval System	X	X				X	Biological effects of water quality (new system)
Defense Documentation Center				X		X	
Distribution Register of Organic Compounds in Water				X	X		New system
Environmental Contaminant Monitoring System				X	X		Fish bioaccumulation studies
Federal Inventory on Environmental Safety and Health Research	X	X	X	X	X	X	2,466 projects
Fish Control Laboratory Data Base Information	X	X		X	X		1,500 chemicals in 8 species manual
Fish Pesticide Research	X	X		X			500 chemicals in 100 species manual
Military Entomology Information Center	X	X		X		X	
National Technical Information Service	X	X	X	X	X	X	Government reports
Oceanic Abstracts	X	X		X		X	
Oceanic and Atmospheric Scientific Information Service	X	X		X	X		
Pollution		X				X	
Research Program of Chemicals that Impact Man	X	X	X	X	X	X	SRI file of 1,500 chemicals
Smithsonian Scientific Information Exchange	X	X	X	X	X	X	Research in progress
Solid Waste Information Retrieval System				X		X	
Toxicology Information On-Line	X	X		X		X	
Inorganic Chemical Computer Toxicology Parameter Data Base	X	X		X			172 inorganics (new system)

[a]Not on original questionnaire.

Table 3-21. Data Systems Applicable to Standards and Regulations

System	Federal	State	Local	International	Bibliographic Only	Comments
Advisory Center on Toxicology	X	X				Manual refers to allowable concentration
Air Pollution Technical Information Center	X	X	X		X	Same as below
Congressional Record Abstracts	X				X	All Congressional publications
Congressional Information Service, Inc.	X				X	
Data Base of U.S. International Trade Commission	X					
Environmental Reports Summaries				X		Foreign regulations
Health Hazard Evaluations	X					Compliance file
National Technical Information Service	X	X			X	Government reports
Pesticides Enforcement Management System	X					Support to pesticide monitoring and enforcement
Pesticide Reporting System	X	X				Sampling results
Registry of Toxic Effects of Chemical Substances	X					NIOSH testing of TWAs
Standards Completion Program	X					400 compounds with TLVs
Technical Data Center	X					OSHA–File of existing standards–20,000 chemicals, 400 compounds with TLVs

Table 3-22. Source of Data and the Proprietary Status of the Primary Systems

Primary Systems	Acronym	Internally Generated Data	Externally Generated Data	Proprietary Information	Mandatory Solicitation Data
Advisory Center on Toxicology		X	X	X	
Aerometric and Emission Reporting System	AEROS	X	X		
Agricultural On-Line Access	AGRICOLA		X		
Air pollution Technical Information Center	APTIC		X		
Annual Survey of Injuries and Illnesses			X	X	X
Astro-4 Drug Information System			X	X	X
Atlas of Cancer Mortality			X		
Biological Data Storage and Retrieval System	BIO-STORCT	X	X		
Biological Sciences Information Service	BIOSIS		X		
Biomedical Studies Group			X		
Cancer Information On-Line	CANCERLINE		X		
Carcinogenesis Bioassay Data System	CBDS	X	X	X	
Census Bureau Foreign Trade Statistics			X	X	X
Census of Manufacturers				X	X
Chemical Abstracts Service Chemical Registry System		X			
Chemical Abstracts Service Information System			X		
Chemical Dictionary of the U.S. ITC		X			
Chemical Dictionary On-Line	CHEMLINE		X		
Chemical Economics Handbook			X		
Chemical Information and Data System	CIDS	X	X		
Chemical Information System	CIS		X		
Chemical Monograph Referral Center	CHEMRIC		X		
Chemical Names File	PHS-149				
Chemical Transportation Emergency Center	CHEMTREC		X		
Clinical Toxicology of Commercial Products	CTCP	X	X		

Data Base	Abbreviation				
Component Information for Chemical Consumer Products			X		
Congressional Information Service Index	CIS INDEX		X	X	X
Congressional Record Abstracts	CRECORD		X		
CPSC Chemical Abstracts		X			
Current Employment Statistics			X	X	X
Data Base of the U.S. ITC			X	X	X
Defense Documentation Center	DDC	X	X		
Directory of Chemical Producers	DCP		X		
Distribution Register of Organic Pollutants in Water	WATERDROP	X	X		
Drug Registration and Listing System			X		
Drug Research and Development Chemical Information System	DR&D CIS	X	X	X	X
Dun's Market Identifiers	DMI	X	X	X	
Environmental Contaminant Monitoring Program			X		
Environmental Mutagen Information Center	EMIC		X		
Environmental Reports Summaries			X	X	
Environmental Teratology Information Center	ETIC	X			
Exposure Dictionary for the National Occupational Hazards Survey	EDNOHS	X			
Federal Inventory of Environmental and Safety Research					
Fish Control Laboratory-Data Base Information		X	X		
Fish-Pesticide Research		X	X		
Health Hazard Evaluations			X		
Index Chemicals Registry System	ICRS	X	X		X
Industrywide Studies					X
Information Bulletin of the Survey of Chemicals Being Tested for Carcinogenicity		X	X		
Information Storage and Referral Section		X			
Inorganic Chemical Computer Toxicology Parameter Data Base			X		
International Cancer Epidemiology Clearinghouse			X		
IPC Chemical Data Base			X		
Kirk-Othmer Encyclopedia of Chemical Technology			X		
Laboratory Animal Data Base	LADB	X	X		

Table 3-22, continued

Primary Systems	Acronym	Internally Generated Data	Externally Generated Data	Proprietary Information	Mandatory Solicitation Data
Mammal Toxicity and Repellency Data Base		X			
Meat & Poultry Inspection Monitoring Program		X		X	X
Medical Literature Analysis and Retrieval System On-Line	MEDLINE	X	X		
Microconstituents in Fish and Fishery Products					
Military Entomology Information Service	MEIS		X		
Mineral Commodity Survey System			X		
NASA Scientific and Technical Information Service		X			
National Center for Health Statistics	NCHS	X	X		
National Center for Toxicology Integrated Research Support System		X			
National Electronic Injury Surveillance System	NEISS		X		
National Occupational Hazard Survey File	NOHS	X			
National Technical Information Service	NTIS		X		
NIOSH Technical Information Center	NIOSHTIC		X		
Oceanic Abstracts			X		
Oceanic and Atmospheric Scientific Information Service	OASIS	X	X		
Office of Standard Reference Data Chemical Files		X	X		
Oil & Hazardous Materials Technical Data System	OHM-TADS	X	X		
Organic Chemical Producers Data Base			X		
Pesticide and Industrial Chemicals					
Pesticide Enforcement Management System	PEMS	X			
Pesticide Reporting System		X			
Pesticides Analysis Retrieval and Control System	PARCS		X	X	
POISINDEX			X		X
Poison Control On-Line Inquiry System			X		
Pollution			X		

Database	Abbreviation			
Pollution				
Population Studies System			X	
Predicasts Marketing Systems			X	X
Registry of Toxic Effects of Chemical Substances	RTECS		X	X
Reporting of Economic Data for Negotiation of International Transportation Conventions	REDNITRAC	X	X	X
Research Program of Chemicals that Impact Man			X	X
Smithsonian Scientific Information Exchange	SSIE		X	
Solid Waste Information Retrieval System	SWIRS		X	
Special Trade Representatives Centralized Data Bank	STRCDB	X	X	X
Standards Completion Program			X	X
Storage and Retrieval for Water Quality Data	STORET		X	X
Subject Content Oriented Retriever for Processing Information On-Line	SCORPIO	X	X	X
Supplementary Data System			X	
Survey of Compounds which have been Tested for Carcinogenic Activity			X	
Technical Data Center	TDC		X	
Thermophysical Properties Research Center			X	X
Toxicology Data Bank	TDB		X	
Toxicology Information On-Line	TOXLINE		X	
Toxicology Testing In Progress	TOX-TIPS		X	
Trade Name Ingredient Clarification	TNIC	X	X	X

SPECIMEN DATA BANK

Environmental data banks do not only contain data. A good example of a most useful environmental data bank is the National Environmental Specimen Bank (NESB) (Van Hook and Huber, 1976). This is a computerized hierarchical information system maintained by the Oak Ridge National Laboratory. Based on a mail survey, it contains information on 650 environmental specimen collections. The data base categories include: animal, atmospheric, geological, microbiological, plant and water.

The following tables classify the collection efforts according to type of collection (Table 3-23), component of interest in specimens (Table 3-24), use of collection (Tables 3-25) and contents (Table 3-26).

Table 3-23. Collections Identified in NESB Survey Classified According to Type of Collection (Van Hook and Huber, 1976)

	Number
Federal	147
State	107
Personal	14
Private Laboratory	30
Private Museum	13
University	347

Table 3-24. Collections Identified in NESB Survey Classified According to Component of Interest in Specimens

	Number
Trace Elements	148
Pesticides	65
Microbiological	58
Mineralogical	78
Organic	64
Radionuclides	34
Medical	33
Other	422
Major Elements	35

Table 3-25. Collections Identified in NESB Survey
Classified According to Use of Collection

Primary Uses		Secondary Uses
96	Chemical Analysis and Baseline Studies	13
9	Personal Collections	
57	Museum Collections	26
50	Environmental Monitoring	13
60	Reference Collections	26
91	Teaching Collections	30
106	Research	118
61	Ecology, population and species diversity	18
51	Systematics, taxonomy, identification and morphology	29
22	Diseases	3
20	Soil characterization	2
7	Physiology	5
16	Seeds	4
11	Specimen Banks	2

CENSUS BUREAU DATA BASES

Probably the major source of information relevant to environmental assessment is the census bureau of the Department of Commerce. The census collects information, builds data bases and reports in summary forms detailed information in the following categories (U.S. Dept. of Commerce, 1969, 1970): general, agriculture, construction, distribution and services, foreign trade, geography, governments, housing, manufacturing and mineral industries, population, and transportation. Geographic areas covered in the statistics include in different cases:

United States
Regions and Divisions
States
Standard Metropolitan Statistical Areas
    a. Criteria for SMSAs
    b. Criteria for central cities
    c. Ring of an SMSA
Standard Consolidated Areas
Counties
Minor Civil Divisions
Census County Divisions
County Subdivisions used in Agriculture Censuses
Congressional Districts
State Economic Areas

Table 3-26. Collections Identified in NESB Survey
Classified According to Collection Contents[a]

	Number
Microorganisms	52
Viruses	15
Bacteria	46
Plants	283
Algae	90
Fungi	66
Lichens	40
Embryophytes	34
Bryophytes	48
Tracheophytes	76
Pteridophytes	83
Spermatophytes	161
Animals	369
Invertebrates	240
Vertebrates	228
Human Tissues	34
Fossils	19
Crustal Materials	170
Soils	79
Bedrock	53
Organic Detritus	16
Bottom Sediments	94
Water	118
Freshwater Lakes	99
Rivers or Streams	105
Groundwater	26
Brackish water	20
Seawater	36
Air	50
Gaseous	13
Particulates	43
Precipitation	17

[a]Each entry was classed as to whether it described: (1) a number of diverse collections in many areas, *i.e.,* water, botanical, geological, etc.; (2) a number of different organisms or types of material in one class such as all geological but including more than one grouping, *i.e.,* soils, organic detritus, bedrock and bottom sediments; or (3) single collections, such as all vertebrates, all spermatophytes, etc.

Table 3-27. Bibliographic Computerized Systems

Name	Source	Operating Period		Number of Records	Update	Description
		From	To			
ABI/INFORM	Data Courier, Inc. Louisville, KY	August 1971	Present	52,000	Monthly	Management and administration
Agricola	National Agriculture Library, Beltsville, MD	1970	Present	920,000	Monthly	Agriculture & related subjects
AIM/ARM	The Ohio State University, Columbus, Ohio	September 1972	Present	17,500	Bimonthly	Manpower, economics, employment, job training, vocational guidance
America	ABC-Clio, Inc., Santa Barbara, CA	1964	Present	43,000	Quarterly	U.S. and Canadian History
APTIC	U.S. Environmental Protection Agency	1966	Present	83,000	Monthly	Air pollution effect, prevention, control
Art Bibliographies Modern	ABC-Clio, Inc. Santa Barbara, CA	1974	Present	21,000	Quarterly	Art & design literature, dissertation, exhibit catalogs
ASFA	FAO, Rome and the Intergovernmental Oceanographic Commission	January 1975	Present	10,000	Monthly	Aquatic sciences and fisheries abstracts, life sciences of the sea and inland waters
BIOSIS Review	Biosciences Information Services of Biological Abstracts, Philadelphia, PA	January 1972	Present	1,200,000	Monthly	Citations from Biological Abstracts & Bioresearch Index, Research in Life-sciences

Name	Source	Operating Period		Number of Records	Update	Description
		From	To			
CA Condensates	Chemical Abstracts Service, Columbus, OH	1970	Present	2,500,000	Monthly	Correspond to printed chemical Abstracts, "K to World's Chemical Literature." Applied chemistry, chemical engineering, biochemistry, macromolecular chemistry, organic chemistry, physical and analytical chemistry
CA Patent Concordance	Chemical Abstracts Service, Columbus, OH	January 1972	Present	75,000	Semiannual	Patents reviewed in Chemical-Abstracts
CAB Abstracts	The Commonwealth Agricultural Bureaus, Farnham House, Farnham Royal, Slough, SL23BN, England	January 1973	Present	480,000	Monthly	Agricultural and biological information e.g., dairy science, breeding, veterinary science
CASIA	Chemical Abstracts Service, Columbus, OH	1972	Present		Monthly	Correspond to records in CA Condensates but better access, e.g., by CAS number or chemical substance
Chemical Industry Notes (CIN)	American Chemical Society, Columbus, OH	1974	Present	170,000	Weekly	Chemical Processing Industries
CHEM NAME	Chemical Abstracts Services, Columbus, OH	1972	Present		Monthly	Derived from CASIA, consisting of lists of chemical subservices in a dictionary type file useful for substance or substructure search

Name	Source	From	To	Records	Update	Description
CLAIMS/CHEM	IFI/Plenum Data Company, Arlington, VA	1950	Present	360,000	Quarterly	U.S. chemical and chemically related patents, plus foreign equivalent from Belgium, France, UK, FRG, Netherlands
CLAIMS/CLASS	IFI/Plenum Data Company, Arlington, VA	1950	Present	15,000		Classification code and title dictionary for all classes and selected subclasses of U.S. Patent Classification System
CLAIMS/GEM	IFI/Plenum Data Company, Arlington, VA	1975	Present	50,000	Quarterly	Electrical and mechanical patents
COMPENDEX	Engineering Index Inc., New York, NY	January 1970	Present	565,000	Monthly	Engineering and technological literature
Comprehensive Dissertation Abstracts	University Microfilms International, Ann Arbor, MI	1861	Present	560,000	Monthly	Subject, title & author guide to every American dissertation since 1861
Current Research Information System (CRIS)	USDA Cooperative State Research Service, Washington, D.C.	July 1974	Present	24,000	Monthly	Current research in agriculture and related sciences sponsored by USDA agencies and other cooperating institutions
Defense Market Measures System (DMMS)	Frost and Sullivan, Inc., New York, NY	January 1975	Present	80,000	Quarterly	U.S. DOD contract awards
ENVIROBIB	Environmental Studies Instate, Santa Barbara, CA	1973	Present	50,000	Bimonthly	Human ecology atmospheric studies, energy, land resources, water resources, and nutrition and health

Name	Source	Operating Period From	Operating Period To	Number of Records	Update	Description
ENVIROLINE®	Environmental Information Center, New York, NY	1971	Present	60,000	Monthly	Environmental information, e.g., planning, law, political sciences, geology, biology, economics, chemistry
ERIC	National Institute of Education, Washington, D.C.	1976	Present	278,000	Monthly	Research in education
Exceptional Child Education Abstracts	The Council for Exceptional Children, Reston, VA	1966	Present	25,000	Quarterly	Education of handicapped and gifted children
Foundation Directory	The Foundation Center, New York, NY	Current Year Data		2,500	Semiannual	Description of 2,500 foundations
Foundation Grants Index	The Foundation Center, New York, NY	January 1973	Present	40,000	Bimonthly	Information on grants awarded by more than 400 major foundations
Historical Abstracts	American Bibliographical Center, Santa Barbara, CA	1973	Present	37,000	Quarterly	Literature on history, related social sciences and humanities
INSPEC	The Institution of Electrical Engineers, Savoy Place, London, WS2R OBL, England	1969	Present	887,000	Monthly	Physics, electrotechnology, computation and control
ISMEC	Data Courier, Inc., Louisville, KY	1973	Present	58,000	Monthly	Information of interest to mechanical engineers in energy, power and transportation and handling

Name	Producer/Source	Start	Coverage	Records	Frequency	Subject
Language and Language Behavior Abstracts (LLBA)	Sociological Abstracts, Inc., San Diego, CA	1973	Present	21,000	Quarterly	Language and language behavior
Metadex (Metals Abstracts/Alloys Index)	American Society for	1974	Present	300,000	Monthly	Metallurgy
Meteorological and Geoastrophysical Abstracts (MGA)	Environmental Science and Information Center, Oceanic and Atmospheric Administration (NOAA) Washington, D.C.	1972	Present	38,000	Irregular	Meteorology, astrophysics, physical oceanography, hydrosphere/jydrology, environmental sciences and glaciology
NICEM	National Information Center for Educational Media, University of Southern California, Los Angeles, CA	January 1964	Present	400,000	Monthly	Nonprint educational material
NTIS	National Technical Information Service, U.S. Department Commerce, Springfield, VA	1964	Present	575,000	Biweekly	Government-sponsored research
Oceanic Abstracts®	Environmental Sciences Information Center, National Oceanic and Atmospheric Administration (NOAA), Washington, D.C.	1964	Present	95,000	Bimonthly	Literature of the seas of the world
Pharmaceutical News Index (PNI)	Data Courier, Inc., Louisville, KY	December 1975	Present	17,000	Monthly	Drug and cosmetic industries
Pollution Abstracts	Data Courier, Inc., Louisville, KY	1970	Present	46,500	Bimonthly	Environmental literature on pollution, its source and control

Name	Source	Operating Period		Number of Records	Update	Description
		From	To			
Psychological Abstracts	American Psychological Association, Washington, D.C.	1967	Present	230,000	Monthly	Psychology and behavioral sciences
PTS Domestic Statistics	Predicasts, Inc., Cleveland, OH	July 1971	Present	160,000	Vary	Business and trade information in government agencies, statistical records and reviews of indsutries, census, handbooks and yearbooks

PREDICASTS statistical Abstracts. More than 70,000 abstracts of published forecasts with historical data for U.S. coverage. Includes general economics, all industries, detailed products and end-use data.

PREDICASTS Composites. Annual historical data (since 1958) and consensus of published forecasts through 1984 for more than 500 key economic, demographic, industrial and product time series. |

PREDICASTS Basebook. Annual data for more than 20,000 time series (1960-1974) on U.S. production, value of shipments, wages, prices, materials, consumption, foreign trade, and end-use distribution for all different types of industries, products, and services.

METROCASTS. Historical and projected (to 1990) data on population, income, employment, earnings and distribution of industrial activity for states, standard business economic areas and standard metropolitan areas.

PREDICASTS Domestic Statistics covers every area of industry and product statistics, government and services statistics, and social economic statistics for the U.S.

PTS EIS Industrial Plants	Economic Information Systems, Inc., New York, NY	Current	117,000	Quarterly

U.S. industrial economy information on 117,000 establishments, and operated

Name	Source	Operating Period		Number of Records	Update	Description
		From	To			
PTS & F&S INDEXES (Funk and Scott)	Predicasts Inc., Cleveland, OH	1972	Present	760,000	Monthly	by 67,000 firms, accounting for more than 90% of U.S. industry Domestic and international product and industry information. Acquisitions, mergers, new products, technological developments and sociological factors
PTS Federal Index	Predicast Inc., Cleveland, OH	October 1976	Present	New	Monthly	Proposed rules and regulations, bills, speeches, roll calls, reports, vetoes, court decisions, executive orders and contract awards
PTS International Statistics	Predicasts, Inc., Cleveland, OH	1972	Present	160,000	Vary	Annual reports of foreign governments, statistical reports of industries and trade associations of foreign countries, publications of United Nations and other international agencies, bank letters, newspapers, and business and trade journals. This essential data base for market development, sales analysis, operations research,

information retrieval, executive decisions, economic forecasting, long-range planning,
diversification study, security
analysis, and market research
includes the following sub-
titles:

Worldcasts Statistical Abstracts. Abstracts of published forecasts with historical data for all countries of
the world (excluding the
United States). Coverage includes general economics,
all industries, detailed products, and end-use data.

Worldcasts Composites.
Annual historical data, SIC
codes, and consensus of published forecasts through 1985
for 2,500 economic, demo-
graphic, industrial and product series for key countries.

Worldcasts Basebook.
Annual data for 20,000 time
series (1960-1974) for all
countries of the world on
production, consumption,

Name	Source	Operating Period		Number of Records	Update	Description
		From	To			
PTS Market Abstracts	Predicasts, Inc., Cleveland, OH	1972	Present	135,000	Monthly	price, foreign trade, and usage statistics for agriculture, mining, manufacturing and services as well as demography and national income. Acquisitions end-uses, capacities environment, foreign trade, market data, new products, production regulations and technology for chemical, communications, computer, electronics, energy, fiber, fuel, instrument & equipment, metals, paper, plastics, and rubber industries.
Search®	The Institute for Scientific Information, Philadelphia, PA	January 1974	Present	1,470,000	Monthly	Cover 90% of world significant scientific and technical literature
Social Scisearch	The Institute for Scientific Information, Philadelphia, PA	1972	Present	420,000	Monthly	Social sciences
Sociological Abstracts	Sociological Abstracts, Inc., San Diego, CA	1963	Present	77,000	Quarterly	Sociology and related disciplines in the social and behavioral sciences
World Aluminum Abstracts	The American Society for Metals, Metals Park, OH	1968	Present	50,000	Monthly	World's literature on Aluminum

Economic Subregions
Agricultural Economic Subregions
Places (cities and other incorporated and unincorporated places)
   a. Incorporated placed
   b. Unincorporated places
Urbanized Areas
Wards
Census Tracts
Enumeration Districts
City Blocks, Block Faces and Block Groupings
Central Business Districts
Major Retail Centers
Foreign Trade Statistical Areas
Government Units (Counties, Municipalities, Townships, School Districts,
   and Special Districts)
Other Special-Purpose Districts
Urban-Rural
Puerto Rico and Other Outlying Areas
International

The standard metropolitan statistical areas (SMSAs) are often used to report statistics. A map of the SMSA is shown as Figure 3-1.

SPECIALIZED DATA BANKS

A number of specialized data banks are summarized below:

Employment and Earnings

The Department of Labor issues a monthly publication entitled *Employment and Earnings,* which presents employment statistics and payroll data by industry, state and selected standard metropolitan statistical areas. The original source is the:

> Information Systems & Data Bank
> Bureau of Labor Statistics
> 441 G. Street, NW
> Washington, D.C.

RECREATION

The Bureau of Outdoor Recreation prepares a "National Inventory of Recreational Facilities," The Inventory presents, on a county-by-county basis, all public facilities (federal, state and local). The Inventory includes acreage and type of recreational function and is provided free on request. Also, the Bureau will run a free computerized search upon request. The Inventory is updated on an irregular basis and its most recent update was

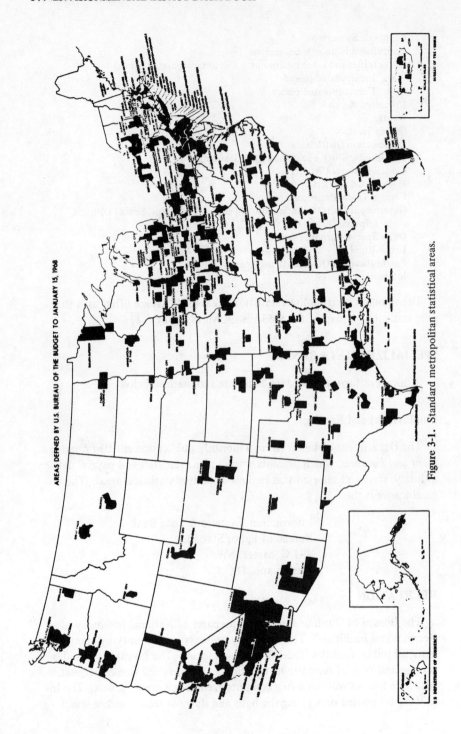

Figure 3-1. Standard metropolitan statistical areas.

in 1972. In 1974, the Bureau will prepare an inventory of private recreational facilities similar to the public inventory. The original source is the:

> Bureau of Outdoor Recreation
> National Inventory of Recreational Facilities
> 18th and C Streets, N.W.
> Washington, D.C. 20240

National Parks and Landmarks

The National Park Service prepares an annual inventory of all national parks and historical and national landmarks recognized by the National Historical Preservation Society. Two key publications, *National Register of Historic Places* and *Registry of National Landmarks,* are updated by the Federal Register. The original source is:

> Inventory of National Parks and Landmarks
> National Park Service
> 1100 L. Street
> Washington, D.C.

Weather and Climate

The principal functions and activities of NOAA include reporting and forecasting weather, issuing warnings against such destructive natural events as hurricanes, tornadoes and floods, and preparation of nautical and aeronautical charts. The following offices are components of NOAA: The National Weather Service, the National Ocean Survey (including the Lakes Survey Center), the National Marine Fisheries Service and the Environmental Data Service (EDS).

ENDEX is a computerized data base developed by EDS. Information is collected from various EDS Data Centers—the National Climatic Center in Washington, the National Geophysical and Solar-Terrestrial Data Center, Boulder, Colorado. In the fully developed system, information on meteorology, oceanography, limnology and geophysics will be available for searching in machine-readable form. Fourteen hundred file descriptions have been received to date. Percentages of total files initially converted to machine-readable form range from 1% of NCCs worldwide meteorological files to 57% of the oceanographic data from the mid-Atlantic states.

In addition to this computer base, NOAA issues a number of publications in print form, including the monthly *Local Climatological* data (with annual summary), *Climates of the States, etc.* The original source is:

> National Oceanic and Atmospheric Administration (NOAA)
> 3300 Whitehaven Street, N.W.
> Washington, D.C.

REFERENCES

Barrett, K., and E. Roberts. "Survey of Information Sources with an Annotated Bibliography on Organic Emissions from the Synthetic Organic Chemical Manufacturing Industry," MTR-7377, The MITRE Corporation, (November 1976).

Bracken, M., J. Dorigan, J. Hushon and J. Overbey, II. "User Requirements for Chemical Information Systems," MRS-7558, The MITRE Corporation, (May 1977).

Brown, P., et al. Energy Information Resources—An Inventory of Energy Research and Development Information Resources in the Continental United States, Hawaii and Alaska, American Society for Information Science, (Washington, D.C.: Information Science, 1975).

Christian, R. W. "The Electronic Library—Bibliographic Data Bases 1975-1976 (White Plains, New York: Knowledge Industry Publications, 1975).

DeForest, J. D. "State Energy Information Systems: A Survey," National Governors' Conference, July 1975.

Energy Program, National Governor's Conference, Washington, D.C., July 1975.

"Energy Information Act Hearings Before Committee on Interior and Insular Affairs," U.S. Senate Pursuant to S. Res 45, A National Fuels and Energy Policy Study, 93rd Congress, 2nd Session, Serial No. 93-24, Report 2 (1974).

Federal Energy Administration. "Preliminary Results of the Interagency Task Force on Energy Information," (July 1974).

Federal Energy Administration. "Federal Energy Information Gathering Activities," A Report to the President of the United States and the Energy Resources Council, December 1975.

Fennelly, P. F., et al. "Environmental Assessment Prospectives," PB-257-911, GCA Corp., Bedford, Massachusetts (March 1976).

General Accounting Office. "Improvements Still Needed in Federal Energy Data Collection, Analysis and Reporting," Report to the Congress, USP-76-21, (June 1976).

Green, K. H., D. A. Blume and J. E. Jones, Jr. A Directory of Computerized Environmental Information Resources, PB 262-486 (Lexington, Kentucky: University of Kentucky, 1976).

Kruzas, A. T. Encyclopedia of Information Systems and Services, (Ann Arbor, Michigan: Edward Brothers, 1974).

Little, A. D. "Nuclear Environmental Information-Resources and Action Plan," prepared for Atomic Industrial Forum (September 1974).

National Technical Information Service. Directory of Computerized Data Files and Related Software Available from Federal Agencies, Washington, D.C. (1974).

Olson, R. J., et al. "Spatial Data on Energy Environmental and Socio-Economic Themes at Oak Ridge National Laboratory," Oak Ridge National Laboratory, ORNL/TM-5746 (1977).

U.S. Department of Commerce, Bureau of the Census. Guide to Census Bureau Data Files and Special Tabulations (1969).

U.S. Department of Commerce, Bureau of the Census. 1970 Census User's Guide (1970).

Van Hook, R. I., and E. E. Huber. "National Environmental Specimen Bank Survey," Oak Ridge National Laboratory, prepared for the Environmental Protection Agency, Report No. EPQ-60011-76-006 (January 1976).

CHAPTER 4

MODELS

INTRODUCTION

An environmental assessment can be completed successfully without the use of any quantitative information and without the aid of models. However, in some cases, the situation is complex enough to warrant the use of computerized models for part of the analysis. Models can be either stochastic or deterministic, they can be analytic or integrative; they can take the form of a simulation of the entire phenomena or can be made to model only a few properties.

The field of models is immense and we could not hope to review it totally. Instead, some detail is presented where models have been demonstrated to be most useful.

We will describe: energy models, noise models, cooling power plume models, transportation models, thermal addition models, models of ambient air quality, and water models. Many other forms of models are left uncovered, including: economic models, population models, social models, ecological models, etc.

ENERGY MODELS

The energy field has spawned a broad range of models. They range in scope from supply-oriented models of a single fuel to models of the overall energy system and its relationship to the economy. A useful classification of energy models is as follows:

- Sectoral models, covering the supply or demand for specific fuels or energy forms.
- Industry market models, which include both supply and demand relationships for individual or related fuels.

147

- Energy system models, which encompass supply and demand relationships for all energy sources.
- Energy/economic models, which model the relationships between the energy system and the overall economy (Hoffman and Wood, 1976).

Several approaches have been followed in developing energy system models. Among the more interesting are those of energy balance, reference energy system and linear programming. The energy balance approach involves a complete accounting of energy flows from original supply sources, through conversion processes, to end-use demands. It accounts for intermediate consumption of energy during conversion processes as well as efficiencies at various points in the energy supply system (Hoffman and Wood, 1976). Energy balance models have been used in forecasting studies. In these applications, independent estimates of energy demand were developed and iterated with expected supply. Human judgment was used to resolve differences in supply and demand (Dupree and West, 1972; National Petroleum Council, 1974).

MAJOR SURVEYS

Four major surveys are discussed below in chronological order. These surveys alone establish the wealth of energy models available or under development, and offer a variety of approaches for classification and evaluation.

Limaye *et al.* (1973) summarize the results of a survey of both "models" and "quantitative studies" performed at Decision Sciences Corporation for the Council on Environmental Quality (final report submitted January 1973). In all, 94 models and quantitative studies are classified and reviewed. The study specifically addressed: demand, supply, supply/demand interaction, environmental impact, technological impact. Found to be most important and relevant for CEQ were 13 specific models, 9 quantitative studies and one qualitative study. Objectives, approach and limitations of the survey are stated clearly.

Stoian (1974) presents a pyramidal classification to a collection of approximately 2,000 distinct models used or proposed in the energy field, and proposes a novel framework for evaluating methods of energy modeling. The greater contribution is the classification; from the top down, this is as follows: "more than seven incremental fundamental-rationalist and empirical-theoretical models . . . more than a dozen large global models a la 'Limits to Growth' . . . more than 30 models covering several sectors of a national and regional economy, and containing an energy or natural resource component . . . about 70 econometric and structural models linking several sub-sectors of the energy industry with each other (*e.g.,* crude oil, natural gas, coal or nuclear energy . . . approximately 450 models depicting one phase of only one sector of the energy industry, *e.g.,* demand for natural gas, oil transportation . . . about 1250 models converging on specific rational or causal aspects of a rather localized process and dealing with supportive actions or functions, *e.g.,* drilling, completion or production of oil wells."

Charpentier (1974, 1975) presents a survey of energy models, drawing attention to the more well-known or more promising ones. The survey is worldwide in scope, classifies each model according to whether it is national or international, applies to the energy sector only or applies to linkage between energy and the general economy, and, within the energy sector, whether one or several kinds of fuel are considered in each model run. A total of 70 models are surveyed, 15 of which are from the United States. Each model is presented in a common format, including goal, modeling techniques, input and output data descriptions, and current status.

FEA (1975) reports a governmental in-house capability of monitoring the status of certain energy models currently under development, inter-networking and running those which are operational. This capacity resides in the Federal Energy Administration, Office of the Assistant Administrator for Policy and Analysis, and is collectively referred to as the Project Independence Evaluation System (PIES). This system is a series of inter-related models which forecast energy supply and demand, prices, capital requirements and cash flows. It is stated in this report that: "The PIES system rapidly became the major analytical tool used in the policy analysis leading to the national energy program presented in President Ford's State of the Union Message in January 1975."

The PIES system, as reported by FEA (1975), consists of 46 models, of which 10 are for short- and mid-range forecasting, 23 support special policy analyses, 8 support economic impact assessment, and 5 are major U.S. macroeconomic forecasting models. For 34 of these models, the report further lists purpose, description of model, policy applications, status and a specific FEA point of contact. These points of contact comprise a staff of over 20 persons at FEA. The total effort involves an FEA staff of approximately 100.

OTHER SURVEYS

Some papers, or collections of papers, which further add to the number of energy models in the literature are: RFF (1973), QMC (1973), RFF (1974), and the paper by Manne (1974) which is found in RFF (1974). In particular, Manne (1974) notes that via his references (which includes the work of Limaye *et al.* (1973) noted earlier, and overlaps with papers in RFF (1973)), approximately 200 different energy models can be found.

Bell's (1974) "Symposium on Analytical Models of Energy Policy," is a collection of four papers describing four different energy models. Although all are econometric models, each is different; one merges econometric production functions to the input/output matrix formulation, and another uses linear programming to characterize but one sector of an econometric model.

Hiatt (1975) presents a survey of energy models, completed in 1974 under the auspices of the Department of Transportation. In this survey, energy models are classified in one aspect as supply, system or demand models, and classified in another aspect as econometric or linear programming (including network) models. The survey then discusses in greater detail nine specific econometric models and three selected linear programming or network models.

Two surveys, one by Argonne National Laboratories and one by Battelle Columbus Laboratories, became available at the end of 1975. The Argonne survey took as criteria for inclusion regional energy models, which (1) look at multiple fuels (interfuel competition), (2) have more than one end-use sector, and (3) are now completed with documentation available. This process of elimination narrowed the field to eight energy models. The Battelle survey is sponsored by NSF. Reviewed will be five specific models, each sponsored by NSF.

Two additional surveys of significant interest appeared in 1976, both under the sponsorship of the Electric Power Research Institute, and are being performed by Charles River Associates (CRA) of Cambridge, Massachusetts. The first of the two to appear was entitled "Performance Tests for State-of-the-Art Models for Electricity Demand." In this study, eight well-known econometric electricity usage forecasting models were tested and compared via estimations from the *same* data base. The second of the EPRI/CRA tasks was a critical survey of large-scale energy models, *i.e.*, models purportedly capable of evaluating energy R&D options or of assessing the impact of introduction of new technology. CRA presented EPRI with a cursory survey of over 30 models, from which EPRI chose ten for further scrutiny. The total effort to be expended by CRA on this critical survey of large-scale energy models will come to approximately one and one-third man-years, with approximately three to four man-weeks on each of the models selected for in-depth scrutiny.

The National Science Foundation Office of R&D Policy is sponsoring a review of energy models by the Stanford Research Institute. This is of interest, as it could be anticipated that the SRI-Gulf Energy Model would be included and placed into the context of this review.

Annual Review, Inc., has published a book in which one chapter is a review of energy models; this chapter was coauthored by Kenneth Hoffman and David Wood.

The reference energy system approach relies on a network description of the energy system (Hoffman and Palmedo, 1972). Each link in the network corresponds to a physical process such as extraction, refining, conversion, transportation, etc., and each is characterized by a conversion efficiency, capital and operating cost, and emissions of air and water pollutants per unit of energy input. The approach facilitates analysis and evaluation of new technologies. One such model accepts regional demand and energy reserve data as input, and produces as output, regional fuel prices, resource production levels, interregional flows and demand for fuels, all over some forecasting time period (Cazelet, 1975). A variation of this approach has been developed, which enables a relatively large number of regions to be considered. This is achieved through use of the Ford-Fulkerson network optimizing algorithm (Deeanne, 1975).

Linear programming has been used in energy system models to optimize allocation of resources and conversion technologies. In such cases, the energy system is represented as a network similar to that used in the reference energy system approach. Among other model inputs, the energy demand must be specified. In effect, the energy sources compete to serve the demand in the linear programming optimization process. Optimization may be performed with respect to a variety of factors. Among them: dollar cost, social cost, resource consumption, environment effects or combinations of these factors (Chermavsky, 1974). A variation of the basic approach accepts time-phased inputs and produces time-phased outputs (Marcuse and Bodin, 1975).

Other approaches have been taken. Of these, one of the more interesting is the difference equation or system dynamics approach which has been used to simulate the flow of resources to the various demand sectors (Baughman, 1972). The model is used to study interfuel competition and as such, it develops the quantities and prices of fuels and energy sources that are used over time as demands for and the availability and cost of resources change. In the integrated energy/economic class of models, an energy system model is integrated with a model of the economy—typically a macroeconomic or an input-output model. Instead of accepting energy demand as an input, these models accept trends in society and the economy such as population, population distribution, household size, GNP, etc., as input, and estimate energy demand endogenously (Hoffman and Wood, 1976).

Use of input-output models requires determination of coefficients indicative of energy input per dollar output for each sector of the economy.

If the number of fuel options and economic sectors is large, the number of coefficients will also be large. Nevertheless, such coefficients have been calculated (Herendeen, 1973; Just, 1973; Just *et al.,* 1975). The fixed nature of these coefficients poses some problems in applying the method to forecasting sutdies. Accordingly, several models have been built which revise or modify the coefficients to reflect new conditions (Bullard and Sebald, 1975; Hudson and Jorgenson, 1974). Such models have been used to predict the impact on energy demand of such alternative tax policies as a uniform Btu tax, a uniform energy sales tax and a sales tax on petroleum.

The model which is perhaps closest to achieving the aims proposed herein, is one developed by the Federal Energy Administration (1974). It is in fact an integration of eight models or submodels. On the input side are four models, including a macroeconomic model, an industrial production model, an annual energy demand model and a supply model indicative of oil and gas production. Coal production at various prices is provided as an input variable. Output of the macroeconomic and industrial production submodels serves as input to the energy demand submodel. The demand model forecasts demand for 47 primary and derived energy products that are conditional on several factors, one of which is assumed energy price. Also of interest, the demand submodel distinguishes transportation as one of three major consuming sectors. Output of the demand submodel and of the oil and gas production submodel, along with predeveloped estimates of coal production as a function of price, serve as inputs to an LP submodel. For the demands and expected prices as determined by the demand model, the LP submodel determines the minimum cost (price) supply which satisfies the demand. If the supply and demand prices differ, demand price adjustments are made internally based on price elasticities. The demand and LP submodels iterate in this fashion until the prices are equal. At this point the LP output is delivered to three output submodels: a macroeconomic submodel, an environmental assessment submodel and an international assessment submodel. The last report in the literature indicates the model's current time frame to be 1973 to 1985.

Specific segments of the energy business have been modeled. The Uranium mining industry (Ahmed, 1977) and the petroleum industry (Jordanides and Meditch, 1977) are cases in point.

The work in transportation energy demand falls into two categories. The first involves determining current and future energy efficiency (or inversely, intensiveness) of the various modes (Hirst, 1972; Rice, 1973; Campbell, 1973; Goss and McGowan, 1973; Pilati, 1974; Hirst, 1974; Fraize *et al.*, 1974; Nutter, 1974; Masey and Paullin, 1974; Fraize, 1974;

DOT, 1976a; Hirst and Stuntz, 1976), while the second deals with the amount of energy required by the modes, and by the transportation sector in total, under various energy conserving actions or policies (Mutch, 1973; Malliaris and Strombotne, 1974; Voorhees, 1974; Faucett, 1974; Pollard *et al.*, 1975; OTA, 1975; Wildhorn *et al.*, 1976; DOT, 1976b; Behhem and Beglinger, 1976; ORNL, 1976; ORNL, 1977). An often cited energy conservation measure is that of shifting traffic from energy-intensive to energy-efficient modes. In a number of cases, the amount of energy saved has been determined as a function of the amount or percent of traffic diverted (Fraize *et al.*, 1974; Hirst and Stuntz, 1976; Malliaris and Strombotne, 1974). In one case the extent of the traffic shift has been estimated for a specified increase in the price of crude oil (Pollard *et al.*, 1975). However, the authors admit that the estimate was little more than a guess.

The expected substantial increased use of coal as an energy source has spawned some controversy about how coal should be transported. Accompanying the controversy are a number of studies that dwell on the transportation of coal (Chuange and Nichols, 1975; Reiber *et al.*, 1975; Armbruster and Candela, 1976; Rifas and White, 1976). Other than the "fallout" from the energy systems and integrated energy/economic models, little has been done to shed light on the future transportation requirements associated with other energy sources or technologies.

NOISE MODELING

The modeling, evaluation and analysis of noise in the living and working environment is better based on the methodology developed in the so-called CHABA (Committee on Bioacaustics and Biomechanics) reports (U.S. Army, 1977), which develop a method for quantifying noise impact.

The impact of noise on people regularly experiencing that insult is the degree to which the noise interferes with various activities such as speech, sleep and, thus, the peaceful pursuit of normal activities, and the degree to which it may impair health through the inducement of hearing loss. CHABA attempts to derive a single number to represent quantitatively the integrated effect of "impact" of the action on the total population experiencing the different sound levels. This single number quantification is defined as the sound level-weighted population, LWP. A second way of describing noise impact is the noise impact index (NII), which is derived as the ratio of sound level-weighted population to the total population.

In some high-level noise environments, people will be exposed to average sound levels in excess of 75 decibels. In these environments, consideration should be given to the potential for noise-induced hearing loss. A measure is defined below, the population-weighted hearing loss (PHL), which provides a measure of the average hearing loss that might be expected for the population under consideration.

Sound Level-Weighted Population

In this method, the "fractional impact" is the product of a sound level weighting value and the increment of population exposed to a specified sound level. Summing the "fractional impacts" over the entire population provides the sound level-weighted population (LWP):

$$LWP = \int P(L_{dn}) \cdot W(L_{dn}) \, d(L_{dn})$$

where:

$P(L_{dn})$ = population distribution function

$W(L_{dn})$ = day-night average sound level weighting function characterizing the severity of the impact as a function of sound level described below

$d(L_{dn})$ = differential change in day-night average sound level.

Sufficient accuracy is usually obtained by taking average values of the weighting function between equal decibel increments, up to 5 decibels in size, and by summations of successive increments in average sound level.

Noise Impact Index

Noise Impact Index (NII) is a useful concept for comparing the relative impact of one noise environment with that of another. It is defined as the sound level-weighted population divided by the total population under consideration:

$$NII = \frac{LWP}{P_{Total}} = \frac{\int P(L_{dn}) \cdot W(L_{dn}) \, d(L_{dn})}{\int P(L_{dn}) \, d(L_{dn})}$$

Population-Weighted Loss of Hearing

The population-weighted loss of hearing (PLH) is a representation of the postential loss of hearing, *i.e.,* the average change in hearing threshold level in decibels that would be expected from a population experiencing the various day-night average sound levels in excess of 75 decibels. This quantity is formed by the ratio of sound level-weighted population to total population (experiencing day-night average sound levels in excess of 75 decibels).

Similar to NII, PHL is computed in decibels as:

$$PHL = \frac{\int_{75}^{x} P(L_{dn})\ H(L_{dn})\ d(L_{dn})}{\int_{75}^{X} P(L_{dn})\ d(L_{dn})}$$

where:

$H(L_{dn})$	=	loss of hearing weighting function described below
$P(L_{dn})$	=	population distribution functions
$d(L_{dn})$	=	differential change in day-night average sound level
NOTE:		PHL is in decibels since the weighting function of loss of hearing has not been normalized.

The integral may be replaced by summation over successive increments of day-night average sound level. It is recommended that increments of day-night average sound level less than five decibels (*e.g.,* 2 decibesl) be used in calculating values of PHL.

Sound Level Weighting Functions

Two different weighting functions are provided in CHABA for use in the analysis of environmental noise impact, one for general application in the majority of analyses, in which the overall impact of the noise on the "Health and Welfare" of residential populations is involved, and one for evaluating the potential for hearing damage when the day-night average sound level exceeds 75 decibels.

Sound level weighting function for overall impact analysis

In the majority of analysis, the primary concern is the effect of noise on the residential population living in the environment under consideration. The weighting function used for this form of analysis is based on the documented reaction of populations to living in noise-impacted **environ**ments and is numerically derived from social survey data relating the fraction of sampled population expressing a high degree of annoyance to various values of day-night average sound level. The weighting function is arbitrarily normalized to unity at L_{dn} = 75 decibels. Values of the function are listed in Table 4-1 and the function is plotted in Figure 4-1. The analytical expression for the function is:

$$W(L_{dn}) = \frac{[3.364 \times 10^{-6}][10^{0.103 L_{dn}}]}{[0.2][10^{0.03 L_{dn}}] + [1.43 \times 10^{-4}][10^{0.08 L_{dn}}]}$$

Table 4-1.   Sound Level Weighting Function for Overall Impact Analysis[a]

L_{dn}·dB	$W(L_{dn})$	$\dfrac{W(L_{dn}) + W(L_{dn} + 5)}{2}$
35	0.006	
40	0.013	0.010
45	0.029	0.021
50	0.061	0.045
55	0.124	0.093
60	0.235	0.180
65	0.412	0.324
70	0.664	0.538
75	1.000	0.832
80	1.428	1.214
85	1.966	1.697
90	2.647	2.307

[a] The right hand column is included for convenience for finding the weighting of certain 5-dB increments (U.S. Army, 1977).

Weighting function for loss of hearing/severe health effects

In those specialized environments in which people are directly exposed, on a regular, continuing, long-term basis, to day-night average sound levels above 75 decibels, there is a potential for producing noise-induced loss of hearing and other potentially severe health effects. The weighting function for loss of hearing/severe health effects, $H(L_{dn})$ or $H(L_{8h})$ is expressed as:

$$H(L_{dn}) = 0.025 \, (L_{dn} - 75)^2$$
$$\text{or } H(L_{8h}) = 0.025 \, (L_{8h} - 75)^2$$

and is shown in Table 4-2.

Airport Noise

Under FAA Order 1050.1B, "Policies and Procedures for Considering Environmental Impacts" (*Federal Register* 42(123)32630, June 27, 1977), the Federal Aviation Administration Requires that noise analysis be conducted using the FAA integrated noise model (INM).

Noise metrics available from the model are Noise Exposure Forecast (NEF), Day-Night Average Sound Level (Ldn), Equivalent Sound Level (Leq), Community Noise Equivalent Leval (CNEL) and time of exposure above a number of user-specified A-weighted sound levels in decibels, dBA (TA_{85}, TA_{95}, etc.).   All these metrics can be displayed in the form of

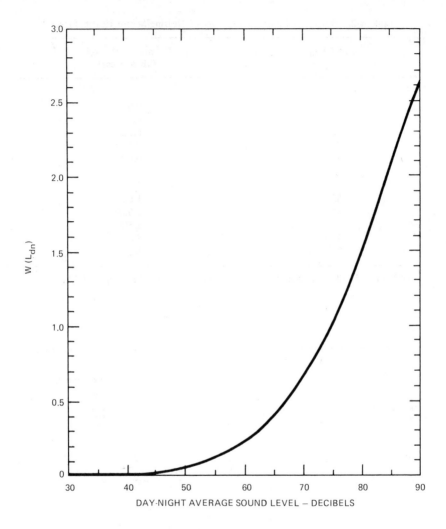

Figure 4-1. Sound level weighting function for overall impact analysis (U.S. Army, 1977).

contours of equal noise exposure to a desired map scale (Figure 4-2). The user normally will choose a single metric of greatest interest for contour plotting, but it is easy to obtain plots in more than one metric. The model also automatically provides numerical listings of the calculated noise values at all intersecting points on a grid which encompasses the airport

Table 4-2. Weighting Function for Loss of Hearing/Severe Health Effects[a]

L_{dn} or L_{8h} (dB)	$H(L_{dn})$ or $H(L_{8h})$ (dB loss/ear)
75	0
76	0.025
77	0.100
78	0.225
79	0.400
80	0.625
81	0.900
82	1.225
83	1.600
84	2.025
85	2.500
90	S.625
95	10.0

[a] Additional details and examples can be found in the CHABA report (U.S. Army, 1977).

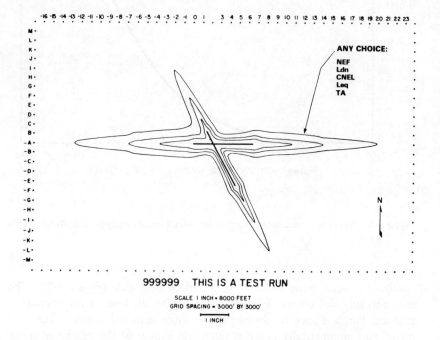

999999   THIS IS A TEST RUN

SCALE 1 INCH = 8000 FEET
GRID SPACING = 3000' BY 3000'

1 INCH

Figure 4-2. Example of computer plot (FAA, 1977).

and its surrounding neighborhoods. This printed output includes computations of the four metrics based on accumulated acoustical energy, and time-above-A-weighted sound levels for six selected noise thresholds, from 65 to 115 decibels. The time of exposure calculations are further broken down into daily periods: for a 24-hour day, for evening hours (7 to 10 PM) and for night hours (10 PM to 7 AM).

The input of certain characteristics of the airport and its operation is a necessary step in the calculations. The user must define runways and flight tracks and allocate the traffic of specific aircraft types. Although the model's data base contains common flight profiles and noise characteristics for many aircraft types, changes to the built-in aircraft noise and performance data base can be accomplished through user option commands. The noise file for each aircraft consists of noise vs distance curves for several thrust settings. Calculations at each grid point are printed in Table 4-3. A letter-number code is being developed to relate the tabular data to grid point intersections on the contour map.

COOLING TOWER PLUME MODELS

The moisture released in the atmosphere contains water droplets over a wide range of sizes. Water droplets with diameters up to about 20μm are considered as fog. Water droplets larger than 20μm are defined as drift or carryover.

A number of models are available (Rioffman, 1974) for predicting the dispersion of vapor plumes from cooling towers. All models are based on one of the following three approaches: (1) Gaussian diffusion, (2) cumulus cloud and fluid-dynamics, or (3) empirical models. All these models were developed for cooling towers. Plume from cooling ponds, lakes or spray canals have been approximated from cooling tower models.

The deposition of water drifts droplets is usually quantified either by: analogy with the deposition of industrial dust; plume rise combined with Gaussian diffusion accounting for droplet fall velocities; trajectories of water droplets taking into account evaporation, size and atmosphere conditions; or diffusion formula describing the rate of change of water droplets concentration as a function of droplet radii, droplet size change due to evaporation, condensation and chemical composition, and atmospheric conditions.

Salt deposition from salt water cooling towers has been studied by Penna and Husler (1975) among many others. No models are available to describe cloud formation or precipitation and snow augmentation. Atmospheric effect, potential impact, model classes and key references are given in Table 4-4. The easy situation described above can become rapidly

Table 4-3. Sample Standard Grid Analysis Printout (FAA, 1977)

Inter-Section	Period	Time in Minutes above indicated A-Weighted Sound Level (dBA)						NEF	LDN	CNEL	LEQ
		85	90	95	100	105	110				
B,-10	24-HR	8.2	4.2	1.0	0.0	0.0	0.0	38.8	74.5	75.1	71.8
	EVENING	1.2	.6	.2	0.0	0.0	0.0				
	NIGHT	.8	.4	.1	0.0	0.0	0.0				
B,-8	24-HR	8.5	4.3	1.1	0.0	0.0	0.0	38.5	74.1	74.7	71.4
	EVENING	1.3	.6	.2	0.0	0.0	0.0				
	NIGHT	.8	.4	.1	0.0	0.0	0.0				
B,-6	24-HR	8.5	4.7	1.9	.4	.0	0.0	41.6	77.0	77.6	71.4
	EVENING	1.2	.7	.2	.1	.0	0.0				
	NIGHT	.8	.4	.2	.0	0.0	0.0				
B,-4	24-HR	7.8	4.1	1.5	.6	.1	0.0	42.3	77.6	78.3	75.0
	EVENING	1.1	.5	.2	.1	.0	0.0				
	NIGHT	.7	.4	.1	.0	.0	0.0				
B,-2	24-HR	6.5	2.5	.3	0.0	0.0	0.0	36.4	71.9	72.3	69.1
	EVENING	.9	.2	.0	0.0	0.0	0.0				
	NI	.6	.2	.0	0.0	0.0	0.0				
B, 0	24-HR	5.6	1.7	.0	0.0	0.0	0.0	34.5	70.0	70.7	67.4
	EVENING	.7	.1	0.0	0.0	0.0	0.0				
	NIGHT	.4	.1	0.0	0.0	0.0	0.0				
B, 2	24-HR	4.8	1.5	.1	0.0	0.0	0.0	35.3	70.7	71.2	67.9
	EVENING	.7	.2	.0	0.0	0.0	0.0				
	NIGHT	.4	.1	.0	0.0	0.0	0.0				

		Con	X-Start	Y-Start	X-Step	NX	NY	Options				
B, 4	24-HR	4.9	1.9	.3	0.0	0.0	0.0	0.0	35.8	71.3	71.8	68.6
	EVENING	.7	.2	0.0	0.0	0.0	0.0	0.0				
	NIGHT	.4	.2	0.0	0.0	0.0	0.0	0.0				
B, 6	24-HR	5.5	2.4	.5	0.0	0.0	0.0	0.0	36.8	72.2	72.8	69.4
	EVENING	.8	.3	.0	0.0	0.0	0.0	0.0				
	NIGHT	.5	.2	.0	0.0	0.0	0.0	0.0				
B, 8	**24**-HR	6.4	3.1	.7	0.0	0.0	0.0	0.0	37.5	73.1	73.7	70.4
	EVENING	1.0	.5	.1	0.0	0.0	0.0	0.0				
	NIGHT	.6	.3	.0	0.0	0.0	0.0	0.0				
B,10	24-HR	7.1	4.1	.7	0.0	0.0	0.0	0.0	38.8	74.4	75.0	71.7
	EVENING	1.1	.6	.1	0.0	0.0	0.0	0.0				
	NIGHT	.7	.4	.0	0.0	0.0	0.0	0.0				

Command	Unit	File	Con	X-Start	Y-Start	X-Step	NX	NY	Options
Nocon	-0	-0	-0	11,000.	0.00	1000.	11	1	*****

Table 4-4. Summary of Cooling Tower Plume Models

Atmospheric Effect	Potential Impact	Model Class	Reference
Visible Plume	Visual intrusion ground shading reduction in visibility	Gaussian diffusion	Bogh et al., 1972 EG&G, 1971 General Public Utilities, 1972 C. H. Hosler, 1971 Kaylor et al., 1972 McVehil, 1970 Roffman, 1973 Travelers Research Corp., 1971 Westinghouse, 1973
		Cumulus-cloud and fluid dynamics	Weinstein, 1968; 1970 England et al., 1973 Westinghouse, 1974
		Empirical models	Currier et al., 1973 Kaylor et al., 1972 Ooms, 1972 Takeda, 1971 Orville, 1968
Ground fog	Hazard to ground and water transportation Nuisance to nearby communities	Psychometric chart	Klanian, 1973 Hansen and Cates, 1972 Landon and Houx, 1973 Veldhuizen and Ledbetter, 1971 Hanna, 1973 Woodruff et al., 1971

Icing	Hazard to ground transportation ice accumulation nearby structures, utility wires	Psychometric chart	
Drift Deposition	Damage to biota including agriculture Acceleration of corrosion Contamination of soil and water	Analogy with industrial dust Plume rise theory with a) Gaussian diffusion b) Estimated trajectories c) Diffusion type equation	Bosanquet, 1950 Hosler, 1972 Roffman, 1973
Cloud Formation	Visual intrusion Weather modification	No model available	
Precipitation and Snow Augmentation	Weather modification Nuisance to nearby communities Hazard to nearby road travelers	No model	

complicated: (1) Multiple sources have been modelled by Briggs (1975); and (2) a combination of calm vs windy atmospheric conditions and moist vs dry plumes have been analyzed and have required the use of different models.

Modeling the effects of a thermal plume discharged from a cooling tower (Watson, 1973) containing a given excess of water vapor over ambient atmosphere may be regarded from the standpoint of two aspects or phases in the generation and progression of the plume:

1. estimating the height to which the plume will rise in its exit from the tower before leveling off and, hence, the distance above ground from which its dispersion into and dilution by the ambient atmosphere will start; and
2. calculating the concentration of water vapor that can be expected at a given point downwind from the tower and, on this basis, predicting the occurrence of fog from the plume.

Height of Plume Rise

For calculating plume rise, a simple model is provided by the so-called Holland equation, in which the height, h, of the plume in meters above the stack is given by the expression:

$$h = Vd/u \left\{ 1.5 + \left[(2.68 \times 10^{-3})p \, \frac{(T_s - T_a)}{T_s} \, d \right] \right\}$$

where:

d = internal diameter of the stack, m
p = atmospheric pressure, mb
V = stack exit velocity, m/sec
u = wind velocity at stack height, m/sec
T_s = stack-gas temperature, $^\circ$K
T_a = ambient temperature, $^\circ$K

Results in a graph from Kennedy (1971) have been published for plume rise as a function of exit diameter.

Water Vapor Content and Length of Visible Plume

The termal plume discharged from a cooling tower contains a considerable mass or concentration of excess water vapor (over that in the surrounding atmosphere) as well as excess heat. If this excess water vapor (Xw) added to the ambient concentration results in a total concentration that equals or exceeds the saturation value at a given temperature, the plume is visible as localized fog. Normally, this visibility continues at an elevation for some distance downwind, the distance depending primarily on atmospheric conditions that govern the rate of dispersion or diffusion of X_W.

The mass of excess water vapor, X_W, in g/m^3 required for saturation can be readily calculated for a given temperature and relative humidity (R) from tables available for that purpose (CRC Handbook of Chemistry and Physics):

Let S_W (t) $\triangleq$ mass of water vapor in saturated air at temperature, t
Let $0 < R < 1 \triangleq$ the relative humidity

then,

R x S_W (t) = mass of water-vapor present in the ambient atmosphere at the given temperature

and,

S_W (t) - R.S_W (L) = D $\triangleq$ the "deficit," or mass of water vapor required to produce saturation

If, at a given point, $X_W \geqslant D$, the plume will be visible at that point. As a matter of practical convenience, a "conservative" assumption may be made that the plume will be visible whenever X_W added to the ambient concentration value, i.e., $X_W + R.S_W$ (t) $\geqslant .95$ S_W (t).

This assumption is conservative in its tendency to underestimate the distance within which the plume will not dissipate. Where there is a question that the plume may have some environmental impact, the assumption is conservative in providing a margin of safety from an environmental point of view; calculations derived from it will tend to overstate the extent of the plume.

To calculate the value of X_W at any three-dimensional point, a conventional or "classical" Gaussian plume model is supplied by the diffusion formula (Slade, 1968):

$$X_W (h,x,y,z) = \frac{Q}{2\pi\sigma_y\sigma_z u} \; e^{-\frac{y^2}{2\sigma_y^2}} \left\{ e^{-\frac{(z-h)^2}{2\sigma_z^2}} + e^{-\frac{(z+h)^2}{2\sigma_z^2}} \right\}$$

where:

$Q \triangleq$ the source-strength (or rate at which water vapor is added to the plume by evaporation) in g/sec
$u \triangleq$ wind velocity in m/sec
$y \triangleq$ horizontal distance (m) from and at right angles to the center line of the plume
$z \triangleq$ vertical distance (m) from and at right angles to the centerline

h $\triangleq$ effective height (m) to which the plume rises before leveling off, representing the height of the tower plus the additional rise (as computed from, for example, the Holland equation)

σ_y and σ_z represent, respectively, the horizontal and vertical dispersion coefficients, expressing (as a function of downwind distance, x), the rate at which the plume idffuses from the centerline. Both coefficients represent exponential functions of x and are generally given in meters. The ratios vary according to atmospheric conditions as defined for the "Pasquill Stability Classes." Application of this formula gives X_W in g/m^3.

To determine the length of the thermal plume, we are concerned with the maximum distance along the centerline at the height, h, at which the concentration X_W exceeds the "deficit" value for a given temperature and humidity. Since, at this point, y = O and Z = h, the Gaussian plume diffusion formula simplifies to:

$$X_W (h,x,o,h) = \frac{Q}{2\pi\sigma_y\sigma_z u} \; 1 + e^{-2(\frac{h}{\sigma_z})}$$

From this expression, the mass of excess water vapor in the plume at the centerline can readily be calculated for any given value of the downwind distance, x, of which the dispersion coefficients are functions. It may be noted that for a ratio of h/σ_z of about 1.5 or more, the contribution of the exponential is negligible. For most ranges of interest, the expression is approximated quite well by $Q/2\pi u \sigma_{zy}$ and the length of the visible plume is essentially independent.

As an example, we calculate X_W for Pasquill stability classes B-F and for a range of distances increasing incrementally up to 20 km. A cut-off feature was supplied to end calculation for a particular stability class when the concentration at any distance fell below a threshold level. The resulting values were then compared to the "deficit" required for 95% saturation at given ambient temperature and humidity to determine the length of the visible plume under varying conditions.

The results of the computer runs are shown in Figures 4-3 and 4-4. These are nomograms by which to determine the maximum length of visible plume (airborne fog) as a function of temperature, relative humidity (R), stability category (Pasquill classes B-F) and associated wind speed in m/sec. Pasquill classes B and D are represented in Figure 4-3, whereas classes C, E and F appear in Figure 4-4. The logarithmic scales along the horizontal and vertical coordinates represent, respectively, distance (km) and mass of water vapor in air (g/m^3).

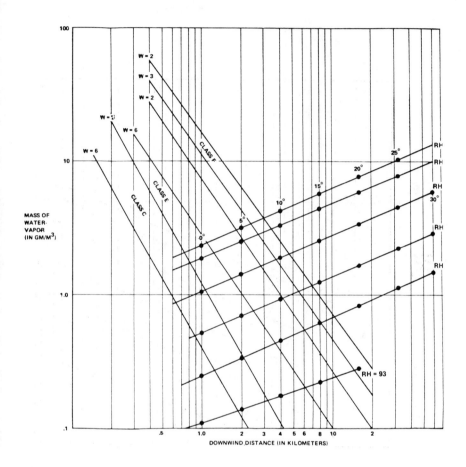

Figure 4-3. Maximum visible distance of plume for Pasquill classes C, E and F (Watson, 1973).

For a given RH, the mass of water vapor required for 95% saturation is plotted as a straight line slanting upward to the right. The deficit mass of water vapor required at selected temperatures (°C) corresponds to the value indicated on the vertical scale at the point where a large dot occurs on each RH plot. For example, at RH = 90, the 15°C dot is placed to denote a reading of 1.27 g/m³, which is the amount of water vapor that the plume must contain so that when added to that already in the atmosphere, 95% of saturation would result (and hence fogging or visible airborne plume is assumed).

The moisutre calculated to be in the plume is plotted for Pasquill stability classes and inclusive wind speeds as straight lines (wind speed lines)

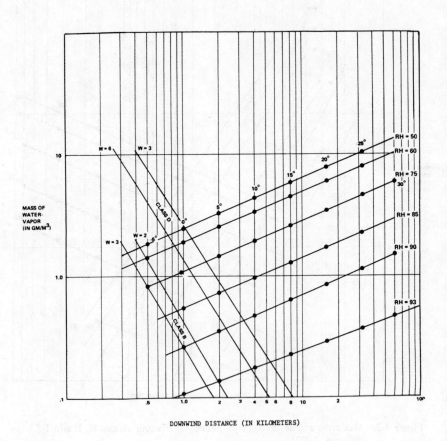

DOWNWIND DISTANCE (IN KILOMETERS)

Figure 4-4. Maximum visible distance of plume for Pasquill classes B and D (Watson, 1973).

slanting downward to the right. The maximum length of visible plume for a given wind condition, temperature and RH can be found as the distance(km) corresponding to the point at which the wind speed line intersects the horizontal extension of the appropriate dot on the RH line. For example, wind speed associated with Pasquill stability class C typically ranges between 2 and 6 m/sec. Wind speed lines for these inclusive velocities have accordingly been plotted. The line for wind speed 2 intersects the 0°C dot for RH = 85 at approximately 1.6 km and the 5° dot for RH = 90 at approximately 2.1 km. The w = 6 line intersects the RH 85 line, 0° dot, at about 850 m (0.85 km). These distance readings represent the computed maximum distances for the visible plume under the specified meteoroligical conditions.

Cooling Lakes

Vogel and Huff (1975) discussed the potential of fog initiation and enhancement due to cooling lakes. Their analysis indicates that natural midwinter fogs occur most frequently within the temperature ranges of -10 to 4° C, while midsummer fogs occur with temperatures of 15 to 20° C. The frequency with which a cooling lake will initiate or intensify existing fog and the density of the lake-related fog are strongly dependent on the nearness to saturation of the layer of air passing over the lake. The important condition for fogging is the saturation deficit of the air under natural conditions. Saturation deficits are defined as grams of water per kilogram of dry air needed to saturate the ambient air.

A typical saturation deficit of 0.5 g/kg or less occurs with winter fogs. Enhancement of existing fog is most likely to occur with deficits of 1 g/kg. In addition to the saturation deficit, minimum temperature difference and vapor pressure deficits are needed to produce heavy fog (30° F and 1 mb for heavy fog, in winter).

The operation of the cooling pond for a moderate-sized fossil fuel plant would favor the initiation of 250 to 300 hours of heavy fog during the winter. At present, there is not an adequate dispersion model to handle the downwind effect of this fog generation for the cooling pond situation.

TRANSPORTATION MODELS

In the transportation field, past efforts have focused on the problems of modeling supply and passenger demand. When energy prices were stable, transportation supply models were relatively easy to develop and keep current (Martin et al., 1964; Meyer et al., 1965; Institute for Defense Analysis, 1972; Gendell, 1973; Roess, 1974; Bhatt, 1976). Adequate passenger demand and intercity modeling has been more elusive. In general, transportation demand can be modeled at a micro- or a macrolevel. Microlevel models divide the physical area under study into subareas or zones, and deal with the amount of inter- and intrazonal travel. Macrolevel models deal only with the total amount of travel within the study area. Clearly, microlevel demand estimates could be summed to provide a macrolevel demand estimate, but as might be suspected, the data required by the former is considerably greater than the latter.

Four classes of microlevel models have evolved over the years: (1) sequential aggregate, (2) direct aggregate, (3) sequential disaggregate, and (4) direct disaggregate.

Traditionally, the travel demand forecasting process has relied on sequential disaggregate models (Schmidt and Campbell, 1956; Federal Highway Administration). Initially, data about the economic activity and socioeconomic makeup of the study are aggregated on a zone-by-zone basis into several variables, and forecasts of these variables are developed for each zone. From the forecasts, total traffic originating in each zone is estimated and subsequently distributed among zone destinations. The modal split model takes the zone-to-zone trips and allocates them to competing modes. Subsequent models allocate the traffic to routes. The approach has two problems. First, the models are run sequentially, with little or no feedback and, as such, are not representative of the decision processes involved in demanding and choosing transportation. Second, it requires large amounts of data.

These difficulties triggered development of other classes of microlevel demand models. One class, known as direct aggregate models, predicts demand by origin, destination and mode with a single equation—that is directly as opposed to a sequence of steps lacking feedback (Systems Analysis and Research Corp., 1963; Domencich et al., 1968; Quandt and Baumol, 1968; McLynn and Woronka, 1969; Billheimer, 1972).

Both the sequential and direct aggregate models rely on aggregated data —data for entire zones, whose sizes range from fractions of a square mile in urban applications to entire metropolitan areas in intercity applications. These kinds of models mask the variations of the individuals who actually make the transport demand decisions being modeled. Accordingly, much recent work has focused on predicting the transport demand decisions of individuals, or of individual households. Initially, the emphases was on sequential disaggregate models and, particularly, on models of the mode choice decision (Lave, 1969; Warner, 1962; Rassam et al., 1970; Watson, P.L., 1973; Spear, 1977). Such models attempt to determine the probability that an individual, or a household, with a particular set of characteristics will chose a particular mode, given the characteristics of all modes. Models of the choice of destination and the choice of making a trip have also been developed (Charles River Assoc., 1972).

The current thrust in microlevel demand modeling development seems pointed toward direct disaggregate models (Manheim, 1972; Stopher and Lavender, 1972; Ben-Akiva, 1973; Talvitie, 1973; McFadden and Reid, 1975), which attempt to determine the probability of an individual or a household making a trip to a particular destination area via a particular mode. The probability is assumed to be a function of the characteristics of the individual or household, of the relative attractiveness of the various destination areas, and of the relative attractiveness of the various modes.

It appears that macrolevel travel demand models have not received nearly as much attention as their microlevel counterparts (Simat *et al.,* 1972; Dot, 1977). One of the more notable efforts, based upon economic input-output analysis, supports the demand forecasts in the U.S. Department of Transportation's recent report: *National Transportation Trends and Choices* (1977).

Freight demand modeling has lagged passenger modeling slightly (Smith and Assoc., 1971; Hedges, 1971; Bolger and Bruck, 1973). Some early efforts, concerned primarily with mode shares on a nationwide basis, produced macrolevel models (Meyer *et al.,* 1959; Perle, 1964; Morton, 1969; Stucker, 1970), while others followed the traditional, or sequential aggregate approach (Hill, 1965; Mathematica, 1967/1969; Sloss and MacAvoy, 1967; Sloss, 1971; Surti and Ebrahami, 1972). Some macrolevel modeling continues (Wang and Epstein, 1975; Carleton *et al.,* 1975; Hutchinson, 1974; Slavin, 1976), but most current efforts focus on disaggregate models (Miklus, 1969; Antle and Haynes, 1971; Kullman, 1973; Hartwig and Linton, 1974; Roberts, 1976; Saski, 1976).

In general, both linear and nonlinear regression methods have been used to calibrate transport demand models. On the linear side, the generalized least squares method and the constrained least squares method have typically been used in macrolevel and in aggregate microlevel models. Limitations on the independent variables in disaggregate models have spawned the use of logit, probit and linear discriminant analysis methods as opposed to linear regression methods. In several well-publicized reports, the demand forecasting methodology is unspecified (FAA, 1977; NASA, 1976).

MODELING AMBIENT AIR QUALITY

This section evaluates available analytical techniques that can be employed to relate emissions to resulting ambient air quality for various points in the future on long- and short-term bases (Overbey *et al.,* 1976a). The purpose in examining the ambient air quality in place of exclusively examining emissions is that EPA has promulgated air quality standards, not emission standards, to protect public health. The setting of emission standards was instituted to achieve the established air quality standards. EPA's philosophy was that all locations within an area must conform to the prescribed standard. No individual location could exceed the standard without the entire area being considered in violation of the standard, even though the majority of locations may have been within compliance. Therefore, any analytical approach must be capable of examining the air quality of a large number of receptor locations since individual locations may change from a state of compliance to a state of noncompliance as growth occurs in emissions or as control techniques are applied.

The analytical technique must also have the capability to distinguish between the contribution to ambient air quality and major categories of emission sources, since control technologies have variations in effectiveness, feasibility, time availability and cost implications across the different emission categories. At a minimum, the technique must be capable of reflecting contributions to ambient air quality from the stationary and mobile emission sectors. Further resolution within each of these sectors is useful.

The relationship between emissions and ambient air quality at a particular point also depends on a number of factors such as emission height, atmospheric chemistry, meteorological condition and topography. These must be accurately reflected in the selected technique. Below, each class of model is examined in light of these criteria, to determine inherent fundamental assumptions, input data requirements, computational effort and basic accuracy for estimating ambient air quality (Table 4-5).

Types of Models Available

The models currently available can be placed in one of the following four categories: (1) rollforward or rollback models; (2) modified rollback models; (3) nonreactive dispersion models; or (4) reactive dispersion models. A description of various model categories follows:

Rollforward or Rollback Models

The simplest technique for relating the changes in emission to changes in ambient air concentration of the pollutant is the so-called "rollback" or "rollforward" technique. The model is generally expressed as follows:

$$C_i = b + K_i \Sigma_j e_j$$

where:

C_i = ambient concentration of the pollutant at receptor location i

b = "irreducible" background concentration; b contains natural background concentrations plus the dispersion of emissions from other geographic areas and is not completely irreducible

K_i = proportionality factor, which takes into account the meteorology and source-receptor distance and the other factors that influence the source-receptor interaction for all sectors simultaneously.

The value of the proportionality factor is determined by solving the equation for a known emission inventory, an ambient pollutant concentration at a point corresponding in time and for a known (or assumed) value of the background concentration.

To develop projections of AAQ for future time periods using this model, one would develop a new estimate of the future emissions (including the effects of controls) and then calculate a new value of pollutant concentration. With this formulation, projections can be made for any geographic location for which the proportionality factor can be determined. Both long- and short-term concentrations could theoretically be developed given adequate and appropriate emission inventories.

An inherent assumption in this model is a linear relationship between changes in emission and ambient air quality. There is an assumption that the geographic deployment of future emissions is at the same location as that used in deriving the proportionality factor. Further, uniform growth between the various emission sectors is assumed.

Although the minimal computational effort and data requirements of this model make it appealing, it does not permit a detailed consideration of nonuniform emission growth or control introductions. Further, the nonavailability of necessary ambient air quality observations at potential locations of interest is a serious drawback.

Modified Rollback Model

The modified rollback model is similar to the rollback except that individual proportionality factors are determined for each emission sector. The model formulation is:

$$C_i = b + \Sigma_j K_{ij} e_j$$

where C_i, b and e_j are as before and K_{ij} is the factor relating emissions from sector j to ambient air concentration at receptor location i.

The modified rollback model represents a major improvement over the simple rollback model by making it possible to consider situations involving nonuniform rates of growth and control applications since the K_{ij} term relates individual emission sectors to the ambient air quality at a receptor point. The increased detail in the model is obtained at the cost of increasing the workload required to obtain the K_{ij} term in the model. As opposed to the simple rollback model, the spatial and meteorological characteristics associated with each emission sector are necessary for this model to obtain a valid K_{ij} term. Each emission sector may have very different characteristics (*e.g.*, height of emissions and location) and a deaggregation of the contributions from each emission sector to the receptor point is

Table 4-5. Comparison of Air Quality Models (Overbey *et al.*, 1976b)

Category Subcategory	Model Name (or relevant document) & Organization/ Individual(s) Involved	Sources Handled	Description of Technique used in Model	Input Data Requirements
Simple Rollback	"Determining Source Reduction Needed to Meet Air Quality Standards R. I. Larson	SP[a], SA, M[b]	This model is based on the assumption of a linear relationship between changes in emission rates and changes in ambient air quality (concentration). The parameters of this relationship are determined empirically	K value for point of AAQ observation Observed concentrations Associated emissions Background concentration (if available)
Modified Rollback Moving cell or box model Emission Plume Model	"Mathematical Modeling of Photochemical Smog Using PICK Method R. C. Sklarew, *et al.* "Workbook of Atmospheric Dispersion Estimates" D. B. Turner Office of Air Programs EPA	SP, SA, M SP, SA, M	The modified rollback models are based on the assumption of a linear relationship between changes in ambient air quality. Individual proportionality factors are estimated for various emittor-receptor pairs The proportionality factors are dependent on the relative locations of emitters and receptors, wind speed and direction, mixing depth, plume height and stability of the atmosphere	K value for point(s) at which AAQ observation is taken Observed concentrations at these receptor points Rates of emissions from various sources and the location of these sources Wind speed, direction and mixing depth Background concentration (if available)
Nonreactive Diffusion Models Gaussian dispersion from a ground level crosswind infinite line source	"An Atmospheric Diffusion Model for Metropolitan Areas" (Miller/ Holzworth model) Marvin E. Miller George C. Holzworth	SP, SA, M[b]	This model is based on the Gaussian dispersion equation for an infinite crosswind tine source emitting at ground level The highest ambient concentration (which occurs at the downwind edge of the community) is obtained by integrating the dispersion equation across the length of the community	Average community-wide emissions rate Average wind speed throughout the mixing layer Average mixing depth

Table 4-5, continued

Output Details	Computing Requirements	Cost of Operation	Advantages Associated with the use of this Model or Merits of the Model	Disadvantages Associated with use of this Model	Underlying Assumptions Comments
Average ambient concentration for one or more points in the community Model can be calibrated for any averaging time	Manual	Low	Very simple Input data requirements are minimal	Purely theoretical with no experimental verification Requires uniform growth rates and uniform reductions in emissions Does not account for meteorological and and chemical variations Cannot model short-lived pollutants except under special conditions.	Assumes a linear relationship between incremental changes in emissions and incremental changes in concentration of the pollutant Assumes constant meteorology
Average ambient air concentrations at various receptor points Proportionality factors for different emittor-receptor pairs The model can be calibrated for any averaging time	Manual or computer Low to medium	Low to medium Low to medium	With the proportionality factors based on diffusion, it is possible to test the underlying assumptions against experimental data It is possible to predict the spatial distribution of various concentrations of pollutants on a given day for some long period of time The computed spatial distribution can be compared with measured air quality and models modified to produce superior agreement These models can be used for making short-term predictions for specific meteorological conditions Source-specific $K_{i, j}$ valves make it possible to estimate contributions by various emittors to to concentration of NO_x at various receptors Overall, these models are suitable for a greater degree of experimental confirmation of their prediction The input data and computational requirements are less tringent than those for reactive models With the exception of a few highly reactive pollutants, these models generate predictions which are not significantly inferior to those made by reactive models	It is usually difficult to get emissions data with sufficient accuracy These models have been experimentally tested for SO_2 and TSP, but they have not been adequately developed and tested for photochemical oxidants, NO_2 or hydrocarbons	A linear relationship is assumed between incremental changes in emissions and incremental changes in the concentration of the pollutant Incremental changes in the pollutant concentration produced by emission changes at various sources are assumed to be additive For a given pattern of emissions, the concentrations of other reactive pollutants and the level of photochemical activity are assumed to remain constant
Average ambient concentration for the community as a whole Hourly or annual averages	Manual (computations are based on reference tables)	Low	Easy and inexpensive to use once the emissions rates have been determined Gives fairly accurate results Although this model is theoretical, empirical validation of the results have been carried out successfully. Results for NO_x concentrations have been unexpectedly good for a nonreactive model	Errors are caused when there are many point sources with high stacks (this model assumes zero emission height for all sources Results are erroneous when there are nonuniformly distributed sources Future projections require assumption of uniform growth rate in emissions	A symetrical shape and uniform distribution of emission sources are assumed for the community under consideration All sources are assumed to discharge emissions at ground level The peak concentration is always assumed to occur at the downwind edge of the community

Table 4-5, continued

Category Subcategory	Model Name (or relevant document) & Organization/ Individual(s) Involved	Sources Handled	Description of Technique used in Model	Input Data Requirements
Atmospheric Dispersion as a function of rate of vertical Plume expansion	Hanna/Gifford models "The Simple ATOL Urban Air Pollution Model", "A Simple Method of Calculating Dispersion from Urban Area Sources" "A Simple Dispersion Model for Analysis of Chemically Reactive Pollutants"[b] E. A. Gifford Steven R. Hanna	SP, SA	The community is divided into equal-sized, two-divisional cells by superimposition of a grid pattern Area source strengths are calculated for each cell The ambient concentration in the cube above any one cell depends only on the emissions in that cell, the average wind speed and the category of atmospheric stability Average community-wide values obtained either by averaging the values for all cubes, or expanding the size of the cells until one cell covers the entire community	Emission rates for stationary area and certain point sources Wind speed Wind direction (for short-term averages)
Nonreactive Diffusion Models Mathematical simulation of atmospheric diffusion processes	"Air Quality Display Model" (AQDM) TRW Systems Group	SP, SA, M	Through a mathematical simulation of the atmospheric diffusion, this model determines the estimated arithmetic average annual concentrations of pollutants at ground level over an annual period The model can generate isopleths of various concentration levels in the region	Emission rates Wind speeds and direction Atmospheric stability Observed air quality concentrations
Semiempirical receptor oriented spatially, disaggregate diffusion simulation	"ERT/MARTIK" Model Environmental Research and Technology, Inc.	SP, M	This model uses a modified Gaussian plume equation which is theoretically more appealing than the conventional Gaussian plume equation The plume diffusion equation is integrated in both X and Y directions for area sources rather than using the virtual point source approach of the AQDM Model	Similar to those of AQDM Model
Semitheoretical spatially disaggregated air diffusion model	"A Transportation and Air Shed Simulation Model" (TASSIM) (combination of Hanna/ Gifford and ERT/ MARTIK Models) Ingram, Fauth and Kroch Harvard University	SP, SA, M	This model is a composite of three sub-models; transportation, vehicle emissions and air diffusion model The air diffusion model is a combination of Hanna/Gifford and the MARTIK Models	Combination of input elements for Hanna/ Gifford and ERT/ MARTIK models for area sources Distribution of trips and speeds for mobile sources Observations at monitoring stations (for calibration)

Table 4-5, continued

Output Details	Computing Requirements	Cost of Operation	Advantages Associated with the use of this Model or Merits of the Model	Disadvantages Associated with use of this Model	Underlying Assumptions Comments
				Entire community is the smallest spatial unit, and only one estimate is generated. Not very satisfactory for reactive pollutants	
Average ambient concentration for 1-mile-square blocks Averages can be generated for selected averaging times	Manual or computer	Low to medium	Simple and inexpensive to use Estimates of long-term averages appear to be quite accurate	Results are not accurate when disparities in emission rates from neighboring area sources are large and/or wind blown predominantly in one direction Short-term concentration estimates are not always accurate Results are not good when there are large point sources having high smoke stacks The "reactive" version does not yield consistently good results	In the nonreactive version, it is assumed that the ambient concentration in the cube above any cell depends only on the emissions in that cell, the average wind speed and the category of atmospheric stability The reactive version is based on a modified form of conservation of mass law and includes terms for mass movement out of this area, emissions within the area and photochemical reaction
Average ambient concentrations Seasonal or annual averages	Computer	Moderate to high	This model is semi-empirical and can be validated This model can handle emissions from all types of sources The estimated concentrations are sensitive to meteorological variations Contributions to ambient concentrations from various sources are computed and these outputs can be used in a modified rollback model	The operating and calibration costs can be high The results are satisfactory for long-term averages only This model has not been proved completely successful for modeling reactive pollutants	The chemical and photochemical reaction rates are assumed to remain constant for a given meteorology The same meteorology is assumed for the entire region
Output is similar to output of the AQDM model	Computer	High	This model is theoretically more sound than the ADQM Model This model can be readily coupled to planning data	The operating and calibrating costs can be quite high The results are satisfactory for long-term averages only This model has not been successful in modeling reactive pollutants	The underlying assumptions are similar to those for the ADQM model
Average ambient concentration for areas as small as 1/2 square mile Concentration averages by hour, day or year	Computer	High	This model has satisfactory accuracy for NO_x The model applicability can be transferred to other communities	In small region, the spatial resolution may be limited Start-up and calibration costs may be high The results have been good for long-term averages only	The diffusion model, being a combination of Hanna/Gifford and AQDM, is based on a combination of the assumptions for these models

Table 4-5, continued

Category Subcategory	Model Name (or relevant document) & Organization/ Individual(s) Involved	Sources Handled	Description of Technique used in Model	Input Data Requirements
Semiempirical receptor oriented diffusion model for two nonreactive pollutants	"Climatological Dispersion Model" (CDM) A. D. Busse J. R. Zimmerman E.P.A. - R.T.P	SP, SA, M	This is a modification of the AQDM A theoretically superior plume rise representation is used, as compared to AQDM Pollutant removal processes are simulated by simple exponential decay functions	Emission Rates Joint wind speed, wind direction and atmospheric stability frequencies Average mixing depth
Semiempirical diffusion model for mobile sources	"Urban Diffusion Model for Vehicular Pollutants" (APRAC) Stanford Research Institute	M^f	For emissions within the region under study, line sources are averaged over segments of sections which radiate out from each receptor point in the wind direction CO transported from surrounding areas is simulated by using simple box model Contributions from each sector within the region are calculated through Gaussian Plume equation A street canyon submodel simulates ground level concentrations in a street bordered by high rise buildings	Vehicle speed and volume per link Average hourly closed cover Temperature, atmospheric stability and mixing depth Wind direction and wind speed
Gaussian steady-state dispersion model	RAM Joan Hrenko Novak D. Bruce Turner EPA	SP, SA	The model makes short-term dispersion estimates using steady-state Gaussian equations Briggs plume rise equations are used for estimation of concentrations from point sources Concentrations from area sources are estimated using a narrow plume hypothesis and using area source squares as given rather than breaking down all area sources to an area of uniform elements	For point sources: source coordinates, emission rates, physical height, stack gas volume flow, stack gas temperature For area sources: coordinate of S-W Corner, area sources emissions rates, effective area source height Wind direction, wind speed, stability class and mixing height (hourly)
Reactive Dispersion Models Fixed coordinate system	"A Simulation Model for Estimating Ground Level Concentrations of Photochemical Pollutants" (SAI) Reynolds, et al. Systems Applications, Inc.	SP, SA, M	This model uses a system of fixed coordinates and computes hourly average concentrations of pollutants in a three-dimensional grid This model is based on the finite difference solution of the equations of conservation of mass using the method of fractional steps Variations in meteorology, as well as photochemical and chemical activity are accounted for through kinetic mechanism factors	Locations of point sources and emission rates including hourly variations Data pertaining to auto usage and aircraft operations Emission rates for area sources Meteorological data including mixing depth Initial ambient concentrations

Table 4-5, continued

Output Details	Computing Requirements	Cost of Operation	Advantages Associated with the use of this Model or Merits of the Model	Disadvantages Associated with use of this Model	Underlying Assumptions Comments
Average ambient concentrations at unlimited number of locations Annual averages	Computer	High	The spatial resolution is as good as that of the emissions inventory Estimates can be made for an unlimited number of receptors The results for annual averages are quite good	The cost of calibration and operation is high Only long-term averages are estimated Incremental contributions from individual sources cannot be ascretained easily	The underlying assumptions are similar to those for the AQDM
Isopleths based on ambient concentration at predetermined receptor points Hourly or annual averages can be generated	Computer	High	The model is well disaggregated spatially For urban areas, the simulation of CO diffusion is more realistic than that obtained by using other models This model can generate short- and long-term estimates	This model can be used for CO only The accuracy of the results of this model is yet to be established	This model is based on the usual assumptions associated with "Gaussian" plume equation models
Ambient concentrations at a number of receptor points Average concentrations for periods ranging from one to 24 hours can be estimated	Computer	Medium to high	Average concentrations for periods as short as one hour can be estimated The algorithm is very efficient The model provides guidance for selecting important receptor points	The results are satisfactory only when the region is level or there is a gently rolling terrain This model gives good results for relatively stable pollutants only (NO_x does not belong to this category) Data for stack gas volume flow and temperature are needed This algorithm cannot handle mobile source emissions Area sources must be squares and the effective area source height must be known	The region under consideration is assumed to be level or gently rolling The pollutant being modeled is assumed to be relatively stable Concentrations from area sources are estimated by using a narrow plume hypothesis
Estimated ambient concentrations at various grid points and/or selected receptor points Estimates of instantaneous and average concentrations	Computer	High	This model accounts for the chemical and photochemical reactions involving reactive pollutants This model can provide short- as well as long-term averages The estimated ambient concentrations are sensitive to variations in the emissions and concentrations of all pollutants The estimated ambient concentrations are sensitive to meteorological variations	Model runs have indicated that there may be inaccuracies in the model due to incomplete understanding of the highly complex processes being simulated Each simulation requires input concerning initial pollutant concentrations and mixing volume, which may be difficult to ascertain Input data requirements are substantial The nature and magnitude of temporal and spatial variations in emissions has to be determined with sufficient accuracy. This	Due to incomplete understanding of the chemical and meteorological processes which affect concentrations of reactive pollutants, numerous assumptions have been made in order to simulate these processes As a better understanding of these processes is developed, many of these assumptions may be relaxed

Table 4-5, continued

Category Subcategory	Model Name (or relevant document) & Organization/ Individual(s) Involved	Sources Handled	Description of Technique used in Model	Input Data Requirements
Fixed coordinate system	"UCLA-Reactive Diffusion Model" C.Y. Lui and Parrine U.C.L.A.	SP, SA, M	This technique can be viewed as a two-dimensional model for the transport of pollutants in an air basin. The dispersion and "conservation of mass" equations are completely independent of vertical diffusivity. Horizontal diffusion also plays a minor role in the transport of pollutants	Distribution of wind speeds and directions Height of inversion base Turbulent diffusivity Inventory of emission sources, including spatial distribution of traffic Initial ambient conditions
Trajectory Approach	"Reactive Environmental Stimulation Model" (REM) L.G. Wayne et al. Pacific Environmental Services, Inc.	SP,SA,M	The model generates estimates of the concentrations of nonreactive and reactive pollutants by utilizing a moving cell approach in which changes within a hypothetical parcel of air are computed as the parcel traverses the air shed.	The input data requirements are similar to those of the SAI and UCLA Models.
Moving Cell Approach	"Diffusion Model for Photochemical Smog Simulation" (DIFKIN) (GRC Model) A. Q. Eschenroeder, et al. General Research Corporation	SP,SA,M	This model uses a technique similar to that used in the REM.	The imput data requirements are similar to those of the SAI Model.

aSP–Starting Point; SA–Stationary Area; M–Mobile
bEmissions from all types of sources are averaged.
cThis is a more complicated version, which treats reactive as well as nonreactive pollutants. However, the model is simpler than the photochemical reactive models. This version of the Hanna/Gifford Model could also be included in the ' reactive" models category.

Table 4-5, continued

Output Details	Computing Requirements	Cost of Operation	Advantages Associated with the use of this Model or Merits of the Model	Disadvantages Associated with use of this Model	Underlying Assumptions Comments
				is not always possible The type of data needed for mobile sources cannot be secured easily The treatment of area sources can create problems due to nonuniform spatial distribution of emissions from these sources The calibration, startup and operating expenses of this model can be very large	
Ambient concentrations of pollutants at a number of receptor points Isopleths	Computer	High	This two-dimensional model is considerably simpler than three-dimensional models Since vertical diffusivity is ignored, knowledge of vertical wind velocity component is not required The computations are simplified significantly by the assumption of zero diffusion in vertical direction	Since the model assumes that advection plays a major role in the transportation of pollutants; the estimates generated by the model may not be accurate when wind speeds are low.	The atmosphere below the inversion base is uniformly mixed along the vertical axis over a time scale on the order of 1 hr. The atmosphere in the layer below the inversion base is similar to that in a well-mixed estuary where horizontal advection is large compared to vertical advection. Horizontal diffusion is much less important than horizontal advection in the transport of the pollutant.
Ambient concentrations are estimated at points along trajectories emanating from the point of origin.	Computer	High	The advantages associated with the use of SAI and UCLA models hold for this model also.	Most of the disadvantages listed in connection with the SAI model are associated with the use of the REM. The validation of a moving cell model is complicated because the cell trajectories rarely pass over a monitoring station. Validation based on spatial interpolation can produce large errors.	The assumptions associated with this model are generally similar to those underlying the SAI model.
Ambient concentrations are estimated at points along the path of a moving cell of air which traverses the air shed.	Computer	High	The advantages listed for the SAI model hold for this model.	The disadvantages associated with the use of the GRC Model are similar to those listed for the REM.	The assumptions underlying this model are similar to the assumptions for the REM.

dStationary sources can be treated by handling them as a composite of a number of line sources.
eThis model is suitable for simulating mobile area sources which are approximately by-line sources for the purpose of developing Gaussian dispersion equations.

present. However, the deaggregation results in a corresponding need for an increasingly accurate description of the transport mechanism and emissions from each emission sector to a receptor point than it does in the simple rollback technique.

The modified rollback model, when applied to future conditions, will reflect changes in growth and controls by individual sectors. However, the limitations imposed by assumptions in the simple rollback technique concerning linear emissions concentration relationship, and temporal and spatial invariance of emissions are still associated with the utilization of this technique. Further, like the simple rollback model, this model does not explicitly account for the reactivity of pollutants. Because of the above constraints, the modified rollback model lacks the capability of making reasonably good future short-term ambient air quality estimates.

Nonreactive Dispersion Models

The nonreactive dispersion/diffusion models are based on mathematical simulation of the physical processes that affect primary pollutants after they are released into the atmosphere. These models are semitheoretical, semiempirical and are generally classified as Gaussian plume models. If the effect of chemical and photochemical reactions is not significant, the Gaussian plume diffusion model gives satisfactory results. If the reactions are significant, the calibration of these models can be expected to account for some of the reactions involving reactive pollutants.

The physical behavior of a plume containing a pollutant is represented mathematically by a Gaussian dispersion equation. The actual dispersion phenomenon is governed by the wind speed and the vertical and horizontal diffusion coefficients, which depend on the atmospheric stability, and the mechanical turbulance from surface roughness. Along the direction of the wind, the wind has the effect of stretching the plume, if convection exceeds the diffusion along this direction. The system of coordinates and equations used in the Gaussian model for a simple source is shown schematically in Figure 4-5.

The Gaussian expression for the ambient concentration at point P is:

$$c(x,y,z,H) = \frac{E}{2\pi\sigma_y \sigma_q U} \exp\left[-\frac{1}{2}\left(\frac{y}{\sigma_y}\right)^2\right] \left[\exp\left(-\frac{1}{2}\left(\frac{z-H}{\sigma_y}\right)^2\right) + \exp\left(-\frac{1}{2}\left(\frac{z+H}{\sigma_z}\right)^2\right)\right]$$

where:

C = concentration, gm/m^3

E = rate of emissions, gm/sec
U = average wind speed, m/sec
σ_y
σ_z = diffusion coefficients in y and z directions, m

H = effective height of the source, m

The ground-level ambient concentration at a receptor located at point G is obtained by setting Z = 0. The diffusion coefficients, σ_y and σ_z, are functions of the wind speed and the atmospheric stability condition. Turner (1970) has prepared tables and charts giving values of σ_y and σ_z as functions of atmospheric stability category and the downwind distance from the source.

The equation can be "solved" for a variety of cases of interest, such as ground-level concentration (z = 0) or integrated for several receptor points. The above equation is for a point source and receptors not further out from the source than 5 km. The model can be modified to handle line sources (*e.g.,* highway traffic) and area sources (*e.g.,* residential area).

Plume Rise

The effective stack height (h) is greater than the actual stack height (h_o) because of the buoyancy of the plume. For stability classes A through D, $h = h_o + h$

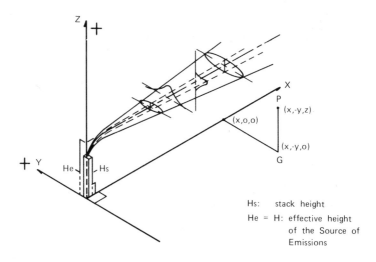

Hs: stack height
He = H: effective height of the Source of Emissions

SOURCE: Harry C. Perkins: "Air Pollution", McGraw Hill Co.

Figure 4-5. Coordinate system showing Gaussian distributions in the horizontal and vertical.

where:

$$\Delta h = 1.6F^{1/3} \; u^{-1} \; x^{2/3} \text{ for } x \leqslant 3.5x^*$$

$$\Delta h = 1.6F^{1/3} \; u^{-1} \; (3.5x^*)^{2/3} \text{ for } x > 3.5x^*$$

$$x^* = 14F^{5/8} \text{ when } F < 55 \text{ m}^4/\text{sec}^3$$

$$x^* = 34F^{2/5} \text{ when } F \geqslant 55 \text{ m}^4/\text{sec}^3$$

$$F = gwr^2 \left(\frac{T_s - T_e}{T_e} \right)$$

g = gravitational acceleration (m/sec^2)
w = stack gas ejection velocity (m/sec)
r = radius of stack (m)
T_s = stack gas temperature ($^\circ$K)
T_e = air temperature ($^\circ$K)

For stability classes E and F the plume rise becomes:

$$\Delta h = 2.9 \left(\frac{F}{us} \right)^{1/3}$$

where:

$$s = \frac{g}{T_e} \frac{d\theta}{dz}$$

$$\frac{d\theta}{dz} = 0.02 \; ^\circ\text{K/m for stability E}$$

$$\frac{d\theta}{dz} = 0.035 \; ^\circ\text{K/m for stability F}$$

For distances greater than 2 x_L, where x_L is given by $\sigma_z (x_L) = 0.47L$, the equation in Figure 4-5 may be approximated by:

$$x_i (x,y,z) = \frac{Q_i (x) \exp \left(\dfrac{-y^2}{2 \; \sigma_y^2 (x)} \right)}{\sqrt{2\pi} \; \sigma_y(x) \; u \; L} \qquad x > 2 \; x_L$$

where:

L = depth of the mixing layer (m).

Chemical Deposition and Washout

The effective source strength can be calculated from a knowledge of deposition and washout.

The deposition rate $W(x,y)$ is evaluated from the following equation:

$$\omega_i (x,y) = v_i \chi_i (x,y,0) + \Lambda_i \int_0^L \chi_i (x,y,z) \; dz$$

where:

ω_i (x,y) = deposition rate of pollutant i (gm/m^2/sec)
v_i = deposition velocity of pollutant i (m/sec)
Λ_i = washout coefficient of pollutant i (sec^{-1})

The depletion of the source strength Q(x) per unit distance is then given by:

$$\frac{\partial Q_i (x)}{\partial x} = - \int_{-\infty}^{\infty} \omega_i (x,y)\,dy$$

Solving for Q_i (x) the following expression is obtained:

$$Q_i (x) = Q_i (0) \exp \left(- \int_0^x \beta_{i} (x')dx' \right)$$

where:

$$\beta_i(x) = \left(\frac{2}{\pi}\right)^{1/2} \frac{v_i}{u\sigma_z(x)} \exp \left(- \frac{h^2(x)}{2\sigma_z^2(x)} \right) + \frac{\Lambda_i}{u}$$

The manner in which most existing dispersion models have been pro-grammed readily permits ambient pollutant concentrations to be calculated for multiple receptor locations and offers a great deal of flexibility of re-solution into the emission sectors. The model formulation adequately ad-dresses the influence of emission height (*e.g.,* stack height or automobile exhaust height) on ground-level receptor concentrations. Also, a number of models permit multiple wind speed, direction and stability conditions. Future estimates can be developed for either short- or long-term projections, depending on the nature of the input parameters.

Developing future projections of ambient pollutant concentrations by use of dispersion models requires specification of all emission inventory parameters. The degree to which meaningful estimates of the large number of these parameters can be specified is low.

These models, developed primarily for application to problems involving inert pollutants such as SO_2, CO or particulates, have been used for model-ing NO_2 dispersion. The assumptions used as an attempt to account for the photochemical reactive nature of NO_x include: (1) considering all NO_x from sources to be considered as NO_2; and (2) alternatively, the specification of an exponential "half-life growth" rate for NO_2. Frequently, model projected concentrations are adjusted by the use of regression to observed pollutant concentration to improve the model accuracy. Sur-prisingly, the results are generally good. The computational costs of using dispersion models are higher than those associated with using rollback types of models and the data collection costs are much greater.

In summary, dispersion models offer significant improvements over the rollback (or modified rollback) category only if an accurate emissions inventory is available for the future time period to be examined. Unfortunately, the results of using the relatively accurate transport model are far overwhelmed by the uncertainties associated with the future location and characteristics of emissions when 10- to 20-year forecasts of ambient air quality are to be examined.

Reactive Diffusion Models

The "reactive" diffusion models are based on a solution of the "conservation of mass" equation and the documented process occurring during dispersion. These models are considerably more complex than the nonreactive models. Such models are most appropriate for estimating the ambient concentration of reactive pollutants because chemical reactions (including processes of accumulation and dispersion) diminish the concentration of some pollutants while the concentrations of other pollutants are increased by these phenomena.

The general form of the "conservation of mass" equation used in reactive diffusion models is presented below:

$$\frac{\partial \chi_i}{\partial t} + \sum_{j=1}^{3} \frac{\partial}{\partial x_j} (u_j \chi_1) = \sum_{j=1}^{3} D_i \frac{\partial^2 \chi_i}{\partial x_j^2}$$
$$+ R_i (\chi_1, \chi_2, \ldots \chi_N)$$
$$+ S_i (x_1, x_2, x_3, t)$$

where:

χ_i	=	concentration of ith species (g/m^3)
u_j	=	jth component of the windspeed (m/sec)
D_i	=	molecular diffusivity of the ith species (m^2/sec) (may be ignored for most applications)
R_i	=	production rate of ith species due to chemical reactions (g/sec)
S_i	=	source term for ith species at (x_1, x_2, x_3) (g/sec)
t	=	time (sec)

Separating the concentrations (χ_i) and windspeeds (u_j) vectors into average ($<\chi_i>$, $<u_j>$) and stochastic components (χ_i', u_j'), and assuming that the term $<u_j'\chi_i'>$ can be linearly related to the gradient of the average concentration, the equation of turbulent diffusion is reconstituted:

$$\frac{\partial <\chi_i>}{\partial t} + \sum_{j=1}^{3} <u_j> \frac{\partial <\chi_i>}{\partial x_j} = \sum_{j=1}^{3} \sum_{k=1}^{3} \frac{\partial}{\partial x_j} K_{jk} \frac{\partial <\chi_i>}{\partial x_k}$$

$$+ R_i \quad <\chi_1 >, \ldots, <\chi_N >$$
$$+ S_i (x_1, x_2, x_3, t)$$

where:

K_{jk} = eddy diffusivity tensor (m^2/sec)

Numerical methods for solving the above equation fall into two categories. The first technique requires that a parcel of air be followed along a calculated trajectory for which time-dependent emissions are specified. Although this scheme is relatively simple, it allows the air quality to be predicted only along certain trajectories. The fixed coordinate or grid solution to the transport-kinetics problem gives a determination of air quality over the entire urban area at a particular instant of time, but requires large amounts of computer storage and time.

To make reasonably accurate estimates of ambient concentrations, the "conservation of mass" equation has to be solved a number of times for every time period (e.g., hour) of simulation. The requirement of frequent solution of this equation along with the collection and preparation of the requisite data input for a reactive model becomes a major task that can be undertaken for simulations involving short time periods only. Consequently, numerous assumptions are frequently made for reducing the input data requirements and simplifying the solution process. It is obvious that these assumptions would lead to a reduced accuracy of the model predictions.

The reactive models developed by Systems Applications Inc. (SAI) (Hecht, 1973) and UCLA (Liu and Goodin, 1976) employ a fixed coordinate system in which ambient concentrations of pollutants are estimated as hourly averages in a two- or three-dimensional grid. The moving cell or trajectory approach is followed in two other reactive models developed by the General Research Corporation (DIFKIN) (Eochenroeder, et al., 1972) and Pacific Environmental Services (REM) (Wayne, et al., 1973). In the DIFKIN and REM models, concentration changes are estimated within a hypothetical cell of air as this cell traverses the airshed being studied.

All existing reactive models are very complex, and require massive data inputs (the SAI model requires 40,000 words of input for simulating a single day for the Los Angeles Air Basin). The computational requirements of these models are also substantial. Perhaps the most demanding requirement of the models is the specification of the "initial conditions" for each simulation run. Despite incomplete understanding of the photochemical kinetics of open system reactions, and the assumptions made for simplifying the solution process, the accuracy of these models tends to be reasonably good. To use these models for making accurate estimates of short-term average ambient concentrations, it is necessary to account for temporal and spatial variations in emissions over exceedingly short periods of time. However, data pertaining to such variations are virtually nonexistent.

At present, existing reactive models should be regarded as effective techniques for simulating complex chemical reactions that can result in the estimation of short-term average concentrations when the emissions inventory, meteorological condition and pollutant mix are relatively well known. The difficulties associated with the collection of input data, and the potential requirement of a rigorous calibration activity, make this category of models unattractive from a cost standpoint for use in situations involving policy decisions concerned with future projections of long-time horizons.

PROGRESS IN AIR POLLUTION MODELING

Recent advances (Knox, 1976) in the simulation of regional air quality and pollutant distributions have emphasized passive and reactive pollutants emitted from distributed sources and/or multiple point sources. The models incorporate transport-diffusion, chemical transformation, deposition and the effect of complex terrain. The major new models are a regional mass-consistent wind field modeling (MATHEW); a three-dimensional Lagrangian-Eulerian transport-diffusion model (ADPIC); and a passive or photochemical-pollutant simulation model (LIRAQ).

Mathew

The MATHEW model (Sherman, 1975) provides a three-dimensional, time-averaged wind field for calculating the regional advective transport of pollutants. The model incorporates the effect of complex terrain. The adjusted wind field satisfies the variable lower boundary condition prescribed by the specified terrain; lateral and upper boundary conditions are open and are satisfied by the velocity potential equal zero. MATHEW is an interpolation scheme for providing estimates of the three-dimensional wind vector. The interpolation scheme includes the influence of topography in shaping the terrain-controlled airflow. With the current implementation of this model, adjusted three-dimensional winds can be obtained on a grid of 30 to 40,000 grid points in a few minutes of CDC 7600 computer time.

ADPIC (Atmospheric Diffusion Particle-in Cell)

ADPIC is a numerical, three-dimensional, particle diffusion model (Lange, 1973, 1974, 1976) for calculating the time-dependent (regional) distribution of air pollutants under conditions of speed and directional wind shear (input to ADPIC grid provided by MATHEW); "calm" or light wind conditions, variable terrain roughness, material deposition, decay, and spatial and temporal diffusion parameters. The method is based on the particle-in-cell technique with the pollutant concentration represented statistically.

The MATHEW/ADPIC computer codes have been verified against several regional field tracer studies (Lange, 1975).

LIRAQ (Livermore Regional Air Quality) Model

LIRAQ (MacCracken, 1975; MacCracken and Sauter, 1975) is an Eulerian (fixed spatial grid) multicell regional air pollution model that incorporates mass-consistent advection, eddy diffusion appropriate to the grid size and photochemical reaction kinetics. The input data include regional topography, meteorology and pollutant source inventory for the region. LIRAQ calculates the temporal and spatial distributions of pollutant concentrations at ground level and the mean concentration between ground level and the base of the inversion layer. The model is modular, with a module (submodel) for each of the major steps, generation of mass-consistent wind fields from meteorological and topographical data, pollutant transport and chemical kinetics. This facilitates the adaptation of the model to new conditions. The chemical kinetics submodel can be modified or expanded without significantly affecting the transport submodel, or the topography and meteorology of one region can be readily replaced by those of another.

The model exists in two versions. LIRAQ-1 is designed to treat the transport of pollutants without detailed photochemical kinetics. LIRAQ-2 has been designed to treat complex chemical reactions (15 active species and 50 reactions) in detail.

WATER MODELS

The general framework for model building in terms of water quality and quantity is displayed as Figure 4-6. Any water model could be mapped onto this general flowchart (Shahane, 1976). From a technical viewpoint, we recognize three kinds of models: (1) water quality, (2) hydraulic, and (3) hydrology. Water quality models analyze the interrelationship between various physical, chemical and biological processes in the equatic system. Hydraulic models are based on and consider the hydrodynamics of a water system. Hydrology models are budgeting and accounting models establishing the balance between precipitation, evapotranspiration, storage, seepage, atmospheric transport and runoff.

A number of groups, agencies and authors have made comparisons of different models in use and are given in the Tables 4-6 to 4-12.

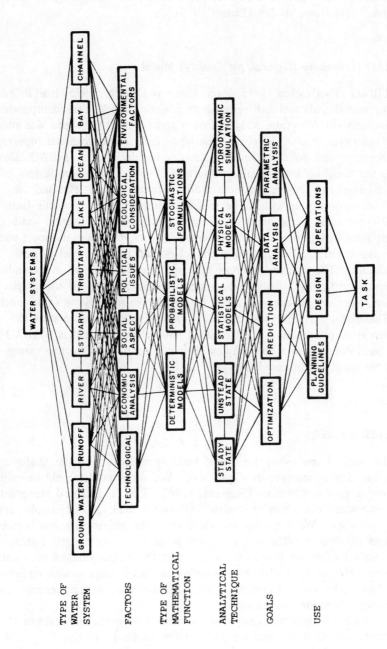

Figure 4-6. Flowchart of the possible model building pathways (Shahane, 1976).

POLLUTANT TRANSPORT MODEL

This group of models attempts to describe the transport of pollutants in aqueous systems. The formulation must take into account such phenomena as advection diffusion and chemical transformation. Further, the model must be somewhat tailored to the physical and geometric characteristics of the body of water under study. Pollutant transport in a system is based on the mass balance equation for each segment of the stream. A vegetation-adsorption-desorption process may be incorporated into the model. Figure 4-7 depicts the material balance for a two-compartment stream sediment system.

The model reduces, in one-dimension, to the following two equations for concentration as a function of time on the liquid and sediment phase:

$$\frac{\partial C}{\partial t} = D_X \frac{\partial^2 C}{\partial_X 2} - U \frac{\partial C}{\partial x} + \frac{k_1}{Ha} (m - K_s C)$$

$$\frac{\partial m}{\partial t} = k_1 (K_s C - m)$$

Values for k_1 and K_s may be estimated from the results of laboratory adsorption-desorption experiments. The diffusivity, D_X, and flow velocity, U, can be taken from field observations. For most flow regimes of interest, D_X has a power law dependence on the flow velocity.

Modeling Pollutant Transport in Soils

While this particular model is only one example of a pollutant transport calculation for the soil, the general procedures apply to most other similar models. By considering the mass balance for a cation within an element of soil of depth, dz, the following expression may be derived, which relates the amount of cation in aqueous solution to that adsorbed on the soil particles:

$$D_0 \frac{\partial^2 C}{\partial z^2} - V_0 \frac{\partial C}{\partial z} = \frac{\partial C}{\partial t} + \frac{\sigma}{\epsilon} \frac{\partial q}{\partial t}$$

where:
D_0 = dispersion coefficient
V_0 = pore velocity
σ = bulk density
ϵ = pore fraction
q = amount of material adsorbed
C = concentration of material in solution

Table 4-6. Comparison of Water Quality Models[a]

Comparison Characteristic	CEM Tributary Model	DOSAG-1	QUAL-11
Basic Modeling Assumptions Application to types of problems & varying environmental conditions	Basic assumptions include complete mixing of all flow additions at the discharge point, steady-state conditions, and no longitudinal dispersion in the direction of the flow. The model is most applicable to periods of dry weather with steady flow.	The model assumptions in DOSAG are quite similar to the CEM Tributary Model.	The basic equation describing the mass transport of conservative and nonconservative parameters assumes steady-state, nonuniform flow. The change in parameter concentration with time is a function of (1) transport due to longitudinal dispersion, (2) transport due to longitudinal advection, and (3) sources and sinks.
Model Structure Structure of River System	A river segment is divided into a fixed number of separate *reaches* of any desired length. All flow additions occur at upstream beginning of reach and all flow withdrawals (and return) occur at downstream end of reach.	The river system is defined by headwater stretches and reaches. A junction, which is the confluence between two streams, will separate two reaches. Each stretch is divided into a fixed number of reaches, which are defined to the nearest river mile. Flow additions and withdrawals are zero-length reaches and must be made to the nearest river mile.	The river system is defined by subdividing the stream into *reaches*. Computational elements within each reach include headwaters, standard, upstream of junction, junction, last in system, input and withdrawal. Branching river system can be simulated.
Data Requirements Volume of data Extent of preprocessing preparation Prior data collection requirements Input data and coefficients needed for physiography, hydrology and water quality	The data requirements for each reach are: equilibrium temperature, rate coefficients (K_1, K_3 and coefficients for temperature and coliforms), velocity and depth for computing K_2, water quality parameters of flow additions (if applicable), and flow extraction and return (if applicable).	The data requirements are: system mean water temperature, K_2 or coefficients for computing it, coefficients for computing depth and velocity K_1 & K_3, DO/BOD of headwater and flow additions. If options are to be exercised some or all of the following is required: minimum DO permissible, headwaters for flow augmentation, and waste discharge treatment levels.	Data requirements include as program inputs reaction rates and physical constants for approximately 23 system parameters. Also required are flowrates and temperature of headwaters and flow additions. Local climatological data are input to compute equilibrium temperature. Initial conditions must be input for each

Water Quality Parameters Modeled Water temperature Dissolved oxygen Biochemical oxygen demand Total dissolved solids Fecal coliforms Nonfecal coliforms	The parameters modeled are: Water temperature - exponential decay to equilibrium temperature DO/BOD—Streeter-Phelps equations with K_1, K_2, and K_3 Total dissolved solids—additive, conservative with mass balance Fecal coliforms—exponential decay Nonfecal coliforms—additive, conservative with mass balance	The parameters modeled are: DO/BOD—Streeter-Phelps Equations with K_1, K_2 and K_3 Water temperature is invariant throughout the river system.	reach. Runoff conditions for inflows and incremental flows are specified and with flow augmentation, the DO target level. The parameters modeled are: Conservative minerals Temperature BOD Chlorophyll a Phosphorus Ammonia, nitrite and nitrate Dissolved oxygen Coliform bacteria Radioactive material Temperature accounts for internal heat generation and all heat transferred across boundaries.
Model Capabilities and Limitations Types of analysis available Model limitations	All parameters are analyzed in same run. A given segment of any size of a river is analyzed but there is no branching. Branching could easily be added. The maximum number of reaches is 20, with a maximum of 100 computational intervals in each reach. These limitations can be greatly expanded and still retain economical core storage requirements. The increment between computation points may be different in each reach.	A variety of analyses may be performed in a single computer run: (1) 12 mos. of year, with corresponding temperatures and flows, (2) 4 permissible DO levels for flow augmentation, and (3) 5 degrees of wastewater treatment. Program limitations include: (1) a maximum of 10 headwater stretches, (2) a maximum of 20 junctions, (3) a maximum of 50 reaches, and (4) a maximum of 20 stretches.	Flow augmentation and wastewater treatment options are available. Capability to simulate dynamic and steady-state temperature, algal productivity, nutrient cycles and benthic oxygen demand major additions over QUAL-1. The model also has capability to dynamically stimulate all water quality constituents, and to operate in metric as well as English units. Dimensional limitations include a maximum

Table 4-6, continued

Comparison Characteristic	CEM Tributary Model	DOSAG-1	QUAL-II
Model Results Degree of temporal and spatial detail possible Presentation of results: tabular and graphical	The spatial detail can be at intervals of 0.1 mi for reaches of 10 mi length and at even smaller intervals for reaches less than 10 mi length and at even smaller intervals for reaches less than 10 mi length. Tabular results include presentation and interpretation of input data, values of all parameters at all computation points in each reach, and a summary of the values at the beginning and end of each reach. A graphical presentation of all computed values of temperature, BOD, DO, DO deficit and fecal coliforms may be obtained by option.	A reach is divided into 10 sub-reaches; therefore, a minimum computation interval of 1 mi is obtained for a reach of 10-mi length. The spatial detail will be at intervals of 0.1 mi for a 1 mi reach. Tabular results include all input data, an intermediate summary which shows, for example, results prior to and after flow augmentation, and a final summary giving DO/BOD at the start and end of each reach & the minimum DO in the reach. No graphical output is obtained.	A reach of a 10-mi length has minimum computational element of 0.5 mi. Tabular results include a highly modified final report, which shows all important hydrologic and biologic parameters, summary of input data, and an intermediate summary of observations. A subroutine to produce plots of water quality vs river mile on the line printer is included.
Characteristics of Computer Program Subroutines Core storage requirements Costs and CPU processing time	The computer program consists of a main program and five subroutines. Storage requirements are approximately 130K on an IMB 360/65 computer. Fully exercising all options and graphing all	The computer program consists of a main program and 12 subroutines. Storage requirements are approximately 132K on an IBM 360/65 computer. The cost will vary greatly depending on the	The computer program consists of a main program and 20 subroutines. Storage requirements are approximately 250 K on an IBM 360/15 computer. Costs of computer runs will vary

(QUAL-II, top cell continued:) of 75 reaches, no more than 20 computational elements per reach nor 500 in total, a maximum of 15 headwater and junction elements, and a maximum of 90 input and withdrawal elements.

	parameters will cost about $1.50 run, with a CPU time of about 12 sec.	the extent to which the various options are exercised. With flow augmentation for a single target level for a single month the cost was $3.00 (40 sec. of CPU). Obviously, multiple use of options in combination would cost much more.	greatly depending on the extent to which the various options are exercised.
Computational Techniques Basic computational procedure Numerical techniques	The computational program is used to calculate the water quality profile reach by reach from upstream to downstream, using a LaGrangian solution technique. The output from the upstream reach will be input to the next downstream reach.	A LaGrangian solution is used to solve the dissolved oxygen equation, which involves a coordinate system which moves with a particle of water in its path down a river. A simple mass balance is performed at the end of each reach and at every junction to arrive at DO/BOD for the next reach downstream.	QUAL-II numerically integrates the set of differential equations using a wholly implicit numerical scheme. Quasi-steady-state conditions are reached in a time equal to the time of flow in a stream reach.

a Federal Power Commission, 1975; Water Resources Engineers, 1974, Texas Water Development Board, 1970a,b, 1971; Ball et al., 1973; Lombardo, 1973)

Table 4-7. Methods and Models for Predicting Flow Changes in Estuaries[a]

Water Quality Characteristic Analytical Approach	Hydraulics
Level I	Louisiana Cooperative Fishery Research Unit, 1974
	EPA, 1971
	EPA, 1972
	Welby. (Personal Communication. N. Carolina State University, 1975
	Alexander et al., 1974
	Asano, 1967
	Bain, 1968
	Battelle, 1974 a,b
	Bella, 1968
	Bella and Dobbins, 1968
	Biswas, 1974
	Callaway et al., 1969
	Clark and Synder, 1969
	Dornhelm and Woolhiser, 1968
	Dresnack and Dobbins, 1968
	Feigner and Harris, 1970
	Fischer, 1970
	Fisher, 1969
	Grenney and Bella, 1970
	Grenney and Bella, 1972
	Hann and Young, 1972
	Harlemann et al., 1968
	Holley, 1969
Level II	Ippen, 1966
	Kadlec, 1971
	King and Sartoris, 1973
	Leeds and Bybee, 1967
	Lehmann, 1974
	Lombardo, 1973
	O'Connor, 1965
	O'Connor et al., 1968
	Orlob et al., 1967
	Pence et al., 1968
	Penumalli et al., 1975
	Riggs, 1972
	Schofield and Krutchkoff, 1974
	Shubinski et al., 1974
	Thayer and Krutchkoff, 1967
	Thomann, 1963
	Thomann, 1967
	Wang et al., 1973
	Wang and Connor, 1974
	Wang and Connor, 1975
	Wastler and Walter, 1968
	Water Resources Engineers, 1965
	Water Resources Engineers, 1966

[a] Stalnaker and Arnette, 1976

Table 4-8. Methods and Models for Predicting Effects of Flow Changes on Water Quality in Estuaries—Literature Matrix[a]

Parameter / Analytical Approach	Dissolved Gases	Temperature	Sediment	Total Dissolved Solids / Nutrient budgets / Microbial Ecology
Level I	EPA, 1971			EPA 1971 / EPA, 1972
Level II	Alexander et al., 1974 / Battelle, 1974 a,b / Bureau of Fisheries, Nacote Creek Res. Sta., 1975 / Callaway et al., 1969 / Dornhelm and Woolhiser, 1968 / Dresnack and Dobbins, 1968 / Feigner and Harris, 1970 / Brenney and Bella, 1972 / Hann and Young, 1972 / Holley, 1969 / Lehmann, 1974 / Lombardo, 1973 / O'Connor, 1960 / Olufeagba and Flake, 1975 / Orlob et al., 1967 / Pence et al., 1968 / Schofield and Krutchkoff, 1974 / Shubinski et al., 1974 / Thayer and Krutchkoff, 1967 / Thomann, 1963 / Thomann, 1967 / Water Resources Engineers, 1965 / Water Resources Engineers, 1966	Alexander et al., 1974 / Battelle, 1974 a,b / Biwas, 1974 / Bureau of Fisheries, Nacote Creek Res. Sta., 1975 / Callaway et al., 1969 / Clark and Snyder, 1969 / Dailey and Harleman, 1972 / Edinger and Geyer, 1968 / Feigner and Harris, 1970 / Gerber, 1967 / Harleman et al., 1968 / Jobson and Yotsukura, 1972 / Lehmann, 1974 / Lombardo, 1973 / O'Connor et al., 1968 / Schofield and Krutchkoff, 1974 / Shubinski et al., 1974 / Water Resources Engineers, 1965 / Water Resources Engineers, 1966	Battelle, 1974 a,b / Biwas, 1974 / Bureau of Fisheries, Nacote Creek Res. Sta., 1975 / Feigner and Harris, 1970 / Lehmann, 1974 / Lombardo, 1973 / O'Connor et al., 1968 / Owens and Odd, 1970 / Schofield and Krutchkoff, 1974 / Shubinski et al., 1974 / Water Resources Engineers, 1965 / Water Resources Engineers, 1966	Armstrong et al., 1975 / Bailey, 1970 / Battelle, 1974 a,b / Bella, 1970 / Biswas, 1974 / Bureau of Fisheries, Nacote Creek Res. Sta., 1975 / Callaway et al., 1969 / DiToro et al., 1970 / Feigner and Harris, 1970 / Fisher, 1969 / Grenney, 1975 / Grenney and Bella, 1972 / Harleman et al., 1968 / Kadlec, 1971 / Lehmann, 1974 / Lombardo, 1973 / Middlebrooks et al., 1973 / O'Connor, 1972 / O'Connor et al., 1968 / Odum et al., 1963 / Orlob et al., 1967 / Patten, 1968 / Riley et al., 1949 / Steele, 1958 / Sverdrup et al., 1942 / Thomann et al., 1970 / Schofield and Krutchkoff, 1974 / Shubinski et al., 1974 / Water Resources Engineers, 1965 / Water Resources Engineers, 1966

[a] Stalnaker and Arnette, 1976

Table 4-9. Low-Resolution Models for Water Quality in Estuaries
(Stalnaker and Arnette, 1976).

Technique	Water Quality Constituents	Linked Constituents	Output	Input Hydraulics
EPA 71 EPA 72	Total dissolved solids:[a] TDS (107)	None	Total dissolved solids concentration resulting from numerous point loads	1. Steady-state flows for all significant inflows and representative points in the estuary 2. Dispersion coefficient (E) for the estuary
	Coliform bacterial COLI (108)	None	Coliform bacteria concentration distributions resulting from numerous point loads	1. Steady-state flows for all significant inflows and at representative points in the estuary 2. Dispersion coefficient (E) for the estuary 3. Estuary travel times for all reaches
	Nutrients NUT (108)	None	Nutrient concentration distributions resulting from numerous point loads	1. Steady-state flows for all significant inflows and at representative points in the estuary
	Biochemical oxygen demand: BOD (108)	Dissolved oxygen	BOD concentration distributions resulting from numerous point loads	1. Steady-state flows for all significant inflows and at representative points in the estuary
	Dissolved oxygen: DO (112)	Biochemical oxygen demand[b]	Dissolved oxygen concentrations distributions resulting from numerous point loads	1. Steady-state flows for all significant inflows and at representative points in the estuary
	Critical dissolved oxygen deficit (45) Photosynthesis and respiration Temperature	Biochemical oxygen demand[b]	Magnitude of the maximum deficit for a given point load	1. Steady-state flows for all significant inflows and at representative points in

[a]Numbers enclosed in parentheses are page numbers.
[b]Indicates that the constituent in column 2 is effected by this linked constituent.

Table 4-9, continued

Input Water Quality	Comments
1. Flows, concentrations and locations of point loads. 2. Background concentration of TDS in the estuary	1. This technique applies for any conservative substance. 2. Maximum concentrations will always occur just downstream from point sources. 3. Tables of average coefficients for dispersion (66, E38)
1. Flows, concentrations and locations of point loads 2. Background concentration of coliforms in the estuary 3. First-order dieoff rate	1. Maximum concentrations will always occur just downstream from point sources. 2. Tables of average coefficients: a) Dieoff rates (111) b) Background concentrations (56) c) Temperature adjustment (70) d) Waste loading estimates (50) e) Dispersion (66, E38)
1. Flows, concentrations and locations of point loads	1. First-order nutrient removal rates are assumed. 2. Maximum concentration will always occur just downstream from point source. 3. Tables of average coefficients: a) Removal rates (111) b) Temperature adjustment (70) c) Water loading estimates (50, 54)
1. Flows, concentrations and locations of point loads	1. Ultimate oxygen demand for the combined effects of carbonaceous and nitrogenous BOD. 2. Tables of average coefficients: a) Decay rates (111, Appendix C) b) Temperature adjustments (70, E35) c) Waste loading estimates (50, 53, E6, E8) 3. Maximum concentrations will always occur just downstream from point sources.
1. Flows, concentrations and locations of point loads 2. Background concentrations of DO in the estuary 3. DO saturation concentration for the existing temperature, elevation and salinity. 4. Reacration coefficient	1. Modeled as dissolved oxygen deficit. 2. Maximum DO deficit as a function of dispersion velocity, deoxygenation rate, and ultimate BOD loading (45). 3. Maximum deficit occurs at some point a distance x_c from waste load (44). 4. Average values for some coefficients: a) Reacration rates (111, 113, 117, Appendix C). b) Temperature effects on reacration rates (E35). c) Assimilation ratios (114, Chart D, Appensix D). d) Saturation concentrations as a function of temperature and salinity (57). 5. Background concentrations (56).
1. Flows, concentrations and locations of point loads	1. Modeled as dissolved oxygen deficit. 2. Solution graph: Critical depth as a function of BOD loading, deoxygenation and reoxygenation rates. Requires a more sophisticated model. Requires a more sophisticated model.

Table 4-10.   Low-Resolution Models for Water Quality in Rivers
(Stalnaker and Arnette, 1976).

Technique	Water Quality Constituents	Linked Constituents	Output	Input Hydraulics
EPA 71 EPA 72	Total dissolved solids: TDS (67)[a]	None	Total dissolved solids concentration distributions resulting from numerous point loads	1. Steady-state river flows for all significant tributaries and at representative points along the river
	Coliform bacteria: COLI (69)	None	Coliform bacteria concentration distributions resulting from numerous point loads	1. Steady-state river flows for all significant tributaries and at representative points along the river 2. River travel times for all reaches
	Nutrients: NUT (69)	None	Nutrients concentration distributions resulting from numerous point loads	1. Steady-state river flows for all significant tributaries and at representative points along the river
	Biochemical oxygen demand	Dissolved oxygen	BOD concentration distributions resulting from numerous point loads	1. Steady-state river flows for all significant tributaries and at representative points along the river
	Dissolved oxygen DO (71)	Biochemical oxygen demand[b]	Dissolved oxygen concentration distributions resulting from numerous point loads	1. Steady-state river flows for all significant tributaries and at representative points along the river
	Critical dissolved deficit (73)	Biochemical oxygen demand[b]	Magnitude of the maximum dissolved oxygen deficit for a given point load	1. Steady-state river flows for all significant tributaries and at representative points along the river
	Reacration over small dam (E25)	Biochemical oxygen demand[b]	Decrease in oxygen deficit over a dam	1. Steady-state river flows for all significant tributaries and at representative points along the river 2. Height through which the water falls
	Photosynthesis and respiration			
	Temperature			

[a]Numbers enclosed in parentheses are page numbers.
[b]Indicates that the constituent in column 2 is effected by this linked constituent.

Table 4-10, continued

Input Water Quality	Comments
1. Flows, concentrations and locations of point loads 2. Background concentration of TDS in the river system	1. This technique applies for any conservative substance. 2. Maximum concentrations will always occur just downstream from point sources.

1. Flows, concentrations and locations of point loads
2. Background concentrations of coliform in the river system
3. First-order dieoff rate
	1. Maximum concentration will always occur just downstream from point sources.
	2. Tables of average coefficients:
	  a) Dieoff rates (70)
	  b) Background concentrations (56)
	  c) Temperature adjustment (70)
	  d) Waste loading estimates (50)

1. Flows, concentration and locations of point loads	1. First-order nutrient removal rates are assumed.
	2. Maximum concentration will always occur just downstream from a point source.
	3. Tables of average coefficients:
	  a) Removal rates (70)
	  b) Temperature adjustment (70)
	  c) Waste loading estimates (50, 54)

1. Flows, concentrations and locations of point loads	1. Ultimate oxygen demand for the combined effects of carbonaceous and nitrogenous BOD.
	2. Tables of average coefficients:
	  a) Decay rates (70, A3, Appensix C)
	  b) Temperature adjustment (70, E35)
	  c) Waste loading estimates (50, 53, E6, E8)
	3. Maximum concentrations will always occur just downstream from a point source

1. Flows, concentrations and locations of point loads
2. Background concentrations of DO in the river system
3. DO saturation concentration for the existing temperature, elevation and salinity.
	1. Modeled as dissolved oxygen deficit
	2. Maximum deficit occurs at some point a distance x_c downstream from waste load (73).
	3. Average values for some coefficients:
	  a) Reacration rates (A3, E18, Appendix C)
	  b) Temperature effects on reacration rates (E35)
	  c) Assimilation ratios (A5)
	  d) Saturation concentration as a function of temperature and salinity
	4. Background concentrations (56).

1. Flows, concentrations and locations of point loads	1. Modeled as dissolved oxygen deficit 2. Solution graph: Critical depth as a function of BOD loading, deoxygenation and reoxygenation rates.

1. Flows, concentrations and locations of point loads	1. Modeled as dissolved oxygen deficit
	2. Solution graphs:
	  a) Decrease in deficit as a function of height
	  b) Effect of a small dam on the dissolved oxygen profile in a river reach

	Requires a more sophisticated model.
	Requires a more sophisticated model.

**Table 4-11.   Summary of Certain Stream and Estuary Models
(Stalnaker and Arnette, 1976)**

Author	Applications	Hydraulics	Mass Transport
Grenney and Porcella (1975)	Water quality for systems of rivers. Applied to the Bear. Virgin, Sevier, Jordan, Weber and Green Rivers in Utah.	RIVER: TYPE One-dimensional simulation, steady-nonuniform flow. Input Boundary conditions (upstream, lateral, tributary) Channel geometry, slope and roughness coefficient. Output Flow distributions	Advection
Battelle, 1974b	Water quality for systems of rivers and estuaries. Applied to the Willamette River Basin	Simulation model, river and estuary Type Two-dimensional (horizontal), unsteady flow. Includes tides and river flows. Input Estuary and/or river configurations and characteristics. Boundary flows. Output Flows, velocities and depths with space and time.	Advection and dispersion
Penumalli, et al., 1975	Estuary: Optimization (nonlinear) water quality simulation model. Minimizes treatment costs subject to constraints: a) physical constraints, b) socioeconomic, c) political/administrative, d) engineering, e) water quality goals. Applied to Corpus Christi Bay on the Gulf Coast of Texas.	Simulation model - estuary. Type Two-dimensional (horizontal), unsteady flow; Includes wind, coriolis accileration, tides and river inflow. Input Estuary configuration and characteristics Output Flows, velocities, and depths with space and time.	Two-dimensional (horizontal) advection and dispersion
Hann and Young. 1972	Estuary: Two-dimensional simulation. Applied to Huston Ship Cannel.	Type Two-dimension, unsteady flow, includes tides and river flows. Input Estuary configurations and characteristics Output Flows, velocities and depths with space and time	Two-dimensional (horizontal) advection and dispersion
Rutherford and O'Sullivan 1974	River: one-dimensional simulation. Applied to Taraw-era River, New Zealand.	Steady - nonuniform as data input	Dispersion and advection, dispersion calculated as a function of hydraulic radius and shear velocity

Table 4-11, continued

DO	Ammonium (Nitrification)	BOD	Temperature	Remarks
Reaeration = $K_2(C_5-C)$, temperature-dependent and linked to BOD, nitrification, photosynthesis	First-order oxidation uptake by algae. Temperature-dependent	First-order oxidation. Temperature-dependent	Air-water surface, radiation	Moderate resolution. User option for exact or numerical solution depending on parameters being modeled.
Reaeration = $K_2(C_5-C)$, K_2 is temperature-dependent, linked to BOD, nitrification, detritus decomposition algae (photo/resp.)	First-order oxidation, uptake by algae. Temperature-dependent	First-order decay. Temperature dependent	Air-water surface, radiation. Steady state or daily variations	Modification and expansion of EPA's Storm Water Management and Dynamic Estuary Model (Feigner and Harris, 1970). High resolution, large data requirement. Solution scheme based on Onlob's link-node technique (WRE 1972).
				Hydraulics: Explicit finite difference solutions technique. Mass Transport: implicit, explicit. Model run for phosphorus only. High resolution, large amounts of detailed data.
a) first-order deficit b) first-order BOD decay		First-order decay	Constant	Explicit and implicit solution techniques are used. High resolution, large amounts of detailed data.
a) First-order deficit; reacration calculated as a function of hydraulic radius and velocity, b) Linked to: Bacteria		Models bacteria biomass, where growth rate is a hyperbolic function of organic substrate availability	Constant	Decomposition of organics is a function of bacteria biomass, which is modeled by saturation kinetics. Explicit and implicit finite difference solution techniques. High resolution, large

Table 4-11, continued

Author	Applications	Hydraulics	Mass Transport
Huck and Farquhar, 1974	River: one-dimensional stochastic simulation. Saint Clair River near Corunna, Canada		
Bayer 1974	Optimization nonlinear objective function, linear constraints: minimum cost of BOD treatment to meet specified stream standards for BOD and DO.	Steady flow input data, average travel times in specific reaches.	Advection
Hwang, *et al.* 1973	Optimization, nonlinear objective function, nonlinear constraints: minimum cost of BOD treatment and cooling to meet stream BOD, DO, and temperature standards. Applied to the Chattahoochee River Basin below Atlanta, Georgia	Steady flow input data. Average travel times in specific reaches.	Advection
Texas Water Development Board. 1974	River: one-dimensional simulation. Applied to the San Antonio River, Texas	<u>Type</u> Steady flow by water balance. <u>Input</u> Constant boundary flows (upstream boundary and lateral); and channel characteristics <u>Output</u> Steady flow, velocity and hydraulic radius along the river. Note: Flows may be augmented from reservoirs to meet target DO values.	Advection and dispersion, dispersion coefficient calculated as a function of velocity, roughness and depth
Jeppson, 1974	River hydraulics. Applied Temple Fork Creek, Logan, Utah	<u>Type</u> One-dimensional simulation, unsteady flow. <u>Input</u> Time varying boundary conditions (upstream, downstream, lateral). Channel geometry, slope and roughness coefficient. <u>Output</u> Hydraulic properties (flow, velocity, depth) at desired downstream locations.	

Table 4-11, continued

DO	Ammonium (Nitrification)	BOD	Temperature	Remarks
				Moderate resolution model. The Box-Jenkins method for time series analysis was used. Water quality parameters not linked or associated explicitly with hydraulics. Long-term records of quality data.
First-order deficit; reaeration constant		First-order decay		Moderate resolution. Moderate data requirements.
First-order deficit; reaeration adjusted for temperature. Net photosynthesis adjusted for temperature.		First-order decay	Surface conduction water temperature, radiation, wind, evaporation	Moderate resolution. Moderate data requirements.
Steady state or daily variations First-order deficit, reaeration may be calculated by one of five options		First-order decay, temperature adjusted	Steady-state or daily variations, surface conduction, radiation, evaporation	High resolution, large detailed data requirements.
				Linear implicit finite difference solution technique. High resolution. Large amounts of detailed data.

Table 4-11, continued

Author	Applications	Hydraulics	Mass Transport
Hydrologic Engineering Center, 1974	Water quality for systems of rivers and impoundments. Applied to California River including Smith Reservoir	RIVER: Type One-dimensional simulation, steady nonuniform flow. Input Boundary conditions (upstream, lateral); Channel geometry, slope and roughness coefficient. RESERVOIR: Type One-dimensional (vertical) simulation, steady flow linked to temperature and density. Input Tributary inflow, dam releases, reservoir properties Output Flow distributions, reservoir level.	Advection and dispersion
Shearman and Swissheim, 1975	River flow simulation and low-flow analysis for systems of rivers and reservoirs. Applied to the Kentucky River.	Type One-dimensional simulation, unsteady flow, based on flow routine equations. Flow may routed downstream, upstream, and through reservoirs. Input Long-term flow and reservoir storage records. Output Average daily flows at desired locations for specified boundary condt.	
Bovee, 1974	River: one-dimensional simulation.	Steady flow, input data	Advection and dispersion
Stochastics, Inc. 1971	river/estuary: one-dimensional stochastic.	Steady average net seaward flow.	Advection and dispersion

Table 4-11, continued

DO	Ammonium (Nitrification)	BOD	Temperature	Remarks
Reaeration = $K_2(C_5\text{-}C)$. K_2 is temperature dependent. Linked to: BOD, nitrification, detritus decomposition, algae photo/resp. zooplankton respiration, fish respiration, benthic animal respiration	First-order decay; detritus recycle uptake or decomposition of algae, zooplankton, fish and benthic animals	First-order decay, temperature dependent	Air-water surface, radiation, evaporation	Linear-implicit finite difference solution technique. High resolu-Large amounts of detailed data. Note: WRE 1972 includes two-dimensional mass transport based on Orlob's link-node technique.
				Moderate resolution. Long-term flow and storatge records.
First-order deficit, Reaeration coefficient calculated as a function of temperature, velocity and depth.		First-order decay	Surface condition, radiation, evaporation.	High resolution. Large detailed data requirements.
First-order deficit.		First order decay	Constant	High resolution. Large detailed data requirements.

Table 4-12. Different Water Models (Fowler and Poh, 1971)

	River Basin Simulation Model	Dynamic Estuary Model	Steady-State and Time-Varying Models	Model for Quantifying Flow Augmentation Benefits
Purpose	To simulate hydrology and water quality and assess the impact of different waste loads and reservoir operating policies on water quality	To simulate a wide variety of hydrologic and water quality conditions	To simulate hydrology and water quality allowing for time variation of certain parameters; to determine the optimum solution of plants and treatment levels to meet water quality goals.	To simulate hydrology and water quality and determine optimum combinations of sewage treatment and low-flow augmentation.
Application	River basins, including reservoirs	Any estuaries wherein vertical stratification is absent or limited to a small area	A stretch of river where bordering populations and industries use the river for water supply, disposal of treated sewage and recreation	Complex river systems, including reservoirs
Simulation Techniques	Statistical methods	A set of differential equations (motion, continuity, advection, diffusion, degradation and reaeration)	Streeter-Phelps oxygen sag equations and other mathematical equations	Statistical methods; differential equations (Streeter-Phelps oxygen sag)
Water Quality Considerations	Handles up to five waste constituents, one of which may be nonconservative	Handles both conservative and nonconservative waste constituents, maximum of 5	BOD, DO, coliforms and chlorides	DO and BOD
Optimization and Economic Aspects	Not considered	Not considered	Path of steepest ascent technique. Cost is function of flow	Linear programming; cost functions for treatment levels from available information, cost curves for reservoirs from cost/volume curves
Output	Historical and simulated flow characteristics; storage level distributions for reservoirs; statistics of deficiencies (failures to meet quality standards for flow requirements)	Hydrologic characteristics at each junction and channel; average concentration of each waste constituent at each junction for each tidal cycle	If treatment levels are specified for each community, program evaluates quality throughout stream; if single-quality criterion is specified for each river section, optimizing routine determines desirable levels of treatment	Flow statistics; water quality predictions for each reach; optimal solution, i.e., combination of treatment and flow-augmentation

	Model 1	Model 2	Model 3	Model 4
Documentation	Fair	Excellent	Fair	Excellent
Includes:				
Program Listing	Yes	Yes	No	Yes
Sample Output	Yes	Yes	No	No
Instructions for User	Yes	Yes	No	Yes
Format of Input	Yes	Yes	No	No
Flow Chart	No	Yes	Yes	Yes
Time Estimate for Each Run	No	Yes	Yes	No
Program	Flexible	Very flexible		In modular form
Machine and Language	IBM 360/65 FORTRAN IV	IBM 7094, CDC 6600, IBM 360/65, FORTRAN IV	CDC 3300 FORTRAN II	IBM 360/65, FORTRAN IV (simulation) MPS package (optimization)
Data Requirements	At least 30 years of historical data	Not excessive	Not excessive, but includes economic and administrative as well as hydrologic and quality data	Large amounts of data required
Comments	Very statistically oriented; enormous program requiring the full computing power of the largest computers	Model verified on San Francisco Bay and Suison Bay network	Flow-routing procedure in time-varying model verified on Susquehanna River in New York and Pennsylvania	Simulation model verified on Farmington River basin in Conn. and Mass.; optimization model used only on hypothetical region; Each step such as checking missing data, normalizing the data, selecting gage stations, synthesizing weekly gage data, water quality prediction, and optimization are all done as separate programs so the user has to submit quite a few programs to obtain the final result.
Advantages	Considers entire river basin as a unit; good for design and operation of reservoir systems; flexible	Data requirements not excessive, initial input can be estimates; very flexible	Allows for time-variation of data by use of time intervals in addition to physical stations; includes optimization technique; considers general community data	Considers reservoirs; includes optimization technique; and provides data for quantification of low-flow augmentation
Disadvantages	Requires large amounts of historical data; does not consider economic aspects	Economic aspects not considered	Optimization depends on cost function	Large amounts of historical data required; optimization dependent on IBM/360 MPS package; numerous programs must be submitted to obtain final result

Table 4-12, Continued

		Regional Water Quality Management Model	Hydro-Quality Simulation Model	Simplified Mathematical Model of Water Quality
Purpose	To simulate hydrology, and allocate water stored in reservoirs to competing demands on the basis of economic efficiency	To estimate the least cost combination of waste treatment alternatives and by-pass piping which will achieve pre-specified water quality goals	To simulate hydrology and water quality considering all types of inflow and outflow	To give reasonable guidelines for evaluating water quality by means of detailed presentation of tables, nomographs and technical data
Application	Rivers and reservoirs allocation of resources	Estuaries or possibly other water bodies	River basins, including reservoirs	Water bodies (rivers, estuaries, tidal rivers) which can be described as approximately 1-dimensional and for which system geometry is relatively simple
Simulation Techniques	Statistical methods		Differential equations	Differential equations used to produce tables and nomographs
Water Quality Considerations	DO and coliforms	DO, BOD	DO, BOD, salinity and temperature	Total dissolved solids, coliforms, DO, nutrients
Optimization and Economic Aspects	Theory of firm steepest ascent	Linear programming—cost is a function of flow	Not considered	Not considered
Output	Reservoir and channel statistics; statistics of benefits received and percent of time water quality targets were met	The solution (lease-cost combination of treatment alternatives and by-pass piping to achieve quality goals), cost for each situation tested	Monthly average values at both ends of each reach and annual time profiles for predesignated points for flow and quality parameters; predicted diurnal variations in DO and temperature; monthly mass balance water budget	Total flow for rivers; minimum DO for rivers assuming single waste source and multiple waste sources; minimum DO for tidal rivers and estuaries, assuming single and multiple waste sources; dilution flow for tidal rivers and estuaries

Documentation	Fair	Fair	Good	Excellent
Includes:				
Program Listing	Yes	No	Yes	No (no program)
Sample Output	No	No	Yes	Yes
Instructions for User	No	No	Yes	Yes
Format of Input	No	No	Yes	No
Flow Chart	Yes	No	Yes	No
Time Estimate for Each Run	No	Yes	Yes	No (no run)
Program		Flexible		
Machine and Language	CDC 6600 FORTRAN, DYNAMO	IBM 360/65 FORTRAN IV	UNIVAC 1108 FORTRAN V	None
Data Requirements	Not excessive	Not excessive; transfer coefficients are calculated prior to applying the model	Coefficients of differential equations are determined by regression analysis of field data prior to applying the model	Minimum
Comments	More work needed in development of benefit functions for various water uses; model tested on Calapooia River in Oregon	The determination of transfer coefficients for in-stream DO changes due to input BOD not included in documentation report. Program listing and deck obtainable from systems analysis and economics branch of Office of Water Programs, Environmental Protection Agency, Washington, D.C. Model applied to Delaware estuary as an example	Developed and verified using data from Little Bear River basin in Utah	A general simplified methodology for the application of mathematical models to the analysis of water quality
Advantages	Considers benefits reaped from various water uses, and allocates limited stored water to competing demands or uses on basis of economic efficiency	Considers all waste treatment alternatives and their costs; good for regional planning	Considers all types of inflow and outflow, including reservoirs	Few data required, no computer required; could be widely used for developing initial rough estimates of water quality and necessary treatment levels
Disadvantages	Depends on benefit functions which are difficult to define and for which the validity may, in some cases, be questionable	Depends on cost functions	Economic aspects not considered	Results must be considered as *trend* indications only and *not* as precise; certain predictions

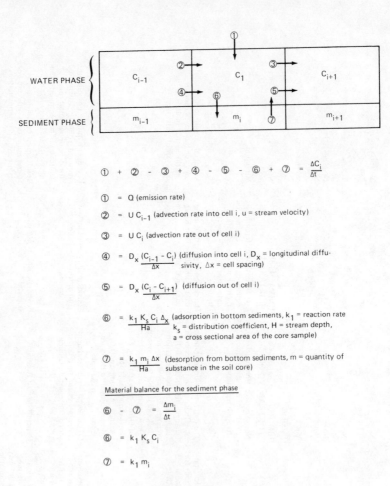

Figure 4-7. Pollutant material balance for water and sediment phases of a stream.

The concentrations in the solid and liquid phases, q and C, may be nondimensionalized by dividing by the cation adsorption capacity (Q) and the initial total concentration in solution (C_0):

$$X = \frac{C}{C_0} \qquad Y = \frac{q}{Q}$$

These nondimensional concentrations are usually related to one another through an adsorption function or adsorption isotherm:

$$Y = f(X)$$

With the transformations indicated in the Equations, the material balance equation may be rewritten as follows:

$$D(X) \frac{\partial^2 X}{\partial z^2} - V(X) \frac{\partial X}{\partial z} = \frac{\partial X}{\partial t}$$

where:

$$D(X) = \frac{Do}{1 + \dfrac{\sigma Q}{\epsilon Co} \dfrac{dY}{dX}}$$

$$V(X) = \frac{Vo}{1 + \dfrac{\sigma Q}{\epsilon Co} \dfrac{dY}{dX}}$$

This may be solved by a finite difference procedure by application of the following boundary conditions:

$$X(z,O) = 0 \qquad 0 \leqslant z \leqslant L$$
$$X(X_o, t) = 1.0 \qquad t > 0$$

$$\frac{\partial X}{\partial z}(L,t) = 0 \qquad t > 0$$

where L is the length of the soil column under study.

COMPARTMENT MODEL

This type of model has been used in the analysis of constituent transport between different identifiable compartments of ecosystems. This technique assumes that the variables of interest are uniform within a volume or region of the compartment.

Compartments are represented schematically as follows:

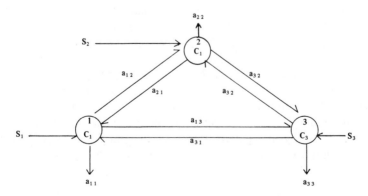

where: S_i = source strength for compartment i
$\quad\quad\quad$ C_i = concentration in compartment i
$\quad\quad\quad$ A_{ij} = transfer rate coefficient between compartments i and j
$\quad\quad\quad$ A_{ii} = decay coefficient associated with compartment i

Then, the rate of change of concentration in each compartment can be described as follows:

$$dC_i/dt = S_i + \sum_{j=i}^{m} (a_{ij}C_j - a_{ji}C_i) - a_{ii}C_i$$

MODELING OF WATER THERMAL DISCHARGE

Purpose of Modeling

Modeling the thermal discharge (Watson, 1972) is part of the process of analyzing the expected environmental impact of a proposed power plant. A prime objective of any such model is, therefore, to map the thermal distribution of the outflow as it mixes with the ambient receiving water. The excess of temperature from the thermal discharge over the ambient temperature is expressed as a function of space coordinates (in two or in three dimensions) and the extent of the isotherms is defined. These predicted thermal distributions then become a tool in estimating whether the effect of the outflow will conform to prescribed standards for water quality and what the impact on biota in the receiving water will be.

Near- and Far-Field Effects

It is known that in a body of water, into which a heated outflow is discharged, the temperature field comprises two zones often termed the "near field" and the "far field" (Policastro, *et al.,* 1972). In the near field, the changes in water temperature are governed primarily by properties of the outflow. This discharge is distinguished not only by an excess of temperature over the cooling water into which it is received, but also by differences in velocity, density, momentum and direction of flow.

Typically, the warm jet experiences vertical motion: usually, its greater buoyancy, resulting from the higher temperature, tends to carry it upward through the ambient water. As a result of mixing between the heated outflow and of entrainment of the diluting water into the discharged jet, the temperature excess of the latter, above the ambient, spreads horizontally and vertically in a pattern that is often termed a "thermal plume." The establishment of a pattern of flow is included within the near-field effects.

In the far field, the outflow is mostly influenced by conditions of the ambient receiving-water. This regime is generally much larger in extent than the near-field zone. In this zone, the plume is envisioned as a passive floating sheet of heated water resting on top of the cooler receiving body of water. However, plumes can exist at submerged positions under specialized circumstances. Within the far-field one must additionally consider surface heat loss and the effects of ambient turbulence. Thus plume spread and dissipation in the far field are determined by complex factors including: ambient advective motions, lateral, longitudinal, and vertical mixing due to ambient turbulence, buoyancy and surface heat loss.

Models of thermal dispersion typically distinguish between the near and the far fields. Some models treat only one or the other of the two zones, whereas others will combine both, sometimes with a transition zone between. In some models, the dispersion calculated for the near field becomes part of the input to calculations for the far-field effects.

VARIABLES GOVERNING CHOICE OF MODEL

There are specific variables which define the specific situation and affect the choice of specific model(s) applicable to a particular use.

Location

Whether the outflow is at surface affects particularly the vertical entrainment of ambient water. With a submerged discharge, there is a need to calculate upward movement. When the jet stream as discharged either reaches the surface or achieves its maximum height, the progress of the plume thereafter tends to be different.

Movement

Depending on the degree of movement in the receiving water, any substantial current affects the rate of movement and of dilution of the outflow. If current is essentially absent or is reversible (as with tidal effects), the result may be to reintroduce some of the heated outflow into the intake system, so that this feature would have to be modeled specifically.

Stratification

This refers to the degree of stratification in the receiving water, which affects particularly the rate and extent of rise of the outflow stream. One study (Koh and Fan, 1970a) showed that under some conditions a small density stratification is all that is necessary to prevent the heated discharge from reaching the surface. In that case, all the temperature excess is assimilated in the subsurface water.

Ports

The number, shape and orientation of the discharge port(s) affect the character of the outflow and, when multiple, cause mixing of the originally distinct streams.

Salinity

The salinity of the water affects the behavior of the jet stream after discharge. Techniques for calculating saline concentration as the outflow mixes with the ambient may be applicable in estimating dilution rates of biocides or other chemicals.

Ratio of Discharge Velocity to Velocity of the Receiving Stream

This relationship significantly affects the mixing between the two streams; specifically, the entrainment of the ambient water and, hence, the dilution of the outflow, may be modeled as a function of this interrelationship.

Angle

These are the angles in the horizontal and the vertical planes made by the jet discharge, relative to the velocity of the receiving water. In the presence of an ambient longshore current flowing perpendicular to the direction of the thermal discharge, the thermal plume will be bent in the down-current direction. When the jet is discharged upwards towards the surface (positive vertical angle, 90°), the plume rise will, other things being equal, rise faster than when the discharge is in the horizontal plane.

Froude Number

This is the initial jet densimetric Froude number, F, which relates the inertia forces to the gravitational effects (Chow, 1964). This parameter may be represented by (EPA, 1972):

$$F = \frac{U_j}{\sqrt{\frac{\rho_o - \rho_j}{\rho_o D}}}$$

where: U_j = initial jet velocity
ρ_o = ambient density
ρ_j = jet density
g = gravitational constant

The Froude number varies directly with the jet velocity and inversely to the square roots of both the jet diameter and the density deficiency of the discharge. Other things being equal, the discharge with the lowest Froude number will rise the fastest.

The Slope of the Bottom Along the Direction of the Center-Line Plume

Several coefficients used in computing center-line temperature and maximum width of a given isotherm may be modeled as partial functions of this variable. A survey of thermal model has been done by Policastro (1972). The major results of this compilation and comparative analysis are contained in Tables 4-13 to 4-15.

EXAMPLES OF THERMAL MODELS

Two frequently used models to be described are: (1) A modified Pritchard-Carpenter Model, and (2) Hirst's Model.

Modified Prichard-Carpenter Model

This model is based on work done previously by Pritchard and Carter.

The mathematical model of the horizontal and vertical dispersion over time of heated outflow (effluent) into a moving body of water takes its point of departure from three sets of differential equations expressing conservation of mass, momentum and energy. The equation of conservation of mass or continuity of flow of a fluid may be given in general form (Jakob, 1959) as follows:

$$\rho \left(\sum_{i=1}^{3} \frac{\partial v_i}{\partial x_i} \right) + \sum_{i=1}^{3} \frac{\partial \rho}{\partial x_i} + \frac{\partial \rho}{\partial t} = 0,$$

where: v_i = velocity along the ith dimension, x_i
ρ = density of the fluid
t = time

For incompressible fluids, this equation (Milne-Thompson, 1968) is often reduced to

$$\sum_{i=1}^{3} \frac{\partial v_i}{\partial x_i} = 0$$

Table 4-13. Summary of the Characteristics of the Jet Models[a] (Policastro, 1972)

	Hoopes et al. 1968	Hayashi and Shuto, 1967	Wada, 1969 (Model No. 4)	Carter, 1969
Direction of Temperature Variation				
Longitudinal	YES	YES	YES	YES
Lateral	YES	YES	YES	YES
Vertical	NO	YES	YES[a]	NO
Initial Mixing (Jet Regime)	YES	YES	YES	YES
Ambient Turbulence (Far-Field Region)	NO	NO	NO	NO
Mathematical Approach				
Numerical	NO	NO	YES	NO
Integral	YES	YES	NO	YES
Closed Form	YES[b]	YES	NO	NO
Semiempirical	YES	YES	YES	YES
Time-Dependent solution	NO	NO	YES	NO
Buoyancy	NO	YES	YES	NO
Crossflow	YES	NO	NO	YES
Bottom Slope	NO[c]	NO	YES	NO
Surface Heat Loss	YES	YES	YES	NO
Provides For Flow Establishment	NO[c]	NO	NO	YES
Ambient Stratification Interaction	NO	NO	NO	NO
Direct Wind Stress Effects	YES	NO	NO	NO
Recirculation of Plume Water	NO	NO	YES	NO
Compared or Fitted With				
Field Data	YES	NO	unknown	NO
Tank Data	NO	YES	unknown	YES
Computer Program	YES[d]	NO[e]	YES[g]	YES[h]

[a]Wada Model No. 3 can also be used for near field or complete-field applications.
[b]A closed form solution has been derived for the case of zero wind stress.
[c]Flow development and bottom effects were considered indirectly via wind speed correlations.
[d]Computer program included with model or available from authors.
[e]Computer code does not exist yet. May be easily written from model equations.

Table 4-13, continued

Motz and Benedict, 1970	Koh and Fan, 1970b (2nd Model)	Koh and Fan (Axisymmetric Model)	Barry and Hoffman, 1971	Stolzenback &Hardleman, 1971	McLay et al., 1972	Stefan, 1971
YES	YES	YES	YES	YES	YES	EYS
YES	NO	YES	YES	YES	YES	YES
NO	YES	YES	YES	YES	YES	YES
YES	YES	YES	YES	YES	NO	YES
NO	NO	NO	NO	NO	YES	NO
NO	NO	NO	YES	NO	YES[c]	NO
YES	YES	YES	NO	YES	YES[c]	YES
NO	NO	NO	NO	NO	NO	NO
YES	YES	YES	YES	YES	NO	YES
NO	NO	NO	NO	NO	NO	NO
NO	YES	YES	YES	YES	NO	YES
YES	NO	NO	YES	YES	YES	YES
NO	NO	NO	YES	YES	NO	NO
NO	YES	YES	YES	YES	YES	YES
YES	NO	NO	NO	YES	YES	NO
NO	NO	NO	NO	NO	NO	NO
NO	NO	NO	NO	NO	YES	YES
NO	NO	NO	NO	NO	NO	NO
YES	NO	NO	YES	NO	YES	NO
YES	NO	NO	NO	YES	NO	YES
YES[d]	YES[d]	NO	YES[g]	YES[d]	YES[d]	YES[d]

[f]The model is actually quasi three-dimensional within a semi-infinite system having two-layer flow. Fluid properties are "averaged" vertically within each layer.
[g]Computer code exists but is presently unavailable from authors.
[h]Computer program written and available at Argonne National Laboratory.
[i]The zone of flow establishment is handled numerically; the established flow region is treated by integral methods.

Table 4-14. Summary of the Characteristics of the Far-Field Models (Policastro, 1972)

	Wada, 1966 (Model No. 1)	Wada, 1968 (Model No. 2)	Wada, 1969c (Model No. 3)	Lawler et al, 1968	Palmer and Izatt[e]
Direction of Temperature Variation					
Longitudinal	YES	YES	YES	YES	YES
Lateral	YES	YES	NO	YES	YES
Vertical	YES	NO	YES	NO	NO
Initial Mixing (Jet Regime)	NO	NO	NO	NO	NO
Ambient Turbulence (Far-Field Region)	YES	YES	YES	YES	YES
Mathematical Approach					
Numerical	YES	YES	YES	NO	NO
Integral	NO	NO	NO	NO	NO
Closed Form	NO	NO	NO	YES	YES
Semiempirical	NO	NO	YES	NO	YES
Time-Dependent Solution	NO	NO	NO	NO	YES
Buoyancy	NO	NO	YES	NO	NO
Crossflow	YES	NO[b]	NO	NO	YES
Bottom Slope	YES	NO	YES	NO	NO
Surface Heat Loss	YES	YES	YES	YES	YES[f]
Discharge Geometry	YES	YES	YES	YES	NO
Provides for Flow Establishment	–	–	–	–	–
Ambient Stratification Interaction	YES	NO	NO	NO	NO
Direct Wind Stress Effects	NO	NO	NO	NO	NO
Recirculation of Plume Water	YES	YES	YES	NO	NO
Compared or Fitted With					
Field Data	YES	–	–	NO	NO
Tank Data	–	–	–	NO	NO
Computer Program	YES[a]	YES[a]	YES[a]	NO[d]	NO[d]

[a]Computer program exists but is presently unavailable from authors.
[b]There is a possibility that this model may be able to handle the effects of ambient cross currents. This is not clear from Wada's papers.
[c]Model can also be used for near-field or complete-field applications.
[d]Computer code does not exist yet is easily written from model equations.
[e]The model is a simple stochastic one based on site current meter data which yield dilution ratios with time.
[f]The model has been extended to incorporate surface heat exchange by Asbury (1970).

Table 4-14, continued

Edinger and Polk (2d Model)	Edinger and Polk (3d Model)	Csandy (Off-shore Model)	Csanady (Shore-line Model)	Koh and Fan[i] (UTD)	Koh and Fan[k] (UTD)	Kolesar and Sonnichsen, 1971	Wnek (In Press)
YES	YES	YES	YES	YES	YES	YES	YES
YES	YES	YES	YES	YES	YES	YES	YES
NO	YES	NO	NO	YES	YES	NO	YES
NO	NO	NO	NO	NO	NO	NO	NO
YES	YES	YES	YES	YES	YES	YES	YES
NO	NO	NO	NO	YES	YES	YES	NO
NO	NO	NO	NO	NO	NO	NO	NO
YES	YES	YES	YES	NO	NO	YES	NO
NO	NO	NO	YES	YES	YES	NO	NO
NO	NO	NO	NO	NO	YES	YES	YES
NO	NO[h]	NO	NO	NO	NO	NO	NO[h]
YES	YES	YES	YES	YES	YES	YES	YES
NO	NO	NO	NO	NO	NO	YES	NO
YES	NO	YES	YES	YES	YES	YES	YES
NO	NO	NO	YES	NO	NO	NO	YES
—	—	—	—	—	—	—	—
NO	NO	NO	NO	NO	NO	NO	YES
NO	NO	NO	NO	NO	NO	NO	NO
NO	NO	NO	NO	NO	NO	NO	YES
YES	YES	NO	NO	NO	NO	YES	NO
NO	NO	NO	NO	NO	NO	NO	NO
YES[g]	YES[g]	NO[d]	YES[g]	YES[j]	YES[j]	YES[j]	NO

[g]Computer program written and available at Argonne National Laboratory.

[h]A constant vertical eddy thermal diffusivity was used in the model. Buoyancy is defined here as being considered if the coupling of flow and energy has been treated.

[i]This model is developed for the case of passive turbulent diffusion from a steady continuous source in a unidirectional steady shear current with constant surface heat exchange (PTD).

[j]Computer code included with model or available from authors.

[k]This model treats the problem of an unsteady continuous source in an unsteady uniform current with unsteady surface exchange (UTD).

Table 4-15. Summary of the Characteristics of the Complete-Field Models[a]
(Policastro, 1972)

	Pritchard, 1970	Sundaram et al., 1969	TSAI[d]	Asbury and Frigo, 1971[f]	Elliott and Harkness, 1972[f]	Giles et al., 1971	Loziuk et al., (In press)
Direction of Temperature Variation							
Longitudinal	YES	YES	YES	YES[c]	YES	YES	YES
Lateral	YES	YES	YES	YES[g]	YES	YES	YES
Vertical	YES	NO	NO[e]	NO	NO	YES	NO
Initial Mixing (Jet Regime)	YES	YES	YES	YES	YES	YES	YES
Ambient Turbulence (Far-Field Region)	YES	YES	YES	YES	YES	YES	YES
Mathematical Approach							
Numerical	NO	NO	NO	NO	NO	YES	YES
Integral	YES	NO	NO	NO	YES	YES	NO
Closed Form	YES	YES	YES	YES	NO	NO	NO
Semiempirical	YES	YES	YES	YES	YES	YES	NO
Time-Dependent Solution	NO	NO	NO	NO	NO	NO	NO
Buoyancy	NO	NO	NO	NO	NO[h]	NO	NO
Crossflow	NO	YES	YES	NO	YES	YES	YES
Bottom Slope	NO	NO	NO	NO	NO	YES	NO
Surface Heat Loss	YES	YES[c]	NO	NO	NO	YES	YES
Discharge Geometry	YES	YES	YES	NO	YES	YES	YES
Provides For Flow Establishment	YES	NO	YES	NO	NO	NO	NO
Ambient Stratification Interaction	NO	NO	NO	NO	NO	NO	NO
Direct Wind Stress Effects	NO	NO	NO	NO	NO	YES	NO
Recirculation of Plume Water	YES	NO	NO	NO	NO	YES	NO
Compared or Fitted With							
Field Data	YES	YES	NO	YES	YES	YES	YES
Tank Data	YES	NO	NO	NO	NO	NO	YES
Computer Program	YES[b]	YES[b]	NO	YES[b]	YES[c]	YES[j]	YES[i]

[a]Wada Model No. 3 may be used for complete-field applications.

[b]Computer program written and available at Argonne National Laboratory.

[c]Surface heat loss was considered only in the far-field regime.

[d]The TSAI Model has been developed for a unique submerged diffuser situation. Because of this, the general applicability of the model is limited. The table description under TSAI applies only to the analytical portion of this model synthesis describing surface spreading. Hydraulic modeling was used in the initial regime of flow.

[e]The cross-current model is strictly two-dimensional. The no-current case uses three-dimensional tank studies for heated surface jets. However, only the surface temperature predictions were utilized in the TSAI Model.

[f]Factors such as buoyancy, bottom slope, surface heat loss, flow establishment region, ambient stratification, wind effects and plume recirculation are implicit in the empirical data utilized for model development yet are not specifically modeled. This also holds true for crossflow and discharge geometry considerations with reference to the Asbury-Frigo Model.

[g]Only plume surface areas are predicted in this model. No temperature distributions are given.

[h]Froude number dependency is included in the model although buoyancy is not specifically modeled.

[i]Computer code exists but is presently unavailable from authors.

[j]Computer program included with model or available from authors.

The three equations of motion expressing conservation of momentum may be given in general form (for $i = 1,2,3$) as:

$$\frac{\partial v_i}{\partial t_i} + \sum_{j=1}^{3} v_j \frac{\partial v_i}{\partial x_i} = -\frac{\partial \Omega}{\partial x_i} - \left(\frac{1}{\rho}\right) \frac{\partial p}{\partial x_i}$$

where: p = pressure on the fluid
Ω = a potential, which is taken variously as a function of turbulent sheer stress, of kinematic viscosity, of eddy momentum diffusivity, etc.

The equation of conservation of energy or, in the present situation, of the equation of heat conduction in a moving fluid is given in general form as:

$$\frac{\partial T}{\partial t} + \sum_{i=1}^{3} \frac{\partial (v_i T)}{\partial x_i} = \alpha \sum_{i=1}^{3} \frac{\partial^2 t}{\partial x_i^2} + \frac{q}{\rho c_p}$$

where: T = temperature
α = the coefficient of thermal diffusivity = $k/\rho c_p$
k = thermal conductivity
c_p = specific heat of the fluid
q = the heat energy developed in unit volume and time

Where thermal conductivity, k, is a function of temperature and may have different values in each dimension, the equation can be represented as:

$$\frac{\partial T}{\partial t} + \sum_{i=1}^{3} \frac{\partial (v_i T)}{\partial x_i} = \frac{1}{\rho c_p} \sum_{i=1}^{3} \frac{\partial}{\partial x_i} \left(k_i \frac{\partial t}{\partial x_i} \right) + q/\rho c_p$$

In the near field, the equations of conservation of mass and of momentum tend to be paramount in defining the establishment of flow. In the far field, the equations of conservation of heat flow predominate, as heat is dissipated both throughout the receiving water and into the atmosphere (especially if the discharge has reached the surface). To render the equations tractable, in any specific model there are necessarily simplifying assumptions, and usually also transformations of variables, that relfect the special conditions modeled. Different models, as set up, calculate dispersion of the thermal plume in terms of a particular set of dimensions and parametric values. Typically, these include a representation of the plume trajectory and/or its dispersion (in two or three dimensions), as well as a measure of temperature excess in form suitable for the derivation of isotherms. But the results are typically given in different terms by different models, often making direct comparison of results somewhat difficult. Also, models may not calculate all the same characteristics.

Hirst's Model

Hirst's model (ORNL, 1976; Benedict *et al.,* 1972) enables the plume and its characteristics to be represented in three-dimensional space. For this purpose, the ordinary (x,y,z) coordinates are transposed to an orthogonal curvilinear system with one of the coordinates, s, representing the distance along the jet axis. A set of six differential equations is established, the solution to which yields values of the following measures as functions of s: (1) centerline velocity, (2) centerline temperature, (3) concentration of a particular foreign substance at the centerline, (4) width, and (5) angular value of the trajectory both with respect to the horizontal planes and to the x-axis within the horizontal plane. Another set of integral equations enables the centerline distance, s, to be represented in terms of the (x,y,z) coordinates.

Two especially interesting features of Hirst's model are the following:

1. Results may be computed according to the angle made by the discharge in the horizontal plane with the direction of the flow of the ambient. Hirst reports results not only for angles of $0°$ and $90°$ (coflow and perpendicular counterflow) but also for angles of $±15°$ and $±45°$.
2. Calculations may be made for the concentration of foreign substances in the discharge as a function of distance traveled along the trajectory. The equation for predicting how such concentration will vary was set up with particular reference to salinity but could be applied to concentrations of any chemical(s) as the discharge is diluted by the receiving water.

The set of differential equations from which the predict the dispersion of the thermal discharge can be solved by numerical means using computer programs that exist for the purpose. Results plotted by Hirst for a large number of jet flows studied experimentally are reported as obtained by an IBM 360/75 computer using Hamming's Modified Predictor-corrector Method (HPCG) of the IBM Scientific Subroutine Package.

Hirst's model has been modified by Shirazi and Davis of the Pacific Northwest Water Laboratory at the National Environmental Research Center under constract to the Environmental Protection Agency. The results have been summarized in the form of nomograms for manual application. By use of the nomograms, vertical rise of the plume, its width and excess temperature at the centerline may be computed as a function of downstream distance (*i.e.*, distance along the x-axis, in the direction of flow of the river). Results are plotted only for specific values of the following parameters: (1) Froude number, (2) ratio of initial jet velocity to that of the river, and (3) vertical angle of discharge (*i.e.*, initial angle made by the jet stream with respect to the horizontal plane). For intermediate values of these parameters, interpolation by eye is necessary.

The particular feature of the Hirst model is the development of a three-dimensional trajectory for a jet stream discharged into a flowing ambient. It also provides for a measure of any concentration of foreign matter in the water. In general, the jet centerline will follow a three-dimensional trajectory because the jet momentum vector, buoyancy force and crossflow vector may all point in different directions. For this purpose, Hirst transposes the trajectory to an orthogonal curvilinear coordinate system (s,r,ϕ), which moves with the jet centerline. The s dimension represents distance along the jet axis, whereas r measures the radial distance from the centerline and ϕ is an azimuthal angle determining the orientation of r. These coordinates are related to the (x,y,z) coordinate system by means of the equations:

$$x = \int_0^s \cos \theta_1 \, \cos \theta_2 \, ds$$

$$y = \int_0^s \sin \theta_1 \, \cos \theta_2 \, ds$$

$$z = \int_0^s \sin \theta_2 \, ds$$

where θ_1 is the angle which the projection of the s-axis onto the horizontal (x,y plane) makes with the x-axis, and θ_2 denotes the angle (in elevation) which the s-axis makes with this plane.

The equations of continuity, energy, concentration and momentum are transformed to the curvilinear coordinate system and written in terms of s, r and ϕ. The assumption is made that the flow is axisymmetric (*i.e.*, the velocity component parallel to the ϕ-axis is assumed to be O, as are the partial derivatives of velocity with respect to ϕ). This assumption leads to a new set of axisymmetric differential equations, which are then integrated in the radial direction from the jet axis to infinity. The resulting set of ordinary differential equations contains the centerline distance, s, as the single independent variable.

Gaussian profiles of velocity and density are assumed and the resulting values inserted to give a final set of ordinary differential equations which can be solved by numerical methods to give values of centerline temperature, velocity and concentration, as well as values of the angles θ_1 and θ_2, as functions of centerline distance, s.

REFERENCES

Ahmed, S. "An Economic Model of the U.S. Uranium Mining Industry," *IEEE Trans Systems, Man, Cybern.* 7(4):231-247 (1977).

Alan M. Voorhees and Assoc., Inc. "Guidelines to Reduce Energy Consumption Through Transportation Actions," McLean, VA: The MITRE Corporation, (1974).

Anderson, D. R., Ed. Truckee-Carson River Basin Modeling Project Data Report, "Environmental Dynamics, Inc. for EPA, Washington, D.C. (1973).

Antle, L. G., and R. W. Haynes. "An Application of Discriminant Analysis to the Division of Traffic Between Transport Models," IWR Report 71-2, Army Corps of Engineers (1971).

Armbruster, F. E., and J. Candela. "Research Analysis of Factors Affecting Transportation of Coal by Rail and Slurry Pipeline, "Report No. HI-2409-RR, Hudson Institute, Inc., Croton-on-Hudson, NY (April 1976).

Armstrong, N., M. Hinson, Jr., J. Collins and E. G. Fruh. "Biogeochemical Cycling of Carbon, Nitrogen and Phosphorus in Saltwater Marshes of Lavaca Bay, Texas, University of Texas, Austin (1975).

Army, U.S. "Guidelines for Preparing Environmental Impact Statement on Noise," Report of CHABA Working Group Number 69 (February 1977).

Asano, T. "Distribution of Pollutional Loadings in Suisun Bay," Nat. Symp. *Estuarine Poll.*, Stanford University, Stanford, CA (1967), pp. 441-461.

Asbury, J. G. "Far-Field Plume Dispersion in the Great Lakes," Intra-Laboratory Memorandum, Argonne National Laboratory, Center for Environmental Studies (April 30, 1970).

Asbury, J. G., and A. A. Frigo. "A Phenomenological Relationship for Predicting the Surface Areas of Thermal Plumes in Lakes," Argonne National Laboratory, ANL/ES-5 (April 1971).

Bailey, T. E. "Estuary Oxygen Resources-Photosynthesis and Reaeration," *J. San. Eng. Div., Am. Soc. Civil Eng.* 96:279 (1970).

Bain, R. C. "Predicting DO Variations Cased by Algae," *J. San. Eng. Div., Am. Soc. Civil Eng.* 94:867-881 (1968).

Ball, J. T., L. E. Johnson and G. M. Northrop. *User's Manual for the Tributary Water Quality Model*, CEM Report 4153-492-1, The Center for the Environment and Man, Inc., Hartford, CT (NSF RANN Grant GI-36580) (1973).

Barry, R. E., and D. P. Hoffman. "Computer Model for a Thermal Plume," Mechanical Division, The Detroit Edison Company, Detroit, Michigan, paper presented at ASCE National Resources Engineering Meeting, Pheonix, AZ, January 11-15, 1971.

Battelle, Pacific Northwest Laboratories. "Pioneer, a Water Quality Simulation Model," Report to the EPA (1974).

Battelle, Pacific Northwest Laboratories. "Explorer, a Water Quality Simulation Model," Report to the EPA (1974).

Baughman, M. L. "Dynamic Energy System Modeling—Interfuel Competition," Report No. 72—1, Energy Analysis and Planning Group, MIT Cambridge, MA (1972).

Bayer, M. B. "Nonlinear Programming in River Basin Modeling," *Water Resources Bull.* 10(2):311-317 (1974).

Behham, J., and R. E. Beglinger. "Effect of Energy Shortage and Land Use on Auto Occupancy," *Transport. Eng. J., Am. Soc. Civil Eng.* 102(TE2)(May 1976).

Bella, D. A. Discussion of "Solution of Estuary Problems and Network Programs" *J. San. Eng. Div., Am. Soc. Civil Eng.* 94:180-181 (1968).

Bella, D. A. "Simulating the Effect of Sinking and Vertical Mixing on Algal Population Dynamics," *J. Water Poll. Control Fed.* 42:R140-R152 (1970).

Bella, D. A., and W. Dobbins. "Difference Modeling of Stream Pollution," *J. San. Eng. Div. Am. Soc. Civil Eng.* 94:995-1016 (1968).

Ben-Akiva, M. E. *Structure of Passenger Travel Demand Models,* PhD Thesis, Department of Civil Engineering, MIT Cambridge, MA (1973).

Benedict, B., J. Anderson and E. Yandell, Jr. "Analytical Modeling of Thermal Discharges: A Review of the State-of-the-Art," performed under contract to Argonne National Laboratory (1972).

Bhatt, K. "Comparative Analysis of Urban Transportation Costs," *Transport. Res. Rec.* No. 559 (1976).

Billheimer, J. W. "Segmented, Multimodal, Intercity Passenger Demand Model," *Transport. Res. Rec.* No. 392 (1972).

Biswas, A. K. "Modeling of Water Resources Systems," Vol. 1,2, and 3. (Montreal: Harvest House, LTD., 1974), pp. 1-292; 296-645; 483-776.

Bogh, P., R. Hopkirk, A. Junod and H. Zuend. "A New Method of Assessing the Environmental Influence of Cooling Towers as First Applied to Kaiseraugst and Leibstadt Nuclear Power Plants," presented at the 3rd International Fair and Technical Meetings of Nuclear Industries (NUCLEX 72), Basel, Switzerland, October 16-21, 1972.

Bolger, F. T., and H. W. Bruck. *An Overview of Urban Goods Movement Projects and Data Sources,* MIT Urban Systems Laboratory (March 1973).

Bosanquet, C. H., W. F. Carey, and E. M. Halton, Dust Deposition from Chimney Stacks, *Proc. Inst. Mech. Eng.* (London), 162:355-367 (1950).

Bovee, K. "The Determination, Assessment, and Design of In-Stream Value Studies for the Northern Great Plains Region," Final Report, University of Montana, Missoula, MT (1974), pp. 55-204.

Bullard, C. W., and A. V. Sebald. "A Model for Analyzing Energy Impact of Technological Change," presented at the Summer Computer Simulation Conference, San Francisco, CA, July, 1975.

Bureau of Fisheries, Nacote Creek Research Station. "Studies of the Great Egg Harbor River and Bay," Miscellaneous Report No. 8M, New Jersey Department of Environmental Protection, Division of Fish, Game and Shellfish, Trenton, NJ (1975).

Callaway, R. J., K. V. Byran and G. R. Ditsworth. "Mathematical model of the Columbia River from the Pacific Ocean to Bonnivelle Dam Part 1, Federal Water Pollution Control Administration, Northwest Region, Corvallis, OR (1969).

Campbell, M. E. "The Energy Outlook for Transportation in the United States," *Traffic Quart.* (April 1973).

Carleton, R., *et al.,* "Intercity Freight Mode Choice," Report No. WP-210-U1-96, Transportation Systems Center, U.S. Department of Transportation (June 1975).

Carter, H. H. "A Preliminary Report on the Characteristics of a Heated Jet Discharged Horizontally into a Transverse Current, Part 1 - Constant Depth," Technical Report No. 61, Chesapeake Bay Institute, The Johns Hopkins University, Baltimore, MD (November 1969).

Cazelet, E. J. *SRI-Gulf Energy Model: Overview of Methodology,* Stanford Research Institute, Menlo Park, CA (1975).

Charles River Associates. *A Disaggregated Behavioral Model of Urban Travel Demands;* U.S. Department of Transportation, Federal Highway Administration (1972).

Charpentier, J.P. "Overview of Techniques and Models Used in the Energy Field," IIASA Research Memorandum RM-75-8 (March 1975).

Charpentier, J.P. "A Review of Energy Models: No. 1 - May 1974," presented at the Working Seminar on Energy Modelling, May 28-29, 1974, of the International Institute for Applied Systems Analysis, Laxenburg, Austria; reissued as IIASA Research Report RR-74-10 (July 1974).

Chermavsky, E. A., *Brookhaven Energy System Optimization Model,* Report No. BNL-19569, Brookhaven National Laboratory, 1974.

Chow, V. T. *Handbook of Applied Hydrology* (New York: McGraw-Hill Book Co., 1964).

Chuang, K. C., and D. G. Nichols. "A Cost Model of Coal Slurry Transport," Department of Chemical Engineering, West Virginia University, Morgantown, WV (1975).

Clark, S. M., and G. R. Snyder. "Timing and Extent of a Flow Reversal in the Lower Columbia River," *Limnol. Oceanog.* 14:960-965 (1969).

Csanady, G. T., Bent-Over Vapor Plumes, *J. Appl. Meteorol.,* 10:36-42, (1971).

Csanady, G. T. "Dispersal of Effluents in the Great Lakes," *Water Res.* 4:70-114 (January 1970).

Currier, E. L., J. B. Knox and T. V. Crawford. "Cooling Pond Steam Fog," in 66th Annual Meeting of the Air Pollution Control Association, Chicago, IL, June 24-28, 1973, Paper 73-126.

Dailey, J. E., and D. R. F. Harleman. "Numerical Model for the Prediction of Transient Water Quality in Estuary Networks," Ralph M Parsons Lab. for Water Resources and Hydrodynamics, Report No. 158, Department of Civil Engineering, MIT, Cambridge, MA (1972).

Deeanne, J. G. "A regional Techno-Economic Energy Supply Distribution Model for North America," Faculty of Management Sciences, University of Ottawa (July 1975).

Ditoro, D. M., D. J. O'Connor and R. V. Thomann. "A Dynamic Model of Phytoplankton Populations in Natural Waters," Manhattan College, Bronx, NY (1970).

Domencich, T. A., G. Kraft, and J. P. Vallette. "Estimation of Urban Passenger Travel Behavior: An Economic Model," Transport. Res. Rec. No. 238 (1968).

Dornhelm, R. B., and D. A. Woolhiser. "Digital Simulation of Estuarine Water Quality," Water Resources Res. 4:1317-1328 (1968).

Dresnack, R., and W. E. Dobbins. "Numerical Analysis of BOD and DO Profiles," J. San. Eng. Div., Am. Soc. Civil Eng. 94:789-807 (1968).

Dupree, W. G., Jr. and J. A. West. "United States Energy Through the Year 2000," U.S. Department of the Interior, Bureau of Mines (December 1972).

Edinger, J. E., and E. M. Polk, Jr., "Intermediate Mixing of Thermal Discharges into a Uniform Current," Water, Air Soil Poll. 1:7-31 (1971).

EG&G, Inc. "Potential Environmental Modifications Produced by Large Evaporative Cooling Towers," prepared for Environmental Protection Agency, Water Pollution Control Research Series, Environmental Services Operation, Boulder, CO, Report 16130 DNH 01/71, Superintendent of Documents, (Washington D. C.: U.S. Government Printing Office, January 1971).

Elliott, R. B., and D. G. Harkness. "A Phenomenological Model for the Prediction of Thermal Plumes in Large Lakes," The Hydro-Electric Power Commission of Ontario, Toronto, paper presented at Fifteenth Conference on Great Lakes Research, Madison, WI, April 5-7, 1972.

Environmental Dynamics, Inc. "Utah Lake-Jordan River Basin modeling Project Documentation and Sensitivity Analysis Report," submitted to the EPA, Office of Water Quality, Washington, D.C. (1971).

Environmental Protection Agency. "Simplified Mathematical Modeling of Water Quality," Hydroscience, Inc., Washington, D.C. (1971).

Environmental Protection Agency. "Addendum to Simplified Mathematical Modeling of Water Quality," Hydroscience, Inc., Washington, D.C. (1972).

Environmental Protection Agency. Workbook of Thermal Plume Prediction, Vol. I., EPA-R2-72-005a (August 1972).

Eochenroeder, A. Q., J. R. Martinez and R. A. Nordsieck. "Evaluation of a Diffusion Model for Photochemical Smog Simulation," Report EPA R4-73-012, General Research Corporation (1972).

Federal Energy Administration. "Energy Analysis and Forecasting Models," Office of the Assistant Administrator for Policy and Analysis, Technical Report 75-19 (October 1975).

Federal Energy Administration. Project Independence Report (Washington, D.C.: U.S. Government Printing Office, 1974).

Federal Highway Administration. Urban Transportation Planning (Washington, D.C.: U.S. Department of Transportation, 1970).

Federal Power Commission. "A Framework for Environmental Impact Evaluation for Electric Power Systems in a River Basin" (1975).

Feigner, K. D., and H. S. Harris. Documentation Report, FWQA Dynamic Estuary Model, Federal Water Quality Administration, (Washington, D.C.: U.S. Dept. of the Interior, 1970).

Fisher, H. B. "A Lagrangian Method for Predicting Dispersion in Bolinas Lagoon, Menlo Park, California, USGS, Water Resources Division, Open File Report (1969).

Fisher, H. B. "A Method for Predicting Pollutant Transport in Tidal Waters," No. 132, Hydraulic Laboratory, University of California, Berkely, (1970).

Fowler, M., and S. Poh. "General Description of Seven Available Mathematical Models for Water Quality Management," WP-7845 (July 1971).

Fraize, W. E., P. Dyson and S. W. Goose, Jr. *Energy and Environmental Aspects of U.S. Transportation,* MTP-391, (McClean, VA: The MITRE Corporation, 1974).

Fread, D. L. "Technique for Implicit Dynamic Routing in Rivers with Tributaries," *Water Resources Res.* 9:4 (1973).

Gendell, D. S. "An Application of the TRANS Approach to Evaluating National Transportation Alternatives," *Proc. Int. Conf. Transport. Res.,* Bruges, Belgium (1973).

General Public Utilities Corporation, Parsippany, N.J. Program to Investigate Feasibility of Natural-Draft Salt Water Cooling Towers, Appendix to Applicant's Environmental Report for Forked River Unit 1, 1972.

Giles, W., N. Johnson, G. McComb, F. Morris, J. Schell and J. Young. "A Thermal Effluent Analysis for Electric Power Generating Plants," Reentry and Environmental Systems Division, General Electric, Technical Information Series No. 71SD257 (September 20, 1971).

Goss, W.P., and J. G. McGowan. "Energy Requirements for Passenger Ground Transportation Systems," ASME Paper 73-ICT-24 (September 1973).

Grenney, W. J., and D. A. Bella. "Finite-difference Convection Errors," *J. San. Eng. Div., Am. Soc. Civil Eng.* 96:1361 (1970).

Grenney, W. J., and D. A. Bella. "Field Study and Mathematical Model of the Slack Water Buildup of a Pollutant in an Estuary," *Limnol. Oceanog.* 17: 229 (1972).

Hann, R., Jr., and P. Young. "Mathematical Models of Water Quality Parameters for Rivers and Estuaries," Technical Report No. 45, Water Resources Institute, Texas A and M University, College Station, TX (1972).

Hanna, S. R. "Fog and Drift Deposition from Evaporative Cooling Towers," paper presented at the Short Course in Applied Ecology at the 1973 Summer Programs in Oak Ridge, Tennessee, for Science and Engineering Faculty held at Oak Ridge Associated Universities, July 16 - August 3, 1973.

Hansen, E. P., and R. E. Cates. "The Parallel Path Wet-Dry Cooling Tower," The Marley Company, Mission, KS (1972).

Harleman, D. R. F., C. Lee and L. C. Hall. "Numerical Studies of Unsteady Dispersion in Estuaries," *J. San. Eng. Div., Am. Soc. Civil Eng.* 94:897-911 (1968).

Hartwig, J. C., and W. E. Linton. *Disaggregate Mode Choice Models of Intercity Freight Movement,* Northwestern University (June 1974).

Hayashi, T., and N. Shuto. "Diffusion of Warm Water Jets Discharged Horizontally at the Water Surface," *Proc. Int. Assoc. Hydraulic Res.,* Colorado State University, Fort Collins, CO, Vol. 4 (1967), pp. 47-59.

Hecht, T. A., *et al.* "Mathematical Simulation of Atmospheric Photochemical Reactions: Model Development, Vaidation and Application," Systems Applications, Inc. (1973).

Hedges, C. A. "Urban Goods Movement: An Overview," *Transportation Research Forum: Proceedings of 12th Annual Meeting* (1971).

Herendeen, R. A. *The Energy Cost of Goods and Services,* Report No. ORNL-NSF-EP-58 (Oak Ridge, TN: Oak Ridge National Laboratory, 1973).

Hiatt, D. B. "Energy Modeling: A Framework and Comparison," U.S. Dept. of Transportation, Transportation Systems Center, working paper WP-210-U2-100 (September 1975).

Hill, D. M. "A Model for Prediction of Truck Traffic in Large Metropolitan Areas," *Transportation Research Forum: Proceedings of 6th Annual Meeting* (1965).

Hirst, E. *Energy Consumption for Transportation in the U.S.,* Report No. ORNL-NSF-EP-15, Oak Ridge National Laboratory, March 1972.

Hirst, E. "Transportation Energy Conservation: Opportunities and Policy Issues," *Transport. J.* 13(3) (Spring 1974).

Hirst, E., and M. S. Stuntz, Jr. "Urban Mass Transit Energy Use and Conservation Potential," *Energy Syst. Pol.* I(4) (1976).

Hoffman, K. C., and D. O Wood. "Energy System Modeling and Forecasting," *Annual Reviews of Energy,* Vol. I (Palo Alto, CA: Annual Reviews, Inc., 1976).

Hoffman, K. C., and P. F. Palmedo. *Reference Energy Systems and Resources Data for Use in the Assessment of Energy Technologies,* Report No. AET-8, Associated Universities, Inc., Upton, NY (1972).

Holley, E. R. "Difference Modeling of Stream Pollution" discussion by D. A. Bella and W. E. Dobbins, *J. San. Eng. Div., Am. Soc. Civil Eng.* 95:968-972 (1969).

Hosler, C., J. Pena, and R. Pena, Determination of Salt Deposition Rates from Drift from Evaporative Cooling Towers, Department of Meteorology, Pennsylvania State University, 1972.

Hudson, E. A., and D. W. Jorgenson. "U.S. Energy Policy and Economic Growth: 1975-2000," *Bell J. Econ. Managemt. Sci.* 5(2)(Autumn 1974).

Huck, P. M., and G. J. Farquhar. "Water Quality Models Using the Box-Jenkins Method." *J. Environ. Eng. Div., Am. Soc. Civil Eng.* 100(EE3):733-752 (1974).

Hutchinson, B. G. "Estimating Urban Goods Movement Demands," *Transport. Res. Rec.* No. 496 (1974).

Hwang, C. L., J. L. Williams, R. Shojalashkari and L. T. Fan. "Regional Water Quality Management of the Generalized Reduced Gradient Method," *Water Resources Bull.* 9(6):1159-1181 (1973).

Hydrologic Engineering Center. "Water Quality for River-Reservoir Systems," No. 401-100 and 401-100A, U.S. Army Corps of Engineers, Davis, CA (1974).

Ippen, A. T. "Estuary and Coastline Hydrodynamics," (New York: McGraw-Hill Book Co., 1966).

Institute for Defense Analysis. *Economic Characteristics of the Urban Public Transportation Industry* (Washington D.C.: U.S. Government Printing Office, Stock No. 5000-0052, 1972).

Jack Faucett Assoc., Inc. "Project Independence and Energy Conservation: Transportation Sectors," Report No. JACKFAU-74-118(2), Chevy Chase, MD (August 1974).

Jeppson, R. W. "Simulation of Steady and Unsteady Flows in Channels and Rivers," PRYNE-070-1. Utah Coop. Fish. Unit, Logan, UT (1974).

Jobson, H. E., and N. Yotsukura. "Mechanics of Heat Transfer in Nonstratified Open-Channel Flows," Institute of River Mechanics, Colorado State University, Fort Collins, CO (1972).

Jordanides, T. and J. S. Meditch. "Some Aspects of Modeling Petroleum Utilization in the United States," *IEEE Trans Systems Man Cybern.* 7(4):217-255 (1977).

Just, J. E. *Impacts of New Energy Technology Using Generalized Input-Output Analysis,* M73-32 (McLean, VA: The MITRE Corporation, 1973).

Just, J., et al. *New Energy Technology Coefficients and Dynamic Energy Models, Volumes I and II,* MTR-6810 (McLean, VA: The MITRE Corporation, 1975).

Kadlec, J. A. "A Partial Annotated Biography of Mathematical Models in Ecology," Analysis of Ecosystems. IBP, University of Michigan, Ann Arbor, MI (1971).

Kaylor, F. B., J. D. Kangos, J. L. Petrillo, and Y. J. Tsai. "Prediction and Verification of Visible Plume Behavior Associated with Wet Plume Discharge," paper presented at 68th Annual Meeting of Air Pollution Control Association, Miami, FL, June 18-22, 1972, Paper 72-132, Air Pollution Control Association, Pittsburgh, PA.

Kennedy, J. F. "Wet Cooling Towers," in *Engineering Aspects of Heat Disposal from River Generation,* Chapter 13, Ralph M. Parkins Laboratory for Water Resources and Hydrodynamics, MIT, Cambridge, MA (1972); "Potential Environmental Modifications Produced by Large Evaporative Cooling Towers," EPA 14-12-542 by EG&C, Inc. (January 1971).

King, D. L., and J. J. Sartoris. "Mathematical Simulation of Temperatures in Deep Impoundments," Engineering and Research Center, REC-ERC-73-20 (Denver, CO: U.S. Bureau of Reclamation, 1973).

Klanian, P. S., and E. G. Noyes. "Economics of Wet/Dry Cooling Towers for Utility Power Plants," *Combustion* 45(4):31-34 (1973).

Knox, J. B. "Recent Advances in the Simulation of Regional Air Quality," Lawrence Livermore Laboratory, UCAL-78176 (August 1976).

Koh, R. C. Y., and L. N. Fan. "Mathematical Models for the Prediction of Temperature Distributions Resulting from The Discharge of Heated Water Into Large Bodies of Water," Tetra Tech., Inc., Report 16130 DWO 10/20 (1970).

Koh, R. C. Y., and L. N. Fan. "Mathematical Models for the Predictions of Temperature Distributions Resulting from the Discharge of Heated Water Into Large Bodies of Water," National Environmental Protection Agency Report, Water Pollution Control Research Series 16130 DWO 10/70 (1970).

Kolesar, D. C., and J. C. Sonnichsen, Jr. "TOPLYR - II—A Two-Dimensional Thermal-Energy Transport Code," Hanford Engineering Development Laboratory, Richland, WA (October 1971).

Kullman, B. C. "A Model of Rail/Truck Competition in the Intercity Freight Market," MIT Report No. 74-35 (December 1973).

Landon, R. D., and J. R. Houx, Jr. "Plume Abatement and Water Conservation with the Wet-Dry Cooling Tower," in *Proc. Am. Power Conf.*, Chicago, IL May 8-10, 1973, Vol. 35 (Chicago, IL: Illinois Institute of Technology, 1973).

Lange, R., and J. B Knox. "Adaptation of a Three-Dimensional Atmospheric Transport and Diffusion Model to Rainout Assessments," Lawrence Livermore Laboratory, UCRL-75731 (1974).

Lange, R. "ADPIC—A Three-Dimensional Computer Code for the Study of Pollutant Dispersal and Deposition Under Complex Conditions," Lawrence Livermore Laboratory, UCRL-51462 (1973).

Lange, R. "ADPIC—A Three-Dimensional Transport-Diffusion Model for the Dispersal of Atmospheric Pollutants and Its Validation Against Regional Tracer Studies," Lawrence Livermore Laboratory, UCRL-76170, Rev. 1, October 10, 1975 (submitted to Journal of Applied Meterology).

Lange, R., M. H. Dickerson, K. R. Peterson, C. A. Sherman and T. J. Sullivan. "Particle-in-Cell vs. Gaussian Calculations of Concentration and Deposition Out to 70 Km for Two Sites," Lawrence Livermore Laboratory (1976).

Lave, C. A. "A Behavioral Approach to Modal Split Forecasting," *Transport. Res.* 3(4) (1969).

Leeds, J. V., and H. H. Bybee. "Solution of estuary problems and network programs," *J. San.Eng. Div., Am Soc. Civil Eng.* 93:29-36 (1967).

Lehmann, E. J. "Water Quality Modeling—A Bibliography with Abstracts," Rep. No. NTIS-WIN-74-036. National Technical Information Service, Springfield, VA (1974).

Limage, D. R., R. Ciliano and J. R. Sharko. "Quantitative Energy Studies and Models: A Review of the State of the Art," in *Energy Policy Evaluation* D. R. Limage, Ed., Workshop on Modeling and Simulation for Energy Policy Evaluation, 44th Joint National Meeting, ORSA/TIMS, San Diego, California, November 1973 (Lexington, MA: D. C. Heath & Co., 1974), Chapter 14.

Lombardo, P. S. "Critical Review of Currently Available Water Quality Models," PB222265, Hydrocomp, Incoporated (DOI Contract No. 12-31-0001-3751) Palo Alto, CA (1973).

Loziuk, L. A., J. C. Anderson and T. Belytschko. "Hydrothermal Analysis by the Finite Element Method," Sargent & Lundy Engineers, Chicago, IL (Submitted for publication).

MacCracken, M. C., and G. D. Sauter, Eds. "Development of an Air Pollution Model for the San Francisco Bay Area," Final Report to the National Science Foundation, Vol. 1 and 2, Lawrence Livermore Laboratory, UCRL-51920 (1975).

MacCracken, M. C., *et al.* "User's Guide to the LIRAQ Model: An Air Pollution Model for the San Francisco Bay Area," Lawrence Livermore Laboratory, UCRL-51983 (1975).

Malliaris, A. C., and R. L. Strombotne. "Demand for Energy by the Transportation Sector and Opportunities for Energy Conservation," *Energy, Demand, Conservation and Institutional Problems,* (Cambridge, MA: MIT Press, 1974).

Manheim, M. L. "Practical Implications of Some Fundamental Properties of Travel-Demand Models," *Transport. Res. Rec.* No. 422 (1972).

Manne, A. S. "Emergency System Modeling," *Energy and the Social Sciences: An Examination of Research Needs,* Resources for the Future, Inc., Washington, D.C. (July 1974).

Marcuse, W., and L. Bodin. "A Dynamic Time-Dependent Model for the Analysis of Alternative Energy Policies," presented at the Summer Computer Simulation Conference, San Francisco, CA, July 1975.

Martin, B. V., F. W. Memmott and J. A. Bone. *Principles and Techniques for Predicting Future Urban Area Transportation* (Cambridge, MA: MIT Press, 1964).

Masey, A. C., and R. Paullin. "Transportation Vehicle Energy Intensities," Report No. DOT-TSC-13-74-1, Transportation Systems Center, U.S. Department of Transportation (June 1974).

McFadden, D., and F. Reid. "Aggregate Travel Demand Forecasting from Disaggregated Behavioral Models," presented at 54th Annual Transportation Research Board Meeting, 1975.

McLay, R. W., M. S. Hundal, F. Martinek and E. B. Henson. "A Mathematical Analysis of Thermal Pollution of Lakes and Estuaries," Department of Mechanical Engineering, University of Vermont, Burlington, VT (1972).

McLynn, J. M., and T. Woronka. *A Family of Demand and Modal Split Models,* Arthur Young and Co. (April 1969).

McVehil, G. E. "Evaluation of Cooling Tower Effects at Zion Nuclear Generating Station," *Final Report to Commonwealth Edison Company,* TR-0824, Sierra Research Corporation, Boulder, CO (1970).

Meyer, J. R., *et al. The Economics of Competition in the Transportation Industries* (Cambridge, MA: Harvard University Press, 1959).

Meyer, J. R., J. F. Kain and M. Wohl. *The Urban Transportation Problem* (Cambridge, MA: Harvard University Press, 1965).

Middlebrooks, E. J., D. H. Falkenborg and T. E. Maloney, Eds. *Modeling the Eutrophication Process* (Ann Arbor, MI: Ann Arbor Science Publishers, Inc., 1974).

Miklius, W. "Estimating Freight Traffic of Competing Transportation Modes: An Application of the Linear Discriminant Function," *Land Econ.* (May 1969).

Milne-Thompson, L. M. *Theoretical Hydrodynamics,* 5th ed. (New York: The MacMillan Company, 1968).

Morton, A. L. "A Statistical Sketch of Intercity Freight Demand," *Transport. Res. Rec.* No. 296 (1969).

Mutch, J. "The Potential for Energy Conservation in Commercial Air Transportation," Report No. R-1360-NSF, RAND Corporation, Santa Monica, CA (October 1973).

National Aeronautics and Space Administration and U.S. Department of Transportation. *Technology Assessment of Future Intercity Passenger Transportation,* Vol. 1-7 (March 1976).

National Petroleum Council. "Emergency Preparedness for Interruption of Petroleum Imports into the United States," Washington, D.C. (1974).

Nutter, R. D. *A Perspective of Transportation Fuel Economy,* MTP-396 (McLean, VA: The MITRE Corporation, 1974).

Oak Ridge National Laboratory. *Transportation Energy Conservation Data Book* (October 1976).

Oak Ridge National Laboratory. *Transportation Energy Conservation Data Book, Supplement II* (February 1977).

O'Connor, D. J. "Estuarine Distribution of Nonconservative Substances," *J. San. Eng. Div., Am. Soc. Civil Eng.* 91:23-24 (1965).

O'Connor, D. J., J. St. John and D. M. Ditoro. "Water Quality Analysis of the Delaware River Estuary," *J. San. Eng. Div., Am. Soc. Civil Eng.* 94:1225-1252 (1968).

Odum, H., W. Siler, R. Beyers and N. Armstrong. "Experiments with Engineering of Marine Eco-systems," Institute of Marine Science, Port Arkansas, TX (1963).

Office of Technology Assessment. "Energy, the Economy, and Mass Transit: Summary Report," U.S. Congress (June 1975).

Olufeagba, B. J., and R. H. Flake. "Modelling and Control of Dissolved Oxygen in an Estuary," *Proc. Sixth Triennial World Cong. Int. Fed. Automatic Control,* Boston/Cambridge, MA.

Ooms, E. "A New Method for the Calculation of the Plume Path of Gases Emitted by a Stack," *Atmos. Environ.* 6:899 (1972).

Orlob, G. T., R. P. Shubinski and K. D. Feigner. "Mathematical Modeling of Water Quality," National Symposium on Estuarine Pollution, Stanford University, Stanford, CA (1967).

Orville, H. D. "Ambient Wind Effects on the Initiation and Development of Cumulus Cloud Over Mountains," *J. Atmos. Sci.* 25:385 (1968).

Overbey, W., *et al. Feasibility Assessment of Study for Need of NO_x Control Technologies,* WP-11893 (McLean, VA: The MITRE Corporation: 1976).

Owens, M. V., and N. V. M. Odd. "A Mathematical Model of the Effect of a Tidal Barrier on Siltation in an Estuary," *Proc. Int. Conf. Utilization of Tidal Power,* Halifax, Nova Scotia, May 24-29 (1970).

Palmer, M. D., and J. B. Izatt. "Great Lakes Nearshore Modeling from Current Meter Data, 1969," Ontario Water Resources Commission, Ontario (November 1969).

Patten, B. C. "Mathematical Models of Plankton Production," *Int. Rev. Gesamten Hydrobiol.* 53:357 (1968).

Pence, G. D., J. Jeglic and R. Thomann. "Time-varying Dissolved Oxygen Model," *J. San. Eng. Div., Am Soc. Civil Eng.* 94:381-401 (1968).

Penna, J. C., and C. L. Husler. "Influence of the Choice of the Plume Diffusions Formula on the Salt Deposition Rate Calculation, Cooling Tower Environment-1974," USAEC, Conf. 740202 (1975).

Penumalli, B. R., R. H. Flake and E. G. Fruh. "Establishment of Operational Guidelines for Texas Coastal Zone Management Studies for Corpus Christi Bay: A Large System Approach," University of Texas, Austin, TX (1975).

Perkins, H. C. *Air Pollution* (New York: McGraw-Hill Book Co.)

Perle, E. D. *The Demand for Transportation—Regional and Commodity Studies in the United States* (Chicago, IL: University of Chicago Press, 1964).

Pilati, D. A. *Airplane Energy Use and Conservation Strategies,* Report No. ORNL-NSF-EP-69, Oak Ridge National Laboratory (May 1974).

Policastro, A. J., and J. V. Tokar. "Heated Effluent Dispersion in Large Lakes," Argonne National Laboratory, Argonne, IL (1972).

Pollard, J., D. Hiatt and D. Rubin. " A Summary of Opportunities to Conserve Transportation Energy," Report No. DOT-TSC-75-22, U.S. Department of Transportation (June 1975).

Pritchard, D. W., and H. H. Carter. "Design and Siting Criteria for Once-Through Cooling Systems," based on a First-Order Thermal Plume Model, Technical Report No. 75.

Pritchard, D. W. "Modeling of Heated Discharges—A Lecture," Westinghouse School for Environmental Management, Colorado State University, Fort Collins, CO, June 25, 1970.

Quandt, R. E., and W. J. Baumol. "The Demand for Abstract Transport Modes: Theory and Measurement," *J. Reg. Sci.* 6(2) (1968).

Queen Mary College, London. *Energy Modelling,* Special Workshop, U.S. National Science Foundation and the Energy Research Unit, October 1973 (Surrey, England: IPC Business Press Ltd., 1974).

Rassam, P. R., R. H. Ellis and J. C. Bennett. "The N-dimensional Logit Model: Development and Application," *Transport. Res. Rec.* No. 322 (1970).

Reiber, M., S. L. Soo and J. Stukel. "The Coal Future: Economic and Technological Analysis of Initiatives and Innovations to Secure Fuel Supply Independence," College of Engineering, University of Illinois at Urbana-Champaign, IL (May 1975).

Rice, R. A. "Energy Efficiencies of the Transport Systems," SAE Paper 730-066 (January 1973).

Rifas, B. E., and S. J. White. "Coal Transportation Capability of the Existing Rail and Barge Network, 1985 and Beyond," Report No. EPRI-EA-237, Electric Power Research Institute, Palo Alto, CA (September 1976).

Riggs, H. C. *Low-Flow Investigations,* USGS, Techniques of Water-Resources Investigations, Book 4, USGS, Washington, D.C.: U.S. Geological Survey, 1972), Chapter 81.

Riley, G. A., H. Stomel and D. F. Bumpas. "Quantitative Ecology of the Plankton of the Western North Atlantic," *Bull. Bingham Oceanog. Coll.* 12(3):1-169 (1949).

Roberts, P. O. "Forecasting Freight Flows Using a Disaggregate Freight Demand Model," MIT CTS Report No. 76-1, MIT (January 1976).

Roess, R. P. "Operating Cost Models for Urban Public Transportation Systems and Their Use in Analysis," *Transport. Res. Rec.* No. 490 (1974).

Roffman, A. "Atmospheric Effects of Wet Cooling Systems," paper presented at the American Geophysical Union Fall Annual Meeting, San Francisco,CA, December 10-14, 1973.

Roffman, A. "Environmental, Economic and Social Considerations in Selecting a Cooling System for a Steam Generating Plant in Cooling Tower Environment," USAEC (1974).

Rutherford, J. C., and M. J. O'Sullivan. "Simulation of Water Quality in Tarawera River," *J. Environ. Eng. Div., Am. Soc. Civil Eng.* 100(EE2):360-390 (1974).

Saski, B. R. "Predicting Transporter's Choice of Mode," *Transport. Res. Rec.* No. 577 (1976).

Schmidt, R. E., and M. E. Campbell. *Highway Traffic Estimation,* Eno Foundation for Highway Traffic Control, Saugatuck, CN (1956).

Schofield, W. R., and R. G. Krutchkoff. "Stochastic Model for a Dynamic Ecosystem," Bull. 60, Virginia Polytechnical Institute and State University, Blacksburg, VA (1974).

Searl, M. F., Ed. "Energy Modeling: Art, Science, Practice," Energy Modeling Seminar, January 1973, Resources for the Future, Inc., Washington, D.C. (March 1973).

Shahane, A. N. "Interdisciplinary Models of Water Systems," *Eco. Model.* 2: 117-145 (1976).

Shearman, J., and R. Swisshelm, Jr. "Derivation of Homogenous Stream Flow Records in the Upper Kentucky River Basin, Southeastern Kentucky, USGS, Water Resources Division, Louisville, KY (1975).

Sherman, C. A. *A Mass-Consistent Model for Wind Fields Over Complex Terrain,* Lawrence Livermore Laboratory, UCRL-76171, Rev. 1 (October 1975).

Shubinski, R. P., J. C. McCarty and M. R. Lindorf. "Computer simulation of Estuarial Networks," *J. Hyd. Div., Am Soc. Civil Eng.* 91(HY5):33-49 (1974).

Slade, D. H., Ed. *Meterology and Atomic Energy* (Washington D.C.: U.S. Atomic Energy Commission, Division of Technical Information, 1968).

Slavin, H. L. "Demand for Urban Goods Vehicle Trips," *Transport. Res. Rec.* No. 591 (1976).

Sloss, J. "The Demand for Intercity Freight Transport," *J. Business* (January 1971).

Sloss, J., and P. W. MacAvoy. *Regulation of Transport Innovation: The ICC and Unit Trains to the East Coast* (New York: Random House, 1967).

Smith, W., and Associates. "State of Research and Data on Urban Goods Movement and Some Comments on the Problem," Transportation Research Board Special Report No. 120 (1971).

Spear, B. D. " Applications of New Travel Demand Forecasting Techniques to Transportation Planning—A Study of Individual Choice Models," Federal Highway Administration, U.S. Department of Transportation (March 1977).

Steele, J. H. "The Quantitative Ecology of Marine Phytoplankton," *Biol. Rev. Camb. Phil. Soc.* 34:129-158 (1958).

Stefan, H. "Surface Discharge of Heated Water, Part I: Three-Dimensional Jet-Type Surface Plumes in Theory and in the Laboratory," Department of Civil and Mineral Engineering, St. Anthony Falls Hydraulic Laboratory, Project Report No. 126, University of Minnesota, Minneapolis, Minnesota (1971).

Stochastics, Inc. "Stochastic Modeling for Water Quality Management," EPA, Office of Water Quality, Washington, D.C. (1971).

Stoian, E. R. "A Novel Framework for Evaluating Methods of Energy Modelling," presented at the 45th Joint National Meeting, ORSA/TIMS, Boston, MA, April 1974.

Stolzenback, K., and D. R. F. Harleman. "An Analytical and Experimental Investigation of Surface Discharges of Heated Water," Ralph M. Parsons Laboratory for Water Resources and Hydrodynamics, Massachusetts Institute of Technology, Report No. 135 (February 1971).

Stopher, P. R., and J. O. Lavender. "Disaggergate Behavioral Travel Demand Models: Empirical Tests of Three Hypotheses," *Transport. Res. Forum Proc.* (1972).

Stucker, J. P. "An Econometric Model of the Demand and Transportation," *Cost Benefit Analysis for Inland Navigation Improvements,* IWR Report 70-4, Army Corps of Engineer (1970).

Studies on the Demand for Freight Transportation; Volume I, II, (Princeton, NJ: Mathematica, 1967; 1969).

Sundaram, T. R., C. C. Easterbrook, K. R. Piech and G. Rudinger. "An Investigation of the Physical Effects of Thermal Discharges Into Cayuga Lake (Analytical Study)," CAL No. VT-2616-0-2, Cornell Aeronautical Laboratory, Inc. (November 1969).

Surti, V. H., and A. Ebrahimi. "Modal Split of Freight Traffic," *Traffic. Quart.* (October 1972).

Sverdrup, H. U., M. W. Johnson and R. H. Fleming. *The Oceans; Their Physics, Chemistry and General Biology* New York: Prentice-Hall, Inc., 1942).

Systems Analysis and Research Corporation. "Demand for Intercity Passenger Travel in the Washington-Boston Corridor," (1963).

Takeda, T. "Numerical Simulation of a Precipitating Convective Cloud. The Formation of a 'Long-Lasting Cloud,'" *J. Atmos. Sci.* 28:350 (1971).

Talvitie, A. P. "Aggregate Travel Demand Forecasts with Disaggregate Travel Demand Models," *Transport. Res. Forum Proc.* XIII (1963).

Texas Water Development Board. "DOSAG-1—Simulation of Water Quality in Streams and Canals—Program Documentation and Users Manual," PB 202 974, Systems Engineering Division of the TWDB (1970).

Texas Water Development Board. "QUAL-1—Simulation of Water Quality in Streams and Canals—Program Documentation and Users Manual," PB 202 973, Systems Engineering Division of the TWDB (1970).

Texas Water Development Board. "Simulation of Water Quality in Streams and Canals," Report 128, PB 202 975, Texas Water Development Board, Austin, TX (1971).

Texas Water Development Board. "Analytical Techniques for Planning Complex Water Resource Systems," Report 183, Texas Water Development Board, Austin, TX (1974).

Thayer, R. P., and R. G. Krutchkoff. "Stochastic Model for BOD and DO in Streams," *J. San. Eng. Div., Am. Soc. Civil Eng.* 93:59-72 (1967).

Thomann, R. V. "Mathematical Model for Dissolved Oxygen," *J. San. Eng. Div., Am; Soc. Civil Eng.* 89:1-30 (1963).

Thomann, R. V. "Time-series Analysis of Water Quality Data," *J. San. Eng. Div., Am. Soc. Civil Eng.* 93:1-23 (1967).

Thomann, R. V., D. J. O'Connor and D. M. Ditoro. "Modeling of the Nitrogen and the Algal Cycles in Estuaries," presented at the Fifth International Association of Water Pollution Research Conference (1970).

Transportation, Department of. "The Report by the Federal Task Force on Motor Vehicle Goals Beyond 1980," (1976).

Transportation, Department of. "Energy Statistics: A Supplement to the Summary of National Transportation Statistics," Report No. DOT-TSC-OST-76-30 (1976).

Transportation, Department of. "National Transportation Trends and Choices," (January 1977).

Travelers Research Corporation, Hartford, CT. "Cooling Tower Effects (Fogging), Vermont Ynakee Generating Station," prepared for Vermont Yankee Company (1971).

Trimble, S. W. "Denudation Studies: Can We Assume Stream Steady State?" *Science* 188(4194):1207-1208 (1972).

Turner, D. B. *Workbook of Atmospheric Dispersion Estimates,* Department of Health, Education and Welfare, NTIS, No. PB-191-482 (1970).

Veldhuizen, H., and J. Ledbetter. "Cooling Tower Fog: Control and Abatement," *J. Air Poll. Control Assoc.* 21(1):21-24. (1971).

Voorhees, A. M. and Assoc., Inc. *Guidelines to Reduce Energy Consumption Through Transportation Actions,* McLean, VA: The MITRE Corporation, 1974.

Wada, A. "Numerical Analysis of Distribution of Flow and Thermal Diffusion Caused by Outfall of Cooling Water," *Proc. Thirteenth Cong. Int. Assoc. Hydraulic Res.* August 31-September 5, 1969 pp. 335-342.

Wada, A. "Numerical Analysis of Distribution and Flow and Thermal Diffusion Caused by Outfall of Cooling Water," *Coastal Eng. in Japan* (11) (1968).

Wada, A. "A Study on Phenomena of Flow and Thermal Diffusion Caused by Outfall of Cooling Water," *Coastal Eng. in Japan* 10 (1966).

Wang, J. D., and J. J. Connor. "Finite Element Model of Two Layer Coastal Circulation," *Proc. 14th Coastal Eng. Conf.* Copenhagen, Denmark (1974).

Wang, J. D., and J. J. Connor. "Mathematical Modeling of Near Coastal Circulation," Report No. 200, School of Engineering, MIT, Cambridge, MA. (1975).

Wang, G. H. K., and R. Epstein. "Econometric Models of Aggregate Freight Transportation Demand," Report No. WP-210-U1-81-A, Transportation Systems Center, U. S. Department of Transportation (May 1975).

Warner, S. L. *Stochastic Choice of Mode in Urban Tranvel: A Study in Binary Choice* (Evanston, IL: Northwestern University Press, 1962).

Wastler, T. A., and C. M. Walter. "Statistical Approach to Estuarine Behavior," *J. San. Eng. Div., Am. Soc. Civil. Eng.* 94:1175-1193 (1968).

Water Resources Engineers Inc. "A Water Quality Model of the Sacramento-San Jaaquin Delta," Report of an Investigation of U.S. Public Health Service, Lafayette, CA (1965).

Water Resources Engineers Inc. "A Hydraulic-Water Quality Model of Suisan and San Pablo Bays," Report of an Investigation for the Federal Water Pollution Control Administration, Lafayette, CA (1966).

Water Resources Engineers. "Computer Program Documentation for the Stream Quality Model QUAL-II," Prepared for EPA Contract No. 68-01-1869, Upper Mississippi River Basin Model Project (1974).

Watson, J. *Possibility of Fogging from Cooling Tower Plume at Grand Gulf: Preliminary Estimate,* WP10187, (McLean, VA: The MITRE Corporation, 1973).

Watson, J. *Preliminary Survey of Thermal Discharge Modeling as Applied to the Grand Gulf Site,* WP-10134 (McLean, VA: The MITRE Corporation, 1972).

Watson, P. L. "Predictions of Intercity Modal Choice from Disaggregate, Behavioral, Stochastic Models," *Transport. Res. Rec.* No. 446 (1973).

Wayne, L. G., A. Kokin and M. I. Weisburd. "Controlled Evaluation of the Reactive Environmental Simulation Model (REM)," Report EPA-R4-73-013, Pacific Environmental Service, Inc. (1973).

Weinstein, A. I. "Numerical Model of Cumulus Dynamics and Microphysics," *J. Atmos. Sci.* 27:246(1970).

Weinstein, A. I., and L. G. Davis. "A Parameterized Numerical Model of Cumulus Convection," Revised Edition, Department of Meteorology, Pennsylvania State University (May 1968).

Westinghouse Environmental Systems Department, Pittsburgh, PA. "Cooling Tower Effects," prepared for Vermont Electric Power Company, Inc., Rutland, VT (June 29, 1973).

Westinghouse Environmental Systems Department, Pittsburgh, PA. "Numerical Model for Cooling Systems Plumes," (1974).

Wildhorn, S., *et al. How to Save Gasoline: Public Policy Alternatives for the Automobile* (Cambridge, MA: Ballinger Publishing Co., 1976).

Wnek, W. "Mathematical Model for the Dispersion of Heat Into a Lake," Illinois Institute of Technology Research Institute (In press).

Woodruff, R. K., D. E. Jenne, C. L. Simpson and J. J. Fuquay. "Final Report on a Meteorological Evaluation of the Effects of the Proposed Cooling Towers at the Hanford Number Two "C" Site on Surrounding Areas," Battelle-Pacific Northwest Laboratory, Richland, WA, Contract No. BR-2808-7 to Burns and Roe, Inc., Hempstead, NY (September 1971).

CHAPTER 5

LEGAL FRAMEWORK

Within the federal system, the Supremacy Clause of the Constitution assigns to the federal government the role of making the Constitution and federal acts "the Supreme Law of the Land" (Art. VI, cl. 2). Within this same clause is also included "all Treaties made . . . under the Authority of the United States." Thus, the highest authority in legal questions is the U.S. Constitution. Under the Constitution, public laws (U.S. Code or Federal Statute) and international treaties have the next ranking—legal status. Federal regulations are written under the authority of public law. Once a regulation is issued as "final," it has the force of public law. Executive Orders and federal court decisions have the same level of authority as federal regulations. Intraagency regulations and state constitutions are considered to be lesser laws. The Constitution gives the states authority to adopt laws in areas not governed by the federal government. Of lesser legal status are state laws (State Code) and state court decisions and opinions. Local city or county ordinances have the least legal power, and do not, as a rule, affect federal decisions or actions. Figure 5-1 summarizes the hierarchy of laws and various court decisions. The EIS process must always include some discussion of these laws and regulations that would be followed to implement the proposed action.

Table 5-1 summarizes some of the more important federal legislation most cited in environmental statements. These laws are grouped according to general subject area (*i.e.,* air, water, noise, etc.). The common name of the legislation, and year passed or amended, are listed. Executive Orders and their numbers are listed along with legislation. Code and public law (PL) are listed by number for quick reference, to enable the user to look up the actual wording in the U.S. Code. Regulations written to implement the law are also listed by number for ready reference, either by *Federal*

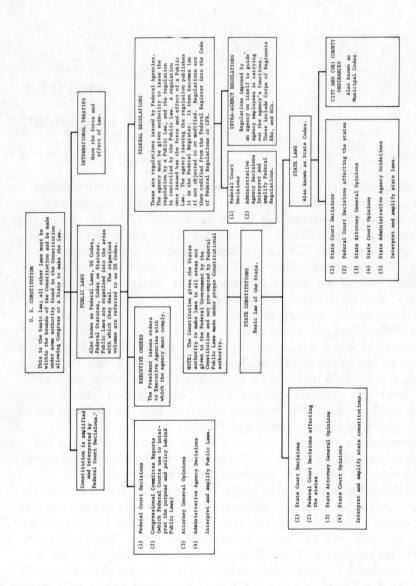

Figure 5-1. Hierarchy of laws and regulations of the federal and state governments.

Table 5-1. Federal Laws/Regulations Relating to Environmental Controls

Subject Area	Legislation Name (Act)	Year	Code	Public Law	Regulations	Agency Authorized	Brief Description of Controls
Air Quality	Clean Air Act or Emission Standards	1970 1973 1975	42USC1857	90-148 91-604 93-15	40CFR50-55 36FR22384 40CFR60-61 36FR24876 38FR8820 40FT18438	Environmental Protection Agency States may set more stringent air standards	Act establishes the Air Pollution Control Agency and duties, and states the federal policy on air pollution control. Bill provides the authority for Environmental Protection Agency to establish federal air quality standards for sulfur dioxide, particulate matter, carbon monoxide, photochemical oxidants, hydrocarbons, nitrogen dioxide. Primary: quality which EPA judges necessary to protect public health. Secondary: level of quality which EPA judges necessary to protect public welfare from known to anticipated adverse effects of pollutants.
Air Administration	Executive Order 11602 Executive Order 11738	1971 1973	— —	— —	36FR12475 38FR25161	Environmental Protection Agency	Provides for administration.
Water Quality	Water Pollution Control Amendments or Pollution Control in Navigable Waters	1972	33USC1251-1376	92-500	40CFR120-131 36FR22489 38FR30982 39FR36176 40FR47714	Environmental Protection Agency States to set standards and enforce, after approval of plan by federal government	Act declares the federal policy to restore and maintain the chemical, physical and biological integrity of the nation's water system. Act provides the authority to prepare comprehensive plans for water pollution control and to establish water quality standards. Act vides funding for construction, research and enforcement of standards. A national system of permits to discharge into U.S. waters is established (NPDES).
	Executive Order 11738 Executive Order 11574	1971 1970	— —	— —	38FR25161 35FR19627	Environmental Protection Agency Secretary of the Army	Define all planned uses of intra- and interstate and coastal waters intended to limit the amount and distribution of pollutants permitted in these waters.
Water Quality	Safe Drinking Water	1974	42USC300	93-523	40CFR131	Environmental Protection Agency States (enforcement)	Federal policy is to protect public water systems and underground water systems. EPA will publish primary drinking water regulations and recommend maximum contaminant levels permissible in drinking water. EPA can require treatment necessary to prevent adverse health effects. States have primary enforcement responsibility.

Table 5-1 (Continued)

Subject Area	Legislation Name (Act)	Year	Code	Public Law	Regulations	Agency Authorized	Brief Description of Controls
Water Quantity	Water Resources Planning	1965	42USC1962	89-80	36FR24144 38FR24778	Water Resources Council	Act establishes council and duties to prepare regional or river basin plans to encourage conservation, development and utilization of water resources. Both economic and environmental costs and benefits will be considered on federally financed water projects and most feasible alternatives.
	Executive Order 11747	1973	—	—	38FR30993	Office Management and Budget	Transfers authority to OMB and Chairman Water Resources Council.
Ocean Dumping	Marine Protection, Research and Sanctuaries Act	1972 1972	33USC1401-1444 16USC1431-1434	92-532 93-254 92-532	42FR10782 41FR47676 40FR41292	Environmental Protection Agency Secretary of the Army	Federal policy is to control dumping of all materials into the ocean. EPA is authorized to establish a dumping permit program and sites for dumping. The Army Corps is authorized to control dredged material disposal by a permit program. Dumping will not degrade health, welfare, marine environment, ecosystems or economic potentialities.
Navigable Waters	Protection of Navigable Waters or River and Harbors Act	1899	33USC403-466	85-802 86-645 88-172	40FR41292 40FR31320 40FR55804	Secretary of the Army Chief of Engineers (Army Corps of Engineers)	Act prohibits obstruction of navigable waters of the U.S. unless authorized by Secretary of the Army. It is also unlawful to excavate to fill in waters of the U.S. without a permit. Section 407 controls deposit of refuse in navigable waters. Section 419 regulates transport of materials for dumping.
River Protection	Wild and Scenic Rivers	1968 1974	16USC1271-1287	5 .-542 92-560 93-279		Secretary of Interior to study Secretary of Agriculture to study States authorized to administer	Act declares the federal policy is to protect wild rivers and to establish a system of national scenic rivers. Bill provides authority to study certain rivers and to control land use adjoining those rivers. Funds are authorized for land acquisition.
Federal Facilities	Executive Order 11752 Control of Pollution on Federal Facilities	1973	—	—	38FR34793	All federal agencies	Order provides that all federal, state and local standards should be met on all federal facilities. These standards include air, noise and water quality regulations. Facilities will install waste collection and disposal systems to prevent pollution of the environment.

Category	Act	Year	USC	Public Law	CFR/FR	Agency	Description
Federal Lands	"BLM Organic Act" or Federal Land Policy and Management	1976	43USC1701-1782	94-579	41FR149	Bureau of Land Management, Department of Interior	Act establishes a federal public land policy and provides authority to manage that land. The federal policy is to retain public lands in federal ownership for management under a multiple-use - sustained yield principle. The Bureau of Land Management is given the authority to manage public lands.
Historic Sites	National Historic Preservation Act Executive Order 11593	1966 1976	16USC470	94-422	36CFR800 40FR5242	National Park Service, Department of Interior	Act states a federal policy for protection of sites of historic interest. The head of the relevant federal agency must inventory sites and take into account the effect of proposed actions on sites listed in the Federal Register, or sites eligible for inclusion on this list.
Military Lands	"Sikes Act" or Fish and Wildlife Conservation on Military Reservations	1974	16USC670	93-452		Department of Defense Department of Interior	Act provides for cooperative plan for fish and wildlife management on military lands between the Department of Defense, Department of Interior and states. Plans include habitat improvement and public access to lands for recre ional use.
National Forests	Multiple-Use Sustained Yield Act	1960	16USC528-531	86-517		Forest Service, Department of Agriculture	Authorizes management of the national forests for sustained yield of timber, recreation, range, watershed, wildlife and fish.
Wetlands	Estuarine areas Protection of Wetlands, Executive Order 11190	1968 1977	16USC1221-1226	90-454	40FR55804	Department of Interior	Federal policy is to protect estuarine areas and balance need for conservation and development. All federal agencies shall consider estuaries and their importance. Department of Interior shall study estuaries and impacts of development upon estuaries.
Energy	Energy Supply and Environmental Coordination Act	1974	15USC791-798	93-319		Federal Energy Administration	Act declares need to meet U.S. Energy needs, while protecting and improving the environment. FEA may prohibit power plants from burning oil or gas, if coal conversion is practicable. Low sulfur fuel will be distributed on priority to minimize adverse impact.
Energy	Research and Development in Nonnuclear Energy	1974	42USC5901-5915	93-577		Energy Research and Development Administration	Act establishes energy goals and authorizes duties of ERDA. Policy is to develop U.S. energy sources and develop technological capabilities for energy use by an environmentally and socially acceptable means. Any program which requires significant use of water will consider the impacts on water resources.

Table 5-1 (Continued)

Subject Area	Legislation Name (Act)	Year	Code	Public Law	Regulations	Agency Authorized	Brief Description of Controls
Wilderness	Wilderness Act	1964 1972 1975	16USC1131-1136	88-577 92-528 93-622 93-632		Department of Agriculture	Act establishes National Wilderness Preservation System and provides for designation of wilderness areas. Act declares specific wilderness areas and limits uses of these areas. Roads and mechanical transport are not allowed in wilderness areas.
Solid Waste	Solid Waste Disposal Act Resource Recovery Act Executive Order 11752	1965 1970 1973 1975 1973	42USC3251-3259 -	89-272 91-512 93-14 93-611 -	40CFR243 38FR34793	Environmental Protection Agency States and localities to develop plans Secretary of Health, Education and Welfare	Act provides for construction, demonstration and application of waste management and resource recovery systems, technical and financial assistance to agencies in planning and developing resource recovery and waste disposal programs, and national research and development programs to develop and test methods of dealing with waste.
Noise	Noise Pollution Control Act Executive Order 11752	1972 1975 1973	42USC4901-4918 49USC1431 -	92-574 -	EPA-550/9-73-002 40CFR203-205 38FR34793	Environmental Protection Secretary of Treasury Secretary of Transportation Federal Aviation Administration	EPA must develop and publish criteria with respect to noise and effects on public health which can be expected from differing qualities and quantities of noise. EPA must publish regulations for major source of noise and noise emission standards for equipment for construction, transportation equipment, any motor or engine, and electrical or electronic equipment.
Noise	Occupational Safety and Health Act	1970	29USC651-656	91-596		Committee on Occupational Safety and Health; National Institute for Occupational Safety and Health (NIOSH) and Secretary of Labor	Authority to Secretary to establish national noise standards to protect health and welfare of employees and to promote occupational safety.
Noise	Noise Abatement and Control	1955 1970	42USC1858	91-604	none	Office of Noise Abatement within Environmental Protection Agency	Report on noise and its effects on public health and welfare by 1971.

Category	Name	Year	USC	Public Law	FR	Agency	Description
Pollutants	Hazardous Substances	1969	15USC1261-1274	86-613 89-756		Secretary Health, Education and Welfare	Act provides definitions of hazardous substances and provides authority to label and control same. Sections 1265(c) and 1273(b) provide for disposition of hazardous substances.
Pollutants	Toxic Substances Act	1976	18USC845	94-469		Environmental Protection Agency	Act defines toxic substances and provides for pre-market testing of new chemicals. Bill provides Environmental Protection Agency authority to define and limit use of toxic chemicals.
Pollutants	Environmental Pesticide Control	1972 1973	7USC136	92-516 93-205		Environmental Protection Agency	All pesticides must be registered with EPA. EPA will register all pesticides that will not cause unreasonable adverse effects on the environment. Pesticides will be classified for general use or restricted use. Applications will be certified.
Pollutants	Oil Pollution Act	1961 1973	33USC1001-1016	87-167 93-119		Coast Guard	Act prohibits discharge of oil at sea except to secure safety of ship and cargo. Coast Guard is given enforcement authority and cleanup.
Policy	National Environmental Policy Act	1969	42USC4321-4347	91-190	38FR30215 39FR35234	Council of Environmental Quality (to review) All federal agencies	Act establishes a federal policy to protect the environment. The Council of Environmental Quality is established to review environmental impact statements on all federal actions and programs having a significant impact on the environment. Section 4332(c) outlines the content of all environmental statements. Authority is given to the council to publish guidelines for environmental statements. (See 38 FR 147, Part II). Section 102(2)(c) requires an impact statement for all major federal actions.
ORVs	Executive Order 11644 Control of Off-Road Vehicles on Public Lands	1972	—	—	37FR2877		Order provides for controls on public lands for off-road recreational vehicles, to protect the resources and to minimize conflicts among users. Section 2(1)(c) applies specifically to military lands. However, Section 2(3)(b) exempts military vehicles when used for emergencies. Section 2(4) provides for official use of vehicles.
Wildlife	Migratory Bird Conservation	1929	16USC701-718			Fish and Wildlife Service, Department of Interior	Act is established to protect and conserve migratory game and insectivorous birds. Bill provides authority for federal regulation and enforcement of certain game laws. Section 715(i) concerns administration of lands in regards to endangered species.
Wildlife	Fish and Wildlife Coordination	1934 1972	16USC661-667	85-624		Fish and Wildlife Service, Department Interior	Act provides for the coordination of fish and wildlife management plans between federal, state, public and private agencies for conservation purposes. Section 661 provides for public access to public lands for hunting and fishing. All agencies must consult with Fish and Wildlife Service on major federal actions.

Table 5-1 (Continued)

Subject Area	Legislation Name (Act)	Year	Code	Public Law	Regulations	Agency Authorized	Brief Description of Controls
Wildlife	Fish and Wildlife Act	1956 1974	16USC742-754	93-271	50CFR19 36FR21034	Fish and Wildlife Service, Department of Interior	Act establishes U.S. Fish and Wildlife Service within the Department of Interior and authorizes the study and management of fish and wildlife resources. Section 742 j-i makes taking by harassment of wildlife from air illegal.
Eagles	Protection of Bald and Golden Eagles	1972	16USC668	86-70 87-884 92-535		Fish and Wildlife Service, Department of Interior	Act protects bald and golden eagles from taking, including pursue, shoot, collect, molest or disturb.
Endangered Species	Endangered Species Act	1973	16USC1531-1543	93-205	40FR17612 40FR27823 40FR44329 40FR49347 41FR18617 41FR22915 41FR24523 41FR24367 41FR27381	Fish and Wildlife Service, Department of Interior	Act states the federal policy is to protect critical habitat for endangered and threatened species. A program is authorized for conservation of these species. The Fish and Wildlife Service is authorized to determine species to be listed and is aauthorized to regulate and enforce the laws. Section 7 of the Act requires federal projects to preserve critical habitat of endangered species.
	Executive Order 11911	1976	—	—			
Planning	Coastal Zone Management Act	1972 1975	16USC1451-1464	89-454 92-583 93-612		Coastal states Department of Commer Commerce	Federal policy is to protect and manage U.S. coastal zone as a high priority planning area. Secretary of Commerce is authorized to make grants to states for coastal zone management planning. All federal actions will comply with state management programs. State certification is necessary for coastal zone projects before a federal permit or license can be granted. Act authorizes estuarine sanctuaries.

Flooding	National Flood Insurance Act	1969 1973	42USC4001-4127	91-152 93-234	Department of Housing and Urban Development; Department of Treasury; Corps of Engineers; Department of Interior (Geological Survey); Soil Conservation Service; National Oceanic and Atmospheric Administration; Tennessee Valley Authority	Bill authorizes flood insurance program through federal government and insurance industry cooperation. Section 4101 authorizes identification of flood plains, flood-risk, mud-slide-prone, and other flood hazard zone mapping. Secretary of HUD is authorized to review adequacy of state management, flood control, zoning and flood damage prevention plans. Flood plans and insurance are mandatory to receive federal financial assistance.
	Executive Order 11988 Flood Plain Management	1977				
Transportation	Federal Highway Act or Department of Transportation	1966 1968	49USC1653	89-670 90-495	39FR35232	Federal Highway Administration; Federal Aviation Administration	Act authorizes a federal transportation network. Regulations outline procedures for considering environmental impacts. Section 4(f) of the Act protects public park and recreation areas.

Register number of by Code of Federal Regulation. The agency authorized to implement the program or to enforce the regulation is then listed. Finally, Table 5-1 provides a brief description of the controls of the Act and subsequent regulations.

Persons employed in environmental fields should also be aware of Committee Prints, which periodically update and compile federal laws on the environment. Two of the best references are: "A Compilation of Federal Laws Relating to Conservation and Development of Our Nation's Fish and Wildlife Resources, Environmental Quality and Oceanography" (Committee on Merchant Marine and Fisheries); and "Treaties and Other International Agreements on Fisheries, Oceanographic Resources, and Wildlife to which the United States is Party" (Committee on Commerce). Both of these committee compilations are available gratis from Congressional Committee offices in Washington, D.C.

Table 5-2 is a chronological listing of federal laws from 1899 to Executive Order 11190 (1977) on protection of wetlands. The table is historical, showing gradually increasing federal concern to protect coastal resources. Acts are listed by common name and cited by code number for reference. A brief summary of action taken or protection granted follows each act. These laws would be used in writing any EIS which pertains to marshes, swamps, waters or wetlands of the U.S.

Table 5-2. Federal Laws/Regulations Pertaining to Wetlands of U.S.

River and Harbors Act—1899 (33 USC 403): dredge and fill requirements and control over navigable waters. Section 10 permits required:

- unlawful to obstruct navigable waters unless approved by COE;
- unlawful to dredge, fill or alter without approval; and
- 101(a)(2) sets goal for protection of fish and shellfish.

Historically only used for navigation . . . however, in 1970, Court ruled that a dredge and fill permit in wetland could be denied based on ecological damages. (*Zabel* v. *Tabb* 430 F 2nd 199, Fifth Circuit decision from Chief Judge Brown.)

Submerged Lands Act—1953 (43 USC 1301 *et seq.*):

- gives ownership of submerged lands under navigable waters to states up to three miles shoreward; and
- federal government still controls uses specifically related to navigation, flood control and power production.

Table 5-2 (Continued)

Fish and Wildlife Coordination Act—1958 (16 USC 661 *et seq.*):

- Law states that any agency of the U.S. or any private interest under federal permit must first consult with Fish and Wildlife Service before issuance of a permit to dredge or fill.

Water Resources Planning Act—1962 (42 USC 1962 *et seq.*): to encourage conservation (and development) of land and water in U.S. on a comprehensive and coordinated basis with federal, state and local governments:

- creates Water Resources Council.
- Title II creates river basin resource commissions; and
- authorizes river basin planning.

In 1967 Council took position that this included coastal, shoreline, island and estuarine areas in study.

Marine Resources and Engineering Development Act—1966 (80 Stat. 203): created National Council on Marine Resources and Engineering Development and NOAA (1970):

- to oversee marine studies and advise President; and
- Commission found that states must have responsibility for coastal zone.

National Estuary Protection Act—1968 (16 USC 1221 *et seq.*): "to protect, conserve and restore these estuaries in a manner that adequately and reasonably maintains a balance between the national need for such protection in the interest of conserving the natural resources and natural beauty of the Nation and the need to develop these estuaries to further growth and development of the Nation."

National Environmental Policy Act—1969 (42 USC 4321 *et seq.*):

- sets out requirements for environmental impact statements by federal agencies; and
- establishes national policy of protecting the environment.

Water Bank Act—1970 (16 USC 1301 *et seq.*): to preserve, restore and improve the wetlands of the U.S. by conserving surface waters, preserving and improving waterfowl habitat, reducing runoff and erosion and contributing to flood control; allows for ten-year contracts between landowner and USDA.

Federal Water Pollution Control Act Amendments—1972 (33 USC 1151):

- regulates discharge of pollutants into U.S. navigable waters including from sources such as a vessel, pipe or floating craft and pollutants such as dredged spoil, rock or sand; and
- enforced by states and/or EPA (except dredge/fill permits which are still under Corps).

Table 5-2 (Continued)

Coastal Zone Management Act–1972 (16 USC 1451 *et seq.*): authorized NOAA to make grants to states to develop coastal zone management program.

- Departments of Commerce and the Interior must approve program.
- Once approved, all permits granted in zone must comply with management program of state

"to preserve, protect, develop and where possible, to restore or enhance the resources of the Nation's coastal zone for this and succeeding generations."

Corps of Engineers Regulation 33 CFR 209; 120(g)(3); 40 FR 144; 40 FR 173–1975:

"Although a particular alteration of wetlands may constitute a minor change, the cumulative effect of numerous such piecemeal changes often results in a major impairment of the wetland resources."

- Thus, the COE will evaluate the permit as part of a complete wetland area and consult with other agencies on cumulative effects of activities.
- It authorizes studies such as the Wetlands Review.

Department of the Interior (FWS) Regulations–1975 (40 FR 231: 55804): guidelines for oil and gas exploration and development in navigable waters and wetlands and review of fish and wildlife aspects of proposals in or affecting navigable waters.

Protection of Wetlands, Executive Order (11190)–1977: All federal agencies will minimize destruction of wetlands. Avoid construction in wetlands unless there is no practicable alternative. The Department of the Interior shall develop plans to protect barrier islands.

Corps of Engineers Regulation 33 CFR 322-323–1977: Regulations define wetlands and functions, values and public interest in wetlands. Provides guidelines and rules for Section 10 and 404 permits in wetlands. Rules prohibit filling of wetlands unless proven to be in the public interest.

Table 5-3 is a compilation of federal noise regulations. The first column refers to the source of the noise (*i.e.,* highways, vehicles, railroads, etc.). The second column is a summary of legal authority for noise control. The third column lists one of ten federal agencies involved in noise regulation of that source. Published and proposed noise controls and references are summarized in the last column.

Table 5-3. Federal Noise-Related Regulations[a]

Source	Legal Authority	Agency	Regulation Published
Highways	23 USC 109	FHWA	Proposed Noise Standard and Procedures 23 CFR 722[b] September 10, 1974[c] Final Regulations: Noise Standards and Procedures for Highway Traffic Noise and Construction Noise, April 23, 1976, Correction Noise Standrads; Compliance July 9, 1976.
Motor Vehicles	NEPA Guidelines, DOT, Order 5610.1B	FHWA	Final Regulations: Design Approval and Environmental Impact 23 CFR 771, etc., December 2, 1974.
Motor Vehicles	Motor Carrier Safety Regulations	FHWA	Final Regulations: Vehicle Interior Noise Levels 49 CFR 393, November 8, 1973.
Motor Vehicles		DOT	Draft Interagency Task Force on Motor Vehicles Goals Beyond 1980, November 10, 1975.
Interstate Motor Carriers 10,000 lb	PL 92-574, Sec. 18	EPA	Final Regulations: Noise Emissions Standards, 40 CFR 202, October 29, 1974. Proposed: Special Local Determinations for Interstate Motor Carrier Noise Emission Standards (40 CFR Part 202), November 29, 1976 and January 11, 1977.
		FHWA	Proposed Compliance Procedures 49 CFR 325, February 28, 1975. Final Regulations, Compliance Procedures 49 CFR 325 September 12, 1975. Corrections and Amendments, March 10, 1976.
Medium- and Heavy-Duty Trucks	PL 92-574, Sec. 5 and 6	EPA	Proposed Standards 40 CFR 205, Oc ober 30, 1974. Final Regulations: Noise Emission Standards for Transportation Equipment, April 28, 1976. Deletion of

[a]Metropolitan Washington Council of Governments. Department of Housing and Urban Development under provisions of Section 701 of the Housing Act of 1954, as amended, 1977.

[b]Indicated that regulation can be found in September 10 *Federal Register* and has been codified under Title 23, Part 772 of *Code of Federal Regulations* (CFR).

[c]Proposed Standards would not be retroactive; therefore, approval actions taken in conformance with 23 CFR 772 as published on June 19, 1973, and 23 CFR 772.30 on February 22, 1974, would remain in effect.

Table 5-3 (Continued)

Source	Legal Authority	Agency	Regulation Published
			40 CFR Sec. 205.54−1(c)(1)(1V) and Sec. 205.54−1(c)(2)(1V) regarding additional passby test for engine brakes March 9, 1977.
Railroads	PL 92-574, Sec. 17	EPA	Proposed Railroad Noise Emission Standards 40 CFR 201, July 3, 1974; January 14, 1976
		DOT/FRA	Proposed Procedures: Railroad Noise Emission Compliance Regulations, 40 CFR 201, November 8, 1976. Proposed: Special Local Determinations for Railroad Noise Emission Standards (40 CFR Part 201), November 29, 1976.
	45 USC 431	FRA	Petition: sleeping quarters for railroad employees 49 CFR 149, February 13, 1975.
Product Standards Identification of Major Sources	PL 92-574, Sec. 5 and 6	EPA	Identification of products as major sources. Publication of report June 21, 1974.
Lawn Mowers		EPA	Identification of Power Lawn Mowers, Report, as Major Sources of Noise, January 12, 1977.
Equipment		EPA	Identification of Pavement Breakers and Rock Drills Report, as Major Sources of Noise, February 3, 1977.
Portable Air Compressors	PL 92-574, Sec. 5 and 6	EPA	Proposed Noise Emission Standards 40 CFR 204, October 29, 1974. Final Regulations regarding Noise Emission Standards 40 CFR 204, January 14, 1976. Correction of January 14, 1976, February 26, 1976.
Low-Noise Products Certification	PL 92-574 Sec. 15	EPA	Final Regulations: Low-Noise Emission Products Certification Procedures 40 CFR 205, February 21, 1974.

Table 5-3 (Continued)

Source	Legal Authority	Agency	Regulation Published
Labeling Hearing	PL 92-574	EPA	Advance notice of Proposed Rulemaking Labeling of Hearing Protectors 40 CFR 211, December 5, 1974.
Housing	PL 89-174	HUD	Final Regulations: Circular 1390.2 Noise Abatement and Control; Department Policy, Implementation and Standards, August 4, 1971.
Military	PL 92-574	DOD	Environmental Protection and En nce-ment Peacetime Responsibilities, December 2, 1975.
	5 USC 552	DOD	Proposed Revisions Air Installations Compatible Use of Zone Policy (AICUZ), August 26, 1976.
Aircraft and Airports	PL 90-411	FAA	Final Regulations by FAA Noise Standards: Aircraft Type and Airworthiness Certification Procedure, 14 FAR 21 and 36. Effective December 1, 1969 as amended. Proposed amendments to 14 CFR Part 36 by FAA, October 28, 1976. Financing of Aircraft Noise Reduction Requirements, November 2, 1976.
	PL 92-574	FAA	Amendments to Noise Standards: Aircraft Type and Airworthiness Certification 14 CFR FAR 36. Effective September 20, 1976. Proposed Alternative Noise Reduc tion Stages and Acoustical Change Require-ments for Subsonic Transport Category Large Airplanes; for Subsonic Turbojet-Powered Airplanes, and for Single Engine Transport Category Airplanes, October 28, 1976. Correction of above, December 9, 1976.
		FAA	Final Amendments to FAR 21 and 36: Acoustical change approvals, December 19, 1974. Noise Standards for Propeller-Driven Small Airplanes, January 6, 1975. Correction of above, January 10, 1975. Correction for January 6, 1975, January 16, 1975. Correction for January 6, 1975, February 11, 1975.

Table 5-3 (Continued)

Source	Legal Authority	Agency	Regulation Published
			Final Regulations: Noise Abatement Operating Restrictions–Limitations for Certain Turbojets, Propeller-Driven Small Airplanes, and Agricultural–Operation and Firefighting Propeller-Driven Aircraft (14 CFR Part 21, 36, 91), December 23, 1976. Correction of above, January 24, 1977. Preamble clarification, March 17, 1977.
		FAA	Proposed Regulations by FAA Civil Air: Sonic Boom, April 10, 1970. Supersonic Aircraft, August 4, 1970. Retrofit Regulations, October 30, 1970. Sonic Boom, April 17, 1973. Short Haul, December 28, 1973. Two-Segment ILS, March 26, 1974. Civil Fleet Regulations, March 27, 1974. Public Hearing Concerning Concorde Supersonic Transport Aircraft Draft Environmental Impact Statement, March 14, 1975. Public Hearing on above, April 4, 1975.
	FAA Act of of 1958 Sec. 604	FAA/DOT	Proposed Noise Reduction Stages and Acoustical Changes Regulations: 14 CFR 36, November 5, 1975. Proposed Noise Reduction and Acoustical Regulations, Supplemental, February 9, 1976. Airport Noise Policy Request Comment on Alternative Policies by January 1, 1976.
	PL 92-574, Sec.7	EPA to FAA	Proposed Regulations by EPA to FAA: Notice of Public Comment Period Noise Regulations: February 19, 1974. Notice of Publication, Proposed Noise Standards, January 3, 1975. Prop-Driven Small Plane Regulations: 14 CFR 36, January 6, 1975. Correction January 28, 1975. Minimum Altitudes for Turbojet Powered Airplanes in Terminal Areas 14 CFR 91, January 6, 1975. Proposed Regulations: Submitted to the FAA by the U.S. EPA, November 22, 1976.

Table 5-3 (Continued)

Source	Legal Authority	Agency	Regulation Published
			Fleet Noise Level Regulations: 14 CFR 121, February 26, 1975. Civil Subsonic Airplanes, Noise Regulations: 14 CFR 19. Aircraft Noise Regulations: Civil Subsonic May 1, 1975. Proposed Noise Abatement: (1) Reduced Flap Setting Noise Abatement Approach; (2) Visual Two-Segment Noise Abatement Approach; (3) Two-Segment ILS Noise Abatement Approach 14 CFR 91, September 15, 1975. Correction of above, September 30, 1975. General Operating and Flight Rules, 14 CFR 91, November 29, 1976.
	(FAA Advisory Circulars Not Listed)		Proposed: Airplane Noise Requirements for Operation to and from an airport within the U.S., February 12, 1976.
	PL 91-190	FAA	Proposed Policies and Procedures for considering environmental impacts, August 12, 1976.
Working Place General	OSHA of 1970, Sec. 7	OSHA	Proposed Requirements and Procedures Occupational Noise Exposure 29 CFR 1910, October 24, 1974.
			Availability of Economic Impact Analysis Hearing, June 18, 1976.
	PL 91-190	OSHA	Notice: Draft Environmental Impact Statement on Proposed Occupational Noise Standards, June 16, 1975.
	OSHA of 1970, Sec. 7	OSHA	Current Regulations for Occupational Noise Exposure (would be superceded by 29 CFR 1910) 29 CFR 1910.95, October 18, 1972.
	OSHA of 1970, Sec. 7	HEW	Proposed: Certification of Industrial Sound Level Meter Sets 42 CFR 82, April 16, 1975. Final Regulations: Certification of Industrial Sound Level Meter Sets, October 8, 1976. Notice: Applications for Certification of Industrial Sound Level Meter Sets being accepted by OSHA, October 26, 1976.

Table 5-3 (Concluded)

Source	Legal Authority	Agency	Regulation Published
	PL 92-574, Sec. 4(c)(2)	EPA	Request for Review and Report on proposed OSHA Regulation, December 18, 1975.
		OSHA/ Labor Department	Response by Secretary of Labor on Proposed OSHA Regulation, March 18, 1975.
Mines	30 USC 725	Bureau of Mines, Department of Interior	Final Regulations Noise Control Standards Metal and Nonmetallic Open Pit Mines, August 7, 1974. Correction, October 7, 1974.

(Requirements for Consideration of Noise in Agency EIS not included)

Table 5-4 is a summary of proposed major environmental regulations under consideration for 1977 to 1979. Regulations are summarized under major headings of "Air," "Water," "Noise," "Pesticide," "Atomic Energy," "Resource Recovery" and "Toxic Substances." A brief description of proposed regulatory controls follows. Anticipated dates for regulation publication follow, but as of 1977, these are not final.

Table 5-4. Major EPA Regulations Under Consideration (Bureau of National Affairs, 1977)

Name	Description	Proposal Date
The Clean Air Act		
Lead Ambient Air Quality Standard	Development of an ambient air quality standard for lead and appropriate reference method	December 1977
Fuel Analysis Regulations for Existing Fossil Fuel-Fired Steam Generators	Establishes procedures for monitoring sulfur dioxide emissions from existing fossil fuel-fired steam generators by analysis of the fueld combusted	November 1977
Revised Regulations for New and Modified Steam Generators	Emissions standards and monitoring procedures for pollutants emitted from fossil fuel- and municipal waste-burning generators	January 1977

Table 5-4 (Continued)

Name	Description	Proposal Date
Indirect Source Regulations	Regulations for the review of planned highway and airport construction projects as indirect sources of air pollution.	December 1977

EPA is now revising the criteria document for photochemical oxidants. After the revision, it may be necessary to change the ambient air quality standard.

Review of the National Ambient Air Quality Standard for Photo-chemical Oxidants	EPA may modify the standard on the basis of new criteria to protect community health and welfare	February 1978

The Administrator has listed benzene as a hazardous pollutant under Section 112 of the Clean Air Act:

National Emission Standards for Hazardous Air Pollutants: Benzene		June 1978

The Administrator is now considering designation of the following source categories under Section 111 of the Clean Air Act for control of air pollutants from new and modified facilities. The dates listed in this section are dates by which a decision is expected on whether to designate a particular source category; regulations may be proposed at the same time.

Stationary Gas Turbines	September 1977
Stationary Internal Combustion Engines	July 1978
Nonmetallic Minerals	August 1978
Glass-Melting Furnaces	June 1978

The following regulations to control emissions from mobile sources of air pollution are now under development:

Aftermarket Parts Guidelines	Guidelines establishing a program program whereby aftermarket parts manufacturers can demonstrate that their parts do not degrade emissions when used as a replacement or add-on part	November 1977
Emissions Control Defects Warranty	Regulations implementing the warranty provisions of Section 207(a) that require manufacturers to produce vehicles free from defects at the time of sale that would cause emission standards to be exceeded.	December 1977

Table 5-4 (Continued)

Name	Description	Proposal Date
Amendment Importation of Motor Vehicles and Motor Vehicle Engines	To improve effectiveness of regulations in preventing importation of vehicles and engines which do not conform to federal emission standards	October 1977
Engine Parameter Adjustment Regulations	This amendment to the certification regulations will provide for certification testing at various engine parameter adjustments; it will help assure that emission levels measured during the certification of new motor vehicles agree with emission levels of vehicles in use	September 1977

The Federal Water Pollution Control Act

Proposed effluent guidelines are now being revised for review of best available technology in the following source categories:

Timber Products Processing	September 1978
Steam Electric Power Plants	September 1978
Leather Tanning and Finishing	September 1978
Iron and Steel Manufacturing	September 1978
Petroleum Refining	September 1978
Nonferrous Metals Manufacturing	December 1978
Paving and Roofing Materials	December 1978
Paint and Ink Formulation	December 1978
Printing and Publishing Services	December 1978
Ore Mining and Dressing	December 1978
Coal Mining	December 1978
Organic Chemical Manufacturing	March 1979
Plastics and Synthetic Material	March 1979
Pulp and Paper	March 1979
Rubber Processing	March 1979
Inorganic Chemicals	March 1979
Textiles	March 1979
Soap and Detergents Manufacturing	June 1979
Auto and Other Laundries	June 1979
Machinery and Mechanical Products	June 1979
Miscellaneous Chemicals—Adhesives and Sealants	June 1979
Miscellaneous Chemicals—Explosives Manufacturing	June 1979
Miscellaneous Chemicals—Gum Wood	June 1979
Miscellaneous Chemicals—Hospitals	June 1979
Miscellaneous Chemicals—Pesticides	June 1979
Miscellaneous Chemicals—Pharmaceuticals	June 1979
Miscellaneous Chemicals—Photographic Processing	June 1979
Miscellaneous Chemicals—Carbon Black	June 1979
Electroplating	June 1979

Table 5-4 (Continued)

Name	Description	Proposal Date

EPA is considering proposal of the following additional action under the Federal Water Pollution Control Act:

Oil Removal	Regulations establishing recommended methods and procedures for the removal of discharged oil	October 1977

The Safe Drinking Water Act

Amended Interim Primary Drinking Water Regulations for Trihalomethanes	Maximum contaminant levels for trihalomethanes in drinking water	September 1977
Revised National Primary Drinking Water Regulations	Regulations to establish treatment techniques or maximum contaminant levels for contaminants in drinking water	February 1978

The Noise Control Act

EPA will propose noise emission standards for the following products under Section 6 of the Noise Control Act:

Truct Transport Refrigeration Units	September 1977
Pavement Breakers and Rock Drills	December 1977
Lawnmowers	December 1977

EPA is also preparing the following regulations for proposal under the Noise Control Act:

Importation of Noise-Emitting Vehicles	Concurrent regulations by the Custom Service and EPA will govern the importation of regulated products under the Noise Control Act	November 1977

The Federal Insecticide, Fungicide and Rodenticide Act

Custom Blending of Pesticides	This regulation will provide relief from the necessity of registration for each possible combination of a specific pesticide with a fertilizer	September 1977
National Pesticide Monitoring Plan	National monitoring plan is required by Section 20 to be established in cooperation with other federal, state and local agencies	September 1977

Table 5-4 (Continued)

Name	Description	Proposal Date
Special Packaging	Establishes standards for pesticide containers to protect children from accidental poisoning	September 1977

EPA will repropose Pesticide Registration Guidelines which detail the information needed in the following areas for the registration process:

Chemistry	November 1977
Hazard Evaluation: Wildlife and Aquatic Organisms	November 1977
Hazard Evaluation: Human and Domestic Animals	January 1978
Product Performance	March 1978
Label Development	May 1978

The Atomic Energy Act

Name	Description	Proposal Date
Guidelines for Plutonium Cleanup	Guidelines for the cleanup of plutonium and other transuranium elements and restoration of contaminated areas	September 1977
Protective Action Guides for Nuclear Incidents	Protective Action Guides will be developed for use by federal agencies, states and local governments in developing emergency plans for accidents at fixed nuclear facilities and for transportatin of nuclear materials	January 1978
Federal Radiation Guidance: Implementation of "As Low As Practicable"	Guidance by which federal agencies can implement the existing requirements that planned radiation exposure be kept as low as practicable	1978
Occupational Limits for Radiation Protection	EPA is considering the need for more stringent federal radiation guidance for occupational exposure	October 1977
Fundamental Environmental Criteria for Radioactive Waste Management	The criteria will provide public health and environmental guidance to federal agencies that have responsibility for developing and regulating various radioactive waste disposal alternatives	September 1977
High Level Radioactive Waste Management	EPA standards will establish public health and environmental requirements to be met for the disposal of high-level radioactive waste	December 1977

Table 5-4 (Continued)

Name	Description	Proposal Date
Resource Conservation and Recovery Act		
Municipal Sanitary Landfill Guidelines	Guidelines under Section 1008 will address the practice of sanitary landfilling	November 1977
Guidelines for Municipal Disposal of Sludge	Guidelines under Section 1008 will be developed on acceptable methods of sludge disposal	May 1978
Hazardous Waste Criteria–Identification and Listing	EPA will develop criteria under Section 3001 for identifying which substances are hazardous for the purposes of the hazardous waste management provisions of the Act	January 1978
Notification System for Hazardous Waste Generators, Transporters, Storers and Disposers	Regulations will establish procedures for notification of EPA, or of a state having an approved program under Section 3006, concerning the identification, location, and general description of hazardous wastes, by transporters, storers, treaters and disposers	September 1977
Standards for Transporters of Hazardous Wastes	Regulations under Section 3003 will make transporters responsible for recordkeeping, transportation to approved facilities and compliance with the manifest system for hazardous wastes	November 1977
Standards for Owners and Operators of Hazardous Waste Treatment Storage and Disposal Facilities	National performance standards for facility owners and operators under Section 3004 will apply to recordkeeping, reporting and monitoring, compliance with operating practices, location and design, contingency plans, and facility maintenance	January 1978
Public Participation Guidelines	Provides mechanisms for public participation in the development, promulgation, revision, implementation, or enforcement of regulations, guidelines, information or programs authorized by the Resource Conservation and Recovery Act	September 1977

Table 5-4 (Continued)

Name	Description	Proposal Date
Permits for Hazardous Waste Treatment, Storage, and Disposal Facilities	To provide a mechanism to assure uniform control by states (or EPA) over hazardous waste facilities, including maintenance of data for compliance monitoring and enforcement	December 1977
Guidelines: State Hazardous Waste Programs	Guidelines to assist states in developing hazardous waste programs authorized under Section 3006	October 1977
Guidelines: State Solid Waste Programs	Regulations under Section 4002(b) will contain guidelines to assist in the development and implementation of state solid waste management plans	October 1977
Criteria: Classification of Disposal Facilities	Regulations will provide criteria for determination of which solid waste disposal facilities shall be classified as sanitary landfills and which shall be classified as open dumps	October 1977
Guidelines: Procurement Practices	Guidelines will assist government procurement agencies in complying with the requirements of Section 6002(e) for procurement of products with the highest practicable percentage of recovered materials	October 1978

Toxic Substances Control Act

Testing of Chemical Substances and Mixtures	Section 4 authorizes EPA to require testing to obtain data on health and environmental effects; an interagency committee will recommend testing priorities; its initial report was due October, 1977	N/A
Premarket Notification	Section 5 requires manufacturers and processors to submit notification before manufacturing new chemicals for commercial purposes and before manufacturing or processing chemicals for significant new uses; exact timetable for rule-making is not certain	N/A
Chlorofluorocarbons— Discharge to the Atmosphere	This phase of rulemaking on chlorofluorocarbons will deal with nonaerosol uses, including refrigerant uses	July 1978

Table 5-4 (Concluded)

Name	Description	Proposal Date
Polychlorinated Biphenyls (PCBs)	This phase of rulemaking will implement the statutory phaseout of production and use of PCBs	October 1977
Reporting and Retention of Information	Section 8(c) and (d) requires the manufacturers, processors, and distributors of chemical substances to keep records of significant adverse reactions to health or the environment and to submit health and safety studies; Section 8(e) requires an immediate notification to the administrator or any information indicating that the chemical may pose a substantial risk to health or the environment	December 1977

The regulations listed below have already been proposed and appear in the *Federal Register* issue of the date indicated.

Name	Description	Date in *Federal Register*	Comment Period Closing Date
Short Test for Emissions Control Warranty	Development of testing methods for exhaust emissions of in-use light-duty vehicles and light-duty trucks to determine whether they exceed applicable emission standards	May 25, 1977	October 7, 1977
Emissions Control (Performance) Warranty	Regulations specifying a short-cycle emissions test for in-use vehicles to determine whether warranty repair by the manufacturer is required	May 25, 1977	October 7, 1977
Testing Retrofit Devices for Fuel Economy Performance	Provides for EPA evaluation of manufacturers' claims for fuel economy retrofit devices	August 10, 1977	November 8, 1977
Classification of Pesticides for Special Use	EPA will classify a significant number of pesticides as special pesticides under Section 3(d)	September 1, 1977	October 3, 1977
Wheel and Crawler Tractor Noise	Noise emission standards for new wheel and track dozers	June 11, 1977	September 30, 1977
Truck-Mounted Solid Waste Compactor Noise	Noise emission standards for new truck-mounted solid waste compactors	August 26, 1977	November 25, 1977

Tables 5-5 through 5-9 are summaries of state laws. Federal agencies, which are considering major actions in state coastal areas, must comply in the future with state Coastal Zone Management Plans, under the Coastal Zone Management Act. Once the plan has been approved by the National Oceanic and Atmospheric Administration, all federal actions must be consistent with state planning. Table 5-5 summarizes major coastal states' legal definitions of "coast." Each state uses different terms in statutes to define coastal area. These terms are listed in the first major column. Landward and seaward boundaries are given in the following columns.

Since there is so much emphasis in federal law to protect wetlands and coastal zones, states have been active in passing wetland and coastal laws too. While most wetlands are located on state submerged lands, the states have been interested in preserving that public resource from degradation. Table 5-6 is a compilation of state law, policy and attitudes regarding placement of dredged material within state boundaries. Thirty-five states with major dredging projects and significant waterways are listed. State laws on coast, wetland, water, environment and land use are listed according to the year they were passed. The state agency having administrative responsibility over water resources is listed by name. A summary of dredge and fill laws, fees charged and state responses to a Corps questionnaire are listed.

Table 5-7 is a summary of state coastal zone management and wetland laws. Coastal states are listed with common names of state statutes. In some cases, the state has both coastal laws and wetland laws. Laws are listed by statute number and year for reference.

Table 5-8 is a summary of 35 states, which have major coastal, river or lake frontage and their applicable environmental laws. Codes are listed by statute number for environmental and water laws. The general subject area of that code is listed in the last column.

Table 5-9 is a summary of federal and state legal sources for periodic update of laws and regulations. By mid-1978, many laws will already have been amended and regulations revised. It is advisable to periodically update legal references. The first column is the legal reference; the second column states how often it is updated; the third column shows the source of these revisions.

Table 5-5. State Statutory Provisions for Boundary-Delineation Techniques on Coast (Robbins, 1974)

Coastal States	Coastal Area or Feature Defined by State Law								Feature Used to Designate Landward Boundaries											Feature Used to Designate Seaward Boundaries						
	Coastal Zone or Area	Wetlands	Marshlands	Shorelands	Shorelines	Estuary	Estuarine Sanctuary or Area	Coastal Waters[a]	Linear Measurement	Areal Measurement[b]	Physical Features[c]	Political Boundaries	Roads and Highways	Vegetation	Elevation	Coastal Mountain Range	Tidal Flow	Marine or Maritime Influence	Wash of Waves	Territorial Jurisdiction	Extent of Defined Feature[d]	Linear Distance	Water Depth	Low Tide	High Water Mark	Unstated
Coastal Management States																										
Alabama	X								X		X									X						
California	X						X	X	X											X						
Delaware	X							X			X									X						
Florida	X							X			X		X							X						
Louisiana	X										X															X
Mississippi		X								X																
New Jersey	X								X	X		X	X							X						
Oregon	X						X		X	X		X				X				X						
Rhode Island	X						X	X	X	X	X	X	X							X	X					
Texas	X									X										X						
Wetlands																										
Connecticut		X									X			X	X		X				X					
Georgia			X				X		X					X	X		X				X					
Hawaii		X	X					X	X							X		X				X				
Maryland		X	X		X			X	X								X	X	X		X			X		
Massachusetts		X						X	X	X	X			X	X		X				X					
New Hampshire		X	X				X		X	X	X			X	X		X				X					
New Jersey		X	X				X	X	X	X	X			X			X				X					
New York		X	X					X	X	X	X			X							X					
North Carolina		X							X	X	X									X						
Rhode Island		X	X		X				X	X	X	X		X	X					X	X	X				
Virginia		X	X						X	X	X			X	X					X		X	X			
Washington					X		X		X											X		X	X			
Shorelands																										
Hawaii				X	X				X										X			X	X			
Maine				X	X				X													X	X		X	X
Michigan				X	X				X																X	
Minnesota				X	X				X																	X
Washington		X						X	X	X	X									X		X				
Wisconsin			X						X	X	X													X	X	

[a] Coastal waters includes one or more of the following terms: coastal and tidal waters, sea, ocean, tidal flow or tidal influences, high and low tides, wave action, marine environment, waters and marine or maritime influences.

[b] This refers to statutes prescribing a minimum area (e.g., ponds of ten acres or more) before the feature is to be included within the application of the law.

[c] Physical features include one or more of the following: marshes, bogs, swamps, floodways, river deltas, flood plains, streams, lakes, tidal waters, rivers, bays, sounds, lagoons, estuaries, inlets, ocean or coastal waters, flood basins, flats, meadows, shrub swamps, wooded swamps, salt marsh, lowlands, flowage, glacial pot-hole lake, bank, salt water, beach, island, soil types, and measurable quantity of seawater.

[d] This term often includes lands under or adjacent to tidal or tidally influenced waters.

Table 5-6. Summary of State Codes and Attitudes Regarding Dredged Material (Wakeford and MacDonald, 1974)

State	Coastal (C), Lake (L) or River (R) State	Coastal Protection	Wetland Protection	Water Quality	Environmental Protection	All Land Use	State Agency Administering Water Quality Laws	Laws Dealing With Dredging and Dredge Disposal Laws	Does State Law Provide a Fee For Dredged Material? What Law Controls?	Creation of New Urban Lands by Filling Shallow Waters or Swampy Tracts	Use Dredged Material to Rehabilitate Strip-Mined Areas or Fill Polluted Wetlands	Use Dredged Material as Soil Builder or Nutrient	Use Dredged Materials to Create Harbor Islands or Wildlife Sanctuaries	Comment
AL	C	73		71		49	Water Improvement Commission	Yes	8-252(2)					
AK	C			73		60	Dept. of Environmental Conservation	No						
AR	R			43,71		39,71	Game & Fish Commission and Pollution Control Commission	Yes						
CA	C	72	70	67		65	Water Resources Control Board	Yes	Pub. Res. Code 6991,6890	Objects	Objects	Maybe	Maybe	
CT	C	72	71,73	35,70			—a	Yes	Yes; No auth.	Objects	Objects	?	Accepts	
DE	C	72	70					Yes	Possible; 7-6402	Objects	Within limits	?	Accepts	
FL	C	60,69,71		72		31	Dept. of Natural Resources	Yes	370.034(3)					
GA	C		70				Water Quality Control Board	C/E exempt from permit requirement	Possible; 91-101	Objects				
HI	C	73		65,72	66	63,69	Department of Health	Yes		Accepts	Accepts	?	?	County takes active role in regulation
IL	R			39,70, 71,72	67,72	59	—b	State & counties developing laws	19 & 65a &	Objects	Accepts	Accepts	Maybe	
IN	L				72		—c	Yes	60-718(10)	Maybe	Accepts	?	?	Regulation is largely at county level
KS	R			65,71			—d	No		Objects	Accepts	Accepts	Objects	
KY	R			68,73	66			Yes	Yes[e]	Objects	?	Accepts	Objects	
LA	C	65	74					Yes		Objects	?	?	Accepts	
ME	C	73						Yes	—g					
MD	C	70	70,72	67,68,71			—f	Yes	Fee $10	Maybe	Maybe	Accepts	Accepts	
MA	C	72	72					Yes		Objects	Accepts	Maybe	Objects	
MI	L		70		67,70			Yes						
MN	L		73	55,69	67,70	69	Pollution Control Agency	No		Objects	Objects	Accepts	Accepts	
MS	R			73			Clean Water Commission	Yes	Possible; 92.50	Objects	Objects	Accepts	Maybe	
MO	R		73				Water Supply & Pollution Control Commission	No	Case 184 M 202					Wants no islands
NH	C	72						Yes		Objects	Objects	Accepts	Maybe	

State	Class	Years	Agency	Ref.						Remarks
NJ	C	73, 73	Water Policy Commission		Yes	Objects	Maybe	Accepts	Accepts	Inventory in progress
NY	C	73, 72	Dept. of Conservation & Development	_h	Yes	Objects	Maybe	Accepts	Maybe	Reclaim strip mines but not wetlands
NC	C	66, 71			Yes	Objects	Accepts	Accepts	Accepts	
OH	L		Director of Environmental Protection	_i	No	Objects	Accepts	Accepts	Accepts	Multiple-agency response
OR	C	71, 69	Dept. of Environmental Resources	274.525 et seq	Yes	Objects	Accepts	Yes	?	
PA	C	70,72, 53		_j	Yes	Objects	Accepts	Maybe	Objects	Urban wetlands only and not to affect wildlife
RI	C	71, 65, 71	Dept. of Natural Resources	_k	Yes	Objects	Maybe	?	?	
SC	C	70	Water Quality Control Board		Yes	Objects	?	Accepts	?	
TN	R	68,71, 69			Yes					
TX	C	73	State Water Control Board	_m	Yes	Objects	Maybe	Accepts	Maybe	Multiple-agency response
VA	C	70, 73, 73	Pollution Control Commission	_n	Yes	Objects	Accepts	Accepts	Accepts	
WA	C	71, 67	Dept. of Natural Resources	_o	Yes	Objects	Accepts	Accepts	Objects	Has current NEPA case and is in court with Corps
WI	L	73, 69,72		_p	Yes	Objects	Maybe			Currently developing a plan
WY	—		Environmental Quality Department			?	?	?	?	
OK	—		Department of Health			Objects	Accepts	Accepts	Accepts	
NM	—		Environmental Improvement Agency			Objects	Accepts	Objects	Objects	
SD	—	73, 73	Board of Environmental Protection			Objects	Objects	Accepts	?	
LA	—		Water Quality Commission			Objects	?	?	N/A	

Note: Numbers in third through seventh columns refer to year in which legislation was first enacted and last revised. Question mark in a box indicates that respondee did not know the answer. "Maybe" indicates that it would be conditional on proven need and strict compliance with regulations.

a Water and Air Resources Commission and Department of Natural Resources and Environmental Control Authority Title 7, Sec. 3911.

b Department of Transportation; Pollution Control Board, Illinois Valley Regional Port District, Natural Resources Department; Ohio River Valley Water Sanitation Compact; Environmental Protection Agency, Department of Conservation; Great Lakes Basin Compact Commission.

c Stream Pollution Control Board.

d Kentucky Department of Environmental Protection; Tennessee River Basin Water Pollution Control Compact; Ohio River Valley Water Sanitation Compact.

e Spoil and fill now sold at 2.5¢/yd^3 royalty with additional severance tax of about 4¢/ton.

f Department of Natural Resources; Susquehanna River Basin Compact.

g Possible via S. 299.2, 322.401, 322.427, and 322.703.

h Possible via S. 146-8, but state discontinued the practice in 1969.

i Possible via S. 1505-07.

j Possible via S. 37-7-2.

k Pollution Control Authority and State Board of Health have permit authority over discharges of waste into any state waters.

l Indirectly through S. 70-330?

m Possible via Art. 4053d and 4053.

n Possible via S. 62.14.

o Possible via S. 79.01.178, 79.16.570, or 79.01.168.

p S. 30.20 (c) (2) and (d).

Table 5-7.　State Coastal and Wetland Laws

State	Coastal Zone Management	Year	Wetland	Year
AL	Coastal Area Act 1274-	1973		
CA	Coastal Zone Conservation, 3 PRC 2700	1972	PRC 6216	1970
CT	Tidal Wetlands Preservation, GSA 22-28	1972	22-7	1973
DE	Coastal Zone Act, 7 Del. C.A. 7001	1972		1970
FL	Coastal Zone Management Act, Fla. Stat. 370.0211	1960 1971		
GA	Coastal Marshlands Protection, Ga. C. Ann 45-136-147	1957		
HI	Shoreline Setback, Hi. Rev. Stat. 205 & 107-73	1950, 1973		
LA	Coast & Marine Resources, La. Rev. Stat. 51:1361	1965		
ME	Shorelands Management, Me. Rev. Stat. 12-4811	1973	Me. Rev. Stat. 12-4701	1974
MD		1970	Md. Ann. Code 66c-718	1970
MA	Coastal Wetlands, Ma. Ann. Ch. 130-105	1972	Ma. Ann. Ch. 130-40	1972
MI	Shorelands Protection, Law Ann. 281.631	1970		
MN	Shorelands Protection, Stat. An. 105.485	1971, 1973		
MS	Swamp Tidewater Land, 4070	1973	Code Ann 49-27-1	1972
NH	Tidal Wetlands, Rev. Stat 483-A:1-a	1972		
NJ	Coastal Area Facility Act 1429	1973	13:9A-1-10	1973
NY	Tidal Wetlands, Environ. Conserv. Law 25-0101	1973	15-0503	
NC		1966	Gen Stat. 113-230	1966 1971
OR	Coastal Zone Act, 191-110-140	1971		
RI	Coastal Zone Management, Gen. Law 46-23-1-6	1971	Gen. Law 2-1-13 to 2-1-18	1965
TX	Coastal Public Lands, Civ. Stat. Art 5415e-1	1973		
VA		1970	Va. Code 62.1-13.1	1970
WA	Shoreline Management Act, Rev. Code Ann. 90.58.010	1971		
WI	Shorelands Zoning, Stat. Ann. 59.971	1973		

Table 5-8. State Environmental and Water Laws

State	Code[a]	Subject
AL	8-252-259	Department of Conservation
	38-1-45	Navigation
	22-140	Water improvement
AK	38.05.135	Department of Natural Resources
	44.37.010	Conservation
	46.03.010	Water pollution
AR	47-801	Water pollution
	82-1904	Pollution control
	10-107	State lands
CA	PR 6201-6203-6370	State lands
	PR 2002-2200	Department of Conservation
	PR 21000	Environmental quality
	PR 8301	Navigable waters
	PR 6890	State permits
	GC 51200	Land conservation
	GC 66600	San Francisco Bay
	FG 5653	Fish and game
	WC 13140	Water quality
CT	25-3-10	Environmental protection
	136-51-54	Navigable waters
DE	7-916	Dredging
	7-1112 & 6303	Water pollution
	7-3911	Air and water resources
		Environmental control
		Department of Natural Resources
	23-1508	Dredge disposal
	7-6401	Submerged land
FL	370.013	Department of Natural Resources
	370.036	Dredge and fill activities
	372.121	State game lands
	373.013	Water resources
	253.123	Restricts filling and controls state tidal lands
	161.011	Beach and shore preservation
	403.061	Air and water pollution
GA	91-101	State properties
	17-507	Water quality control
HI	171-2	Public lands
	171-3	Department of Natural Resources
	201-30	Submerged lands
	266-1	Navigable waters, harbors
	321-16	Sanitation, sewage and protection of waters
	342-33	Disposal of wastes in state waters

[a]PR—Public Resources, GC—Government Code, FG—Fish and Game, WC—Water Code.

Table 5-8 (Continued)

State	Code	Subject
IL	Title 19-52	Rivers and lakes
	Title 19-61-65	Use of waters and water permits
	Title 19-829	Fill and small structures permits
	Title 19-1077.08	Navigation
	Title 111½-1001	Environmental protection
	Title 127-63	Department of Conservation, Fish and Game, Pollution
IN	35-5201	Environmental policy
	35-5212	Air and water pollution
	35-5235	Permits for pollution, disposal and construction
	48-5211 (10741)	Rivers and harbors
	60-719 (4742.1)	State shorelands
	60-718 (4742)	Department of Conservation
	68-523-536	Water Pollution Agency and Controls
KS	65-171	Stream pollution
	12-3105	Sewage systems
KY	224.005-033	Department of Environmental Protection
	224.190	Ohio River Valley water
	224.195	Tennessee River Basin water
	146.110	Soil and water conservation
	150.460	Inuurious substances in water
	151.250	Filling of lands
LA	Title 38-3	Navigation
	Title 9-1101	Public lands
	Title 30-179-1	Submerged lands
ME	12-514	Dredging and filling
	12-504	State-owned lands
	38-422	Environmental protection permits
MD	66C-6-30	Chesapeake Bay
	66C-33	Conservation, hunting and fishing
	66C-722	Dredging and filling
	66C-759-763	Scenic River Policy
	96A-26	Pollution of state waters and permits required
	96A-60	Susquehanna River
MA	130-25	Dredge material disposal
MI	16.352	Department of Natural Resources
	281.501	State waterways
	281.632	Water resources
	281.761	Natural rivers
	281.951	Inland lakes and streams
	281.953	State permits
	299.1-3	Department of Conservation
	322.401	State bottom lands
	322.701	Great Lakes submerged land and filling of same

Table 5-8 (Continued)

State	Code	Subject
MN	1.21	Great Lakes Basin
	84.03	Department of Natural Resources
	84.033	Natural areas
	92.45	State public lands
	465.18	State navigable rivers
	115.01	Water pollution control
MS	5956-01	Water resources
	5974-04	Submerged lands and parks
	4095	Submerged state lands
	7567	Local Permit Authority for Dredging
	5948	State mineral lands
	Mississippi Coastal Wetlands Act of 1973	
MO	40(a)	Conservation Commission
	204.006-.051	Water pollution
	241.290	River beds and islands
	241.291	Mississippi and Missouri River islands
NH	149:8-a	Dredge and fill permits
	483-A:1	Water resources
NJ	12:6-1-20	Navigation
	12:3-21-22	Dredge and fill permits in tidal waters
	58:1-34	Water resources
NY	3-0101	Department of Environmental Conservation
	21-0101-21-0723	Delaware River
	21-0301-21-0321	Susquehanna River
	11-0305(8)	Fish and wildlife
	15-0501	Streambed modification
	75	Navigation jurisdiction
NC	104-25	Inland waterway lands
	146-6-8	Filling lands and dredging
	113-229	Permits to dredge and fill
OH	721-04	Lake Erie soil and water
	721-11	Waterfront development
	1501-01	Department of Natural Resources
	1501-16	Scenic rivers
	1501-17	River modification
	1531-07	Public parks and lakes
	6111-01	Water pollution
	6111-03	Environmental protection
	6111.41	Water resources
	6161.01	Great Lakes Basin
OR	174.005	State lands
	274.025	Submerged lands
	274.280	Reclamation
	174.525-550	Streambed material

Table 5-8 (Concluded)

State	Code	Subject
	390.815	Scenic waterways
	449.075-083	Water pollution
	541.605-615	Dredge and fill permits
PA	3-849-852	Soil conservation
	30-200	Water pollution
	35-691.1-5	Clear streams and permit review
	35-691.402	Potential pollution
	32-751	Schuylkill River
	55-361	Erie Harbor
RI	2-1-21	Freshwater wetlands
	11-46.1-1	Intertidal salt marsh
	46-6-1	Navigation
	46-17.1-1-2	Dredge material
SC	63-195.12	Water pollution
	63-195.13	Dredge material
TN	11-1401	Scenic rivers
	11-1416	Water pollution
	12-201	Natural resources
	70-324-330	Water quality control
	70-1901	Tennessee River Basin
TX	Art. 4026	Public rivers, fish, wildlife
	Art. 4054	Dredging Corpus Christi
	Art. 4051	All islands, rivers, bays, etc., are state property
	Art. 4053	Dredging permits
	Art. 5421	Taking parkland
	Art. 969a-1	Submerged lands
VA	62.1-3	Dredging and filling
	62.1-44.47	Discharge into waters
	45.1-219	Reclamation of land
		Scenic rivers
WA	43.21.130	Water resources
	43.21A.040-190	Department of Ecology
	43.27A.020-090	Department of Water Resources
	43.51.240-650	Tidelands, beaches
	43.51.655	Seashore conservation
	79.01.004-084	Public lands (tidelands, shorelands defined)
	79.01.178	Use of dredged material
	79.70.010	Natural area preserves
	90.48.021-160	Water pollution
	90.58.140	Development permits
	WAC 173-16-060	Regulations
	(14)	Landfill
	(16)	Dredging
WI	24.39	Leases of public lands
	30.05	Submerged lands
	30.12-20	Navigable waters
	144.26	Navigable waters protection

Table 5-9. Data Update Regulations

Item	Revisions	Source[a]
Federal and State Statutes	Annual	Pocket Parts U.S. Code and State Codes
Federal Code	Annual	CFR and Supplements
Federal Register	Daily	Office of Federal Register, National Archives and Records Service
Engineering Regulations	Periodically	DMRP, WES, Corps of Engineers
Engineering Circulars	Periodically	DMRP, WES, Corps of Engineers
Laws, Court Decisions	Weekly	Environmental Reporter (BNA)
Environment Index (Federal legislation)	Annual	Environment Information Center
NEPA 102 Reporter	Biweekly	CEQ
Abstract Literature	Bimonthly	Environment Information Access

[a]CFR—Code of Federal Regulations, DMRP—Dredged Material Research Program, WES—Waterways Experiment Station, BNA—Bureau National Affairs, CEQ—Council of Environmental Quality.

REFERENCES

Bureau of National Affairs. *Chemical Regulation Reporter* (September 30, 1977).

Robbins, J. M. "Boundaries of the Coastal Zone," *Coastal Zone Managemt. J.* 1(3):305-331 (1974).

Wakeford, R. C., and D. MacDonald. "Legal, Policy and Institutional Constraints Associated with Dredged Material Marketing and Land Enhancement," U.S. Army Engineer Waterways Experiment Station, Vicksburg, MS, 3918C (1974).

CHAPTER 6

AIR QUALITY

To estimate the impact of a particular project on the quality of the surrounding air, one must have an estimate of the emissions to the air and the resulting ambient concentration. Generally, five pollutants are analyzed, for which standards are set (although other specific pollutants are considered when appropriate). These pollutants are: sulfur dioxide (SO_2), particulates, carbon monoxide (CO), oxides of nitrogen (NO_x), and oxidants.

Table 6-1 gives the national standards, along with the appropriate averaging time. To estimate the quantities of the pollutants emitted as a result of a specific activity, "emission factors" are used, which are average estimates of the rate at which a pollutant is released to the atmosphere as a result of some activity. Table 6-2 gives a list of emission factors available from the U.S. Environmental Protection Agency (EPA). The emission factors given by EPA are identified or ranked as for their accuracy. Each process is ranked A, B, C, D or E. For a process with an A ranking, the emission factor should be considered excellent. A process ranked B should be considered above average. A rank of C is considered average; D, below average; and E, poor. Tables 6-3 through 6-14 present several emission factors as an example of the data that can be obtained for specific activities.

The United States is divided into 247 Air Quality Control Regions (AQCRs). Table 6-15 gives a listing of the AQCRs along with the designation of that area. The designations are based upon the ambient air quality of the region. Values used for designation are given in Table 6-16.

To estimate the effect of additional loading due to the specific activity under consideration, a knowledge of the existing emissions is necessary. The National Emissions Report, prepared by EPA, estimates by source

277

category and by criteria pollutant, the emissions within each AQCR. The Appendix for Chapter 6 presents the 1973 data (latest available data) for the entire United States. This same information is available for each AQCR.

A summary of values of federal standards of performance for new stationary sources of air pollution promulgated by the EPA in the period from December 1971 through June 1976 is given in Table 6-17.

Table 6-1. National Ambient Air Quality Standards[a]

Contaminant	Averaging Interval	Primary Standard		Secondary Standard	
		μg/m^3	ppm[b] (by vol)	μg/m^3	ppm[b] (by vol)
Suspended	1 year[c]	75	–	60	–
Particulates	24 hr	260	–	150	–
Sulfur Dioxide	1 year[c]	80	0.03	–	–
Dioxide	24 hr	365	0.14	–	–
	3 hr	–	–	1,300	0.5
Carbon	8 hr	10,000	9.0	10,000	9.0
Monoxide	1 hr	40,000	35.0	40,000	35.0
Photochemical Oxidant	1 hr	160	0.08	160	0.08
Hydrocarbons (nonmethane)	3 hr (6-9 AM)	160	0.24	160	0.24
Nitrogen Dioxide	1 year[c]	100	0.05	100	0.05

[a] All values other than annual values are maximum concentrations *not to be exceeded more than once per year*. All concentrations relate to air at standard conditions of 25°C temperature and 760 mm of mercury pressure.

[b] PPM values are approximate only.

[c] Annual average refers to arithmetic mean for gases and geometric mean for particulates.

Table 6-2. List of Sources for which Emission Factors are Available (EPA, 1976a)

External Combustion Sources	Wood waste combustion in boilers
Bituminous coal combustion	Lignite combustion
Anthracite coal combustion	
Fuel oil combustion	Solid Waste Disposal
Natural gas combustion	Refuse incineration
Liquified petroleum gas consumption	Automobile body incineration

Table 6-2 (Continued)

Conical burners
Open burning
Sewage sludge incineration
Internal Combustion Engine Sources
Definitions Used in Chapter 3
    Highway vehicles
    Off-highway mobile sources
    Off-highway stationary sources
Evaporation Loss Sources
    Dry cleaning
    Surface coating
    Petroleum storage
    Gasoline marketing
Chemical Process Industry
    Adipic acid
    Ammonia
    Carbon black
    Charcoal
    Chloralkali
    Explosives
    Hydrochloric acid
    Hydrofluoric acid
    Nitric acid
    Paint and varnish
    Phosphoric acid
    Phthalic anhydride
    Plastics
    Printing ink
    Soap and detergents
    Sodium carbonate
    Sulfuric acid
    Sulfur
    Synthetic fibers
    Synthetic rubber
    Terephthalic acid
Food and Agricultural Industry
    Alfalfa dehydrating
    Coffee roasting
    Cotton ginning
    Feed and grain mills and elevators
    Fermentation
    Fish processing
    Meat smokehouses
    Nitrate fertilizers
    Orchard heaters
    Phosphate fertilizers
    Starch manufacturing
    Sugar cane processing

Metallurgical Industry
    Primary aluminum production
    Metallurgical coke manufacturing
    Copper smelters
    Ferroalloy production
    Iron and steel mills
    Lead smelting
    Zinc smelting
    Secondary aluminum operations
    Brass and bronze ingots
    Gray iron foundry
    Secondary lead smelting
    Secondary magnesium smelting
    Steel foundries
    Secondary zinc processing
Mineral Products Industry
    Asphaltic concrete plants
    Asphalt roofing
    Bricks and related clay products
    Calcium carbide manufacturing
    Castable refractories
    Portland cement manufacturing
    Ceramic clay manufacturing
    Clay and fly-ash sintering
    Coal cleaning
    Concrete batching
    Fiberglass manufacturing
    Frit manufacturing
    Glass manufacturing
    Gypsum manufacturing
    Lime manufacturing
    Mineral wool manufacturing
    Perlite manufacturing
    Phosphate rock processing
    Sand and gravel processing
    Stone quarrying and processing
Petroleum Industry
    Petroleum refining
    Natural gas processing
Wood Processing
    Chemical wood pulping
    Pulpboard
    Plywood veneer and layout operations
    Woodworking operations
Miscellaneous Sources
    Forest wildfires
    Fugitive dust sources

Table 6-3. Emissions from Anthracite Coal Combustion Without Control Equipment—Emission Factor Rating: B (EPA, 1976a)

Type of Furnace	Particulate[a]		Sulfur Dioxide[b]		Sulfur Trioxide		Hydrocarbons[c]		Carbon Monoxide		Nitrogen Oxides	
	(lb/ton)	(kg/MT)	(lb/ton)	(kg/MT)	(lb/ton)	(kg/MT)	(lb/ton)	(kg/MT)	(lb/ton)	(kg/MT)	(lb/ton)	(kg/MT)
Pulverized (dry bottom), no flyash reinjection	17A	8.5A	38S	19S	0.5S	0.25S	0.03	0.015	1	0.5	18	9
Overfeed stokers, no flyash reinjection	2A	1A	38S	19S	0.5S	0.25S	0.2	0.1	(2-10)	(1-5)	(6-15)	(3-7.5)
Hand-fired units	10	5	36S	18S	0.8S	0.4S	2.5	1.25	90	45	3	1.5

NOTE: Approximate efficiencies of control devices used for anthracite are: cyclone, 75-85%; and electrostatic precipitator, 85%.
aA is the ash content expressed as wt %.
bS is the sulfur content expressed as wt %.
cExpressed as methane.

Table 6-4. Emission Factors for Heavy-Duty Construction Equipment

Type of Equipment	Emission Factor (lb/hr)					
	CO	Exhaust HC	NO_X as NO_2	RCHO as HCHO	SO_X as SO_2	Particulate
Gasoline-Powered						
Wheeled tractor	9.52	0.362	0.430	0.0176	0.0155	0.0240
Motor grader	12.10	0.410	0.320	0.0194	0.0167	0.0207
Wheeled loader	15.60	0.531	0.518	0.0213	0.0234	0.0298
Roller	13.40	0.611	0.362	0.0167	0.0185	0.0260
Miscellaneous	17.00	0.560	0.412	0.0198	0.0234	0.0258
Diesel-Powered						
Tracklaying tractor	0.386	0.110	1.470	0.027	0.137	0.112
Wheeled tractor	2.150	0.148	0.994	0.030	0.090	0.136
Wheeled dozer	0.739	0.234	5.050	0.065	0.348	0.165
Scraper	1.460	0.626	6.220	0.143	0.463	0.406
Motor grader	0.215	0.054	1.050	0.012	0.086	0.061
Wheeled loader	0.553	0.187	2.400	0.041	0.182	0.172
Tracklaying loader	0.160	0.032	0.584	0.009	0.076	0.058
Off-highway truck	1.340	0.437	7.630	0.112	0.454	0.256
Roller	0.184	0.054	1.040	0.016	0.067	0.050
Miscellaneous	0.414	0.157	2.270	0.031	0.143	0.139

Table 6-5. Emission Factors for Refuse Incinerators Without Controls—Emission Factor Rating: A

Incinerator Type	Particulates		Sulfur Oxides[a]		Carbon Monoxide		Hydrocarbons[b]		Nitrogen Oxides[c]	
	(lb/ton)	(kg/MT)	(lb/ton)	(kg/MT)	(lb/ton)	(kg/MT)	(lb/ton)	(kg/MT)	(lb/ton)	(kg/MT)
Municipal										
Multiple chamber, uncontrolled	30	15	2.5	1.25	35	17.5	1.5	0.75	3	1.5
With settling chamber and water spray system	14	7	2.5	1.25	35	17.5	1.5	0.75	3	1.5
Industrial/commercial										
Multiple chamber	7	3.5	2.5	1.25	10	5	3	1.5	3	1.5
Single chamber	15	7.5	2.5	1.25	20	10	15	7.5	2	1
Trench										
Wood	13	6.5	0.1	0.05	NA	NA	NA	NA	4	2
Rubber tires	138	69	NA	NA	NA	NA	NA	NA	NA	NA
Municipal refuse	37	18.5	2.5	1.25	NA	NA	NA	NA	NA	NA
Controlled air	1.4	0.7	1.5	0.75	Neg	Neg	Neg	Neg	10	5
Flue-fed single chamber	30	15	0.5	0.25	20	10	15	7.5	3	1.5
Flue-fed (modified)	6	3	0.5	0.25	10	5	3	1.5	10	5
Domestic single chamber										
Without primary burner	35	17.5	0.5	0.25	300	150	100	50	1	0.5
With primary burner	7	3.5	0.5	0.25	Neg	Neg	2	1	2	1
Pathological	8	4	Neg	Neg	Neg	Neg	Neg	Neg	3	1.5

aExpressed as sulfur dioxide.
bExpressed as methane.
cExpressed as nitrogen dioxide.

Table 6-6. Average Emission Factors for Highway Vehicles,
Calendar Year 1972–Emission Factor Rating: B

Vehicle Weight Mix	Scenario						Emission Factors for Highway Vehicles									
	Average Route Speed		Ambient Temperature		Cold Operation	Carbon Monoxide		Hydrocarbons		Nitrogen Oxides		Particulate		Sulfur Oxides	
	(mi/hr)	(km/hr)	(°F)	(°C)	(%)	(g/mi)	(g/km)	(g/mi)	(g/km)	(g/mi)	(g/km)	(g/mi)	(g/km)	(g/mi)	(g/km)
National Average	19.6	31.6	75	24	20	76.5	47.5	10.8	6.7	4.9	3.0	0.60	0.37	0.23	0.14
			50	10	20	97.1	60.3	13.0	8.1	5.4	3.4	0.60	0.37	0.23	0.14
			75	24	100	145	90.0	14.6	9.1	4.6	2.9	0.60	0.37	0.23	0.14
			50	10	100	228	142	22.4	13.9	4.6	2.9	0.60	0.37	0.23	0.14
No heavy-Duty Travel	19.6	31.6	75	24	20	70.6	43.8	9.6	6.0	4.2	2.6	0.54	0.34	0.13	0.08
			50	10	20	92.9	57.7	11.3	7.0	4.7	2.9	0.54	0.34	0.13	0.08
			75	24	100	146	90.7	13.8	8.6	3.8	2.4	0.54	0.34	0.13	0.08
			50	10	100	234	145	22.1	13.7	3.8	2.4	0.54	0.34	0.13	0.08
Central City	19.6	31.6	75	24	20	78.2	48.6	11.2	7.0	4.8	3.0	0.60	0.37	0.20	0.12
			50	10	20	101	62.7	13.7	8.5	5.3	3.3	0.60	0.37	0.20	0.12
			75	24	100	154	95.6	15.6	9.7	4.5	2.8	0.60	0.37	0.20	0.12
			50	10	100	245	152	24.5	15.2	4.5	2.8	0.60	0.37	0.20	0.12
National Average	45	72.5	75	24	0	29.8	18.5	4.7	2.9	8.0	5.0	0.60	0.37	0.23	0.14

Table 6-7. Average Emission Factors for Highway Vehicles Based on Nationwide Statistics[a]

Year	Carbon Monoxide (g/mi)	(g/km)	Hydrocarbons Exhaust (g/mi)	(g/km)	Crankcase and Evaporation (g/mi)	(g/km)	Nitrogen Oxides (NO$_x$ as NO$_2$) (g/mi)	(g/km)	Particulates Exhaust (g/mi)	(g/km)	Tire Wear (g/mi)	(g/km)	Sulfur Oxides (SO$_2$) (g/mi)	(g/km)
1965	89	55	9.2	5.7	5.8	3.6	4.8	3.0	0.38	0.24	0.20	0.12	0.20	0.12
1970	78	48	7.8	4.8	3.9	2.4	5.3	3.3	0.38	0.24	0.20	0.12	0.20	0.12
1971	74	46	7.2	4.5	3.5	2.2	5.4	3.4	0.38	0.24	0.20	0.12	0.20	0.12
1972	63	42	6.6	4.1	2.9	1.8	5.4	3.4	0.38	0.24	0.20	0.12	0.20	0.12
1973	62	39	6.1	3.8	2.4	1.5	5.4	3.4	0.38	0.24	0.20	0.12	0.20	0.12
1974	56	35	5.5	3.4	2.0	1.2	5.2	3.2	0.38	0.24	0.20	0.12	0.20	0.12
1975	50	31	5.0	3.1	1.5	0.93	5.0	3.1	0.38	0.24	0.20	0.12	0.20	0.12
1976	44	27	4.3	2.7	1.3	0.81	4.8	3.0	0.38	0.24	0.20	0.12	0.20	0.12
1977	37	23	3.7	2.3	1.0	0.62	4.3	2.7	0.38	0.24	0.20	0.12	0.20	0.12
1978	31	19	3.2	2.0	0.83	0.52	3.8	2.4	0.38	0.24	0.20	0.12	0.20	0.12
1979	27	17	2.7	1.7	0.67	0.42	3.4	2.1	0.38	0.24	0.20	0.12	0.20	0.12
1980	23	14	2.4	1.5	0.53	0.33	3.1	1.9	0.38	0.24	0.20	0.12	0.20	0.12
1990	12	7.5	1.3	0.81	0.38	0.24	1.8	1.1	0.38	0.24	0.20	0.12	0.20	0.12

[a]This table reflects interim standards promulgated by EPA in 1973.

Table 6-8. Emission Factors for Motorcycles—Emission Factor Rating: B

Pollutant	Emissions			
	Two-Stroke Engine		Four-Stroke Engine	
	(g/mi)	(g/km)	(g/mi)	(g/km)
Carbon Monoxide	27	17	33	20
Hydrocarbons				
Exhaust	16	9.9	2.9	1.8
Crankcase	–	–	0.60	0.37
Evaporative	0.36	0.22	0.36	0.22
Nitrogen Oxides (NO$_X$ as NO$_2$)	0.12	0.075	0.24	0.15
Particulates	0.33	0.21	0.046	0.029
Sulfur Oxides (SO$_2$)	0.038	0.024	0.022	0.014
Aldehydes (RCHO as HCHO)	0.11	0.068	0.047	0.029

Table 6-9. Emission Factors per Aircraft Landing-Takeoff Cycle (lb/engine and kg/engine)—Emission Factor Rating: B

Aircraft	Solid Particulates (lb)	(kg)	Sulfur Oxides (lb)	(kg)	Carbon Monoxide (lb)	(kg)	Hydrocarbons (lb)	(kg)	Nitrogen Oxides (NO$_X$ as NO$_2$) (lb)	(kg)
Jumbo Jet	1.30	0.59	1.82	0.83	46.8	21.2	12.2	5.5	31.4	14.2
Long-Range Jet	1.21	0.55	1.56	0.71	47.4	21.5	41.2	18.7	7.9	3.6
Medium-Range Jet	0.41	0.19	1.01	0.46	17.0	7.71	4.9	2.2	10.2	4.6
Air Carrier Turboprop	1.1	0.49	0.40	0.18	6.6	3.0	2.9	1.3	2.5	1.1
Business Jet	0.11	0.05	0.37	0.17	15.8	7.17	3.6	1.6	1.6	0.73
General Aviation Turboprop	0.20	0.09	0.18	0.08	3.1	1.4	1.1	0.5	1.2	0.54
General Aviation Piston	0.02	0.01	0.014	0.006	12.2	5.5	0.40	0.18	0.047	0.021
Piston Transport	0.56	0.25	0.28	0.13	304.0	138.0	40.7	18.5	0.40	0.18
Helicopter	0.25	0.11	0.18	0.08	5.7	2.6	0.52	0.24	0.57	0.26
Military Transport	1.1	0.49	0.41	0.19	5.7	2.6	2.7	1.2	2.2	1.0
Military Jet	0.31	0.14	0.76	0.35	15.1	6.85	9.93	4.5	3.29	1.49
Military Piston	0.28	0.13	0.14	0.04	152.0	69.0	20.4	9.3	0.20	0.09

Table 6-10. Average Emission Factors for Inboard Pleasure Craft[a]–Emission Factor Rating: D

	Based on Fuel Consumption				Based on Operating Time			
	Diesel Engine		Gasoline Engine		Diesel Engine		Gasoline Engine	
Pollutant	$(kg/10^3)$	$(lb/10^3/gal)$	$(kg/10^3/l)$	$(lb/10^3/gal)$	(kg/hr)	(lb/hr)	(kg/hr)	(lb/hr)
Sulfur Oxides (SO_X as SO_2)	3.2	27	0.77	6.4	—	—	0.008	0.019
Carbon Monoxide	17	140	149	1240	—	—	1.69	3.73
Hydrocarbons	22	180	10.3	86	—	—	0.117	0.258
Nitrogen Oxides (NO_X as NO_2)	41	340	15.7	131	—	—	0.179	0.394

[a]Average emission factors are based on the duty cycle developed for large outboards ($\geq$ 48 kW or $\geq$ 65 hp).

Table 6-11. Emission Factors for Snowmobiles—
Emission Factor Rating: B

Pollutant	(g/unit-year)[a]	Emissions		
		(g/gal)[b]	(g/l)[b]	(g/hr)[b]
Carbon Monoxide	58,700	1,040	275	978
Hydrocarbons	37,800	670	177	630
Nitrogen Oxides	600	10.6	2.8	10.0
Sulfur Oxides[c]	51	0.90	0.24	0.85
Solid Particulate	1,670	29.7	7.85	27.9
Aldehydes (RCHO)	552	9.8	2.6	9.2

[a]Based on 60 hr/yr of operation and 362 cm^3 displacement.
[b]Based on 362 cm^3 displacement and average fuel consumption of 0.94 gph.
[c]Based on sulfur content of 0.043 % by weight.

Table 6-12. Emission Factors for Wheeled Farm Tractors and Nontractor Agricultural Equipment—Emission Factor Rating: C

Pollutant	Diesel Farm Tractor	Gasoline Farm Tractor	Diesel Farm Equipment (nontractor)	Gasoline Farm Equipment (nontractor)
Carbon Monoxide				
g/hr	161	3,380	95.2	4,360
lb/hr	0.355	7.46	0.210	9.62
Exhaust Hydrocarbons				
g/hr	77.8	128	38.6	143
lb/hr	0.172	0.282	0.085	0.315
Crankcase Hydrocarbons				
g/hr	—	26.0	—	28.6
lb/hr	—	0.057	—	0.063
Evaporative Hydrocarbons				
g/unit-year	—	15,600	—	1,600
lb/unit-year	—	34.4	—	3.53
Nitrogen Oxides (NO_X as NO_2)				
g/hr	452	157	210	105
lb/hr	0.996	0.346	0.463	0.231
Aldehydes (RCHO as HCHO)				
g/hr	16.3	7.07	7.23	4.76
lb/hr	0.036	0.016	0.016	0.010
Sulfur Oxides (SO_X as SO_2)				
g/hr	42.2	5.56	21.7	6.34
lb/hr	0.093	0.012	0.048	0.014
Particulate				
g/hr	61.8	8.33	34.9	7.94
lb/hr	0.136	0.018	0.077	0.017

Table 6-13. Organic Compound Evaporative Emission Factors for Petroleum, Transportation and Marketing Sources—Emission Factor Rating: A

Emission Source	Gasoline	Crude Oil	Naphtha Jet Fuel (JP-4)	Kerosene	Distillate Oil
Tank Cars/Trucks					
Splash loading					
$lb/10^3$ gal transferred	12.4	10.6	1.8	0.88	0.93
Submerged loading					
$lb/10^3$ gal transferred	4.1	4.0	0.91	0.45	0.48
Unloading					
$lb/10^3$ gal transferred	2.1	2.0	0.45	0.23	0.24
Marine Vessels					
Loading					
$lb/10^3$ gal transferred	2.9	2.6	0.60	0.27	0.29
Unloading					
$lb/10^3$ gal transferred	2.5	2.3	0.52	0.24	0.25
Transit					
lb/wk, 10-gal load	3.6	3.2	0.74	0.34	0.36
Underground Gasoline Storage Tanks					
Splash loading					
$lb/10^3$ gal transferred	11.5	NU[a]	NU	NU	NU
Uncontrolled submerged loading					
$lb/10^3$ gal transferred	7.3	NU	NU	NU	NU
Submerged loading with open-vapor return system					
$lb/10^3$ gal transferred	0.80	NU	NU	NU	NU
Submerged loading with closed-vapor return system					
$lb/10^3$ gal transferred	Neg	NU	NU	NU	NU
Unloading					
$lb/10^3$ gal transferred	1.0	NU	NU	NU	NU
Filling Motor Vehicle Gasoline Tanks					
Vapor displacement loss					
$lb/10^3$ gal pumped	11.0	NU	NU	NU	NU
Liquid spillage loss					
$lb/10^3$ gal pumped	0.67	NU	NU	NU	NU

[a]Not used.

Table 6-14. Emission Factors and Fuel Loading Factors for Open Burning of Agricultural Materials—Emission Factor Rating: B (Resources Research, Inc., 1970; Gerstle and Kemnitz, 1967)

| | Emission Factors | | | | | | Fuel Loading Factors (waste production) | |
| | Particulate | | Carbon Monoxide | | Hydrocarbons (as C_6H_{14}) | | | |
Refuse Category	(lb/ton)	(kg/MT)	(lb/ton)	(kg/MT)	(lb/ton)	(kg/MT)	(ton/ac)	(MT/ha)
Field Crops								
Unspecified (burning technique not significant)								
Asparagus	21	11	117	58	23	12	2.0	4.5
Barley	40	20	150	75	85	42	1.5	3.4
Corn	22	11	157	78	19	10	1.7	3.8
Cotton	14	7	108	54	16	8	4.2	9.4
Grasses	8	4	176	88	6	3	1.7	3.8
Pineapple	16	8	101	50	19	10		
Rice	8	4	112	56	8	4		
Safflower	9	4	83	41	10	5	3.0	6.7
Sorghum	18	9	144	72	26	13	1.3	2.9
Sugar Beets	18	9	77	38	9	4	2.9	6.5
Sugar Cane	7	4	71	35	10	5	11.0	24.0
Headfire Burning								
Alfalfa	45	23	106	53	36	18	0.8	1.8
Bean (red)	43	22	186	93	46	23	2.5	5.6
Hay (wild)	32	16	139	70	22	11	1.0	2.2
Oats	44	22	137	68	33	16	1.6	3.6
Pea	31	16	147	74	38	19	2.5	5.6
Wheat	22	11	128	64	17	9	1.9	4.3

aFactors expressed as weight of pollutant emitted per weight of refuse material burned.

Table 6-14 (Continued)

Refuse Category	Emission Factors						Fuel Loading Factors (waste production)	
	Particulate		Carbon Monoxide		Hydrocarbons (as C_6H_{14})			
	(lb/ton)	(kg/MT)	(lb/ton)	(kg/MT)	(lb/ton)	(kg/MT)	(ton/ac)	(MT/ha)
Backfire Burning								
Alfalfa	29	14	119	60	37	18	0.8	1.8
Bean (red), pea	14	7	148	72	25	12	2.5	5.6
Hay (wild)	17	8	150	75	17	8	1.0	2.2
Oats	21	11	136	68	18	9	1.6	3.6
Wheat	13	6	108	54	11	6	1.9	4.3
Vine Crops								
Weeds								
Unspecified	15	8	85	42	12	6	3.2	7.2
Russian thistle (tumbleweed)	22	11	309	154	2	1	0.1	0.2
Tules (wild reeds)	5	3	34	17	27	14		
Orchard Crops								
Unspecified	6	3	52	26	10	5	1.6	3.6
Almond	6	3	46	23	8	4	1.6	3.6
Apple	4	2	42	21	4	2	2.3	5.2
Apricot	6	3	49	24	8	4	1.8	4.0
Avocado	21	10	116	58	32	16	1.5	3.4

Cherry	8	4	44	22	10	5	1.0	2.2
Citrus (orange, lemon)	6	3	81	40	12	6	1.0	2.2
Date palm	10	5	56	28	7	4	1.0	2.2
Fig	7	4	57	28	10	5	2.2	4.9
Nectarine	4	2	33	16	4	2	2.0	4.5
Olive	12	6	114	57	18	9	1.2	2.7
Peach	6	3	42	21	5	2	2.5	5.6
Pear	9	4	57	28	9	4	2.6	5.8
Prune	3	2	42	21	3	2	1.2	2.7
Walnut	6	3	47	24	8	4	1.2	2.7
Forest residues								
Unspecified	17	8	140	70	24	12	70	157
Hemlock, Douglas fir, cedar	4	2	90	45	5	2		
Ponderosa pine	12	6	195	98	14	7		

Table 6-15. Classification of Air Quality Control Regions[a]

Air Quality Control Region	Particulate Matter	Sulfur Oxides	Nitrogen Dioxide	Carbon Monoxide	Photochemical Oxidants
ALABAMA					
Alabama & Tombigbee Rivers Intrastate	II	III	III	III	III
Columbus (Georgia)- Phenix City (Alabama) Interstate	I	III	III	III	III
East Alabama Intrastate	I	III	III	III	III
Metropolitan Birmingham Intrastate	I	II	III	I	I
Mobile (Alabama)-Pnesacola- Panama City (Florida)- Southern Mississippi Interstate	I	I	III	III	I
Southeast Alabama Intrastate	II	III	III	III	III
Tennessee River Valley (Alabama)-Cumberland Mountains (Tennessee) Interstate	I	I	III	III	III
ALASKA					
Cook Inlet Intrastate	I	III	III	III	III
Northern Alaska Intrastate	I	III	III	I	III
South Central Alaska Intrastate	III	III	III	III	III
Southeastern Alaska Intrastate	III	IA*	III	III	III
ARIZONA					
New Mexico Southern Border Interstate	IA	IA	III	III	III
Clark-Mohave Interstate	IA	IA	III	I	I
Phoenix-Tucson Intrastate	I	I	III	I	I
Four Corners Interstate	IA	IA	III	III	III
ARKANSAS					
Central Arkansas Intrastate	II	III	III	III	III
Metropolitan Fort Smith Interstate	II	III	III	III	III
Metropolitan Memphis Interstate	II	III	III	III	III
Monroe (Louisiana)-El Dorado (Arkansas) Interstate	II	III	III	III	III
Northeast Arkansas Intrastate	III	III	III	III	III

*A signifies one point source
[a]CFR 40 Part 52, July 1, 1975

Table 6-15 (Continued)

Air Quality Control Region	Particulate Matter	Sulfur Oxides	Nitrogen Dioxide	Carbon Monoxide	Photochemical Oxidants
Northwest Arkansas Intrastate	III	III	III	III	III
Shreveport-Texarkana-Tyler Interstate	II	III	III	III	III
CALIFORNIA					
North Coast Intrastate	II	III	III	III	III
San Francisco Bay Area Intrastate	II	II	III	I	I
North Central Coast Intrastate	II	III	III	III	I
South Central Coast Intrastate	III	III	III	III	III
Metropolitan Los Angeles Intrastate	I	II	I	I	I
Northeast Plateau Intrastate	III	III	III	III	III
Sacramento Valley Intrastate	II	III	III	I	I
San Joaquin Valley Intrastate	I	III	III	I	I
Great Basin Valley Intrastate	III	III	III	III	III
Southeast Desert Intrastate	I	III	III	III	I
San Diego Intrastate	II	III	III	I	I
COLORADO					
Pawnee Intrastate	I	III	III	III	III
Metropolitan Denver Intrastate	I	III	III	I	I
Comanche Intrastate	III	III	III	III	III
San Isabel Intrastate	I	III	III	III	III
San Luis Intrastate	III	III	III	III	III
Four Corners Interstate	IA	IA	III	III	III
Grand Mesa Intrastate	III	III	III	III	III
Yampa Intrastate	III	III	III	III	III
CONNECTICUT					
New Jersey-New York-Connecticut Interstate	I	I	I	I	I
Hartford-New Haven-Springfield Interstate	I	I	III	I	I
Northwestern Intrastate	III	III	III	III	III
Eastern Intrastate	II	III	III	III	III
DELAWARE					
Metropolitan Philadelphia Interstate	I	I	III	I	I
Eastern Intrastate	III	III	III	III	III

Table 6-15 (Continued)

Air Quality Control Region	Particulate Matter	Sulfur Oxides	Nitrogen Dioxide	Carbon Monoxide	Photochemical Oxidants
DISTRICT OF COLUMBIA					
National Capital Interstate	I	I	III	I	I
FLORIDA					
Mobile (Alabama)-Pensacola-Panama City (Florida)-Southern Mississippi Interstate	I	I	III	III	I
Jacksonville (Florida)-Brunswick (Georgia) Interstate	I	II	III	III	I
West Central Florida Intrastate	I	I	III	III	III
Central Florida Intrastate	II	III	III	III	III
Southwest Florida Intrastate	III	III	III	III	III
Southeast Florida Intrastate	II	III	III	III	III
GEORGIA					
Augusta (Georgia)-Aiken (South Carolina) Interstate	I	II	III	III	III
Metropolitan Atlanta Intrastate	I	I	III	III	III
Chattanooga Interstate	I	II	III	III	III
Columbus (Georgia)-Phenix City (Alabama) Interstate	I	III	III	III	III
Central Georgia Intrastate	I	I	III	III	III
Jacksonville (Florida)-Brunswick (Georgia) Interstate	I	II	III	III	I
Northeast Georgia Intrastate	II	III	III	III	III
Savannah (Georgia)-Beaufort (South Carolina) Interstate	I	I	III	III	III
Southwest Georgia Intrastate	II	II	III	III	III
HAWAII					
State of Hawaii	II	III	III	III	III
IDAHO					
Eastern Idaho Intrastate	I	IA	III	III	III
Eastern Washington-Northern Idaho Interstate	I	IA	III	I	III
Idaho Intrastate	I	III	III	III	III
Metropolitan Boise Intrastate	II	III	III	III	III

Table 6-15 (Continued)

Air Quality Control Region	Particulate Matter	Sulfur Oxides	Nitrogen Dioxide	Carbon Monoxide	Photochemical Oxidants
ILLINOIS					
Burlington-Keokuk					
Interstate	I	I	III	III	III
East Central Illinois					
Intrastate	III	II	III	III	III
Metropolitan Chicago					
Interstate (Indiana-					
Illinois)	I	I	I	I	I
Metropolitan Dubuque					
Interstate	I	III	III	III	III
Metropolitan Quad Cities					
Interstate	I	III	III	III	III
Metropolitan St. Louis					
Interstate (Missouri-					
Illinois)	I	I	III	I	I
North Central Illinois					
Intrastate	II	IA	III	III	III
Paducah (Kentucky)-Cairo					
(Illinois) Interstate	I	II	III	III	III
Rockford (Illinois)-					
Janesville-Beloit					
(Wisconsin) Interstate	II	III	III	III	III
Southeast Illinois					
Intrastate	III	II	III	III	III
West Central Illinois					
Intrastate	I	IA	III	III	III
INDIANA					
East Central Indiana					
Intrastate	II	II	III	III	III
Evansville (Indiana)-					
Owensboro-Henderson					
(Kentucky) Interstate	I	II	III	III	III
Louisville Interstate	I	I	III	III	I
Metropolitan Chicago					
Interstate (Indiana-					
Illinois)	I	I	I	I	I
Metropolitan Cincinnati					
Interstate	I	II	III	III	I
Metropolitan Indianapolis					
Intrastate	I	I	I	I	I
Northeast Indiana					
Intrastate	II	III	III	III	III
South Bend-Elkhart					
(Indiana)-Benton Harbor					
(Michigan) Interstate	I	IA	III	III	III

Table 6-15 (Continued)

Air Quality Control Region	Particulate Matter	Sulfur Oxides	Nitrogen Dioxide	Carbon Monoxide	Photochemical Oxidants
Southern Indiana Intrastate	IA	IA	III	III	III
Wabash Valley Intrastate	I	I	III	III	III
IOWA					
Metropolitan Omaha- Council Bluffs					
Interstate	I	II	III	III	III
Metropolitan Sioux Falls					
Interstate	II	III	III	III	III
Metropolitan Sioux City					
Interstate	III	III	III	III	III
Metropolitan Dubuque					
Interstate	I	III	III	III	III
Metropolitan Quad Cities					
Interstate	I	III	III	III	III
Burlington-Keokuk					
Interstate	I	I	III	III	III
Northwest Iowa Intrastate	III	III	III	III	III
North Central Iowa					
Intrastate	IA	III	III	III	III
Northeast Iowa Intrastate	I	III	III	III	III
Southwest Iowa Intrastate	III	III	III	III	III
South Central Iowa					
Intrastate	I	III	III	III	I
Southwest Iowa Intrastate	III	III	III	III	III
KANSAS					
Metropolitan Kansas City					
Interstate	I	III	III	I	I
South Central Kansas					
Intrastate	I	III	III	III	I
Northeast Kansas					
Intrastate	I	III	III	III	III
Southeast Kansas					
Intrastate	III	III	III	III	III
North Central Kansas					
Intrastate	I	III	III	III	III
Northwest Kansas					
Intrastate	I	III	III	III	III
Southwest Kansas					
Intrastate	I	III	III	III	III
KENTUCKY					
Appalachian Intrastate	II	III	III	III	III
Bluegrass Intrastate	II	III	III	III	III

Evansville (Indiana)-
  Owensboro-Henderson
  (Kentucky) Interstate
	I	II	III	III	III

Table 6-15 (Continued)

Air Quality Control Region	Particulate Matter	Sulfur Oxides	Nitrogen Dioxide	Carbon Monoxide	Photochemical Oxidants
Huntington, Ashland Portsmith, Ironton Interstate	I	III	III	III	III
Louisville Interstate	I	I	III	III	I
Metropolitan Cincinnati Interstate	I	II	III	III	I
North Central Kentucky Intrastate	II	III	III	III	III
Paducah (Kentucky)-Cairo (Illinois) Interstate	I	II	III	III	III
South Central Kentucky Intrastate	III	III	III	III	III
LOUISIANA Southern Louisiana- Southeast Texas Interstate	II	I	III	III	I
Shreveport-Texarkana- Tyler Interstate	II	III	III	III	III
Monroe-El Dorado Interstate	II	III	III	III	III
MAINE Metropolitan Portland Intrastate	I	II	III	III	III
Androscoggin Valley Interstate	IA	IA	III	III	III
Down East Intrastate	IA	IA	III	III	III
Aroostook Intrastate	III	III	III	III	III
Northwest Maine Intrastate	III	III	III	III	III
MARYLAND Cumberland-Keyser Interstate	I	I	III	III	III
Central Maryland Intrastate	II	II	III	III	III
Metropolitan Baltimore Intrastate	I	I	I	I	I
National Capital Interstate	I	I	III	I	I
Southern Maryland Intrastate	III	III	III	III	III
Eastern Shore Intrastate	II	III	III	III	III
MASSACHUSETTS Metropolitan Boston Intrastate	I	I	III	I	I
Merrimack Valley-Southern New Hampshire Interstate	I	I	III	III	III
Metropolitan Providence Interstate	I	I	III	III	III

Table 6-15 (Continued)

Air Quality Control Region	Particulate Matter	Sulfur Oxides	Nitrogen Dioxide	Carbon Monoxide	Photochemical Oxidants
Central Massachusetts Intrastate	I	II	III	III	III
Hartford-New Haven- Springfield Interstate	I	I	III	I	I
Berkshire Intrastate	II	III	III	III	III
MICHIGAN					
Metropolitan Detroit- Port Huron Intrastate	I	I	III	III	III
Metropolitan Toledo Interstate	I	I	III	III	I
South Central Michigan Intrastate	II	II	III	III	III
South Bend-Elkhart (Indiana)-Benton Harbor (Michigan) Interstate	I	IA	III	III	III
Central Michigan Intrastate	II	III	III	III	III
Upper Michigan Intrastate	III	III	III	III	III
MINNESOTA					
Central Minnesota Intrastate	II	III	III	III	III
Southeast Minnesota-La Crosse (Wisconsin) Interstate	II	IA	III	III	III
Duluth (Minnesota)- Superior (Wisconsin) Interstate	I	II	III	III	III
Metropolitan Fargo- Moorhead Interstate	II	III	III	III	III
Minneapolis-St. Paul Intrastate	I	I	III	I	III
Northwest Minnesota Intrastate	II	III	III	III	III
Southwest Minnesota Intrastate	III	III	III	III	III
MISSISSIPPI					
Mobile (Alabama)-Pensacola- Panama City (Florida)- Gulfport (Mississippi) Interstate	I	I	III	III	I
Metropolitan Memphis Interstate	I	III	III	III	I
Mississippi Delta Intrastate	III	III	III	III	III
Northeast Mississippi Intrastate	II	III	III	III	III

Table 6-15 (Continued)

Air Quality Control Region	Particulate Matter	Sulfur Oxides	Nitrogen Dioxide	Carbon Monoxide	Photochemical Oxidants
MISSOURI					
Metropolitan Kansas City					
Interstate	I	III	III	I	I
Southwest Missouri					
Intrastate	I	III	III	III	III
Southeast Missouri					
Intrastate	III	III	III	III	III
Northern Missouri					
Intrastate	II	III	III	III	III
Metropolitan St. Louis					
Interstate	I	I	III	I	I
MONTANA					
Billings Intrastate	II	II	III	III	III
Great Falls Intrastate	III	IA	III	III	III
Helena Intrastate	IA	IA	III	III	III
Miles City Intrastate	III	III	III	III	III
Missoula Intrastate	I	III	III	III	III
NEBRASKA					
Metropolitan Omaha-					
Council Bluffs Interstate	I	II	III	III	III
Lincoln-Beatrice-Fairbury					
Intrastate	II	III	III	III	III
Metropolitan Sioux City					
Interstate	III	III	III	III	III
Nebraska Intrastate	III	III	III	III	III
NEVADA					
Clark-Mohave Interstate	I	IA	III	I	I
Northwest Nevada					
Intrastate	I	III	III	III	III
Nevada Intrastate	IA	IA	III	III	III
NEW HAMPSHIRE					
Androscoggin Valley					
Interstate	IA	IA	III	III	III
Central New Hampshire					
Intrastate	III	III	III	III	III
Merrimack Valley-Southern					
New Hampshire					
Interstate	I	I	III	III	III
NEW JERSEY					
New Jersey-New York-					
Connecticut Interstate	I	I	I	I	I
Metropolitan Philadelphia					
Interstate	I	I	III	I	I

Table 6-15 (Continued)

Air Quality Control Region	Particulate Matter	Sulfur Oxides	Nitrogen Dioxide	Carbon Monoxide	Photochemical Oxidants
Northeast Pennsylvania- Upper Delaware Valley Interstate	I	II	III	III	III
New Jersey Intrastate	III	IA	III	I	III
NEW MEXICO					
Albuquerque-Mid-Rio Grande Intrastate	I	III	III	III	I
Arizona-New Mexico Southern Border Interstate	IA	IA	III	III	III
El Paso-Las Cruces- Alamogordo Interstate	I	I	III	I	I
Four Corners Interstate	IA	IA	III	III	III
Northeastern Plains Intrastate	III	III	III	III	III
Pecos-Permian Basin Intrastate	III	III	III	III	III
Southwestern Mountains- Augustine Plains Intrastate	III	III	III	III	III
Upper Rio Grande Valley Intrastate	III	III	III	III	III
NEW YORK					
Niagara Frontier Intrastate	I	I	III	III	I
Champlain Valley Interstate	II	II	III	III	III
Central New York Intrastate	I	II	III	I	I
Genesee-Finger Lakes Intrastate	II	II	III	III	I
Hudson Valley Intrastate	I	II	III	III	III
Southern Tier East Intrastate	II	II	III	III	III
Southern Tier West Intrastate	II	II	III	III	III
New Jersey-New York- Connecticut Interstate	I	I	I	I	I
NORTH CAROLINA					
Western Mountain Intrastate	I	III	III	III	III
Eastern Mountain Intrastate	I	III	III	III	III
Metropolitan Charlotte Interstate	I	II	III	III	I
Northern Piedmont Intrastate	I	III	III	III	III

Table 6-15 (Continued)

Air Quality Control Region	Particulate Matter	Sulfur Oxides	Nitrogen Dioxide	Carbon Monoxide	Photochemical Oxidants
Eastern Piedmont Intrastate	I	III	III	III	III
Northern Coastal Intrastate	I	III	III	III	III
Southern Coastal Intrastate	II	III	III	III	III
Sandhills Intrastate	II	III	III	III	III
NORTH DAKOTA					
Metropolitan Fargo-					
Moorhead Interstate	II	III	III	III	III
North Dakota Intrastate	II	III	III	III	III
OHIO					
Greater Metropolitan					
Cleveland Intrastate	I	I	III	III	I
Huntington (West Virginia)-					
Ashland (Kentucky)-					
Portsmouth-Ironton					
(Ohio) Interstate	I	III	III	III	III
Mansfield-Marion Intrastate	II	II	III	III	III
Metropolitan Cincinnati					
Interstate	I	II	III	III	I
Metropolitan Columbus					
Intrastate	I	III	III	III	I
Metropolitan Dayton					
Intrastate	I	II	III	III	I
Metropolitan Toledo					
Interstate	I	I	III	III	I
Northwest Ohio Intrastate	II	I	III	III	III
Northwest Pennsylvania-					
Youngstown Interstate	I	II	III	III	III
Parkersburg (West Virginia)-					
Marietta (Ohio) Interstate	I	II	III	III	III
Sandusky Intrastate	III	III	III	III	III
Steubenville-Weirton-					
Wheeling Interstate	I	I	III	III	III
Wilmington-Chillicothe-					
Logan Intrastate	III	III	III	III	III
Zanesville-Cambridge					
Intrastate	II	IA	III	III	III
OKLAHOMA					
Central Oklahoma					
Intrastate	I	III	III	III	I
Northeastern Oklahoma					
Intrastate	I	III	III	III	I
Southeastern Oklahoma					
Intrastate	III	III	III	III	III
North Central Oklahoma					
Intrastate	III	III	III	III	III

Table 6-15 (Continued)

Air Quality Control Region	Particulate Matter	Sulfur Oxides	Nitrogen Dioxide	Carbon Monoxide	Photochemical Oxidants
Southwestern Oklahoma Intrastate	III	III	III	III	III
Northwestern Oklahoma Intrastate	III	III	III	III	III
Metropolitan Fort Smith Interstate	II	III	III	III	III
Shreveport-Texarkana-Tyler Interstate	II	III	III	III	III
OREGON					
Portland Interstate	I	IA	III	I	I
Southwest Oregon Intrastate	II	III	III	III	III
Northwest Oregon Intrastate	III	III	III	III	III
Central Oregon Intrastate	II	III	III	III	III
Eastern Oregon Intrastate	II	III	III	III	III
PENNSYLVANIA					
Metropolitan Philadelphia Interstate	I	I	III	I	I
Northeast Pennsylvania-Upper Delaware Valley Interstate	I	II	III	III	III
South Central Pennsylvania Intrastate	I	II	III	III	III
Central Pennsylvania Intrastate	I	III	III	III	III
Southwest Pennsylvania Intrastate	I	I	III	I	I
Northwest Pennsylvania-Youngstown Interstate	I	II	III	III	III
RHODE ISLAND					
Metropolitan Providence Interstate	I	I	III	I	I
SOUTH CAROLINA					
Augusta (Georgia)-Aiken (South Carolina) Interstate	I	II	III	III	III
Metropolitan Charlotte Interstate	I	II	III	III	I
Camden-Sumter Intrastate	II	III	III	III	III
Charleston Intrastate	I	I	III	III	III
Columbia Intrastate	II	III	III	III	III
Florence Intrastate	III	III	III	III	III
Georgetown Intrastate	II	III	III	III	III

Table 6-15 (Continued)

Air Quality Control Region	Particulate Matter	Sulfur Oxides	Nitrogen Dioxide	Carbon Monoxide	Photochemical Oxidants
Greenville-Spartanburg					
Intrastate	I	III	III	III	III
Greenwood Intrastate	III	III	III	III	III
Savannah (Georgia)-Beaufort					
(South Carolina)					
Interstate	I	I	III	III	III
SOUTH DAKOTA					
Metropolitan Sioux City					
Interstate	III	III	III	III	III
Metropolitan Sioux Falls					
Interstate	II	III	III	III	III
Black Hills-Rapid City					
Intrastate	III	III	III	III	III
South Dakota Intrastate	III	III	III	III	III
TENNESSEE					
Eastern Tennessee-					
Southwestern Virginia					
Interstate	I	I	III	III	III
Tennessee River Valley-					
Cumberland Mountains					
Intrastate	I	I	III	III	III
Middle Tennessee					
Intrastate	I	II	III	III	I
Western Tennessee					
Intrastate	I	III	III	III	III
Chattanooga Interstate	I	II	III	III	III
Metropolitan Memphis					
Interstate	I	III	III	III	I
TEXAS					
Abilene-Wichita Falls					
Intrastate	II	II	III	III	III
Amarillo-Lubbock					
Intrastate	II	I	III	III	III
Austin-Waco Intrastate	II	III	III	III	I
Brownsville-Laredo					
Intrastate	I	III	III	III	III
Corpus Christi-Victoria					
Intrastate	I	I	III	III	I
Midland-Odessa-San					
Angelo Intrastate	II	II	III	III	III
Metropolitan Houston-					
Galveston Intrastate	I	I	III	III	I
Metropolitan Dallas-					
Fort Worth Intrastate	II	III	III	III	I

Table 6-15 (Continued)

Air Quality Control Region	Particulate Matter	Sulfur Oxides	Nitrogen Dioxide	Carbon Monoxide	Photochemical Oxidants
Metropolitan San Antonio Intrastate	II	III	III	III	I
Southern Louisiana-Southeast Texas Interstate	II	I	III	III	I
El Paso-Las Cruces Alamogordo Interstate	I	I	III	I	I
Shreveport-Texarkana-Tyler Interstate	II	III	III	III	III
UTAH					
Wasatch Front Intrastate	I	I	I	I	I
Four Corners Interstate	IA	IA	III	III	III
Utah Intrastate	III	III	III	III	III
VERMONT					
Champlain Valley Interstate	II	II	III	III	III
Vermont Intrastate	II	II	III	III	III
VIRGINIA					
Eastern Tennessee-Southwestern Virginia Interstate	I	I	III	III	III
Valley of Virginia Intrastate	I	III	III	III	III
Central Virginia Intrastate	I	III	III	III	III
Northeastern Virginia Intrastate	IA	III	III	III	III
State Capital Intrastate	I	III	III	III	I
Hampton Roads Intrastate	I	II	III	III	I
National Capital Interstate	I	I	III	I	I
WASHINGTON					
Eastern Washington-Northern Idaho Interstate	I	IA	III	I	III
Northern Washington Intrastate	II	III	III	III	III
Olympic-Northwest Washington Intrastate	II	II	III	III	III
Portland Interstate	I	IA	III	I	I
Puget Sound Intrastate	I	IA	III	I	I
South Central Washington Intrastate	I	III	III	III	III
WEST VIRGINIA					
Steubenville-Weirton-Wheeling Interstate	I	I	III	III	III
Parkersburg-Marietta Interstate	I	II	III	III	III

Table 6-15 (Continued)

Air Quality Control Region	Particulate Matter	Sulfur Oxides	Nitrogen Dioxide	Carbon Monoxide	Photochemical Oxidants
Huntington-Ashland-Portsmouth Ironton Interstate	I	III	III	III	III
Kanawha Valley Intrastate	I	III	III	III	III
Southern West Virginia Intrastate	III	III	III	III	III
North Central West Virginia Intrastate	I	III	III	III	III
Cumberland-Keyser Interstate	I	I	III	III	III
Central West Virginia Intrastate	III	III	III	III	III
Allegheny Intrastate	III	III	III	III	III
Eastern Panhandle Intrastate	III	III	III	III	III
WISCONSIN					
Duluth (Minnesota)-Superior (Wisconsin) Interstate	I	II	III	III	III
North Central Wisconsin Intrastate	II	III	III	III	III
Lake Michigan Intrastate	II	III	III	III	III
Southeast Minnesota-La Crosse (Wisconsin) Interstate	II	IA	III	III	III
Southern Wisconsin Intrastate	II	III	III	III	III
Southeastern Wisconsin Intrastate	I	II	III	III	I
Rockford (Illinois)-Jamesville-Beloit (Wisconsin) Interstate	II	III	III	III	III
Metropolitan Dubuque Interstate	I	III	III	III	III
WYOMING					
Cheyenne Intrastate	II	III	III	III	III
Casper Intrastate	II	III	III	III	III
Wyoming Intrastate	III	III	III	III	III
GUAM	III	II	III	III	III
PUERTO RICO	IA	IA	III	III	III
U.S. VIRGIN ISLANDS	IA	IA	III	III	III
AMERICAN SAMOA	III	III	III	III	III

Table 6-16. Pollutant Values for Determining Air Quality Control Region Classifications (EPA, 1975)

	I	II	III
Sulfur Oxides			
Annual arithmetic mean	$> 100\ \mu g/m^3$	$60\text{-}100\ \mu g/m^3$	$< 60\ \mu g/m^3$
24-hr maximum	$> 455\ \mu g/m^3$	$260\text{-}455\ \mu g/m^3$	$< 260\ \mu g/m^3$
3-hr minimum	—	$\geqslant 1300\ \mu g/m^3$	$< 1300\ \mu gm/^3$
Particulate Matter			
Annual geometric mean	$> 95\ \mu g/m^3$	$60\text{-}95\ \mu g/m^3$	$< 60\ \mu g/m^3$
24-hr maximum	$> 325\ \mu g/m^3$	$150\text{-}325\ \mu g/m$	$< 150\ \mu g/m^3$
Carbon Monoxide			
1-hr maximum	$> 55\ mg/m^3$	—	$< 55\ mg/m^3$
8-hr maximum	$\geqslant 14\ mg/m^3$	—	$< 14\ mg/m^3$
Nitrogen Dioxide			
Annual arithmetic mean	$\geqslant 110\ \mu g/m$	—	$< 110\ \mu g/m^3$
Photochemical Oxidants			
1-hr maximum	$\geqslant 195\ \mu g/m^3$	—	$< 195\ \mu g/m^3$

Table 6-17. Standards of Performance (Chaput, 1976)

Source Category	Affected Facility	Pollutant	Emission Level
Steam Generators (> 250 million Btu/hr)	Coal-fired boilers	Particulate	0.10 lb/10^6 Btu
		Opacity	20%
		SO_2	1.2 lb/10^6 Btu
		NO_x (except lignite and coal refuse)	0.70 lb/10^6 Btu
Promulgated December 23, 1971 (36 FR 24876)			
Revised July 26, 1972 (37 FR 14877)	Oil-fired boilers	Particulate	0.10 lb/10^6 Btu
June 14, 1974 (39 FR 20790)		Opacity	20%; 40% 2 min/hr
January 16, 1975 (40 FR 2803)		SO_2	0.80 lb/10^6 Btu
October 6, 1975 (40 FR 46250)		NO_x	0.30 lb/10^6 Btu
	Gas-fired boilers	Particulate	0.10/10^6 Btu
		Opacity	20%
		NO_x	0.20 lb/10^6 Btu
Incinerators (> 50 tons/day)	Incinerators	Particulate	0.08 g/dsct corrected to 10% CO_2
Promulgated December 23, 1971 (36 FR 24876)			
Revised June 14, 1974 (36 FR 20790)			
Portland Cement Plants	Kiln	Particulate	0.30 lb/ton
		Opacity	20%
Promulgated December 23, 1971 (36 FR 24876)			
Revised June 14, 1974 (39 FR 20790)	Clinker cooler	Particulate	0.10 lb/ton
November 12, 1974 (39 FR 39874)		Opacity	10%
October 6, 1975 (40 FR 46250)	Fugitive Emission points	Opacity	10%

Table 6-17, Continued.

Source Category	Affected Facility	Pollutant	Emission Level
Nitric Acid Plants	Process equipment	Opacity	10%
Promulgated December 23, 1971 (36 FR 24876)		NO_x	3.0 lb/ton
Revised May 23, 1973 (38 FR 13562) June 14, 1974 (39 FR 20790) October 6, 1975 (40 FR 46250)			
Sulfuric Acid Plants	Process equipment	SO_2	4.0 lb/ton
Promulgated December 23, 1971 (36 FR 24876)		Acid mist	0.15 lb/ton
Revised May 23, 1973 (38 FR 13562) June 14, 1974 (39 FR 20790) October 6, 1975 (40 FR 46250)		Opacity	10%
Asphalt Concrete Plants	Dryers; screening and weighing systems; storage, transfer, and loading systems; and dust handling equipment.	Particulate	0.04 g/dscf (90 mg/dscm)
Promulgated March 8, 1974 (39 FR 9308)		Opacity	20%
Revised October 6, 1975 (40 FR 46250)			
Petroleum Refineries	Catalytic cracker	Particulate	1.0 lb/1000 lb
Promulgated March 8, 1974 (39 FR 9308)		Opacity	30% (3-min exemption)
		CO	0.05%
Revised October 6, 1975 (40 FR 26250)	Fuel gas combination	SO_2	0.1 g H_2S/dscf (230 mg/dscm)

Source		Pollutant	Standard
Storage Vessels for Petroleum Liquids *Promulgated* March 8, 1974 (39 FR 9308) *Revised* April 17, 1974 (39 FR 13776) June 14, 1974 (39 FR 20790)	Storage tanks > 40,000-gal capacity	Hydrocarbons	For vapor pressure **78-570** mm Hg. equipment with floating roof, vapor recovery system, or equivalent; for vapor pressure > 570 mm Hg. equipment with vapor recovery system or equivalent
Secondary Lead Smelters *Promulgated* March 8, 1974 (39 FR 9308) *Revised* April 17, 1974 (39 FR 13776) October 6, 1975 (40 FR 46250)	Reverberatory and blast furnaces	Particulate Opacity	0.022 g/dscf (50 mg/dscm) 20%
	Pot furnaces	Opacity	10%
Secondary Brass and Bronze Plants *Promulgated* March 8, 1974 (39 FR 9308)	Reverberatory furnace	Particulate Opacity	0.022 g/dscf (50 mg/dscm) 20%
	Blast and electric furnaces	Opacity	10%
Iron and Steel Plants *Revised* October 6, 1975 (40 FR 46250)	Basic oxygen process furnace	Particulate	0.022 g/dscf (50 mg/dscm)
Sewage Treatment Plants *Promulgated* March 8, 1974 (39 FR 9308)	Sludge incinerators	Particulate Opacity Mercury	1.30 lb/ton 20% 3200 g/24 hr

Table 6-17, Continued.

Source Category	Affected Facility	Pollutant	Emission Level
Revised April 17, 1974 (39 FR 13776) May 3, 1974 (39 FR 15396) October 6, 1975 (40 FR 46250)			
Primary Copper Smelters	Dryer	Particulate Opacity	0.022 g/dscf (50 mg/dscm) 20%
Promulgated January 15, 1976 (41 FR 2331)	Roaster, smelting furnace, copper converter	SO_2 Opacity	0.065% 20%
Revised February 26, 1976 (41 FR 8346)	Reverberatory furnaces that process high-impurity feed materials are exempt from SO_2 standard.		
Primary Zinc Smelters Promulgated January 15, 1976 (41 FR 2331)	Sintering machine	Particulate Opacity 20%	0.022 g/dscf (50 mg/dscm)
	Roaster	SO_2 Opacity	0.065% 20%
Primary Lead Smelters Promulgated January 15, 1976 (41 FR 2331)	Blast or reverberatory furnace, sintering machine discharge end.	Particulate Opacity	0.022 g/dscf (50 mg/dscm) 20%
	Sintering machine, electric smelting furnace, converter.	SO_2 Opacity	0.065% 20%
Primary Aluminum Reduction Plants Promulgated January 26, 1976 (41 FR 3825)	Potroom group (a) Soderberg plant (b) Prebake plant	(a) Total fluorides Opacity (b) Total fluorides Opacity	2.0 lb/ton 10% 1.9 lb/ton 10%
	Anode bake plants	Total fluorides Opacity	0.1 lb/ton 20%

Phosphate Fertilizer Plants		
Promulgated August 6, 1975 (40 FR 3315)		
Wet process phosphoric acid	Total fluorides	0.02 lb/ton
Superphosphoric acid	Total fluorides	0.01 lb/ton
Diammonium phosphate	Total fluorides	0.06 lb/ton
Triple superphosphate	Total fluorides	0.2 lb/ton
Granular triple superphosphate	Total fluorides	5.0×10^{-4} lb/hr/ton
Coal Preparation Plants		
Promulgated January 15, 1976 (41 FR 2232)		
Thermal dryer	Particulate Opacity	0.031 g/dscf (0.070 g/dscm) 20%
Pneumatic coal cleaning equipment	Particulate	0.018 g/dscf (0.040 g/dscm)
	Opacity	10%
Processing and conveying equipment, storage systems, transfer and loading systems.	Opacity	20%
Ferroalloy Production Facilities		
Promulgated May 4, 1976 (41 FR 18497)		
Revised May 20, 1976 (41 FR 10659)		
Electric submerged arc furnaces	Particulate	0.99 lb/MWh (0.45 kg/MWh) ("high silicon alloys") 0.51 lb/MWh (0.23 kg/MWh) (chrome and manganese alloys)
		No visible emissions may escape furnace capture system
		No visible emission may escape tapping system for >| 40% of each tapping period
	Opacity	15%
	CO	20% volume basis

Table 6-17, Continued.

Source Category	Affected Facility	Pollutant	Emission Level
Iron and Steel Plants	Dust handling equipment	Opacity	10%
	Electric arc furnaces	Particulate	0.0052 g/dscf (12 mg/dscm)
		Opacity (a) Control	3%
		(a) Control devise	3%
Promulgated		(b) Shop roof	0 except 20%—charging
September 23, 1975 (40 FR 43850)			40%—tapping
	Dust handling equipment	Opacity	10%

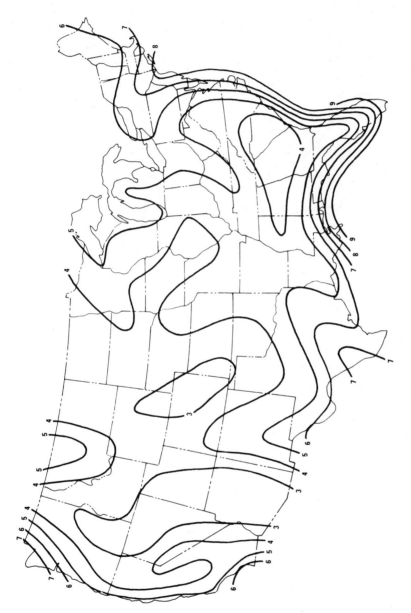

Figure 6-1. Isopleths (m x 10²) of mean annual morning mixing heights (Holzworth, 1972).

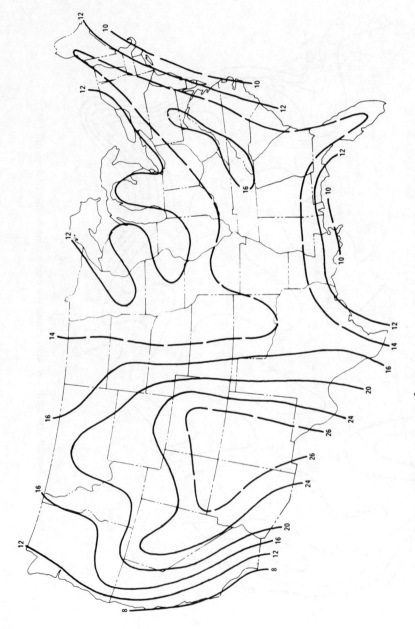

Figure 6-2. Isopleths (m x 10^2) of mean annual afternoon mixing heights (Holzworth, 1972).

APPENDIX

National Emissions Report (EPA, 1976b)

UNITED STATES

Emission categories	Pollutant, tons per year				
	Particulates	Sulfur oxides	Nitrogen oxides	Hydro-carbons	Carbon monoxide
GRAND TOTAL	15,922,841	32,696,630	21,746,991	23,778,764	97,020,190
-AREA	3,552,561	3,092,889	11,538,783	17,437,958	81,777,365
-POINT	12,395,280	29,603,741	10,208,208	6,340,806	15,242,825
FUEL COMBUSTION-AREA	1,457,099	2,408,098	1,678,329	211,050	640,343
-POINT	5,194,234	23,059,049	9,276,864	253,540	754,361
External Combustion-area	1,457,099	2,408,098	1,678,329	211,050	640,343
-point	5,181,936	23,024,825	8,952,840	195,321	698,613
Residential Fuel-area	235,944	504,115	364,793	148,012	504,261
Anthracite Coal	14,385	38,553	4,315	3,596	129,462
Bituminous Coal	51,873	194,152	7,781	51,873	233,430
Distillate Oil	73,788	234,749	88,546	22,136	36,894
Residual Oil	9,427	31,472	16,395	1,230	1,639
Natural Gas	28,048	1,683	224,388	22,439	56,097
Wood	58,423	3,505	23,369	46,738	46,738
Electric Generation-point	3,569,763	19,386,428	6,963,105	85,208	260,129
Anthracite Coal	21,808	48,108	32,071	177	4,279
Bituminous Coal	3,375,096	17,001,079	4,538,178	57,117	185,171
Lignite	58,513	127,170	61,886	1,134	3,878
Residual Oil	78,600	1,983,635	1,023,678	20,219	29,701
Distillate Oil	5,375	106,206	64,099	1,241	1,568
Natural Gas	21,522	61,292	1,181,259	3,137	34,676
Process Gas	311	3,024	17,854	30	310
Coke	287	3,435	362	1	20
Solid Waste/Coal	0	0	0	0	0
Other	8,251	52,481	43,718	2,153	527
Industrial Fuel-area	982,645	1,127,816	746,555	29,062	69,274
-point	1,530,760	3,452,358	1,903,538	104,812	428,162
Anthracite Coal-area	106	154	86	1	11
-point	10,759	66,184	37,765	45	1,345
Bituminous Coal-area	876,683	649,803	120,916	8,061	16,122
-point	1,030,615	2,061,975	495,101	16,331	39,398
Lignite-point	9,640	11,511	7,058	545	1,105
Residual Oil-area	49,118	401,560	128,135	6,407	8,542
-point	98,933	983,785	269,974	15,244	30,695
Distillate Oil-area	34,868	74,984	139,473	6,974	9,298
-point	23,415	109,652	129,160	4,918	5,442
Natural Gas-area	19,838	1,19.	357,086	5,951	33,725
-point	35,370	52,322	747,938	20,992	112,701
Process Gas-area	62	6	71	93	0
-point	17,585	115,609	65,190	2,041	9,815
Coke-point	1,016	1,569	246	12	46
Wood-area	1,969	118	788	1,575	1,575
-point	248,894	24,237	138,917	35,571	200,220
Liquid Petroleum Gas-point	272	2,403	1,930	53	224
Bagasse-point	42,949	3	5,981	6,004	7,163
Other-point	11,312	23,108	4,277	3,055	20,008
Commercial-Institutional Fuel-area	238,510	776,168	566,980	33,976	66,808
-point	81,412	186,039	86,197	5,301	10,322
Anthracite Coal-area	1,163	3,576	1,327	27	796
-point	5,401	2,288	631	37	231
Bituminous Coal-area	101,809	163,058	18,965	4,123	14,842
-point	56,000	98,009	22,379	1,420	3,587
Lignite-point	3,761	2,607	1,062	85	225
Residual Oil-area	66,920	490,435	174,574	8,729	11,638
-point	7,722	69,466	20,632	1,043	1,390
Distillate Oil-area	56,327	118,361	225,307	11,265	15,020
-point	1,669	8,319	6,928	369	463
Natural Gas-area	12,232	734	146,783	9,786	24,464
-point	6,474	5,073	29,809	1,915	3,823
Wood-area	59	4	24	47	47
-point	266	98	655	298	577
Liquid Petroleum Gas-point	5	1	32	2	4
Miscellaneous-point	1	0	0	0	0
Internal Combustion-point	12,297	34,224	324,025	58,219	55,748
Electric Generation	6,363	20,051	110,687	7,087	17,540
Distillate Oil	3,879	17,176	51,837	2,471	6,173
Natural Gas ft	24683	1,355	43,980	2,085	4,779
Diesel Fuel	1,626	1,208	12,084	1,374	6,486
Industrial Fuel	4,241	13,985	212,641	50,305	37,115
Distillate Oil	167	817	2,629	222	459
Natural Gas	1,995	10,245	185,146	46,341	28,616
Gasoline	8	4	164	259	2,142
Diesel Fuel	1,553	2,877	21,909	2,530	4,753

Emission categories	Pollutant, tons per year				
	Particulates	Sulfur oxides	Nitrogen oxides	Hydro-carbons	Carbon monoxide
Other	518	42	2,792	954	1,145
Commercial-Institutional	0	0	0	0	0
Diesel Fuel	0	0	0	0	0
Other	0	0	0	0	0
Engine-Testing	1,693	187	697	828	1,093
Aircraft 2	275	187	621	816	928
Other	1,418	0	76	12	165
Miscellaneous	0	0	0	0	0
INDUSTRIAL PROCESS-POINT	7,051,905	6,499,974	899,296	5,925,396	13,493,979
Chemical Manufact..ing	270,908	759,401	170,687	1,508,326	3,806,084
Food/Agriculture	663,752	905	762	44,827	1,455
Primary Metal	1,446,618	3,495,797	23,974	101,739	2,582,572
Secondary Metals	163,860	102,401	22,623	4,790	1,242,971
Mineral Products	3,855,212	816,635	201,839	13,420	298,053
Petroleum Industry	151,994	1,060,254	390,408	756,204	4,327,103
Wood Products	386,343	122,258	19,040	21,186	822,027
Evaporation	11,704	2,743	3,942	3,232,541	6,152
Metal Fabrication	2,758	1,122	11,796	78,079	3,985
Leath. Products	64	27	4	899	1
Textile Manufacturing	716	38	24	14,038	2
Inprocess Fuel	84,547	112,701	41,582	32,800	372,775
Other/Not Classified	13,430	25,692	12,614	116,547	30,802
SOLID WASTE DISPOSAL-AREA	420,298	37,224	124,499	801,016	2,294,074
-POINT	147,491	43,074	31,629	161,113	991,771
Government-point	75,788	10,464	15,621	61,095	225,117
Municipal Incineration	53,293	9,023	7,328	18,042	108,355
Open Burning	21,597	1,316	8,041	42,670	115,374
Other	898	124	252	382	1,388
Residential-area	316,952	15,294	85,744	684,593	1,984,833
On Site Incineration	96,329	1,505	3,010	270,926	812,777
Open Burning	220,622	13,789	82,733	413,667	1,172,057
Commercial-Institutional-area	66,062	15,075	24,773	69,136	181,289
-point	2,955	2,808	3,442	4,036	19,713
On Site Incineration-area	43,784	13,683	16,419	27,365	62,939
-point	1,412	2,805	3,225	3,510	15,463
Open Burning-area	22,278	1,392	8,354	41,771	118,350
-point	1,435	1	170	341	4,227
Apartment-point	25	1	11	12	21
Other-point	83	1	36	172	1
Industrial-area	37,285	6,855	13,982	47,288	127,951
-point	68,722	29,802	12,566	95,982	746,941
On Site Incineration-area	18,097	5,655	6,786	11,311	26,015
-point	55,500	21,644	9,768	61,509	710,094
Open Burning-area	19,188	1,199	7,195	35,978	101,936
-point	9,232	482	2,190	34,164	36,274
Auto Body Incineration-point	103	0	5	32	101
Other-point	3,888	7,676	604	278	472
Miscellaneous-point	26	0	0	0	0
TRANSPORTATION-AREA	1,156,240	646,539	9,649,050	14,209,967	75,987,164
Land Vehicles	969,651	506,896	9,299,987	12,163,167	74,067,627
Gasoline	778,847	214,670	6,839,263	11,754,694	73,002,802
Light Vehicles	687,560	172,415	5,844,508	9,117,521	54,507,863
Heavy Vehicles	71,268	27,018	766,501	1,993,572	11,198,300
Off Highway	20,019	10,477	228,254	643,601	7,296,639
Diesel Fuel	190,804	292,226	2,460,724	408,473	1,054,825
Heavy Vehicles	83,743	117,241	1,061,788	133,003	601,739
Off Highway	49,898	44,653	552,921	60,537	155,837
Rail	57,163	130,332	846,016	214,934	297,249
Aircraft	161,795	37,764	155,390	485,516	835,726
Military	145,872	27,855	70,077	339,391	364,313
Civil	10,507	2,087	9,492	46,535	265,913
Commercial	5,416	7,823	75,821	99,590	205,499
Vessels	24,794	101,878	193,673	367,411	1,083,811
Bituminous Coal	1,273	3,183	191	1,273	5,729
Diesel Fuel	18,573	23,217	173,352	45,505	60,673
Residual Oil	4,947	73,313	10,715	743	359
Gasoline	0	2,165	9,415	319,890	1,017,050
Gas Handling Evaporation Loss	0	0	0	1,193,872	0
MISCELLANEOUS-AREA	518,923	29	86,905	2,215,924	2,865,784
Forest Fires	223,808	0	52,661	315,965	1,843,128
Structural Fires	15,500	29	1,349	4,018	35,018
Slash Burning	279,608	0	32,895	328,951	986,852
Frost Control	7	0	0	1,536	786
Solvent Evaporation Loss	0	0	0	1,565,454	0

ALABAMA

Emission categories	Pollutant, tons per year				
	Particulates	Sulfur oxides	Nitrogen oxides	Hydro-carbons	Carbon monoxide
GRAND TOTAL	1,187,950	977,433	438,197	729,076	2,113,380
-AREA	92,061	45,435	214,554	339,370	1,581,510
-POINT	1,095,889	931,998	223,644	389,706	531,870
FUEL COMBUSTION-AREA	30,374	31,868	19,426	5,366	11,520
-POINT	652,025	797,050	208,899	3,329	8,186
External Combustion-area	30,374	31,868	19,426	5,366	11,520
-point	651,997	795,865	208,282	3,270	8,023
Residential Fuel-area	5,198	2,970	4,454	4,402	9,700
Anthracite Coal	0	0	0	0	0
Bituminous Coal	1,389	2,640	208	1,389	6,252
Distillate Oil	70	106	83	21	35
Residual Oil	0	0	0	0	0
Natural Gas	351	21	2,806	281	702
Wood	3,389	203	1,356	2,711	2,711
Electric Generation-point	596,309	677,284	172,010	1,858	5,519
Anthracite Coal	0	0	0	0	0
Bituminous Coal	596,273	676,258	167,632	1,833	5,432
Lignite	0	0	0	0	0
Residual Oil	0	0	0	0	0
Distillate Oil	25	1,022	1,252	20	7
Natural Gas	11	3	3,126	5	80
Process Gas	0	0	0	0	0
Coke	0	0	0	0	0
Solid Waste/Coal	0	0	0	0	0
Other	0	0	0	0	0
Industrial Fuel-area	24,399	25,053	10,497	697	1,259
-point	55,688	118,582	36,271	1,412	2,503
Anthracite Coal-area	0	0	0	0	0
-point	2,826	3,916	0	0	0
Bituminous Coal-area	23,833	20,490	8,088	539	1,078
-point	23,591	81,823	24,123	549	1,362
Lignite-point	0	0	0	0	0
Residual Oil-area	272	4,356	710	35	47
-point	1,451	15,630	602	39	41
Distillate Oil-area	202	199	807	40	54
-point	58	488	194	10	13
Natural Gas-area	47	3	840	14	79
-point	2,903	1,870	7,423	67	340
Process Gas-area	45	4	52	68	0
-point	674	10,763	96	0	0
Coke-point	0	0	0	0	0
Wood-area	0	0	0	0	0
-point	22,701	2,796	3,738	748	748
Liquid Petroleum Gas-point	0	0	0	0	0
Bagasse-point	0	0	0	0	0
Other-point	1,484	1,296	96	0	0
Commercial-Institutional Fuel-area	777	3,845	4,476	268	562
-point	0	0	0	0	0
Anthracite Coal-area	0	0	0	0	0
-point	0	0	0	0	0
Bituminous Coal-area	3	6	1	0	1
-point	0	0	0	0	0
Lignite-point	0	0	0	0	0
Residual Oil-area	266	3,543	694	35	46
-point	0	0	0	0	0
Distillate Oil-area	289	283	1,156	58	77
-point	0	0	0	0	0
Natural Gas-area	219	13	2,624	175	437
-point	0	0	0	0	0
Wood-area	0	0	0	0	0
-point	0	0	0	0	0
Liquid Petroleum Gas-point	0	0	0	0	0
Miscellaneous-point	0	0	0	0	0
Internal Combustion-point	28	1,184	617	59	163
Electric Generation	28	1,184	617	59	163
Distillate Oil	13	362	176	14	40
Natural Gas	15	823	441	45	123
Diesel Fuel	0	0	0	0	0
Industrial Fuel	0	0	0	0	0
Distillate Oil	0	0	0	0	0
Natural Gas	0	0	0	0	0
Gasoline	0	0	0	0	0
Diesel Fuel	0	0	0	0	0

Emission categories	Pollutant, tons per year				
	Particulates	Sulfur oxides	Nitrogen oxides	Hydro-carbons	Carbon monoxide
Other	0	0	0	0	0
Commercial-Institutional	0	0	0	0	0
Diesel Fuel	0	0	0	0	0
Other	0	0	0	0	0
Engine-Testing	0	0	0	0	0
Aircraft	0	0	0	0	0
Other	0	0	0	0	0
Miscellaneous	0	0	0	0	0
INDUSTRIAL PROCESS-POINT	442,448	134,913	14,432	384,697	506,939
Chemical Manufacturing	3,541	30,155	3,427	15,823	29,882
Food/Agriculture	3,519	0	.0	0	0
Primary Metal	178,076	9,202	91	9,058	284,370
Secondary Metals	23,523	1	21	140	178,271
Mineral Products	209,500	73,593	10,835	4	4
Petroleum Industry	41	30	0	159	0
Wood Products	18,319	13,501	11	22	14,312
Evaporation	8	0	0	359,042	0
Metal Fabrication	280	0	0	0	0
Leather Products	0	0	0	0	0
Textile Manufacturing	0	0	0	0	0
Inprocess Fuel	4,879	8,431	48	448	101
Other/Not Classified	760	0	0	0	0
SOLID WASTE DISPOSAL-AREA	18,772	1,173	7,039	35,198	99,726
-POINT	1,416	35	312	1,680	16,746
Government-point	0	0	0	0	0
Municipal Incineration	0	0	0	0	0
Open Burning	0	0	0	0	0
Other	0	0	0	0	0
Residential-area	16,662	1,041	6,248	31,241	88,515
On Site Incineration	0	0	0	0	0
Open Burning	16,662	1,041	6,248	31,241	88,515
Commercial-Institutional-area	1,729	108	648	3,242	9,184
-point	0	0	0	0	0
On Site Incineration-area	0	0	0	0	0
-point	0	0	0	0	0
Open Burning-area	1,729	108	648	3,242	9,184
-point	0	0	0	0	0
Apartment-point	0	0	0	0	0
Other-point	0	0	0	0	0
Industrial-area	382	24	143	716	2,027
-point	1,416	35	312	1,680	16,746
On Site Incineration-area	0	0	0	0	0
-point	1,092	30	277	1,510	16,198
Open Burning-area	382	24	143	716	2,027
-point	208	5	35	171	548
Auto Body Incineration-point	2	0	0	0	0
Other-point	114	0	0	0	0
Miscellaneous-point	0	0	0	0	0
TRANSPORTATION-AREA	30,321	12,394	185,125	277,365	1,366,551
Land Vehicles	18,225	9,846	177,290	227,395	1,314,840
Gasoline	14,302	3,977	127,048	219,246	1,293,545
Light Vehicles	12,164	3,154	103,940	159,538	942,575
Heavy Vehicles	2,047	776	22,062	56,760	317,553
Off Highway	92	48	1,045	2,948	33,417
Diesel Fuel	3,923	5,869	50,242	8,149	21,295
Heavy Vehicles	1,695	2,374	21,520	2,684	12,085
Off Highway	1,144	1,024	12,675	1,388	3,572
Rail	1,084	2,472	16,047	4,077	5,638
Aircraft	11,970	2,353	6,501	28,865	33,528
Military	11,840	2,261	5,688	27,548	29,571
Civil	77	15	69	340	1,941
Commercial	53	77	744	977	2,015
Vessels	125	194	1,334	5,897	18,183
Bituminous Coal	0	0	0	0	0
Diesel Fuel	125	157	1,169	307	409
Residual Oil	0	0	0	0	0
Gasoline	0	38	165	5,590	17,773
Gas Handling Evaporation Loss	0	0	0	15,209	0
MISCELLANEOUS-AREA	12,594	0	2,963	21,441	103,712
Forest Fires	12,594	0	2,963	17,779	103,712
Structural Fires	0	0	0	0	0
Slash Burning	0	0	0	0	0
Frost Control	0	0	0	0	0
Solvent Evaporation Loss	0	0	0	3,662	0

ALASKA

Emission categories	Pollutant, tons per year				
	Particulates	Sulfur oxides	Nitrogen oxides	Hydro-carbons	Carbon monoxide
GRAND TOTAL	64,165	20,543	63,211	109,370	534,089
–AREA	46,485	11,711	39,138	86,976	511,046
–POINT	17,681	8,833	24,072	22,394	23,043
FUEL COMBUSTION–AREA	3,388	9,319	6,077	1,133	2,486
–POINT	7,924	8,702	23,227	3,605	4,367
External Combustion–area	3,388	9,319	6,077	1,133	2,486
–point	7,647	8,357	11,043	1,513	1,040
Residential Fuel–area	1,178	1,104	965	849	1,927
Anthracite Coal	0	0	0	0	0
Bituminous Coal	276	210	41	276	1,243
Distillate Oil	298	858	357	89	149
Residual Oil	0	0	0	0	0
Natural Gas	43	3	342	34	85
Wood	561	34	225	449	449
Electric Generation–point	3,959	1,458	2,179	101	245
Anthracite Coal	0	0	0	0	0
Bituminous Coal	3,738	1,457	1,472	100	225
Lignite	0	0	0	0	0
Residual Oil	0	0	0	0	0
Distillate Oil	0	0	0	0	0
Natural Gas	12	1	707	1	20
Process Gas	0	0	0	0	0
Coke	0	0	0	0	0
Solid Waste/Coal	0	0	0	0	0
Other	209	0	0	0	0
Industrial Fuel–area	594	6,826	2,113	92	152
–point	3,178	5,726	7,781	1,314	654
Anthracite Coal–area	0	0	0	0	0
–point	0	0	0	0	0
Bituminous Coal–area	0	0	0	0	0
–point	1,770	1,202	2,372	158	316
Lignite–point	0	0	0	0	0
Residual Oil–area	410	6,513	1,068	53	71
–point	0	0	0	0	0
Distillate Oil–area	163	312	650	33	43
–point	282	4,183	1,249	62	82
Natural Gas–area	22	1	394	7	37
–point	63	3	3,056	34	88
Process Gas–area	0	0	0	0	0
–point	0	0	0	0	0
Coke–point	0	0	0	0	0
Wood–area	0	0	0	0	0
–point	976	113	732	146	146
Liquid Petroleum Gas–point	0	0	0	0	0
Bagasse–point	0	0	0	0	0
Other–point	88	225	371	913	21
Commercial-Institutional Fuel–area	1,616	1,389	2,999	192	407
–point	510	1,173	1,084	98	141
Anthracite Coal–area	0	0	0	0	0
–point	0	0	0	0	0
Bituminous Coal–area	1,062	253	153	33	120
–point	458	1,089	875	61	127
Lignite–point	0	0	0	0	0
Residual Oil–area	16	254	42	2	3
–point	0	0	0	0	0
Distillate Oil–area	456	877	1,826	91	122
–point	51	85	206	37	13
Natural Gas–area	82	5	979	65	163
–point	0	0	2	0	1
Wood–area	0	0	0	0	0
–point	0	0	0	0	0
Liquid Petroleum Gas–point	0	0	0	0	0
Miscellaneous–point	0	0	0	0	0
Internal Combustion–point	277	345	12,184	2,092	3,327
Electric Generation	207	323	8,852	1,321	3,081
Distillate Oil	13	8	168	1	2
Natural Gas	24	49	3,869	163	156
Diesel Fuel	169	266	4,808	480	2,922
Industrial Fuel	70	22	3,332	771	246
Distillate Oil	0	0	0	0	0
Natural Gas	1	0	927	0	0
Gasoline	0	0	0	0	0
Diesel Fuel	5	1	68	5	15

Emission categories	Pollutant, tons per year				
	Particulates	Sulfur oxides	Nitrogen oxides	Hydro-carbons	Carbon monoxide
Other	64	21	2,337	766	231
Commercial-Institutional	0	0	0	0	0
Diesel Fuel	0	0	0	0	0
Other	0	0	0	0	0
Engine-Testing	0	0	0	0	0
Aircraft	0	0	0	0	0
Other	0	0	0	0	0
Miscellaneous	0	0	0	0	0
INDUSTRIAL PROCESS-POINT	8,614	102	622	16,918	172
Chemical Manufacturing	464	0	0	0	0
Food/Agriculture	0	0	0	0	0
Primary Metal	0	0	0	0	0
Secondary Metals	0	0	0	0	0
Mineral Products	8,107	2	0	0	0
Petroleum Industry	43	19	622	3,842	172
Wood Products	0	80	0	0	0
Evaporation	0	0	0	13,076	0
Metal Fabrication	0	0	0	0	0
Leather Products	0	0	0	0	0
Textile Manufacturing	0	0	0	0	0
Inprocess Fuel	0	2	0	0	0
Other/Not Classified	0	0	0	0	0
SOLID WASTE DISPOSAL-AREA	819	48	270	1,625	4,652
-POINT	1,142	29	224	1,871	18,505
Government-point	215	14	80	399	1,132
Municipal Incineration	3	0	0	0	3
Open Burning	212	13	80	398	1,129
Other	0	0	0	0	0
Residential-area	718	40	232	1,446	4,147
On Site Incineration	107	2	3	301	904
Open Burning	610	38	229	1,145	3,243
Commercial-Institutional-area	60	6	22	103	288
-point	0	0	0	0	1
On Site Incineration-area	8	3	3	5	11
-point	0	0	0	0	1
Open Burning-area	52	3	19	98	276
-point	0	0	0	0	0
Apartment-point	0	0	0	0	0
Other-point	0	0	0	0	0
Industrial-area	41	3	15	77	217
-point	927	15	144	1,472	17,373
On Site Incineration-area	0	0	0	0	1
-point	889	13	134	1,470	17,373
Open Burning-area	41	3	15	77	217
-point	0	0	0	0	0
Auto Body Incineration-point	0	0	0	0	0
Other-point	38	2	10	2	0
Miscellaneous-point	0	0	0	0	0
TRANSPORTATION-AREA	3,049	2,343	23,561	27,796	180,851
Land Vehicles	1,432	1,163	15,343	19,128	161,300
Gasoline	848	300	7,953	17,837	158,621
Light Vehicles	519	135	4,249	7,341	46,867
Heavy Vehicles	43	16	448	1,315	7,669
Off Highway	286	149	3,256	9,181	104,085
Diesel Fuel	584	863	7,390	1,291	2,679
Heavy Vehicles	88	123	1,091	145	684
Off Highway	283	253	3,136	343	884
Rail	214	487	3,162	803	1,111
Aircraft	862	220	1,105	3,247	9,658
Military	557	106	268	1,296	1,392
Civil	262	52	237	1,162	6,639
Commercial	43	62	601	789	1,628
Vessels	755	959	7,114	4,185	9,892
Bituminous Coal	0	0	0	0	0
Diesel Fuel	755	943	7,045	1,849	2,466
Residual Oil	0	0	0	0	0
Gasoline	0	16	69	2,336	7,427
Gas Handling Evaporation Loss	0	0	0	1,235	0
MISCELLANEOUS-AREA	39,228	0	9,230	56,421	323,057
Forest Fires	39,228	0	9,230	55,381	323,057
Structural Fires	0	0	0	0	0
Slash Burning	0	0	0	0	0
Frost Control	0	0	0	0	0
Solvent Evaporation Loss	0	0	0	1,040	0

ARIZONA

Emission categories	Pollutant, tons per year				
	Particulates	Sulfur oxides	Nitrogen oxides	Hydro-carbons	Carbon monoxide
GRAND TOTAL	122,795	2,051,745	169,119	241,985	1,171,580
–AREA	30,968	9,424	130,705	231,374	1,147,458
–POINT	91,827	2,042,321	38,414	10,611	24,121
FUEL COMBUSTION–AREA	1,851	927	5,998	1,325	1,860
–POINT	6,549	8,361	32,421	237	1,100
External Combustion–area	1,851	927	5,998	1,325	1,860
–point	6,508	8,204	31,514	180	1,013
Residential Fuel–area	1,404	84	2,000	1,123	1,350
Anthracite Coal	0	0	0	0	0
Bituminous Coal	0	0	0	0	0
Distillate Oil	0	0	0	0	0
Residual Oil	0	0	0	0	0
Natural Gas	189	11	1,514	151	378
Wood	1,215	73	486	972	972
Electric Generation–point	6,325	5,042	27,971	144	879
Anthracite Coal	0	0	0	0	0
Bituminous Coal	5,740	2,778	3,133	52	174
Lignite	0	0	0	0	0
Residual Oil	99	1,280	1,302	25	37
Distillate Oil	121	963	1,584	30	45
Natural Gas	366	22	21,954	37	622
Process Gas	0	0	0	0	0
Coke	0	0	0	0	0
Solid Waste/Coal	0	0	0	0	0
Other	0	0	0	0	0
Industrial Fuel–area	190	511	1,562	44	133
–point	160	763	3,535	36	134
Anthracite Coal–area	0	0	0	0	0
–point	0	0	0	0	0
Bituminous Coal–area	0	0	0	0	0
–point	0	0	0	0	0
Lignite–point	0	0	0	0	0
Residual Oil–area	0	0	0	0	0
–point	52	479	136	7	9
Distillate Oil–area	132	507	528	26	35
–point	42	281	192	10	13
Natural Gas–area	57	3	1,034	17	98
–point	66	4	3,206	20	112
Process Gas–area	0	0	0	0	0
–point	0	0	0	0	0
Coke–point	0	0	0	0	0
Wood–area	0	0	0	0	0
–point	0	0	0	0	0
Liquid Petroleum Gas–point	0	0	0	0	0
Bagasse–point	0	0	0	0	0
Other–point	0	0	0	0	0
Commercial–Institutional Fuel–area	258	332	2,435	157	377
–point	22	2,399	8	0	1
Anthracite Coal–area	0	0	0	0	0
–point	0	0	0	0	0
Bituminous Coal–area	0	0	0	0	0
–point	0	0	0	0	0
Lignite–point	0	0	0	0	0
Residual Oil–area	17	81	44	2	3
–point	0	0	0	0	0
Distillate Oil–area	62	240	250	12	17
–point	0	0	0	0	0
Natural Gas–area	178	11	2,142	143	357
–point	22	2,399	8	0	1
Wood–area	0	0	0	0	0
–point	0	0	0	0	0
Liquid Petroleum Gas–point	0	0	0	0	0
Miscellaneous–point	0	0	0	0	0
Internal Combustion–point	42	157	907	57	86
Electric Generation	33	137	771	15	37
Distillate Oil	13	137	177	7	15
Natural Gas	20	0	595	8	22
Diesel Fuel	0	0	0	0	0
Industrial Fuel	9	10	125	9	26
Distillate Oil	0	1	2	0	0
Natural Gas	0	0	6	0	0
Gasoline	0	0	0	0	0
Diesel Fuel	8	9	117	9	26

Emission categories	Pollutant, tons per year				
	Particulates	Sulfur oxides	Nitrogen oxides	Hydro-carbons	Carbon monoxide
Other...	0	0	0	0	0
Commercial-Institutional...	0	0	0	0	0
Diesel Fuel...	0	0	0	0	0
Other...	0	0	0	0	0
Engine-Testing...	0	9	10	33	23
Aircraft...	0	9	10	33	23
Other...	0	0	0	0	0
Miscellaneous...	0	0	0	0	0
INDUSTRIAL PROCESS-POINT...	82,258	2,033,793	4,982	4,878	216
Chemical Manufacturing...	21	2,190	730	212	0
Food/Agriculture...	3,585	1	0	0	0
Primary Metal...	50,053	2,031,596	550	22	72
Secondary Metals...	649	6	6	0	0
Mineral Products...	27,852	0	2,592	12	0
Petroleum Industry...	0	0	0	0	0
Wood Products...	0	0	0	0	0
Evaporation...	0	0	0	0	0
Metal Fabrication...	0	0	3	4,587	0
Leather Products...	0	0	0	0	0
Textile Manufacturing...	0	0	0	0	0
Inprocess Fuel...	98	1	1,100	45	144
Other/Not Classified...	0	0	0	0	0
SOLID WASTE DISPOSAL-AREA...	7,300	800	1,871	13,741	39,498
-POINT...	3,020	167	1,011	5,495	22,806
Government-point...	2,491	156	934	4,671	13,235
Municipal Incineration...	0	0	0	0	0
Open Burning...	2,491	156	934	4,671	13,235
Other...	0	0	0	0	0
Residential-area...	3,490	100	442	8,908	26,420
On Site Incineration...	2,521	39	79	7,090	21,269
Open Burning...	970	61	364	1,818	5,151
Commercial-Institutional-area...	532	86	200	736	2,015
-point...	2	1	1	4	11
On Site Incineration-area...	210	66	79	131	302
-point...	0	0	0	0	0
Open Burning-area...	322	20	121	605	1,713
-point...	2	1	1	4	11
Apartment-point...	0	0	0	0	0
Other-point...	0	0	0	0	0
Industrial-area...	3,278	614	1,229	4,098	11,063
-point...	526	10	76	820	9,559
On Site Incineration-area...	1,638	512	614	1,024	2,355
-point...	525	9	75	819	9,557
Open Burning-area...	1,639	102	615	3,074	8,708
-point...	1	1	1	1	2
Auto Body Incineration-point...	0	0	0	0	0
Other-point...	0	0	0	0	0
Miscellaneous-point...	0	0	0	0	0
TRANSPORTATION-AREA...	15,695	7,697	121,439	193,896	1,056,617
Land Vehicles...	12,293	6,936	118,695	166,238	1,023,623
Gasoline...	9,473	2,698	82,604	160,466	1,006,822
Light Vehicles...	7,648	1,983	63,390	106,035	663,771
Heavy Vehicles...	1,663	630	17,364	49,215	283,919
Off Highway...	162	85	1,850	5,216	59,132
Diesel Fuel...	2,820	4,238	36,091	5,772	16,801
Heavy Vehicles...	1,522	2,131	19,171	2,460	11,330
Off Highway...	616	551	6,821	747	1,922
Rail...	682	1,556	10,099	2,566	3,548
Aircraft...	3,402	729	2,605	9,588	18,096
Military...	3,015	576	1,448	7,014	7,530
Civil...	325	65	294	1,440	8,226
Commercial...	62	89	863	1,134	2,340
Vessels...	0	32	138	4,686	14,899
Bituminous Coal...	0	0	0	0	0
Diesel Fuel...	0	0	0	0	0
Residual Oil...	0	0	0	0	0
Gasoline...	0	0	0	0	0
Gas Handling Evaporation Loss...	0	32	138	4,686	14,899
MISCELLANEOUS-AREA...	6,121	0	0	13,384	0
Forest Fires...	5,837	1	1,398	22,413	49,483
Structural Fires...	277	0	1,373	8,241	48,072
Slash Burning...	0	1	24	72	625
Frost Control...	7	0	0	1,536	786
Solvent Evaporation Loss...	0	0	0	12,564	0

ARKANSAS

Emission categories	Pollutant, tons per year				
	Particulates	Sulfur oxides	Nitrogen oxides	Hydro-carbons	Carbon monoxide
GRAND TOTAL	145,841	72,242	216,790	189,896	874,913
-AREA	34,050	12,445	131,257	170,881	835,677
-POINT	111,791	59,797	85,533	19,014	39,235
FUEL COMBUSTION-AREA	4,986	5,301	15,642	3,461	4,749
-POINT	24,382	54,921	84,767	1,319	2,367
External Combustion-area	4,986	5,301	15,642	3,461	4,749
-point	24,381	54,921	84,745	1,282	2,143
Residential Fuel-area	3,860	293	4,198	3,081	3,501
Anthracite Coal	0	0	0	0	0
Bituminous Coal	0	0	0	0	0
Distillate Oil	14	63	17	4	2
Residual Oil	0	0	0	0	0
Natural Gas	348	21	2,782	278	695
Wood	3,498	210	1,399	2,798	2,798
Electric Generation-point	3,148	54,072	77,322	223	1,004
Anthracite Coal	0	0	0	0	0
Bituminous Coal	1,980	36,968	42,000	0	0
Lignite	0	0	0	0	0
Residual Oil	535	14,580	6,980	133	199
Distillate Oil	178	2,498	2,335	44	63
Natural Gas	456	26	26,007	45	73
Process Gas	0	0	0	0	0
Coke	0	0	0	0	0
Solid Waste/Coal	0	0	0	0	0
Other	0	0	0	0	0
Industrial Fuel-area	788	4,589	8,198	170	744
-point	21,225	848	7,417	1,056	1,13
Anthracite Coal-area	0	0	0	0	0
-point	0	0	0	0	0
Bituminous Coal-area	0	0	0	0	0
-point	0	0	0	0	0
Lignite-point	0	0	0	0	0
Residual Oil-area	388	4,565	1,013	51	6
-point	394	10	2	0	0
Distillate Oil-area	342	0	0	0	0
-point	0	0	0	0	0
Natural Gas-area	399	24	7,185	120	67
-point	395	3	2,230	16	8
Process Gas-area	0	0	0	0	0
-point	0	0	0	0	0
Coke-point	0	0	0	0	0
Wood-area	0	0	0	0	0
-point	20,094	835	5,186	1,040	1,04
Liquid Petroleum Gas-point	0	0	0	0	0
Bagasse-point	0	0	0	0	0
Other-point	0	0	0	0	0
Commercial-Institutional Fuel-area	339	418	3,246	210	50
-point	8	1	7	3	0
Anthracite Coal-area	0	0	0	0	0
-point	0	0	0	0	0
Bituminous Coal-area	0	0	0	0	0
-point	0	0	0	0	0
Lignite-point	0	0	0	0	0
Residual Oil-area	13	151	34	2	0
-point	3	0	0	0	0
Distillate Oil-area	88	252	350	18	2
-point	0	0	0	0	0
Natural Gas-area	238	14	2,862	191	47
-point	0	0	0	0	0
Wood-area	5	1	7	3	0
-point	0	0	0	0	0
Liquid Petroleum Gas-point	0	0	0	0	0
Miscellaneous-point	0	0	0	0	0
Internal Combustion-point	1	0	22	37	22
Electric Generation	0	0	0	0	0
Distillate Oil	0	0	0	0	0
Natural Gas	0	0	0	0	0
Diesel Fuel	0	0	0	0	0
Industrial Fuel	1	0	22	37	22
Distillate Oil	0	0	0	0	0
Natural Gas	0	0	0	0	0
Gasoline	0	0	7	12	2
Diesel Fuel	0	0	7	12	0

Emission categories	Pollutant, tons per year				
	Particulates	Sulfur oxides	Nitrogen oxides	Hydro-carbons	Carbon monoxide
Other.........	0	0	7	12	75
Commercial-Institutional.............	0	0	0	0	0
Diesel Fuel........	0	0	0	0	0
Other.........	0	0	0	0	0
Engine-Testing.........	0	0	0	0	0
Aircraft.........	0	0	0	0	0
Other.........	0	0	0	0	0
Miscellaneous.........	0	0	0	0	0
INDUSTRIAL PROCESS-POINT.............	84,629	4,485	166	14,136	10,125
Chemical Manufacturing.............	8,864	2,312	0	3,234	6,677
Food/Agriculture.............	13,564	0	0	0	0
Primary Metal.........	7,975	0	0	0	0
Secondary Metals.............	724	147	0	1,315	123
Mineral Products.............	42,378	1	8	73	17
Petroleum Industry.............	15	1,750	157	20	0
Wood Products.............	10,976	276	0	146	3,308
Evaporation.............	0	0	0	9,348	0
Metal Fabrication.............	3	0	0	0	0
Leather Products.............	0	0	0	0	0
Textile Manufacturing.............	0	0	0	0	0
Inprocess Fuel.............	131	0	0	0	0
Other/Not Classified.............	0	0	0	0	0
SOLID WASTE DISPOSAL-AREA.............	2,605	220	737	5,090	14,629
-POINT	2,780	391	600	3,560	26,743
Government-point.............	948	63	321	1,561	4,480
Municipal Incineration.............	118	11	10	5	72
Open Burning.............	830	52	311	1,556	4,408
Other.............	0	0	0	0	0
Residential-area.............	2,051	95	529	4,498	13,072
On Site Incineration.............	697	11	22	1,960	5,881
Open Burning.............	1,354	85	508	2,538	7,191
Commercial-Institutional-area.............	379	87	142	396	1,038
-point.............	0	0	0	0	0
On Site Incineration-area.............	252	79	94	158	362
-point.............	0	0	0	0	0
Open Burning-area.............	127	8	48	239	676
-point.............	0	0	0	0	0
Apartment-point.............	0	0	0	0	0
Other-point.............	0	0	0	0	0
Industrial-area.............	176	38	66	196	519
-point.............	1,832	329	279	1,999	22,263
On Site Incineration-area.............	107	33	40	67	154
-point.............	1,235	44	220	1,881	20,787
Open Burning-area.............	69	4	26	129	366
-point.............	597	0	59	118	1,476
Auto Body Incineration-point.............	0	0	0	0	0
Other-point.............	0	285	0	0	0
Miscellaneous-point.............	0	0	0	0	0
TRANSPORTATION-AREA.............	11,444	6,924	111,406	136,086	695,134
Land Vehicles.............	10,791	6,661	109,987	116,087	675,638
Gasoline.............	7,783	2,168	70,948	109,970	661,369
Light Vehicles.............	6,902	1,789	61,017	85,226	468,107
Heavy Vehicles.............	568	215	6,357	14,668	79,014
Off Highway.............	313	164	3,574	10,077	114,249
Diesel Fuel.............	3,008	4,493	39,039	6,117	14,269
Heavy Vehicles.............	1,188	1,664	15,651	1,702	6,785
Off Highway.............	953	853	10,561	1,156	2,976
Rail.............	867	1,976	12,828	3,259	4,507
Aircraft.............	584	143	629	1,834	3,216
Military.............	520	99	250	1,211	1,300
Civil.............	39	8	35	173	986
Commercial.............	25	35	343	451	931
Vessels.............	69	120	790	5,218	16,280
Bituminous Coal.............	0	0	0	0	0
Diesel Fuel.............	69	86	642	168	225
Residual Oil.............	0	0	0	0	0
Gasoline.............	0	34	149	5,050	16,055
Gas Handling Evaporation Loss.............	0	0	0	12,946	0
MISCELLANEOUS-AREA.............	15,014	1	3,471	26,244	121,165
Forest Fires.............	14,599	0	3,435	20,610	120,227
Structural Fires.............	415	1	36	108	938
Slash Burning.............	0	0	0	0	0
Frost Control.............	0	0	0	0	0
Solvent Evaporation Loss.............	0	0	0	5,526	0

CALIFORNIA

Emission categories	Pollutant, tons per year				
	Particulates	Sulfur oxides	Nitrogen oxides	Hydro-carbons	Carbon monoxide
GRAND TOTAL	**534,614**	**539,582**	**1,371,104**	**2,115,039**	**9,118,296**
-AREA	**178,203**	**177,737**	**978,814**	**1,820,317**	**8,626,967**
-POINT	**356,411**	**361,845**	**392,290**	**294,722**	**491,330**
FUEL COMBUSTION-AREA	20,634	119,347	83,959	8,052	14,552
-POINT	44,991	180,852	291,947	18,087	66,391
External Combustion-area	20,634	119,347	83,959	8,052	14,552
-point	42,206	179,990	281,745	13,722	65,838
Residential Fuel-area	6,600	927	27,625	5,207	9,306
Anthracite Coal	0	0	0	0	0
Bituminous Coal	40	69	6	40	181
Distillate Oil	163	475	196	49	82
Residual Oil	0	0	0	0	0
Natural Gas	3,272	196	26,174	2,617	6,543
Wood	3,125	187	1,250	2,500	2,500
Electric Generation-point	14,880	102,649	224,110	5,278	10,154
Anthracite Coal	0	0	0	0	0
Bituminous Coal	0	0	0	0	0
Lignite	0	0	0	0	0
Residual Oil	6,996	57,011	73,442	2,617	3,411
Distillate Oil	20	805	377	273	1
Natural Gas	3,181	362	126,262	660	6,741
Process Gas	0	0	0	0	0
Coke	0	0	0	0	0
Solid Waste/Coal	0	0	0	0	0
Other	4,682	44,472	24,029	1,728	1
Industrial Fuel-area	5,203	41,971	20,835	849	1,550
-point	27,167	77,158	53,293	8,289	55,661
Anthracite Coal-area	0	0	0	0	0
-point	0	0	0	0	0
Bituminous Coal-area	0	0	0	0	0
-point	3,424	905	1,053	13	41
Lignite-point	0	0	0	0	0
Residual Oil-area	3,216	38,720	8,391	420	559
-point	8,433	55,691	20,468	2,345	1,210
Distillate Oil-area	1,666	3,232	6,663	333	444
-point	2,382	2,279	10,278	574	769
Natural Gas-area	321	19	5,781	96	546
-point	560	7,008	12,632	259	593
Process Gas-area	0	0	0	0	0
-point	140	4,054	2,737	389	22
Coke-point	35	0	22	6	5
Wood-area	0	0	0	0	0
-point	12,090	350	5,491	4,653	53,010
Liquid Petroleum Gas-point	0	10	2	0	0
Bagasse-point	0	0	0	0	0
Other-point	103	6,860	610	51	10
Commercial-Institutional Fuel-area	8,831	76,449	35,499	1,996	3,696
-point	159	183	4,343	155	23
Anthracite Coal-area	0	0	0	0	0
-point	0	0	0	0	0
Bituminous Coal-area	0	0	0	0	0
-point	0	0	0	0	0
Lignite-point	0	0	0	0	0
Residual Oil-area	6,243	73,460	16,285	814	1,086
-point	0	0	0	0	0
Distillate Oil-area	1,481	2,922	5,922	296	395
-point	2	6	24	1	0
Natural Gas-area	1,108	66	13,292	886	2,215
-point	58	2	250	23	2
Wood-area	0	0	0	0	0
-point	0	0	0	0	0
Liquid Petroleum Gas-point	1	0	4	1	0
Miscellaneous-point	0	0	0	0	0
Internal Combustion-point	2,785	862	10,202	4,365	553
Electric Generation	1,483	271	6,402	221	62
Distillate Oil	212	179	3,808	97	2
Natural Gas	47	31	1,892	50	6
Diesel Fuel	1,184	54	581	61	46
Industrial Fuel	43	583	3,719	4,139	185
Distillate Oil	7	43	166	2	2
Natural Gas	17	539	2,935	3,296	124
Gasoline	0	0	0	0	0
Diesel Fuel	19	1	619	811	59

Emission categories	Pollutant, tons per year				
	Particulates	Sulfur oxides	Nitrogen oxides	Hydro-carbons	Carbon monoxide
Other	0	0	0	29	0
Commercial-Institutional	0	0	0	0	0
Diesel Fuel	0	0	0	0	0
Other	0	0	0	0	0
Engine-Testing	1,258	8	80	5	306
Aircraft	8	8	80	5	306
Other	1,250	0	0	0	0
Miscellaneous	0	0	0	0	0
INDUSTRIAL PROCESS-POINT	291,148	179,098	96,187	249,443	157,590
Chemical Manufacturing	10,921	51,810	3,484	8,353	42,270
Food/Agriculture	19,967	2	420	1,647	169
Primary Metal	1,799	22,759	6,762	107	1,766
Secondary Metals	4,516	2,581	528	110	3,681
Mineral Products	215,785	20,539	43,326	411	7,290
Petroleum Industry	6,958	76,023	34,607	28,578	47,629
Wood Products	11,878	496	549	1,459	19,141
Evaporation	8,490	1,119	46	202,673	239
Metal Fabrication	238	0	3	274	0
Leather Products	0	0	0	0	0
Textile Manufacturing	37	0	6	70	1
Inprocess Fuel	10,554	3,770	6,454	5,743	35,406
Other/Not Classified	5	0	4	18	0
SOLID WASTE DISPOSAL-AREA	48,276	1,874	8,141	116,613	343,701
-POINT	20,243	1,895	4,074	26,892	267,345
Government-point	4,667	234	1,596	10,283	23,978
Municipal Incineration	0	0	0	0	0
Open Burning	4,304	221	1,562	10,270	23,578
Other	363	13	34	13	400
Residential-area	44,776	1,440	6,828	111,125	328,440
On Site Incineration	28,982	453	906	81,512	244,536
Open Burning	15,794	987	5,923	29,613	83,904
Commercial-Institutional-area	1,774	213	665	2,816	7,842
-point	11	1	5	13	130
On Site Incineration-area	408	128	153	255	587
-point	10	1	3	13	130
Open Burning-area	1,366	85	512	2,561	7,255
-point	0	0	0	0	0
Apartment-point	0	0	0	0	0
Other-point	1	0	3	0	0
Industrial-area	1,726	221	647	2,672	7,419
-point	15,539	1,659	2,473	16,596	243,236
On Site Incineration-area	452	141	169	282	649
-point	13,791	40	2,063	14,240	235,595
Open Burning-area	1,274	80	478	2,390	6,770
-point	1,641	41	347	2,319	7,570
Auto Body Incineration-point	46	0	2	23	57
Other-point	61	1,579	60	13	14
Miscellaneous-point	26	0	0	0	0
TRANSPORTATION-AREA	109,292	56,516	886,714	1,461,184	8,268,714
Land Vehicles	94,412	44,987	860,807	1,270,927	8,095,860
Gasoline	78,975	21,576	665,387	1,236,963	8,004,541
Light Vehicles	71,496	18,536	586,463	1,009,024	6,426,218
Heavy Vehicles	6,051	2,293	62,641	182,024	1,057,784
Off Highway	1,428	747	16,284	45,914	520,539
Diesel Fuel	15,437	23,411	195,420	33,964	91,319
Heavy Vehicles	6,019	8,426	73,453	10,482	52,073
Off Highway	4,684	4,192	51,905	5,683	14,629
Rail	4,734	10,793	70,061	17,799	24,616
Aircraft	13,308	3,177	13,623	41,279	75,621
Military	11,727	2,239	5,634	27,285	29,288
Civil	1,080	214	975	4,782	27,323
Commercial	501	724	7,014	9,213	19,010
Vessels	1,573	8,351	12,284	32,230	97,233
Bituminous Coal	0	0	0	0	0
Diesel Fuel	1,118	1,397	10,431	2,738	3,651
Residual Oil	456	6,755	987	68	33
Gasoline	0	199	866	29,424	93,549
Gas Handling Evaporation Loss	0	0	0	116,748	0
MISCELLANEOUS-AREA	0	0	0	234,468	0
Forest Fires	0	0	0	0	0
Structural Fires	0	0	0	0	0
Slash Burning	0	0	0	0	0
Frost Control	0	0	0	0	0
Solvent Evaporation Loss	0	0	0	234,468	0

COLORADO

Emission categories	Pollutant, tons per year				
	Particulates	Sulfur oxides	Nitrogen oxides	Hydro-carbons	Carbon monoxide
GRAND TOTAL	232,178	47,643	185,396	224,797	1,164,010
–AREA	37,860	19,373	143,128	213,639	1,109,215
–POINT	194,317	28,270	42,268	11,158	54,795
FUEL COMBUSTION–AREA	21,903	11,994	18,421	2,220	7,027
–POINT	26,517	24,011	41,103	887	2,211
External Combustion–area	21,903	11,994	18,421	2,220	7,027
–point	26,501	24,011	40,619	838	2,077
Residential Fuel–area	1,589	1,250	4,280	1,407	4,921
Anthracite Coal	0	0	0	0	0
Bituminous Coal	829	944	124	829	3,730
Distillate Oil	61	264	73	18	31
Residual Oil	0	0	0	0	0
Natural Gas	500	30	4,002	400	1,001
Wood	199	12	80	159	159
Electric Generation–point	20,426	21,444	30,805	574	1,510
Anthracite Coal	0	0	0	0	0
Bituminous Coal	20,296	19,317	14,746	500	1,117
Lignite	0	0	0	0	0
Residual Oil	34	501	451	9	13
Distillate Oil	25	1,498	1,249	24	36
Natural Gas	70	129	14,360	41	344
Process Gas	0	0	0	0	0
Coke	0	0	0	0	0
Solid Waste/Coal	0	0	0	0	0
Other	0	0	0	0	0
Industrial Fuel–area	16,991	7,167	8,054	335	847
–point	5,624	2,121	8,893	213	457
Anthracite Coal–area	0	0	0	0	0
–point	0	0	0	0	0
Bituminous Coal–area	16,367	4,784	3,147	210	420
–point	5,255	853	1,082	137	176
Lignite–point	0	0	0	0	0
Residual Oil–area	285	1,971	743	37	50
–point	127	943	402	20	27
Distillate Oil–area	139	401	556	28	37
–point	63	316	252	13	17
Natural Gas–area	200	12	3,607	60	341
–point	140	8	7,146	41	235
Process Gas–area	0	0	0	0	0
–point	0	0	0	0	0
Coke–point	0	0	0	0	0
Wood–area	0	0	0	0	0
–point	39	2	11	2	2
Liquid Petroleum Gas–point	0	0	0	0	0
Bagasse–point	0	0	0	0	0
Other–point	0	0	0	0	0
Commercial-Institutional Fuel–area	3,323	3,577	6,087	479	1,260
–point	450	446	921	51	110
Anthracite Coal–area	0	0	0	0	0
–point	0	0	0	0	0
Bituminous Coal–area	2,543	1,665	672	146	526
–point	317	76	30	2	4
Lignite–point	0	0	0	0	0
Residual Oil–area	134	929	350	18	23
–point	62	284	161	8	11
Distillate Oil–area	335	964	1,339	67	89
–point	28	83	110	6	7
Natural Gas–area	310	19	3,725	248	621
–point	44	3	620	35	88
Wood–area	0	0	0	0	0
–point	0	0	0	0	0
Liquid Petroleum Gas–point	0	0	0	0	0
Miscellaneous–point	0	0	0	0	0
Internal Combustion–point	16	0	483	49	135
Electric Generation	16	0	483	49	135
Distillate Oil	0	0	0	0	0
Natural Gas	16	0	483	49	135
Diesel Fuel	0	0	0	0	0
Industrial Fuel	0	0	0	0	0
Distillate Oil	0	0	0	0	0
Natural Gas	0	0	0	0	0
Gasoline	0	0	0	0	0
Diesel Fuel	0	0	0	0	0

Emission categories	Pollutant, tons per year				
	Particulates	Sulfur oxides	Nitrogen oxides	Hydro-carbons	Carbon monoxide
Other	0	0	0	0	0
Commercial–Institutional	0	0	0	0	0
Diesel Fuel	0	0	0	0	0
Other	0	0	0	0	0
Engine–Testing	0	0	0	0	0
Aircraft	0	0	0	0	0
Other	0	0	0	0	0
Miscellaneous	0	0	0	0	0
INDUSTRIAL PROCESS–POINT	166,834	4,210	998	9,255	40,937
Chemical Manufacturing	0	0	34	222	7
Food/Agriculture	2,236	0	32	12	0
Primary Metal	7,569	2,104	21	2,157	23,007
Secondary Metals	526	65	0	0	102
Mineral Products	156,345	1	9	61	49
Petroleum Industry	134	2,039	835	937	17,772
Wood Products	10	0	0	6	0
Evaporation	10	0	0	5,770	0
Metal Fabrication	0	0	0	0	0
Leather Products	0	0	0	0	0
Textile Manufacturing	0	0	0	0	0
Inprocess Fuel	4	0	68	14	0
Other/Not Classified	0	0	0	78	0
SOLID WASTE DISPOSAL–AREA	871	78	207	1,762	5,104
–POINT	966	49	168	1,016	11,647
Government–point	0	0	0	0	0
Municipal Incineration	0	0	0	0	0
Open Burning	0	0	0	0	0
Other	0	0	0	0	0
Residential–area	636	23	119	1,518	4,465
On Site Incineration	347	5	11	977	2,931
Open Burning	289	18	108	542	1,534
Commercial–Institutional–area	218	50	82	226	590
–point	377	21	63	100	1,021
On Site Incineration–area	147	46	55	92	212
–point	59	21	25	25	84
Open Burning–area	71	4	27	134	378
–point	319	0	38	75	938
Apartment–point	0	0	0	0	0
Other–point	17	4	6	19	49
Industrial–area	589	28	105	916	10,626
–point	10	3	4	7	15
On Site Incineration–area	581	28	105	916	10,626
–point	6	0	2	12	34
Open Burning–area	0	0	0	0	0
–point	8	0	0	0	0
Auto Body Incineration–point	0	0	0	0	0
Other–point	0	0	0	0	0
Miscellaneous–point	15,086	7,301	124,500	197,620	1,097,084
TRANSPORTATION–AREA	12,798	6,727	121,980	174,893	1,078,304
Land Vehicles	10,341	2,928	90,510	169,421	1,064,120
Gasoline	8,561	2,220	71,561	116,943	721,250
Light Vehicles	1,544	585	16,264	44,905	257,014
Heavy Vehicles	236	123	2,686	7,573	85,857
Off Highway	2,457	3,799	31,470	5,472	14,184
Diesel Fuel	980	1,372	12,143	1,648	7,916
Heavy Vehicles	678	607	7,518	823	2,119
Off Highway	798	1,819	11,809	3,000	4,149
Rail	2,289	559	2,453	7,108	11,637
Aircraft	2,083	398	1,000	4,845	5,201
Military	109	22	99	484	2,765
Civil	97	140	1,354	1,779	3,670
Commercial	0	15	66	2,247	7,142
Vessels	0	0	0	0	0
Bituminous Coal	0	0	0	0	0
Diesel Fuel	0	0	0	0	0
Residual Oil	0	15	66	2,247	7,142
Gasoline	0	0	0	13,373	0
Gas Handling Evaporation Loss	0	0	0	12,036	0
MISCELLANEOUS–AREA	0	0	0	0	0
Forest Fires	0	0	0	0	0
Structural Fires	0	0	0	0	0
Slash Burning	0	0	0	0	0
Frost Control	0	0	0	0	0
Solvent Evaporation Loss	0	0	0	12,036	0

CONNECTICUT

Emission categories	Pollutant, tons per year				
	Particulates	Sulfur oxides	Nitrogen oxides	Hydro-carbons	Carbon monoxide
GRAND TOTAL	44,721	160,689	174,503	221,736	993,002
-AREA	25,104	38,734	130,590	205,686	989,936
-POINT	19,617	121,955	43,913	16,050	3,066
FUEL COMBUSTION-AREA	12,358	32,957	24,034	2,232	4,096
-POINT	11,414	120,632	43,722	1,758	2,976
External Combustion-area	12,358	32,957	24,034	2,232	4,096
-point	11,244	120,546	41,652	1,524	2,458
Residential Fuel-area	3,990	10,666	5,868	1,339	2,715
Anthracite Coal	49	127	15	12	444
Bituminous Coal	0	0	0	0	0
Distillate Oil	3,652	10,521	4,383	1,096	1,826
Residual Oil	0	0	0	0	0
Natural Gas	178	11	1,427	143	357
Wood	110	7	44	88	88
Electric Generation-point	9,586	110,570	36,529	1,285	2,117
Anthracite Coal	0	0	0	0	0
Bituminous Coal	6,681	32,294	5,097	97	323
Lignite	0	0	0	0	0
Residual Oil	2,856	77,687	30,585	1,174	1,757
Distillate Oil	37	589	590	13	19
Natural Gas	11	1	257	1	19
Process Gas	0	0	0	0	0
Coke	0	0	0	0	0
Solid Waste/Coal	0	0	0	0	0
Other	0	0	0	0	0
Industrial Fuel-area	6,574	16,215	12,011	568	861
-point	1,518	9,176	4,753	220	315
Anthracite Coal-area	0	0	0	0	0
-point	0	0	10	0	0
Bituminous Coal-area	2,862	2,509	413	28	55
-point	0	0	1	0	0
Lignite-point	0	0	0	0	0
Residual Oil-area	3,006	12,473	7,843	392	523
-point	1,481	9,139	4,311	216	287
Distillate Oil-area	640	1,229	2,560	128	171
-point	0	0	0	0	0
Natural Gas-area	66	4	1,196	20	113
-point	12	1	380	4	20
Process Gas-area	0	0	0	0	0
-point	0	0	0	0	0
Coke-point	21	37	26	0	4
Wood-area	0	0	0	0	0
-point	4	0	25	1	3
Liquid Petroleum Gas-point	0	0	0	0	0
Bagasse-point	0	0	0	0	0
Other-point	0	0	0	0	0
Commercial-Institutional Fuel-area	1,794	6,076	6,154	326	520
-point	140	799	370	19	26
Anthracite Coal-area	0	0	0	0	0
-point	0	0	0	0	0
Bituminous Coal-area	0	0	0	0	0
-point	0	0	0	0	0
Lignite-point	0	0	0	0	0
Residual Oil-area	1,257	5,214	3,279	164	219
-point	138	799	360	18	24
Distillate Oil-area	446	856	1,783	89	119
-point	0	0	0	0	0
Natural Gas-area	91	5	1,093	73	182
-point	0	0	1	0	0
Wood-area	0	0	0	0	0
-point	0	0	0	0	0
Liquid Petroleum Gas-point	2	0	9	1	2
Miscellaneous-point	0	0	0	0	0
Internal Combustion-point	170	86	2,070	234	518
Electric Generation	102	44	1,470	113	313
Distillate Oil	102	44	1,469	113	313
Natural Gas	0	0	1	0	0
Diesel Fuel	0	0	0	0	0
Industrial Fuel	39	28	562	43	119
Distillate Oil	32	22	465	36	97
Natural Gas	0	0	2	0	0
Gasoline	0	0	0	0	0
Diesel Fuel	7	6	95	8	21

Emission categories	Pollutant, tons per year				
	Particulates	Sulfur oxides	Nitrogen oxides	Hydro-carbons	Carbon monoxide
Other	0	0	0	0	0
Commercial-Institutional	0	0	0	0	0
Diesel Fuel	0	0	0	0	0
Other	0	0	0	0	0
Engine-Testing	30	14	38	78	86
Aircraft	30	14	38	78	86
Other	0	0	0	0	0
Miscellaneous	0	0	0	0	0
INDUSTRIAL PROCESS-POINT	8,185	26	186	14,288	76
Chemical Manufacturing	1	0	1	57	0
Food/Agriculture	3	0	0	0	0
Primary Metal	113	0	8	0	0
Secondary Metals	10	0	0	0	0
Mineral Products	2,275	0	0	0	0
Petroleum Industry	0	0	0	0	0
Wood Products	0	0	0	0	0
Evaporation	231	0	0	3,393	0
Metal Fabrication	1	0	0	0	0
Leather Products	0	0	0	0	0
Textile Manufacturing	0	0	0	0	0
Inprocess Fuel	0	0	0	0	0
Other/Not Classified	5,551	26	177	10,838	76
SOLID WASTE DISPOSAL-AREA	594	40	186	1,174	3,365
-POINT	18	1,297	4	4	15
Government-point	0	0	0	0	0
Municipal Incineration	0	0	0	0	0
Open Burning	0	0	0	0	0
Other	0	0	0	0	0
Residential-area	527	28	161	1,088	3,132
On Site Incineration	106	2	3	297	892
Open Burning	422	26	158	791	2,240
Commercial-Institutional-area	67	12	25	86	232
-point	16	4	4	4	15
On Site Incineration-area	32	10	12	20	45
-point	16	4	4	4	15
Open Burning-area	35	2	13	66	187
-point	0	0	0	0	0
Apartment-point	0	0	0	0	0
Other-point	0	0	0	0	0
Industrial-area	0	0	0	0	0
-point	2	1,293	0	0	0
On Site Incineration-area	0	0	0	0	0
-point	2	1,293	0	0	0
Open Burning-area	0	0	0	0	0
-point	0	0	0	0	0
Auto Body Incineration-point	0	0	0	0	0
Other-point	0	0	0	0	0
Miscellaneous-point	0	0	0	0	0
TRANSPORTATION-AREA	12,152	5,737	106,370	175,458	982,475
Land Vehicles	11,891	4,692	105,366	156,223	967,392
Gasoline	10,584	2,807	89,007	153,718	958,603
Light Vehicles	10,105	2,620	83,955	139,502	869,623
Heavy Vehicles	439	166	4,598	12,934	74,452
Off Highway	40	21	454	1,281	14,527
Diesel Fuel	1,307	1,885	16,359	2,505	8,789
Heavy Vehicles	863	1,208	10,683	1,452	6,982
Off Highway	243	218	2,694	295	759
Rail	202	459	2,982	758	1,048
Aircraft	177	75	550	1,057	2,930
Military	86	16	41	199	214
Civil	59	12	53	259	1,482
Commercial	33	47	456	598	1,235
Vessels	84	970	454	3,862	12,153
Bituminous Coal	0	0	0	0	0
Diesel Fuel	22	28	208	55	73
Residual Oil	62	917	134	9	4
Gasoline	0	26	112	3,798	12,075
Gas Handling Evaporation Loss	0	0	0	14,316	0
MISCELLANEOUS-AREA	0	0	0	26,822	0
Forest Fires	0	0	0	0	0
Structural Fires	0	0	0	0	0
Slash Burning	0	0	0	0	0
Frost Control	0	0	0	0	0
Solvent Evaporation Loss	0	0	0	26,822	0

DELAWARE

Emission categories	Pollutant, tons per year				
	Particulates	Sulfur oxides	Nitrogen oxides	Hydro-carbons	Carbon monoxide
GRAND TOTAL	39,584	177,304	56,484	64,813	268,125
-AREA	17,060	9,024	32,990	53,795	252,272
-POINT	22,524	168,281	23,494	11,017	15,853
FUEL COMBUSTION-AREA	12,553	7,595	4,166	442	1,270
-POINT	3,315	47,954	19,687	526	1,004
External Combustion-area	12,553	7,595	4,166	442	1,270
-point	3,315	47,954	19,687	526	1,004
Residential Fuel-area	721	1,689	1,104	279	916
Anthracite Coal	53	138	16	13	481
Bituminous Coal	0	0	0	0	0
Distillate Oil	536	1,543	643	161	268
Residual Oil	0	0	0	0	0
Natural Gas	52	3	413	41	103
Wood	80	5	32	64	64
Electric Generation-point	1,410	30,665	13,131	232	575
Anthracite Coal	0	0	0	0	0
Bituminous Coal	1,074	25,207	7,325	122	407
Lignite	0	0	0	0	0
Residual Oil	328	5,439	5,688	108	163
Distillate Oil	6	19	77	1	2
Natural Gas	1	0	41	0	3
Process Gas	0	0	0	0	0
Coke	0	0	0	0	0
Solid Waste/Coal	0	0	0	0	0
Other	0	0	0	0	0
Industrial Fuel-area	11,382	4,982	1,943	99	225
-point	1,671	16,047	5,940	263	387
Anthracite Coal-area	36	49	27	0	4
-point	0	0	0	0	0
Bituminous Coal-area	11,266	4,834	1,193	80	159
-point	0	0	0	0	0
Lignite-point	0	0	0	0	0
Residual Oil-area	0	0	0	0	0
-point	1,533	15,666	4,659	233	311
Distillate Oil-area	51	98	204	10	14
-point	110	379	440	22	29
Natural Gas-area	29	2	519	9	49
-point	28	2	832	8	47
Process Gas-area	0	0	0	0	0
-point	0	0	6	0	0
Coke-point	0	0	0	0	0
Wood-area	0	0	0	0	0
-point	0	0	0	0	0
Liquid Petroleum Gas-point	0	0	3	0	0
Bagasse-point	0	0	0	0	0
Other-point	0	0	0	0	0
Commercial-Institutional Fuel-area	451	924	1,119	63	128
-point	234	1,243	616	31	42
Anthracite Coal-area	44	60	22	0	13
-point	0	0	0	0	0
Bituminous Coal-area	167	160	24	5	19
-point	0	0	0	0	0
Lignite-point	0	0	0	0	0
Residual Oil-area	36	351	94	5	6
-point	233	1,242	607	30	40
Distillate Oil-area	183	352	733	37	49
-point	1	0	4	0	0
Natural Gas-area	20	1	245	16	41
-point	0	0	6	0	1
Wood-area	0	0	0	0	0
-point	0	0	0	0	0
Liquid Petroleum Gas-point	0	0	0	0	0
Miscellaneous-point	0	0	0	0	0
Internal Combustion-point	0	0	0	0	0
Electric Generation	0	0	0	0	0
Distillate Oil	0	0	0	0	0
Natural Gas	0	0	0	0	0
Diesel Fuel	0	0	0	0	0
Industrial Fuel	0	0	0	0	0
Distillate Oil	0	0	0	0	0
Natural Gas	0	0	0	0	0
Gasoline	0	0	0	0	0
Diesel Fuel	0	0	0	0	0

Emission categories	Pollutant, tons per year				
	Particulates	Sulfur oxides	Nitrogen oxides	Hydro-carbons	Carbon monoxide
Other	0	0	0	0	0
Commercial-Institutional	0	0	0	0	0
Diesel Fuel	0	0	0	0	0
Other	0	0	0	0	0
Engine-Testing	0	0	0	0	0
Aircraft	0	0	0	0	0
Other	0	0	0	0	0
Miscellaneous	0	0	0	0	0
INDUSTRIAL PROCESS–POINT	19,205	120,324	3,804	10,488	14,841
Chemical Manufacturing	550	10,955	765	4,726	5,785
Food/Agriculture	1,959	0	0	0	0
Primary Metal	438	0	0	0	6,948
Secondary Metals	59	0	0	0	32
Mineral Products	283	0	9	1	0
Petroleum Industry	15,666	101,178	3,003	770	2,076
Wood Products	0	0	0	0	0
Evaporation	31	0	0	4,484	0
Metal Fabrication	0	0	0	0	0
Leather Products	12	0	0	380	0
Textile Manufacturing	0	0	0	0	0
Inprocess Fuel	204	8,191	28	56	0
Other/Not Classified	3	0	0	72	0
SOLID WASTE DISPOSAL–AREA	478	94	169	598	1,622
–POINT	4	2	3	3	8
Government-point	0	0	0	0	0
Municipal Incineration	0	0	0	0	0
Open Burning	0	0	0	0	0
Other	0	0	0	0	0
Residential-area	199	11	64	403	1,156
On Site Incineration	31	0	1	88	263
Open Burning	168	10	63	315	893
Commercial-Institutional-area	134	38	50	105	258
–point	0	0	0	0	0
On Site Incineration-area	118	37	44	74	169
–point	0	0	0	0	0
Open Burning-area	17	1	6	32	89
–point	0	0	0	0	0
Apartment-point	0	0	0	0	0
Other-point	0	0	0	0	0
Industrial-area	145	45	54	91	208
–point	4	2	3	3	8
On Site Incineration-area	145	45	54	91	208
–point	4	2	3	3	8
Open Burning-area	0	0	0	0	0
–point	0	0	0	0	0
Auto Body Incineration-point	0	0	0	0	0
Other-point	0	0	0	0	0
Miscellaneous-point	0	0	0	0	0
TRANSPORTATION–AREA	3,473	1,335	28,590	50,342	247,389
Land Vehicles	2,750	1,123	28,071	44,659	242,671
Gasoline	2,471	773	24,555	44,267	241,410
Light Vehicles	1,396	362	12,411	16,916	90,799
Heavy Vehicles	1,048	397	11,845	26,508	141,053
Off Highway	26	14	299	843	9,559
Diesel Fuel	279	350	3,516	392	1,261
Heavy Vehicles	172	241	2,300	239	909
Off Highway	97	87	1,077	118	304
Rail	9	21	139	35	49
Aircraft	711	140	412	1,830	3,213
Military	650	124	312	1,512	1,623
Civil	58	11	52	256	1,461
Commercial	3	5	48	63	129
Vessels	13	72	107	487	1,504
Bituminous Coal	0	0	0	0	0
Diesel Fuel	9	11	85	22	30
Residual Oil	4	57	8	1	0
Gasoline	0	3	14	464	1,474
Gas Handling Evaporation Loss	0	0	0	3,367	0
MISCELLANEOUS–AREA	555	0	66	2,413	1,991
Forest Fires	15	0	3	21	120
Structural Fires	30	0	3	8	67
Slash Burning	511	0	60	601	1,803
Frost Control	0	0	0	0	0
Solvent Evaporation Loss	0	0	0	1,784	0

DISTRICT OF COLUMBIA

Emission categories	Pollutant, tons per year				
	Particulates	Sulfur oxides	Nitrogen oxides	Hydro-carbons	Carbon monoxide
GRAND TOTAL	10,846	50,606	46,068	33,187	162,483
-AREA	7,538	22,080	29,281	32,411	155,877
-POINT	3,309	28,526	16,787	777	6,606
FUEL COMBUSTION-AREA	4,448	20,829	10,686	904	2,462
-POINT	2,036	28,113	16,456	464	873
External Combustion-area	4,448	20,829	10,686	904	2,462
-point	2,036	28,113	16,456	464	873
Residential Fuel-area	583	1,062	1,052	396	1,621
Anthracite Coal	22	49	7	6	201
Bituminous Coal	250	380	37	250	1,125
Distillate Oil	218	628	261	65	109
Residual Oil	0	0	0	0	0
Natural Gas	93	6	746	75	187
Wood	0	0	0	0	0
Electric Generation-point	1,387	23,240	14,148	300	515
Anthracite Coal	0	0	0	0	0
Bituminous Coal	317	4,528	2,072	53	144
Lignite	0	0	0	0	0
Residual Oil	1,070	18,711	12,074	247	371
Distillate Oil	0	1	2	0	0
Natural Gas	0	0	0	0	0
Process Gas	0	0	0	0	0
Coke	0	0	0	0	0
Solid Waste/Coal	0	0	0	0	0
Other	0	0	0	0	0
Industrial Fuel-area	326	1,914	1,257	49	95
-point	434	3,606	1,760	116	227
Anthracite Coal-area	0	0	0	0	0
-point	0	0	0	0	0
Bituminous Coal-area	0	0	0	0	0
-point	422	3,344	1,650	110	220
Lignite-point	0	0	0	0	0
Residual Oil-area	267	1,844	696	35	46
-point	12	262	110	6	7
Distillate Oil-area	36	69	143	7	10
-point	0	0	0	0	0
Natural Gas-area	23	1	418	7	39
-point	0	0	0	0	0
Process Gas-area	0	0	0	0	0
-point	0	0	0	0	0
Coke-point	0	0	0	0	0
Wood-area	0	0	0	0	0
-point	0	0	0	0	0
Liquid Petroleum Gas-point	0	0	0	0	0
Bagasse-point	0	0	0	0	0
Other-point	0	0	0	0	0
Commercial-Institutional Fuel-area	3,539	17,852	8,377	460	745
-point	215	1,267	548	48	131
Anthracite Coal-area	0	0	0	0	0
-point	0	0	0	0	0
Bituminous Coal-area	737	678	205	45	161
-point	20	30	3	20	90
Lignite-point	0	0	0	0	0
Residual Oil-area	2,374	16,413	6,192	310	413
-point	190	1,231	496	25	33
Distillate Oil-area	395	759	1,581	79	105
-point	2	5	7	0	0
Natural Gas-area	33	2	400	27	67
-point	4	0	43	3	8
Wood-area	0	0	0	0	0
-point	0	0	0	0	0
Liquid Petroleum Gas-point	0	0	0	0	0
Miscellaneous-point	0	0	0	0	0
Internal Combustion-point	0	0	0	0	0
Electric Generation	0	0	0	0	0
Distillate Oil	0	0	0	0	0
Natural Gas	0	0	0	0	0
Diesel Fuel	0	0	0	0	0
Industrial Fuel	0	0	0	0	0
Distillate Oil	0	0	0	0	0
Natural Gas	0	0	0	0	0
Gasoline	0	0	0	0	0
Diesel Fuel	0	0	0	0	0

Emission categories	Pollutant, tons per year				
	Particulates	Sulfur oxides	Nitrogen oxides	Hydro-carbons	Carbon monoxide
Other	0	0	0	0	0
Commercial-Institutional	0	0	0	0	0
Diesel Fuel	0	0	0	0	0
Other	0	0	0	0	0
Engine-Testing	0	0	0	0	0
Aircraft	0	0	0	0	0
Other	0	0	0	0	0
Miscellaneous	0	0	0	0	0
INDUSTRIAL PROCESS-POINT	1,143	0	0	60	0
Chemical Manufacturing	0	0	0	0	0
Food/Agriculture	0	0	0	0	0
Primary Metal	0	0	0	0	0
Secondary Metals	0	0	0	0	0
Mineral Products	1,143	0	0	0	0
Petroleum Industry	0	0	0	0	0
Wood Products	0	0	0	0	0
Evaporation	0	0	0	60	0
Metal Fabrication	0	0	0	0	0
Leather Products	0	0	0	0	0
Textile Manufacturing	0	0	0	0	0
Inprocess Fuel	0	0	0	0	0
Other/Not Classified	0	0	0	0	0
SOLID WASTE DISPOSAL-AREA	1,104	345	414	690	1,588
-POINT	130	412	331	252	5,732
Government-point	120	408	326	245	5,713
Municipal Incineration	120	408	326	245	5,713
Open Burning	0	0	0	0	0
Other	0	0	0	0	0
Residential-area	0	0	0	0	0
On Site Incineration	0	0	0	0	0
Open Burning	0	0	0	0	0
Commercial-Institutional-area	1,104	345	414	690	1,588
-point	10	4	5	8	19
On Site Incineration-area	1,104	345	414	690	1,588
-point	10	4	5	8	19
Open Burning-area	0	0	0	0	0
-point	0	0	0	0	0
Apartment-point	0	0	0	0	0
Other-point	0	0	0	0	0
Industrial-area	0	0	0	0	0
-point	0	0	0	0	0
On Site Incineration-area	0	0	0	0	0
-point	0	0	0	0	0
Open Burning-area	0	0	0	0	0
-point	0	0	0	0	0
Auto Body Incineration-point	0	0	0	0	0
Other-point	0	0	0	0	0
Miscellaneous-point	0	0	0	0	0
TRANSPORTATION-AREA	1,985	907	18,181	27,904	151,828
Land Vehicles	1,985	903	18,164	24,965	150,522
Gasoline	1,711	456	14,561	24,346	148,775
Light Vehicles	1,619	420	13,578	21,689	131,451
Heavy Vehicles	79	30	842	2,258	12,796
Off Highway	12	7	142	399	4,528
Diesel Fuel	274	447	3,603	619	1,747
Heavy Vehicles	163	228	2,050	263	1,221
Off Highway	24	22	271	30	76
Rail	87	198	1,282	326	450
Aircraft	0	0	0	0	0
Military	0	0	0	0	0
Civil	0	0	0	0	0
Commercial	0	0	0	0	0
Vessels	0	3	17	411	1,305
Bituminous Coal	0	0	0	0	0
Diesel Fuel	0	1	4	1	2
Residual Oil	0	0	0	0	0
Gasoline	0	3	12	410	1,304
Gas Handling Evaporation Loss	0	0	0	2,528	0
MISCELLANEOUS-AREA	0	0	0	2,912	0
Forest Fires	0	0	0	0	0
Structural Fires	0	0	0	0	0
Slash Burning	0	0	0	0	0
Frost Control	0	0	0	0	0
Solvent Evaporation Loss	0	0	0	2,912	0

FLORIDA

Emission categories	Pollutant, tons per year				
	Particulates	Sulfur oxides	Nitrogen oxides	Hydro-carbons	Carbon monoxide
GRAND TOTAL	290,720	1,173,550	761,560	1,140,776	3,293,972
-AREA	112,780	30,196	356,597	1,118,670	3,193,656
-POINT	177,941	1,143,354	404,963	22,106	100,316
FUEL COMBUSTION-AREA	2,805	10,737	8,959	1,017	1,539
-POINT	83,118	993,995	379,812	8,465	15,868
External Combustion-area	2,805	10,737	8,959	1,017	1,539
-point	81,173	989,863	364,763	7,644	13,985
Residential Fuel-area	905	76	1,385	603	824
Anthracite Coal	0	0	0	0	0
Bituminous Coal	11	37	2	11	52
Distillate Oil	246	0	295	74	123
Residual Oil	0	0	0	0	0
Natural Gas	109	7	873	87	218
Wood	539	32	216	431	431
Electric Generation-point	56,423	922,177	331,133	4,425	10,193
Anthracite Coal	0	0	0	0	0
Bituminous Coal	32,471	536,039	100,631	1,097	3,658
Lignite	0	0	0	0	0
Residual Oil	22,141	360,854	160,018	3,203	4,805
Distillate Oil	386	5,718	1,301	25	37
Natural Gas	1,425	19,565	69,184	100	1,694
Process Gas	0	0	0	0	0
Coke	0	0	0	0	0
Solid Waste/Coal	0	0	0	0	0
Other	0	0	0	0	0
Industrial Fuel-area	22	0	89	4	6
-point	24,430	64,550	32,591	3,154	3,682
Anthracite Coal-area	0	0	0	0	0
-point	0	0	0	0	0
Bituminous Coal-area	0	0	0	0	0
-point	0	0	0	0	0
Lignite-point	0	0	0	0	0
Residual Oil-area	0	0	0	0	0
-point	5,293	56,552	11,924	575	765
Distillate Oil-area	22	0	89	4	6
-point	453	5,598	1,734	88	112
Natural Gas-area	0	0	0	0	0
-point	215	13	9,276	66	374
Process Gas-area	0	0	0	0	0
-point	0	0	0	0	0
Coke-point	0	0	4	0	6
Wood-area	0	0	0	0	0
-point	11,206	1,155	8,433	1,687	1,687
Liquid Petroleum Gas-point	0	0	0	0	0
Bagasse-point	5,486	0	729	738	738
Other-point	1,778	1,233	490	0	0
Commercial-Institutional Fuel-area	1,878	10,661	7,485	409	709
-point	319	3,136	1,039	65	110
Anthracite Coal-area	0	0	0	0	0
-point	0	0	0	0	0
Bituminous Coal-area	0	0	0	0	0
-point	0	0	0	0	0
Lignite-point	0	0	0	0	0
Residual Oil-area	1,027	10,651	2,679	134	179
-point	264	2,793	632	40	54
Distillate Oil-area	676	0	2,704	135	180
-point	29	209	112	6	7
Natural Gas-area	175	11	2,102	140	350
-point	26	134	295	19	49
Wood-area	0	0	0	0	0
-point	0	0	0	0	0
Liquid Petroleum Gas-point	0	0	0	0	0
Miscellaneous-point	1	0	0	0	0
Internal Combustion-point	1,945	4,132	15,049	822	1,883
Electric Generation	1,562	4,038	14,937	470	1,633
Distillate Oil	1,409	3,444	10,527	117	323
Natural Gas	79	288	2,169	247	662
Diesel Fuel	37	18	1,065	106	648
Industrial Fuel	294	18	0	0	0
Distillate Oil	0	0	0	0	0
Natural Gas	0	0	0	0	0
Gasoline	0	0	0	0	0
Diesel Fuel	0	0	0	0	0

Emission categories	Pollutant, tons per year				
	Particulates	Sulfur oxides	Nitrogen oxides	Hydro-carbons	Carbon monoxide
Other	294	18	0	0	0
Commercial-Institutional	0	0	0	0	0
Diesel Fuel	0	0	0	0	0
Other	0	0	0	0	0
Engine-Testing	90	76	111	351	250
Aircraft	90	76	111	351	250
Other	0	0	0	0	0
Miscellaneous	0	0	0	0	0
INDUSTRIAL PROCESS-POINT	86,141	148,098	24,259	11,456	62,166
Chemical Manufacturing	7,238	75,615	18,070	4,832	1,771
Food/Agriculture	1,776	16	11	29	0
Primary Metal	1,145	0	0	0	0
Secondary Metals	75	4,134	1	0	1,036
Mineral Products	31,875	45,898	3,697	2	1
Petroleum Industry	42	11,351	0	0	0
Wood Products	29,594	3,746	84	2,001	59,357
Evaporation	0	0	1	4,229	0
Metal Fabrication	0	0	0	0	0
Leather Products	0	0	0	0	0
Textile Manufacturing	0	0	0	0	0
Inprocess Fuel	14,390	7,338	2,396	356	0
Other/Not Classified	6	0	0	8	0
SOLID WASTE DISPOSAL-AREA	347	55	119	507	1,404
-POINT	8,681	1,261	893	2,185	22,283
Government-point	5,447	655	524	393	5,188
Municipal Incineration	5,445	655	524	393	5,188
Open Burning	0	0	0	0	0
Other	2	0	1	0	0
Residential-area	155	8	47	321	923
On Site Incineration	31	0	1	88	265
Open Burning	124	8	46	233	659
Commercial-Institutional-area	65	17	24	57	143
-point	232	47	84	85	437
On Site Incineration-area	52	16	19	33	75
-point	186	47	65	82	434
Open Burning-area	13	1	5	24	68
-point	0	0	0	0	0
Apartment-point	5	0	1	3	3
Other-point	40	0	19	0	0
Industrial-area	127	30	48	130	338
-point	3,003	559	284	1,707	16,657
On Site Incineration-area	87	27	33	55	125
-point	1,363	159	283	1,707	16,657
Open Burning-area	40	2	15	75	213
-point	0	0	0	0	0
Auto Body Incineration-point	0	0	0	0	0
Other-point	1,640	401	1	0	0
Miscellaneous-point	0	0	0	0	0
TRANSPORTATION-AREA	48,036	19,404	338,414	572,512	2,898,964
Land Vehicles	36,036	15,394	328,133	486,594	2,804,511
Gasoline	31,708	8,591	270,523	477,080	2,776,337
Light Vehicles	27,586	7,070	228,846	364,648	2,199,476
Heavy Vehicles	3,960	1,436	39,835	107,239	607,983
Off Highway	162	85	1,842	5,193	58,878
Diesel Fuel	4,556	6,803	57,610	9,514	28,174
Heavy Vehicles	2,287	3,202	28,251	3,874	18,733
Off Highway	1,135	1,016	12,579	1,377	3,545
Rail	1,134	2,585	16,779	4,263	5,895
Aircraft	11,582	2,487	8,714	31,548	48,829
Military	10,830	2,068	5,203	25,196	27,047
Civil	537	107	485	2,376	13,580
Commercial	216	312	3,026	3,975	8,202
Vessels	190	1,523	1,567	14,507	45,624
Bituminous Coal	0	0	0	0	0
Diesel Fuel	103	128	958	251	335
Residual Oil	88	1,298	190	13	6
Gasoline	0	96	419	14,242	45,282
Gas Handling Evaporation Loss	0	0	0	39,863	0
MISCELLANEOUS-AREA	61,591	0	9,105	117,634	291,750
Forest Fires	15,804	0	3,719	22,311	130,149
Structural Fires	0	0	0	0	0
Slash Burning	45,787	0	5,387	53,867	161,600
Frost Control	0	0	0	0	0
Solvent Evaporation Loss	0	0	0	41,456	0

GEORGIA

Emission categories	Pollutant, tons per year				
	Particulates	Sulfur oxides	Nitrogen oxides	Hydro-carbons	Carbon monoxide
GRAND TOTAL	383,715	520,688	438,377	467,461	2,366,747
-AREA	92,803	46,339	277,791	453,440	2,193,714
-POINT	290,912	474,348	160,587	14,021	173,033
FUEL COMBUSTION–AREA	19,463	32,262	30,151	4,440	9,322
-POINT	86,177	433,152	152,315	5,161	10,807
External Combustion–area	19,463	32,262	30,151	4,440	9,322
-point	86,172	433,152	152,315	5,161	10,807
Residential Fuel–area	4,287	2,987	5,408	3,519	6,939
Anthracite Coal	0	0	0	0	0
Bituminous Coal	798	2,579	120	798	3,593
Distillate Oil	139	208	167	42	70
Residual Oil	0	0	0	0	0
Natural Gas	498	30	3,980	398	995
Wood	2,851	171	1,141	2,281	2,281
Electric Generation–point	58,778	370,709	110,024	1,572	5,588
Anthracite Coal	0	0	0	0	0
Bituminous Coal	58,669	365,673	91,349	1,517	5,058
Lignite	0	0	0	0	0
Residual Oil	47	4,914	1,342	26	38
Distillate Oil	0	0	0	0	0
Natural Gas	62	122	17,333	29	491
Process Gas	0	0	0	0	0
Coke	0	0	0	0	0
Solid Waste/Coal	0	0	0	0	0
Other	0	0	0	0	0
Industrial Fuel–area	13,033	8,570	16,133	443	1,526
-point	26,546	62,242	34,896	2,998	3,752
Anthracite Coal–area	0	0	0	0	0
-point	0	0	0	0	0
Bituminous Coal–area	11,759	7,896	1,834	122	244
-point	3,199	4,786	2,116	52	131
Lignite–point	0	0	0	0	0
Residual Oil–area	2	24	4	0	0
-point	3,046	52,821	9,522	476	635
Distillate Oil–area	615	610	2,461	123	164
-point	61	828	311	15	21
Natural Gas–area	657	39	11,834	197	1,118
-point	606	539	11,304	125	636
Process Gas–area	0	0	0	0	0
-point	0	0	0	0	0
Coke–point	0	0	0	0	0
Wood–area	0	0	0	0	0
-point	19,576	3,191	11,641	2,329	2,329
Liquid Petroleum Gas–point	1	77	2	0	1
Bagasse–point	0	0	0	0	0
Other–point	58	0	0	0	0
Commercial-Institutional Fuel–area	2,143	20,705	8,610	478	857
-point	848	201	7,396	591	1,468
Anthracite Coal–area	0	0	0	0	0
-point	0	0	0	0	0
Bituminous Coal–area	0	0	0	0	0
-point	62	46	28	4	15
Lignite–point	0	0	0	0	0
Residual Oil–area	1,328	20,101	3,464	173	231
-point	7	85	19	1	1
Distillate Oil–area	580	589	2,320	116	155
-point	62	27	248	12	17
Natural Gas–area	235	14	2,826	188	471
-point	717	43	7,101	574	1,435
Wood–area	0	0	0	0	0
-point	0	0	0	0	0
Liquid Petroleum Gas–point	0	0	0	0	0
Miscellaneous–point	0	0	0	0	0
Internal Combustion–point	4	0	0	0	0
Electric Generation	0	0	0	0	0
Distillate Oil	0	0	0	0	0
Natural Gas	0	0	0	0	0
Diesel Fuel	0	0	0	0	0
Industrial Fuel	4	0	0	0	0
Distillate Oil	0	0	0	0	0
Natural Gas	0	0	0	0	0
Gasoline	0	0	0	0	0
Diesel Fuel	0	0	0	0	0

Emission categories	Pollutant, tons per year				
	Particulates	Sulfur oxides	Nitrogen oxides	Hydro-carbons	Carbon monoxide
Other	4	0	0	0	0
Commercial-Institutional	0	0	0	0	0
Diesel Fuel	0	0	0	0	0
Other	0	0	0	0	0
Engine-Testing	0	0	0	0	0
Aircraft	0	0	0	0	0
Other	0	0	0	0	0
Miscellaneous	0	0	0	0	0
INDUSTRIAL PROCESS-POINT	203,149	40,981	8,062	8,078	155,136
Chemical Manufacturing	3,080	10,810	6,287	1,279	12,500
Food/Agriculture	5,512	0	3	1	12
Primary Metal	2,415	5,888	0	0	6,120
Secondary Metals	460	540	0	966	5,879
Mineral Products	132,762	6,308	1,674	355	170
Petroleum Industry	26	71	95	5	0
Wood Products	52,557	16,456	0	5	130,455
Evaporation	2	0	0	5,048	0
Metal Fabrication	0	0	0	0	0
Leather Products	0	0	0	0	0
Textile Manufacturing	0	0	0	0	0
Inprocess Fuel	6,335	910	3	75	0
Other/Not Classified	0	0	0	344	0
SOLID WASTE DISPOSAL-AREA	4,458	317	1,671	8,166	23,086
-POINT	1,321	205	210	522	7,089
Government-point	966	199	159	142	2,768
Municipal Incineration	966	199	159	141	2,766
Open Burning	0	0	0	0	1
Other	0	0	0	0	0
Residential-area	1,459	91	546	2,736	7,754
On Site Incineration	2	0	0	5	15
Open Burning	1,457	91	546	2,732	7,739
Commercial-Institutional-area	1,106	107	415	1,882	5,282
-point	61	3	11	88	1,002
On Site Incineration-area	153	48	57	96	220
-point	61	3	11	88	1,002
Open Burning-area	953	60	357	1,787	5,062
-point	0	0	0	0	0
Apartment-point	0	0	0	0	0
Other-point	0	0	0	0	0
Industrial-area	1,893	119	710	3,547	10,050
-point	295	3	40	292	3,320
On Site Incineration-area	2	1	1	1	3
-point	193	3	28	268	3,020
Open Burning-area	1,891	118	709	3,546	10,047
-point	102	0	12	24	300
Auto Body Incineration-point	0	0	0	0	0
Other-point	0	0	0	0	0
Miscellaneous-point	0	0	0	0	0
TRANSPORTATION-AREA	26,494	13,758	240,526	376,693	1,993,503
Land Vehicles	24,041	12,793	235,732	320,112	1,930,752
Gasoline	19,160	5,519	173,025	310,258	1,903,968
Light Vehicles	15,263	3,957	130,610	199,742	1,177,095
Heavy Vehicles	3,306	1,253	35,680	91,526	511,585
Off Highway	591	309	6,735	18,989	215,288
Diesel Fuel	4,881	7,274	62,707	9,854	26,784
Heavy Vehicles	2,407	3,369	30,752	3,744	16,522
Off Highway	1,253	1,122	13,889	1,521	3,915
Rail	1,221	2,783	18,065	4,590	6,347
Aircraft	2,427	736	4,235	9,892	22,228
Military	1,838	351	883	4,276	4,590
Civil	374	74	338	1,657	9,469
Commercial	215	311	3,014	3,959	8,169
Vessels	26	229	559	12,772	40,524
Bituminous Coal	0	0	0	0	0
Diesel Fuel	18	22	167	44	58
Residual Oil	8	120	18	1	1
Gasoline	0	86	375	12,727	40,465
Gas Handling Evaporation Loss	0	0	0	33,916	0
MISCELLANEOUS-AREA	42,388	2	5,443	64,141	167,803
Forest Fires	4,131	0	972	5,832	34,021
Structural Fires	977	2	85	253	2,208
Slash Burning	37,279	0	4,386	43,858	131,573
Frost Control	0	0	0	0	0
Solvent Evaporation Loss	0	0	0	14,198	0

HAWAII

Emission categories	Pollutant, tons per year				
	Particulates	Sulfur oxides	Nitrogen oxides	Hydro-carbons	Carbon monoxide
GRAND TOTAL	**73,971**	**51,805**	**54,084**	**94,405**	**329,931**
-AREA	**27,144**	**3,664**	**30,128**	**79,781**	**322,401**
-POINT	**46,827**	**48,141**	**23,956**	**14,624**	**7,530**
FUEL COMBUSTION-AREA	197	860	644	69	95
-POINT	11,189	42,421	22,825	5,868	4,803
External Combustion-area	197	860	644	69	95
-point	10,995	41,540	20,269	5,757	4,108
Residential Fuel-area	53	7	82	42	51
Anthracite Coal	0	0	0	0	0
Bituminous Coal	0	0	0	0	0
Distillate Oil	1	4	2	0	1
Residual Oil	0	0	0	0	0
Natural Gas	8	0	63	6	16
Wood	44	3	18	35	35
Electric Generation-point	1,056	26,823	13,750	272	382
Anthracite Coal	0	0	0	0	0
Bituminous Coal	0	0	0	0	0
Lignite	0	0	0	0	0
Residual Oil	1,056	26,823	13,750	272	382
Distillate Oil	0	0	0	0	0
Natural Gas	0	0	0	0	0
Process Gas	0	0	0	0	0
Coke	0	0	0	0	0
Solid Waste/Coal	0	0	0	0	0
Other	0	0	0	0	0
Industrial Fuel-area	2	0	36	1	3
-point	9,939	14,717	6,519	5,485	3,726
Anthracite Coal-area	0	0	0	0	0
-point	0	0	0	0	0
Bituminous Coal-area	0	0	0	0	0
-point	0	0	0	0	0
Lignite-point	0	0	0	0	0
Residual Oil-area	0	0	0	0	0
-point	643	14,167	2,758	122	154
Distillate Oil-area	0	0	0	0	0
-point	113	212	389	23	26
Natural Gas-area	2	0	36	1	3
-point	0	0	0	0	0
Process Gas-area	0	0	0	0	0
-point	0	0	0	0	0
Coke-point	0	0	0	0	0
Wood-area	0	0	0	0	0
-point	0	0	0	0	0
Liquid Petroleum Gas-point	0	0	0	0	0
Bagasse-point	9,106	0	3,315	3,337	3,337
Other-point	78	339	57	2,003	209
Commercial-Institutional Fuel-area	142	853	526	27	40
-point	0	0	0	0	0
Anthracite Coal-area	0	0	0	0	0
-point	0	0	0	0	0
Bituminous Coal-area	0	0	0	0	0
-point	0	0	0	0	0
Lignite-point	0	0	0	0	0
Residual Oil-area	52	689	137	7	9
-point	0	0	0	0	0
Distillate Oil-area	85	164	342	17	23
-point	0	0	0	0	0
Natural Gas-area	4	0	47	3	8
-point	0	0	0	0	0
Wood-area	0	0	0	0	0
-point	0	0	0	0	0
Liquid Petroleum Gas-point	0	0	0	0	0
Miscellaneous-point	0	0	0	0	0
Internal Combustion-point	194	881	2,556	111	695
Electric Generation	183	881	2,556	111	695
Distillate Oil	104	623	608	0	1
Natural Gas	0	0	0	0	0
Diesel Fuel	79	257	1,948	111	694
Industrial Fuel	11	0	0	0	0
Distillate Oil	0	0	0	0	0
Natural Gas	0	0	0	0	0
Gasoline	0	0	0	0	0
Diesel Fuel	11	0	0	0	0

Emission categories	Pollutant, tons per year				
	Particulates	Sulfur oxides	Nitrogen oxides	Hydro-carbons	Carbon monoxide
Other	0	0	0	0	0
Commercial-Institutional	0	0	0	0	0
Diesel Fuel	0	0	0	0	0
Other	0	0	0	0	0
Engine-Testing	0	0	0	0	0
Aircraft	0	0	0	0	0
Other	0	0	0	0	0
Miscellaneous	0	0	0	0	0
INDUSTRIAL PROCESS-POINT	35,045	5,462	925	7,212	668
Chemical Manufacturing	30	833	0	0	0
Food/Agriculture	227	0	0	0	0
Primary Metal	12	0	0	0	450
Secondary Metals	8	0	0	0	9
Mineral Products	34,601	3,150	525	0	0
Petroleum Industry	90	1,141	343	430	0
Wood Products	0	0	0	0	0
Evaporation	0	0	0	4,778	0
Metal Fabrication	0	0	0	0	0
Leather Products	0	0	0	0	0
Textile Manufacturing	0	0	0	0	0
Inprocess Fuel	0	0	0	0	0
Other/Not Classified	78	339	57	2,003	209
SOLID WASTE DISPOSAL-AREA	749	45	263	1,451	4,135
-POINT	593	257	206	1,544	2,058
Government-point	593	257	206	1,544	2,058
Municipal Incineration	593	257	206	1,544	2,058
Open Burning	0	0	0	0	0
Other	0	0	0	0	0
Residential-area	659	39	230	1,284	3,662
On Site Incineration	51	1	2	144	432
Open Burning	608	38	228	1,140	3,230
Commercial-Institutional-area	46	3	17	85	239
-point	0	0	0	0	0
On Site Incineration-area	1	0	0	1	1
-point	0	0	0	0	0
Open Burning-area	45	3	17	84	238
-point	0	0	0	0	0
Apartment-point	0	0	0	0	0
Other-point	0	0	0	0	0
Industrial-area	44	3	17	83	234
-point	0	0	0	0	0
On Site Incineration-area	0	0	0	0	1
-point	0	0	0	0	0
Open Burning-area	44	3	16	83	234
-point	0	0	0	0	0
Auto Body Incineration-point	0	0	0	0	0
Other-point	0	0	0	0	0
Miscellaneous-point	0	0	0	0	0
TRANSPORTATION-AREA	4,005	2,759	26,610	44,471	239,844
Land Vehicles	2,675	1,013	23,684	36,331	230,062
Gasoline	2,312	629	19,526	35,830	228,291
Light Vehicles	2,101	545	17,306	29,439	186,211
Heavy Vehicles	183	69	1,899	5,486	31,823
Off Highway	28	15	321	905	10,257
Diesel Fuel	363	384	4,158	501	1,771
Heavy Vehicles	118	165	1,438	203	1,005
Off Highway	245	220	2,720	298	766
Rail	0	0	0	0	0
Aircraft	1,123	310	1,583	3,905	6,252
Military	1,014	194	487	2,359	2,532
Civil	33	7	30	145	830
Commercial	76	110	1,066	1,401	2,890
Vessels	207	1,436	1,343	1,293	3,529
Bituminous Coal	0	0	0	0	0
Diesel Fuel	121	151	1,127	296	394
Residual Oil	86	1,278	187	13	6
Gasoline	0	7	29	984	3,129
Gas Handling Evaporation Loss	0	0	0	2,942	0
MISCELLANEOUS-AREA	22,193	0	2,611	33,789	78,327
Forest Fires	0	0	0	0	0
Structural Fires	0	0	0	0	0
Slash Burning	22,193	0	2,611	26,109	78,327
Frost Control	0	0	0	0	0
Solvent Evaporation Loss	0	0	0	7,680	0

IDAHO

Emission categories	Pollutant, tons per year				
	Particulates	Sulfur oxides	Nitrogen oxides	Hydro-carbons	Carbon monoxide
GRAND TOTAL	**74,747**	**55,661**	**78,418**	**118,532**	**525,828**
-AREA	**39,771**	**6,753**	**61,096**	**111,378**	**474,359**
-POINT	**34,976**	**48,908**	**17,322**	**7,154**	**51,469**
FUEL COMBUSTION-AREA	2,772	3,752	6,144	1,847	5,602
-POINT	19,014	5,298	16,964	2,648	4,249
External Combustion-area	2,772	3,752	6,144	1,847	5,602
-point	19,014	5,298	16,964	2,648	4,249
Residential Fuel-area	2,169	2,354	1,438	1,678	5,144
Anthracite Coal	0	0	0	0	0
Bituminous Coal	943	896	142	943	4,246
Distillate Oil	491	1,414	589	147	245
Residual Oil	0	0	0	0	0
Natural Gas	54	3	435	44	109
Wood	680	41	272	544	544
Electric Generation-point	83	104	129	8	1,494
Anthracite Coal	0	0	0	0	0
Bituminous Coal	83	104	129	8	1,494
Lignite	0	0	0	0	0
Residual Oil	0	0	0	0	0
Distillate Oil	0	0	0	0	0
Natural Gas	0	0	0	0	0
Process Gas	0	0	0	0	0
Coke	0	0	0	0	0
Solid Waste/Coal	0	0	0	0	0
Other	0	0	0	0	0
Industrial Fuel-area	375	474	3,358	88	290
-point	18,931	5,194	16,835	2,641	2,755
Anthracite Coal-area	0	0	0	0	0
-point	0	0	0	0	0
Bituminous Coal-area	0	0	0	0	0
-point	4,522	2,225	1,446	26	83
Lignite-point	0	0	0	0	0
Residual Oil-area	0	0	0	0	0
-point	70	964	245	12	16
Distillate Oil-area	243	466	970	49	65
-point	18	50	76	4	4
Natural Gas-area	133	8	2,388	40	226
-point	40	2	2,128	11	64
Process Gas-area	0	0	0	0	0
-point	0	0	0	0	0
Coke-point	0	0	0	0	0
Wood-area	0	0	0	0	0
-point	13,878	1,941	12,939	2,588	2,588
Liquid Petroleum Gas-point	0	0	0	0	0
Bagasse-point	0	0	0	0	0
Other-point	403	12	0	0	0
Commercial-Institutional Fuel-area	227	924	1,348	80	168
-point	0	0	0	0	0
Anthracite Coal-area	0	0	0	0	0
-point	0	0	0	0	0
Bituminous Coal-area	0	0	0	0	0
-point	0	0	0	0	0
Lignite-point	0	0	0	0	0
Residual Oil-area	58	719	151	8	10
-point	0	0	0	0	0
Distillate Oil-area	105	202	420	21	28
-point	0	0	0	0	0
Natural Gas-area	65	4	777	52	129
-point	0	0	0	0	0
Wood-area	0	0	0	0	0
-point	0	0	0	0	0
Liquid Petroleum Gas-point	0	0	0	0	0
Miscellaneous-point	0	0	0	0	0
Internal Combustion-point	0	0	0	0	0
Electric Generation	0	0	0	0	0
Distillate Oil	0	0	0	0	0
Natural Gas	0	0	0	0	0
Diesel Fuel	0	0	0	0	0
Industrial Fuel	0	0	0	0	0
Distillate Oil	0	0	0	0	0
Natural Gas	0	0	0	0	0
Gasoline	0	0	0	0	0
Diesel Fuel	0	0	0	0	0

Emission categories	Pollutant, tons per year				
	Particulates	Sulfur oxides	Nitrogen oxides	Hydro-carbons	Carbon monoxide
Other	0	0	0	0	0
Commercial-Institutional	0	0	0	0	0
Diesel Fuel	0	0	0	0	0
Other	0	0	0	0	0
Engine-Testing	0	0	0	0	0
Aircraft	0	0	0	0	0
Other	0	0	0	0	0
Miscellaneous	0	0	0	0	0
INDUSTRIAL PROCESS-POINT	14,952	43,574	0	558	569
Chemical Manufacturing	6,946	18,500	0	0	0
Food/Agriculture	3,247	0	0	0	0
Primary Metal	1,213	25,058	0	0	0
Secondary Metals	0	0	0	0	0
Mineral Products	2,206	0	0	0	0
Petroleum Industry	0	0	0	0	0
Wood Products	620	12	0	0	569
Evaporation	0	0	0	558	0
Metal Fabrication	0	0	0	0	0
Leather Products	0	0	0	0	0
Textile Manufacturing	0	0	0	0	0
Inprocess Fuel	721	4	0	0	0
Other/Not Classified	0	0	0	0	0
SOLID WASTE DISPOSAL-AREA	2,344	149	879	4,383	12,415
-POINT	1,010	36	359	3,947	46,651
Government-point	0	0	0	0	0
Municipal Incineration	0	0	0	0	0
Open Burning	0	0	0	0	0
Other	0	0	0	0	0
Residential-area	2,334	146	875	4,377	12,402
On Site Incineration	0	0	0	0	0
Open Burning	2,334	146	875	4,377	12,402
Commercial-Institutional-area	10	3	4	6	14
-point	0	0	0	0	0
On Site Incineration-area	10	3	4	6	14
-point	0	0	0	0	0
Open Burning-area	0	0	0	0	0
-point	0	0	0	0	0
Apartment-point	0	0	0	0	0
Other-point	0	0	0	0	0
Industrial-area	0	0	0	0	0
-point	1,010	36	359	3,947	46,651
On Site Incineration-area	0	0	0	0	0
-point	1,010	36	359	3,947	46,651
Open Burning-area	0	0	0	0	0
-point	0	0	0	0	0
Auto Body Incineration-point	0	0	0	0	0
Other-point	0	0	0	0	0
Miscellaneous-point	0	0	0	0	0
TRANSPORTATION-AREA	5,643	2,852	50,665	69,809	354,143
Land Vehicles	4,934	2,678	49,942	60,154	342,609
Gasoline	3,814	1,105	35,743	57,979	337,766
Light Vehicles	2,999	778	26,532	36,707	199,728
Heavy Vehicles	683	259	7,709	17,037	90,025
Off Highway	132	69	1,502	4,235	48,013
Diesel Fuel	1,120	1,573	14,199	2,175	4,843
Heavy Vehicles	317	444	4,195	445	1,718
Off Highway	507	454	5,616	615	1,583
Rail	297	676	4,388	1,115	1,542
Aircraft	709	161	671	2,282	5,896
Military	539	103	259	1,255	1,347
Civil	150	30	136	665	3,801
Commercial	20	28	276	363	748
Vessels	0	12	52	1,774	5,639
Bituminous Coal	0	0	0	0	0
Diesel Fuel	0	0	0	0	0
Residual Oil	0	0	0	0	0
Gasoline	0	12	52	1,774	5,639
Gas Handling Evaporation Loss	0	0	0	5,599	0
MISCELLANEOUS-AREA	29,012	0	3,408	35,339	102,200
Forest Fires	0	0	0	0	0
Structural Fires	154	0	13	40	348
Slash Burning	28,858	0	3,395	33,951	101,852
Frost Control	0	0	0	0	0
Solvent Evaporation Loss	0	0	0	1,349	0

ILLINOIS

Emission categories	Pollutant, tons per year				
	Particulates	Sulfur oxides	Nitrogen oxides	Hydro-carbons	Carbon monoxide
GRAND TOTAL	931,059	2,618,468	1,311,572	1,831,465	3,814,291
-AREA	171,582	191,710	548,616	894,263	3,375,242
-POINT	759,477	2,426,758	762,957	937,203	439,049
FUEL COMBUSTION-AREA	86,234	161,844	90,160	16,723	63,296
-POINT	334,646	2,332,860	731,886	8,320	24,387
External Combustion-area	86,234	161,844	90,160	16,723	63,296
-point	334,586	2,332,472	730,528	8,020	24,307
Residential Fuel-area	16,239	68,141	25,542	13,786	56,823
Anthracite Coal	226	499	68	57	2,036
Bituminous Coal	10,698	56,916	1,605	10,698	48,143
Distillate Oil	2,442	10,553	2,931	733	1,221
Residual Oil	0	0	0	0	0
Natural Gas	2,604	156	20,831	2,083	5,208
Wood	269	16	108	215	215
Electric Generation-point	232,415	1,997,854	629,754	5,285	17,346
Anthracite Coal	0	0	0	0	0
Bituminous Coal	230,937	1,984,067	578,760	4,835	15,891
Lignite	0	0	0	0	0
Residual Oil	1,190	13,641	20,257	386	579
Distillate Oil	53	116	728	14	20
Natural Gas	236	30	30,009	51	856
Process Gas	0	0	0	0	0
Coke	0	0	0	0	0
Solid Waste/Coal	0	0	0	0	0
Other	0	0	0	0	0
Industrial Fuel-area	63,656	68,285	36,161	1,336	3,506
-point	88,653	315,345	93,703	2,288	5,888
Anthracite Coal-area	0	0	0	0	0
-point	0	0	0	0	0
Bituminous Coal-area	60,394	61,788	8,711	581	1,161
-point	84,096	271,709	57,983	1,444	3,754
Lignite-point	0	0	0	0	0
Residual Oil-area	0	0	0	0	0
-point	3,419	40,782	10,322	509	655
Distillate Oil-area	2,234	6,436	8,936	447	596
-point	235	1,237	937	47	61
Natural Gas-area	1,029	62	18,514	309	1,749
-point	738	44	23,394	259	1,274
Process Gas-area	0	0	0	0	0
-point	0	0	0	0	0
Coke-point	0	0	0	0	0
Wood-area	0	0	0	0	0
-point	7	1	4	1	3
Liquid Petroleum Gas-point	159	1,572	1,063	27	141
Bagasse-point	0	0	0	0	0
Other-point	0	0	0	0	0
Commercial-Institutional Fuel-area	6,338	25,418	28,457	1,601	2,967
-point	13,518	19,273	7,070	447	1,073
Anthracite Coal-area	0	0	0	0	0
-point	0	0	0	0	0
Bituminous Coal-area	0	0	0	0	0
-point	12,970	17,294	2,520	182	411
Lignite-point	0	0	0	0	0
Residual Oil-area	2,895	18,014	7,551	378	503
-point	106	919	279	13	17
Distillate Oil-area	2,551	7,350	10,206	510	680
-point	136	1,044	544	10	36
Natural Gas-area	892	54	10,700	713	1,783
-point	306	15	3,727	243	609
Wood-area	0	0	0	0	0
-point	0	0	0	0	0
Liquid Petroleum Gas-point	0	1	1	0	0
Miscellaneous-point	0	0	0	0	0
Internal Combustion-point	59	388	1,358	300	80
Electric Generation	59	387	1,353	300	79
Distillate Oil	54	365	1,079	148	34
Natural Gas	5	21	268	151	41
Diesel Fuel	0	1	7	1	4
Industrial Fuel	0	1	5	0	1
Distillate Oil	0	0	0	0	0
Natural Gas	0	0	0	0	0
Gasoline	0	0	0	0	0
Diesel Fuel	0	1	5	0	1

Emission categories	Pollutant, tons per year				
	Particulates	Sulfur oxides	Nitrogen oxides	Hydro-carbons	Carbon monoxide
Other	0	0	0	0	0
Commercial-Institutional	0	0	0	0	0
Diesel Fuel	0	0	0	0	0
Other	0	0	0	0	0
Engine-Testing	0	0	0	0	0
Aircraft	0	0	0	0	0
Other	0	0	0	0	0
Miscellaneous	0	0	0	0	0
INDUSTRIAL PROCESS-POINT	409,374	91,394	29,075	923,113	390,608
Chemical Manufacturing	6,544	16,388	13,808	13,023	2,859
Food/Agriculture	28,431	0	0	12,360	0
Primary Metal	11,983	894	69	2,462	37,439
Secondary Metals	9,571	4,975	53	176	72,240
Mineral Products	339,807	7,087	1,041	692	256
Petroleum Industry	11,354	60,329	14,014	22,417	277,797
Wood Products	83	0	0	0	0
Evaporation	103	0	0	868,505	0
Metal Fabrication	1,069	0	0	0	0
Leather Products	0	0	0	0	0
Textile Manufacturing	0	0	0	0	0
Inprocess Fuel	423	1,715	90	15	17
Other/Not Classified	6	6	0	3,462	0
SOLID WASTE DISPOSAL-AREA	38,211	3,819	10,716	71,882	206,027
-POINT	15,457	2,504	1,996	5,769	24,054
Government-point	10,730	1,209	968	1,849	15,686
Municipal Incineration	10,730	1,209	968	1,849	15,685
Open Burning	0	0	0	0	0
Other	0	0	0	0	0
Residential-area	24,839	1,060	5,701	56,428	164,807
On Site Incineration	10,512	164	329	29,566	88,698
Open Burning	14,326	895	5,372	26,862	76,109
Commercial-Institutional-area	5,076	1,241	1,904	4,901	12,654
-point	1,184	631	448	299	3,135
On Site Incineration-area	3,694	1,154	1,385	2,309	5,310
-point	124	630	324	46	49
Open Burning-area	1,382	86	518	2,592	7,344
-point	1,046	0	123	246	3,077
Apartment-point	13	0	1	7	9
Other-point	0	0	0	0	0
Industrial-area	8,296	1,519	3,111	10,553	28,566
-point	3,544	664	581	3,621	5,234
On Site Incineration-area	4,002	1,251	1,501	2,501	5,752
-point	3,537	664	580	3,621	5,234
Open Burning-area	4,294	268	1,610	8,052	22,814
-point	7	0	1	0	0
Auto Body Incineration-point	0	0	0	0	0
Other-point	0	0	0	0	0
Miscellaneous-point	0	0	0	0	0
TRANSPORTATION-AREA	47,137	26,046	447,740	606,755	3,105,919
Land Vehicles	44,698	23,769	436,213	526,659	3,043,401
Gasoline	37,036	10,083	330,513	507,292	3,002,003
Light Vehicles	34,172	8,859	298,497	426,597	2,382,558
Heavy Vehicles	1,910	724	21,132	50,008	271,542
Off Highway	955	500	10,883	30,687	347,903
Diesel Fuel	7,662	13,686	105,700	19,367	41,398
Heavy Vehicles	3,604	5,045	47,281	5,232	21,213
Off Highway	442	395	4,893	536	1,379
Rail	3,617	8,246	53,526	13,599	18,806
Aircraft	1,792	761	5,455	10,003	21,609
Military	1,225	234	588	2,850	3,059
Civil	234	47	212	1,038	5,933
Commercial	333	480	4,655	6,114	12,617
Vessels	647	1,517	6,072	13,728	40,908
Bituminous Coal	0	0	0	0	0
Diesel Fuel	601	752	5,612	1,473	1,964
Residual Oil	46	682	100	7	3
Gasoline	0	83	360	12,248	38,940
Gas Handling Evaporation Loss	0	0	0	56,366	0
MISCELLANEOUS-AREA	0	0	0	198,903	0
Forest Fires	0	0	0	0	0
Structural Fires	0	0	0	0	0
Slash Burning	0	0	0	0	0
Frost Control	0	0	0	0	0
Solvent Evaporation Loss	0	0	0	198,903	0

INDIANA

Emission categories	Pollutant, tons per year				
	Particulates	Sulfur oxides	Nitrogen oxides	Hydro-carbons	Carbon monoxide
GRAND TOTAL	598,559	2,262,141	1,242,209	603,771	6,298,642
-AREA	145,348	172,027	332,315	454,923	2,284,020
-POINT	453,210	2,090,114	909,895	148,848	4,014,621
FUEL COMBUSTION-AREA	100,433	152,382	50,741	7,092	23,450
-POINT	269,788	1,904,297	884,033	13,124	33,529
External Combustion-area	100,433	152,382	50,741	7,092	23,450
-point	269,662	1,904,096	856,444	12,016	33,132
Residential Fuel-area	6,946	28,909	11,116	5,005	18,073
Anthracite Coal	96	212	29	24	863
Bituminous Coal	3,037	19,040	456	3,037	13,665
Distillate Oil	2,213	9,562	2,655	664	1,106
Residual Oil	0	0	0	0	0
Natural Gas	965	58	7,722	772	1,930
Wood	635	38	254	508	508
Electric Generation-point	202,766	1,602,036	480,709	4,666	15,699
Anthracite Coal	0	0	0	0	0
Bituminous Coal	200,650	1,560,049	408,619	4,421	14,368
Lignite	0	0	0	0	0
Residual Oil	217	2,404	8,517	16	67
Distillate Oil	812	29,949	7,623	126	374
Natural Gas	432	2,426	30,379	54	684
Process Gas	221	2,403	8,540	16	70
Coke	0	0	0	0	0
Solid Waste/Coal	0	0	0	0	0
Other	434	4,806	17,030	32	135
Industrial Fuel-area	79,966	89,638	26,385	1,047	2,794
-point	59,121	276,399	372,067	7,104	16,955
Anthracite Coal-area	0	0	0	0	0
-point	0	0	0	0	0
Bituminous Coal-area	78,324	83,947	10,042	669	1,339
-point	24,678	80,708	15,867	727	1,733
Lignite-point	0	0	0	0	0
Residual Oil-area	341	4,007	889	44	59
-point	16,462	132,255	56,263	2,299	3,031
Distillate Oil-area	569	1,640	2,278	114	152
-point	9,725	32,936	48,781	1,943	2,814
Natural Gas-area	732	44	13,177	220	1,244
-point	2,929	3,104	199,812	1,424	7,802
Process Gas-area	0	0	0	0	0
-point	4,705	24,498	49,768	528	1,294
Coke-point	0	0	0	0	0
Wood-area	0	0	0	0	0
-point	489	88	543	158	253
Liquid Petroleum Gas-point	7	220	248	1	7
Bagasse-point	0	0	0	0	0
Other-point	126	2,590	786	25	21
Commercial-Institutional Fuel-area	13,521	33,834	13,240	1,040	2,583
-point	7,774	25,661	3,667	246	479
Anthracite Coal-area	0	0	0	0	0
-point	0	0	0	0	0
Bituminous Coal-area	11,155	26,798	1,966	427	1,539
-point	7,703	25,202	3,380	221	453
Lignite-point	0	0	0	0	0
Residual Oil-area	102	1,204	267	13	18
-point	44	379	109	6	8
Distillate Oil-area	2,019	5,817	8,077	404	538
-point	18	76	81	5	4
Natural Gas-area	244	15	2,930	195	488
-point	8	3	95	13	11
Wood-area	2	0	2	1	2
-point	0	0	0	0	0
Liquid Petroleum Gas-point	0	0	0	0	0
Miscellaneous-point	0	0	0	0	0
Internal Combustion-point	126	201	27,590	1,107	397
Electric Generation	5	43	25,316	0	0
Distillate Oil	2	43	6,369	0	0
Natural Gas	3	0	18,947	0	0
Diesel Fuel	0	0	0	0	0
Industrial Fuel	103	98	1,997	865	309
Distillate Oil	2	2	15	0	0
Natural Gas	0	0	563	752	0
Gasoline	0	0	0	0	0
Diesel Fuel	101	96	1,419	113	309

Emission categories	Pollutant, tons per year				
	Particulates	Sulfur oxides	Nitrogen oxides	Hydro-carbons	Carbon monoxide
Other	0	0	0	0	0
Commercial-Institutional	0	0	0	0	0
Diesel Fuel	0	0	0	0	0
Other	0	0	0	0	0
Engine-Testing	18	60	277	242	88
Aircraft	18	60	277	242	88
Other	0	0	0	0	0
Miscellaneous	0	0	0	0	0
INDUSTRIAL PROCESS-POINT	183,120	185,765	25,734	135,535	3,980,192
Chemical Manufacturing	2,946	7,756	218	3,217	6,198
Food/Agriculture	33,116	94	0	8,742	13
Primary Metal	47,578	64,254	1,616	25,874	3,663,290
Secondary Metals	8,701	2,163	333	127	64,533
Mineral Products	85,273	13,805	3,963	523	296
Petroleum Industry	1,737	37,690	6,523	723	210,865
Wood Products	934	1	8	308	1
Evaporation	178	0	31	94,279	2,724
Metal Fabrication	4	24	10	4	2
Leather Products	0	0	0	0	0
Textile Manufacturing	0	0	0	0	0
Inprocess Fuel	1,185	51,195	8,056	302	2,356
Other/Not Classified	1,469	8,785	4,978	1,436	29,913
SOLID WASTE DISPOSAL-AREA	15,626	1,411	4,106	30,711	88,509
-POINT	302	51	127	189	901
Government-point	225	27	37	33	36
Municipal Incineration	222	27	36	27	18
Open Burning	3	0	1	6	18
Other	0	0	0	0	0
Residential-area	11,327	469	2,494	26,021	76,117
On Site Incineration	5,102	80	159	14,349	43,047
Open Burning	6,225	389	2,334	11,672	33,069
Commercial-Institutional-area	2,488	607	933	2,409	6,224
-point	19	16	73	6	18
On Site Incineration-area	1,805	564	677	1,128	2,594
-point	19	16	73	6	18
Open Burning-area	683	43	256	1,281	3,630
-point	0	0	0	0	0
Apartment-point	0	0	0	0	0
Other-point	0	0	0	0	0
Industrial-area	1,811	336	679	2,282	6,168
-point	58	8	17	150	847
On Site Incineration-area	891	278	334	557	1,281
-point	48	8	16	142	811
Open Burning-area	920	57	345	1,725	4,888
-point	10	0	1	8	36
Auto Body Incineration-point	0	0	0	0	0
Other-point	0	0	0	0	0
Miscellaneous-point	0	0	0	0	0
TRANSPORTATION-AREA	29,290	18,234	277,468	388,733	2,172,061
Land Vehicles	28,486	15,404	274,647	348,852	2,154,159
Gasoline	22,071	6,144	193,640	336,361	2,116,599
Light Vehicles	19,381	5,025	164,378	257,776	1,546,345
Heavy Vehicles	1,996	757	21,353	56,285	317,439
Off Highway	694	363	7,909	22,300	252,816
Diesel Fuel	6,415	9,260	81,007	12,491	37,560
Heavy Vehicles	3,387	4,742	42,595	5,492	25,390
Off Highway	1,723	1,542	19,088	2,090	5,380
Rail	1,306	2,977	19,323	4,909	6,789
Aircraft	512	182	1,182	2,431	5,457
Military	366	70	176	852	914
Civil	79	16	72	352	2,010
Commercial	67	96	934	1,227	2,533
Vessels	291	2,647	1,639	4,114	12,446
Bituminous Coal	0	0	0	0	0
Diesel Fuel	125	156	1,167	306	408
Residual Oil	166	2,465	360	25	12
Gasoline	0	26	111	3,782	12,025
Gas Handling Evaporation Loss	0	0	0	33,337	0
MISCELLANEOUS-AREA	0	0	0	28,386	0
Forest Fires	0	0	0	0	0
Structural Fires	0	0	0	0	0
Slash Burning	0	0	0	0	0
Frost Control	0	0	0	0	0
Solvent Evaporation Loss	0	0	0	28,386	0

IOWA

Emission categories	Pollutant, tons per year				
	Particulates	Sulfur oxides	Nitrogen oxides	Hydro-carbons	Carbon monoxide
GRAND TOTAL	**391,112**	**323,551**	**326,216**	**353,844**	**1,848,567**
-AREA	48,735	26,068	184,819	292,049	1,536,013
-POINT	342,377	297,483	141,397	61,795	312,554
FUEL COMBUSTION-AREA	5,904	14,381	11,729	1,825	4,890
-POINT	149,274	259,375	121,010	2,496	4,731
External Combustion-area	5,904	14,381	11,729	1,825	4,890
-point	148,997	259,211	120,062	2,412	4,430
Residential Fuel-area	2,416	7,907	6,364	1,397	3,711
Anthracite Coal	0	0	0	0	0
Bituminous Coal	388	2,409	58	388	1,744
Distillate Oil	1,227	5,450	1,473	368	614
Residual Oil	0	0	0	0	0
Natural Gas	594	36	4,750	475	1,187
Wood	208	12	83	166	166
Electric Generation-point	125,300	237,744	80,392	1,622	2,972
Anthracite Coal	0	0	0	0	0
Bituminous Coal	116,990	227,454	56,352	1,237	2,396
Lignite	0	0	0	0	0
Residual Oil	1,833	2,512	714	12	21
Distillate Oil	1,857	2,029	756	27	22
Natural Gas	2,396	2,886	21,760	323	511
Process Gas	0	0	0	0	0
Coke	0	0	0	0	0
Solid Waste/Coal	0	0	0	0	0
Other	2,225	2,863	810	24	21
Industrial Fuel-area	0	0	0	0	0
-point	23,674	21,440	39,508	763	1,452
Anthracite Coal-area	0	0	0	0	0
-point	473	7	2	0	0
Bituminous Coal-area	0	0	0	0	0
-point	21,922	18,942	3,201	187	372
Residual Oil-area	0	0	0	0	0
-point	350	1,823	659	35	40
Distillate Oil-area	0	0	0	0	0
-point	255	634	542	63	27
Natural Gas-area	0	0	0	0	0
-point	625	35	34,746	457	968
Process Gas-area	0	0	0	0	0
-point	4	0	39	9	9
Coke-point	0	0	10	4	6
Wood-area	0	0	0	0	0
-point	0	0	0	0	0
Liquid Petroleum Gas-point	45	0	300	9	39
Bagasse-point	0	0	0	0	0
Other-point	0	0	9	0	0
Commercial-Institutional Fuel-area	3,488	6,474	5,365	428	1,179
-point	22	27	161	27	6
Anthracite Coal-area	0	0	0	0	0
-point	0	0	0	0	0
Bituminous Coal-area	3,069	6,403	473	103	370
-point	0	0	0	0	0
Lignite-point	0	0	0	0	0
Residual Oil-area	0	0	0	0	0
-point	0	0	0	0	0
Distillate Oil-area	16	47	63	3	4
-point	13	26	47	7	0
Natural Gas-area	402	24	4,829	322	805
-point	10	0	114	19	5
Wood-area	0	0	0	0	0
-point	0	0	0	0	0
Liquid Petroleum Gas-point	0	0	0	0	0
Miscellaneous-point	0	0	0	0	0
Internal Combustion-point	277	164	948	84	301
Electric Generation	126	157	836	79	270
Distillate Oil	18	136	170	13	28
Natural Gas	18	0	466	46	121
Diesel Fuel	7	19	201	20	122
Industrial Fuel	152	7	112	5	31
Distillate Oil	1	6	9	1	2
Natural Gas	0	0	0	0	0
Gasoline	0	0	1	1	22
Diesel Fuel	1	0	20	2	4

Emission categories	Pollutant, tons per year				
	Particulates	Sulfur oxides	Nitrogen oxides	Hydro-carbons	Carbon monoxide
Other	150	1	83	2	3
Commercial-Institutional	0	0	0	0	0
Diesel Fuel	0	0	0	0	0
Other	0	0	0	0	0
Engine-Testing	0	0	0	0	0
Aircraft	0	0	0	0	0
Other	0	0	0	0	0
Miscellaneous	0	0	0	0	0
INDUSTRIAL PROCESS-POINT	191,612	36,448	19,964	59,198	307,569
Chemical Manufacturing	14,735	8,307	392	20,679	5,824
Food/Agriculture	78,532	6	19	12	63
Primary Metal	43,576	0	0	0	0
Secondary Metals	5,315	77	16,960	66	42,189
Mineral Products	45,744	28,051	2,497	318	259,493
Petroleum Industry	0	0	0	0	0
Wood Products	87	0	26	6	0
Evaporation	996	0	0	38,104	0
Metal Fabrication	1	0	0	0	0
Leather Products	0	0	0	0	0
Textile Manufacturing	0	0	0	0	0
Inprocess Fuel	2,580	2	12	2	0
Other/Not Classified	45	5	59	13	0
SOLID WASTE DISPOSAL-AREA	24,548	2,226	9,205	42,566	119,682
-POINT	155	26	86	84	245
Government-point	3	0	0	0	0
Municipal Incineration	0	0	0	0	0
Open Burning	0	0	0	0	0
Other	3	0	0	0	0
Residential-area	21,774	1,361	8,165	40,826	115,672
On Site Incineration	0	0	0	0	0
Open Burning	21,774	1,361	8,165	40,826	115,672
Commercial-Institutional-area	1,989	620	746	1,250	2,881
-point	82	13	56	76	235
On Site Incineration-area	1,983	620	744	1,240	2,851
-point	82	13	56	76	235
Open Burning-area	6	0	2	11	30
-point	0	0	0	0	0
Apartment-point	0	0	0	0	0
Other-point	0	0	0	0	0
Industrial-area	785	245	294	491	1,129
-point	70	13	30	8	10
On Site Incineration-area	785	245	294	491	1,129
-point	19	7	5	3	10
Open Burning-area	0	0	0	0	0
-point	0	0	0	0	0
Auto Body Incineration-point	0	0	0	0	0
Other-point	51	5	26	5	0
Miscellaneous-point	0	0	0	0	0
TRANSPORTATION-AREA	17,408	9,459	163,781	240,806	1,408,361
Land Vehicles	16,356	9,114	161,764	210,759	1,378,085
Gasoline	12,587	3,697	113,986	203,553	1,356,757
Light Vehicles	10,164	2,635	87,188	132,326	775,406
Heavy Vehicles	1,427	541	15,444	39,213	218,393
Off Highway	996	521	11,354	32,015	362,957
Diesel Fuel	3,769	5,417	47,778	7,206	21,328
Heavy Vehicles	2,008	2,811	25,492	3,176	14,282
Off Highway	1,018	911	11,286	1,236	3,181
Rail	743	1,695	11,000	-2,795	3,865
Aircraft	1,052	315	1,883	4,785	15,737
Military	526	101	253	1,225	1,315
Civil	438	87	395	1,938	11,076
Commercial	88	127	1,235	1,622	3,347
Vessels	0	31	135	4,573	14,540
Bituminous Coal	0	0	0	0	0
Diesel Fuel	0	0	0	0	0
Residual Oil	0	0	0	0	0
Gasoline	0	31	135	4,573	14,540
Gas Handling Evaporation Loss	0	0	0	20,689	0
MISCELLANEOUS-AREA	876	1	103	6,852	3,080
Forest Fires	161	0	38	228	1,330
Structural Fires	606	1	53	157	1,370
Slash Burning	108	0	13	127	380
Frost Control	0	0	0	0	0
Solvent Evaporation Loss	0	0	0	6,340	0

KANSAS

Emission categories	Pollutant, tons per year				
	Particulates	Sulfur oxides	Nitrogen oxides	Hydro-carbons	Carbon monoxide
GRAND TOTAL	213,966	96,906	302,745	336,756	1,217,824
-AREA	49,631	35,019	184,100	262,870	1,070,960
-POINT	164,335	61,887	118,645	73,887	146,864
FUEL COMBUSTION-AREA	9,558	23,472	24,601	1,869	6,462
-POINT	7,623	26,720	107,063	743	3,842
External Combustion-area	9,558	23,472	24,601	1,869	6,462
-point	7,485	26,411	103,166	611	3,296
Residential Fuel-area	1,311	5,935	4,791	1,156	4,227
Anthracite Coal	0	0	0	0	0
Bituminous Coal	676	5,655	101	676	3,044
Distillate Oil	57	246	68	17	28
Residual Oil	0	0	0	0	0
Natural Gas	578	35	4,621	462	1,155
Wood	0	0	0	0	0
Electric Generation-point	6,555	24,618	88,961	494	2,760
Anthracite Coal	0	0	0	0	0
Bituminous Coal	5,838	23,277	38,150	391	1,304
Lignite	0	0	0	0	0
Residual Oil	45	1,278	954	18	27
Distillate Oil	7	17	46	1	1
Natural Gas	666	45	49,811	84	1,427
Process Gas	0	0	0	0	0
Coke	0	0	0	0	0
Solid Waste/Coal	0	0	0	0	0
Other	0	0	0	0	0
Industrial Fuel-area	6,375	13,524	14,892	365	1,349
-point	904	1,563	14,098	110	523
Anthracite Coal-area	0	0	0	0	0
-point	0	0	0	0	0
Bituminous Coal-area	4,825	5,492	493	33	66
-point	465	303	41	1	2
Lignite-point	0	0	0	0	0
Residual Oil-area	607	7,136	1,584	79	106
-point	116	1,022	309	15	21
Distillate Oil-area	298	858	1,191	60	79
-point	34	217	138	7	9
Natural Gas-area	646	39	11,625	194	1,098
-point	289	17	13,606	87	491
Process Gas-area	0	0	0	0	0
-point	0	0	0	0	0
Coke-point	0	0	0	0	0
Wood-area	0	0	0	0	0
-point	0	0	0	0	0
Liquid Petroleum Gas-point	1	3	4	0	1
Bagasse-point	0	0	0	0	0
Other-point	0	0	0	0	0
Commercial-Institutional Fuel-area	1,872	4,012	4,918	348	886
-point	25	231	107	7	12
Anthracite Coal-area	0	0	0	0	0
-point	0	0	0	0	0
Bituminous Coal-area	1,387	3,538	195	42	152
-point	0	0	15	1	2
Lignite-point	0	0	0	0	0
Residual Oil-area	7	81	18	1	1
-point	19	205	49	2	3
Distillate Oil-area	129	372	516	26	34
-point	4	25	15	1	1
Natural Gas-area	349	21	4,189	279	698
-point	3	0	28	2	6
Wood-area	0	0	0	0	0
-point	0	0	0	0	0
Liquid Petroleum Gas-point	0	0	0	0	0
Miscellaneous-point	0	0	0	0	0
Internal Combustion-point	138	309	3,897	132	546
Electric Generation	101	309	2,158	113	531
Distillate Oil	51	245	693	17	47
Natural Gas	19	0	674	18	48
Diesel Fuel	31	64	790	79	436
Industrial Fuel	38	0	1,739	19	15
Distillate Oil	0	0	0	0	0
Natural Gas	38	0	1,735	19	14
Gasoline	0	0	0	0	0
Diesel Fuel	0	0	4	0	1

Emission categories	Pollutant, tons per year				
	Particulates	Sulfur oxides	Nitrogen oxides	Hydro-carbons	Carbon monoxide
Other	0	0	0	0	0
Commercial-Institutional	0	0	0	0	0
Diesel Fuel	0	0	0	0	0
Other	0	0	0	0	0
Engine-Testing	0	0	0	0	0
Aircraft	0	0	0	0	0
Other	0	0	0	0	0
Miscellaneous	0	0	0	0	0
INDUSTRIAL PROCESS-POINT	156,647	35,165	11,572	73,094	142,465
Chemical Manufacturing	583	5,309	0	21,863	135,066
Food/Agriculture	109,155	0	11	7	1
Primary Metal	0	0	0	0	0
Secondary Metals	399	20	0	0	3,488
Mineral Products	44,072	19,303	4,430	1	1
Petroleum Industry	2,232	10,534	7,129	25,353	3,908
Wood Products	0	0	0	0	0
Evaporation	0	0	0	25,868	0
Metal Fabrication	0	0	0	0	0
Leather Products	0	0	0	0	0
Textile Manufacturing	0	0	0	0	0
Inprocess Fuel	206	0	2	4	0
Other/Not Classified	0	0	0	0	0
SOLID WASTE DISPOSAL-AREA	16,499	980	4,756	34,118	98,426
-POINT	65	2	10	50	557
Government-point	0	0	0	0	0
Municipal Incineration	0	0	0	0	0
Open Burning	0	0	0	0	0
Other	0	0	0	0	0
Residential-area	14,880	735	4,149	31,801	92,054
On Site Incineration	4,161	65	130	11,704	35,112
Open Burning	10,718	670	4,019	20,097	56,942
Commercial-Institutional-area	1,348	203	505	1,934	5,320
-point	0	1	1	1	3
On Site Incineration-area	475	149	178	297	683
-point	0	1	1	1	3
Open Burning-area	873	55	327	1,637	4,637
-point	0	0	0	0	0
Apartment-point	0	0	0	0	0
Other-point	0	0	0	0	0
Industrial-area	271	42	102	383	1,053
-point	65	1	9	49	554
On Site Incineration-area	100	31	37	62	143
-point	25	1	4	38	447
Open Burning-area	171	11	64	321	910
-point	36	0	4	10	107
Auto Body Incineration-point	0	0	0	0	0
Other-point	4	0	0	0	0
Miscellaneous-point	0	0	0	0	0
TRANSPORTATION-AREA	14,479	10,568	153,673	174,335	933,971
Land Vehicles	14,244	10,449	152,927	157,114	921,567
Gasoline	9,527	2,791	90,256	146,131	899,504
Light Vehicles	7,567	1,962	67,944	92,246	496,052
Heavy Vehicles	1,359	515	15,458	34,559	184,344
Off Highway	601	315	6,854	19,326	219,108
Diesel Fuel	4,717	7,658	62,671	10,983	22,063
Heavy Vehicles	1,424	1,994	18,884	1,992	7,704
Off Highway	1,332	1,192	14,756	1,616	4,159
Rail	1,962	4,472	29,030	7,375	10,200
Aircraft	215	73	470	1,032	2,808
Military	129	25	62	301	323
Civil	60	12	55	268	1,529
Commercial	25	36	353	463	956
Vessels	20	45	276	3,047	9,597
Bituminous Coal	0	0	0	0	0
Diesel Fuel	20	25	188	49	66
Residual Oil	0	0	0	0	0
Gasoline	0	20	88	2,998	9,531
Gas Handling Evaporation Loss	0	0	0	13,142	0
MISCELLANEOUS-AREA	9,095	0	1,070	52,548	32,100
Forest Fires	0	0	0	0	0
Structural Fires	0	0	0	0	0
Slash Burning	9,095	0	1,070	10,700	32,100
Frost Control	0	0	0	0	0
Solvent Evaporation Loss	0	0	0	41,848	0

KENTUCKY

Emission categories	Pollutant, tons per year				
	Particulates	Sulfur oxides	Nitrogen oxides	Hydro-carbons	Carbon monoxide
GRAND TOTAL	540,810	1,626,535	534,767	352,382	1,387,632
-AREA	62,511	60,298	180,520	235,828	1,196,942
-POINT	478,299	1,566,238	354,247	116,555	190,690
FUEL COMBUSTION-AREA	38,822	51,159	29,488	6,861	20,953
-POINT	189,700	1,555,950	351,080	5,096	14,624
External Combustion-area	38,822	51,159	29,488	6,861	20,953
-point	189,671	1,555,949	350,201	4,479	13,472
Residential Fuel-area	6,443	10,396	5,805	5,611	17,626
Anthracite Coal	0	0	0	0	0
Bituminous Coal	3,243	8,564	486	3,243	14,592
Distillate Oil	385	1,662	462	115	192
Residual Oil	0	0	0	0	0
Natural Gas	491	29	3,927	393	982
Wood	2,325	139	930	1,860	1,860
Electric Generation-point	168,971	1,481,038	330,474	3,615	11,800
Anthracite Coal	0	0	0	0	0
Bituminous Coal	168,849	1,479,415	319,186	3,441	11,469
Lignite	0	0	0	0	0
Residual Oil	111	1,586	8,821	168	252
Distillate Oil	9	34	124	2	4
Natural Gas	2	3	2,343	4	75
Process Gas	0	0	0	0	0
Coke	0	0	0	0	0
Solid Waste/Coal	0	0	0	0	0
Other	0	0	0	0	0
Industrial Fuel-area	24,291	24,592	13,661	466	1,376
-point	19,810	73,377	18,603	781	1,474
Anthracite Coal-area	0	0	0	0	0
-point	0	0	0	0	0
Bituminous Coal-area	23,242	19,675	3,526	235	470
-point	17,110	68,497	10,954	518	1,091
Lignite-point	0	0	0	0	0
Residual Oil-area	360	4,227	938	47	63
-point	202	2,050	664	37	39
Distillate Oil-area	230	662	920	46	61
-point	197	338	793	40	53
Natural Gas-area	460	28	8,276	138	782
-point	154	388	5,305	40	211
Process Gas-area	0	0	0	0	0
-point	1,282	1,681	475	78	16
Coke-point	0	0	0	0	0
Wood-area	0	0	0	0	0
-point	839	47	324	65	65
Liquid Petroleum Gas-point	0	0	1	0	0
Bagasse-point	0	0	0	0	0
Other-point	25	377	87	3	0
Commercial-Institutional Fuel-area	8,087	16,171	10,022	784	1,951
-point	891	1,534	1,124	83	198
Anthracite Coal-area	0	0	0	0	0
-point	0	0	0	0	0
Bituminous Coal-area	6,338	11,219	1,444	314	1,130
-point	824	1,462	522	49	124
Lignite-point	0	0	0	0	0
Residual Oil-area	56	662	147	7	10
-point	0	0	0	0	0
Distillate Oil-area	1,485	4,278	5,940	297	396
-point	28	68	111	6	7
Natural Gas-area	208	12	2,491	166	415
-point	27	2	478	22	55
Wood-area	0	0	0	0	0
-point	12	2	12	6	12
Liquid Petroleum Gas-point	0	0	0	0	0
Miscellaneous-point	0	0	0	0	0
Internal Combustion-point	29	1	879	617	1,151
Electric Generation	1	0	38	4	11
Distillate Oil	0	0	0	0	0
Natural Gas	1	0	38	4	11
Diesel Fuel	0	0	0	0	0
Industrial Fuel	28	1	841	614	1,141
Distillate Oil	0	1	4	0	1
Natural Gas	24	0	694	418	383
Gasoline	0	0	49	70	665
Diesel Fuel	0	0	0	0	0

Emission categories	Pollutant, tons per year				
	Particulates	Sulfur oxides	Nitrogen oxides	Hydro- carbons	Carbon monoxide
Other....................	4	0	94	126	92
Commercial-Institutional....................	0	0	0	0	0
Diesel Fuel	0	0	0	0	0
Other....................	0	0	0	0	0
Engine-Testing....................	0	0	0	0	0
Aircraft....................	0	0	0	0	0
Other....................	0	0	0	0	0
Miscellaneous....................	0	0	0	0	0
INDUSTRIAL PROCESS-POINT	287,084	10,161	2,781	110,771	170,952
Chemical Manufacturing....................	8,609	0	0	44,968	1,194
Food/Agriculture....................	5,558	0	0	21,180	2
Primary Metal....................	41,689	0	0	3	124,130
Secondary Metals....................	2,851	64	82	50	25,331
Mineral Products....................	222,682	286	42	5	3
Petroleum Industry....................	1,908	7,734	2,525	20,142	7,296
Wood Products....................	2,256	2,034	0	89	12,988
Evaporation	170	0	4	23,122	0
Metal Fabrication....................	53	0	0	601	0
Leather Products....................	0	0	0	0	0
Textile Manufacturing....................	0	0	0	0	0
Inprocess Fuel....................	1,199	1	111	224	9
Other/Not Classified	110	42	16	388	0
SOLID WASTE DISPOSAL-AREA	4,237	439	1,526	7,204	20,254
-POINT....................	1,515	127	385	688	5,114
Government-point....................	0	0	0	0	0
Municipal Incineration....................	0	0	0	0	0
Open Burning....................	0	0	0	0	0
Other....................	0	0	0	0	0
Residential-area....................	2,913	173	1,029	5,634	16,048
On Site Incineration....................	184	3	6	517	1,551
Open Burning....................	2,729	171	1,023	5,117	14,497
Commercial-Institutional-area....................	569	110	213	695	1,869
-point....................	9	2	3	3	9
On Site Incineration-area....................	298	93	112	186	428
-point....................	9	2	3	3	9
Open Burning-area....................	271	17	102	509	1,441
-point....................	0	0	0	0	0
Apartment-point....................	0	0	0	0	0
Other-point....................	0	0	0	0	0
Industrial-area....................	755	155	283	876	2,337
-point....................	1,505	125	383	685	5,105
On Site Incineration-area....................	432	135	162	270	620
-point....................	1,465	125	381	675	5,053
Open Burning-area....................	323	20	121	606	1,717
-point....................	1	0	0	0	2
Auto Body Incineration-point	20	0	1	0	25
Other-point....................	20	0	1	5	25
Miscellaneous-point....................	0	0	0	0	0
TRANSPORTATION-AREA....................	16,406	8,698	148,905	204,285	1,135,260
Land Vehicles....................	14,568	7,669	142,090	179,561	1,119,417
Gasoline....................	11,574	3,270	103,704	173,765	1,102,453
Light Vehicles....................	10,031	2,601	86,600	129,002	745,427
Heavy Vehicles....................	956	362	10,417	25,908	143,255
Off Highway....................	586	307	6,687	18,856	213,771
Diesel Fuel....................	2,994	4,399	38,386	5,796	16,964
Heavy Vehicles....................	1,698	2,377	21,709	2,638	11,623
Off Highway....................	674	603	7,467	817	2,104
Rail....................	622	1,419	9,211	2,340	3,236
Aircraft....................	1,311	360	1,853	4,688	8,989
Military....................	1,108	212	532	2,579	2,768
Civil....................	116	23	104	512	2,924
Commercial....................	87	125	1,216	1,598	3,296
Vessels....................	526	669	4,961	2,905	6,855
Bituminous Coal	0	0	0	0	0
Diesel Fuel....................	526	658	4,913	1,290	1,720
Residual Oil....................	0	0	0	0	0
Gasoline....................	0	11	48	1,615	5,136
Gas Handling Evaporation Loss....................	0	0	0	17,130	0
MISCELLANEOUS-AREA	3,047	1	602	17,478	20,474
Forest Fires....................	2,253	0	530	3,181	18,554
Structural Fires....................	696	1	61	180	1,572
Slash Burning....................	99	0	12	116	348
Frost Control....................	0	0	0	0	0
Solvent Evaporation Loss....................	0	0	0	14,001	0

LOUISIANA

Emission categories	Pollutant, tons per year				
	Particulates	Sulfur oxides	Nitrogen oxides	Hydro-carbons	Carbon monoxide
GRAND TOTAL	446,447	538,818	748,774	1,228,769	4,177,99
–AREA	62,507	22,372	247,720	335,610	1,650,30
–POINT	383,940	516,446	501,054	893,159	2,527,69
FUEL COMBUSTION–AREA	4,482	6,001	41,021	1,873	5,05
–POINT	63,544	298,013	419,674	11,828	67,68
External Combustion–area	4,482	6,001	41,021	1,873	5,05
–point	63,259	297,985	409,957	9,799	65,63
Residential Fuel–area	1,065	84	3,900	845	1,39
Anthracite Coal	0	0	0	0	
Bituminous Coal	0	0	0	0	
Distillate Oil	14	21	17	4	
Residual Oil	0	0	0	0	
Natural Gas	456	27	3,645	364	91
Wood	595	36	238	476	47
Electric Generation–point	15,886	158,580	150,478	691	2,13
Anthracite Coal	0	0	0	0	
Bituminous Coal	0	0	0	0	
Lignite	0	0	0	0	
Residual Oil	12,905	125,482	54,639	151	22
Distillate Oil	0	2,082	1	0	
Natural Gas	2,707	30,333	91,527	534	1,81
Process Gas	86	621	4,311	6	9
Coke	0	0	0	0	
Solid Waste/Coal	0	0	0	0	
Other	187	62	0	0	
Industrial Fuel–area	2,445	1,924	30,701	634	2,79
–point	47,373	139,405	257,944	9,108	63,50
Anthracite Coal–area	0	0	0	0	
–point	1,343	55,581	34,549	0	
Bituminous Coal–area	0	0	0	0	
–point	0	0	0	0	
Lignite–point	0	0	0	0	
Residual Oil–area	76	1,002	199	10	1
–point	8,625	29,161	12,236	309	50
Distillate Oil–area	867	832	3,466	173	23
–point	4,320	34,743	42,821	999	14
Natural Gas–area	1,502	90	27,036	451	2,55
–point	10,956	10,055	160,432	5,506	33,52
Process Gas–area	0	0	0	0	
–point	210	3,889	1,606	711	10
Coke–point	0	0	0	0	
Wood–area	0	0	0	0	
–point	15,891	3,723	4,601	841	14,93
Liquid Petroleum Gas–point	0	0	0	0	
Bagasse–point	4,914	3	736	729	1,88
Other–point	1,114	2,249	962	14	12,39
Commercial–Institutional Fuel–area	972	3,993	6,420	394	8
–point	0	0	1,535	0	
Anthracite Coal–area	0	0	0	0	
–point	0	0	0	0	
Bituminous Coal–area	0	0	0	0	
–point	0	0	0	0	
Lignite–point	0	0	0	0	
Residual Oil–area	278	3,655	726	36	4
–point	0	0	0	0	
Distillate Oil–area	329	316	1,317	66	8
–point	0	0	0	0	
Natural Gas–area	365	22	4,378	292	73
–point	0	0	1,535	0	
Wood–area	0	0	0	0	
–point	0	0	0	0	
Liquid Petroleum Gas–point	0	0	0	0	
Miscellaneous–point	0	0	0	0	
Internal Combustion–point	285	28	9,717	2,029	2,04
Electric Generation	47	1	1,760	183	4
Distillate Oil	0	0	0	0	
Natural Gas	47	1	1,760	183	4
Diesel Fuel	0	0	0	0	
Industrial Fuel	234	27	7,903	1,833	1,6
Distillate Oil	0	0	0	0	
Natural Gas	232	25	7,633	1,814	1,5
Gasoline	0	0	0	0	
Diesel Fuel					

Emission categories	Pollutant, tons per year				
	Particulates	Sulfur oxides	Nitrogen oxides	Hydro-carbons	Carbon monoxide
Other	2	2	270	19	87
Commercial-Institutional	0	0	0	0	0
Diesel Fuel	0	0	0	0	0
Other	0	0	0	0	0
Engine-Testing	4	0	54	12	0
Aircraft	0	0	0	0	0
Other	4	0	54	12	0
Miscellaneous	0	0	0	0	0
INDUSTRIAL PROCESS-POINT	314,772	212,072	80,331	876,660	2,415,648
Chemical Manufacturing	16,374	113,253	17,073	585,926	1,791,130
Food/Agriculture	3,208	63	50	17	57
Primary Metal	178,386	4,056	1,259	6,000	8
Secondary Metals	1,313	1,373	2,622	28	40
Mineral Products	47,441	9,870	6,658	29	2,846
Petroleum Industry	19,138	75,209	48,729	212,500	587,305
Wood Products	45,780	5,932	1,237	144	32,550
Evaporation	8	0	138	69,752	975
Metal Fabrication	0	0	0	0	0
Leather Products	0	0	0	0	0
Textile Manufacturing	0	0	0	0	0
Inprocess Fuel	3,124	2,316	2,555	2,264	739
Other/Not Classified	2	0	12	0	0
SOLID WASTE DISPOSAL-AREA	11,604	725	4,351	21,758	61,646
-POINT	5,624	6,360	1,049	4,671	44,363
Government-point	961	200	160	120	2,803
Municipal Incineration	961	200	160	120	2,803
Open Burning	0	0	0	0	0
Other	0	0	0	0	0
Residential-area	11,604	725	4,351	21,758	61,646
On Site Incineration	0	0	0	0	0
Open Burning	11,604	725	4,351	21,758	61,646
Commercial-Institutional-area	0	0	0	0	0
-point	33	5	32	172	1
On Site Incineration-area	0	0	0	0	0
-point	3	4	22	0	0
Open Burning-area	0	0	0	0	0
-point	0	0	0	0	0
Apartment-point	0	0	0	0	0
Other-point	30	1	10	172	1
Industrial-area	0	0	0	0	0
-point	4,630	6,155	857	4,379	41,559
On Site Incineration-area	0	0	0	0	0
-point	3,952	3,948	550	3,712	39,559
Open Burning-area	0	0	0	0	0
-point	424	14	124	545	1,598
Auto Body Incineration-point	0	0	0	0	0
Other-point	254	2,193	183	122	401
Miscellaneous-point	0	0	0	0	0
TRANSPORTATION-AREA	24,275	15,645	197,205	264,331	1,403,977
Land Vehicles	17,509	8,955	167,205	216,913	1,346,445
Gasoline	13,738	3,830	120,529	209,865	1,326,846
Light Vehicles	12,050	3,124	102,157	160,419	963,229
Heavy Vehicles	1,226	464	13,102	34,587	195,163
Off Highway	462	242	5,270	14,859	168,455
Diesel Fuel	3,771	5,125	46,676	7,048	19,599
Heavy Vehicles	1,434	2,008	18,034	2,327	10,765
Off Highway	1,595	1,428	17,679	1,936	4,983
Rail	741	1,689	10,963	2,785	3,852
Aircraft	3,792	833	3,036	10,463	15,331
Military	3,583	684	1,721	8,336	8,948
Civil	123	25	111	546	3,123
Commercial	86	124	1,203	1,580	3,260
Vessels	2,974	5,857	26,965	17,306	42,201
Bituminous Coal	0	0	0	0	0
Diesel Fuel	2,821	3,526	26,329	6,911	9,215
Residual Oil	153	2,261	330	23	11
Gasoline	0	70	305	10,371	32,974
Gas Handling Evaporation Loss	0	0	0	19,650	0
MISCELLANEOUS-AREA	22,147	1	5,142	47,648	179,622
Forest Fires	21,684	0	5,102	30,613	178,578
Structural Fires	462	1	40	120	1,044
Slash Burning	0	0	0	0	0
Frost Control	0	0	0	0	0
Solvent Evaporation Loss	0	0	0	16,915	0

MAINE

Emission categories	Pollutant, tons per year				
	Particulates	Sulfur oxides	Nitrogen oxides	Hydro-carbons	Carbon monoxide
GRAND TOTAL	57,243	151,204	88,711	125,390	413,944
–AREA	12,824	22,933	54,246	76,643	331,802
–POINT	44,419	128,271	34,466	48,747	82,143
FUEL COMBUSTION–AREA	4,163	20,257	5,702	1,629	2,322
–POINT	10,113	115,454	31,627	2,286	2,955
External Combustion–area	4,163	20,257	5,702	1,629	2,322
–point	10,093	115,404	31,195	2,245	2,739
Residential Fuel–area	3,006	5,372	2,719	1,482	2,101
Anthracite Coal	28	72	8	7	253
Bituminous Coal	0	0	0	0	0
Distillate Oil	1,815	5,230	2,178	545	908
Residual Oil	0	0	0	0	0
Natural Gas	9	1	71	7	18
Wood	1,154	69	462	923	923
Electric Generation–point	296	37,461	11,585	221	331
Anthracite Coal	0	0	0	0	0
Bituminous Coal	0	0	0	0	0
Lignite	0	0	0	0	0
Residual Oil	295	37,459	11,575	220	331
Distillate Oil	1	3	10	0	0
Natural Gas	0	0	0	0	0
Process Gas	0	0	0	0	0
Coke	0	0	0	0	0
Solid Waste/Coal	0	0	0	0	0
Other	0	0	0	0	0
Industrial Fuel–area	38	25	91	2	9
–point	9,439	74,133	18,602	1,983	2,343
Anthracite Coal–area	14	19	11	0	1
–point	0	0	0	0	0
Bituminous Coal–area	19	6	4	0	0
–point	0	0	0	0	0
Lignite–point	0	0	0	0	0
Residual Oil–area	0	0	0	0	0
–point	3,990	73,094	'2,166	608	811
Distillate Oil–area	0	0	0	0	0
–point	11	81	44	2	3
Natural Gas–area	4	0	76	1	7
–point	0	0	1	0	0
Process Gas–area	0	0	0	0	0
–point	0	0	0	0	0
Coke–point	0	0	0	0	0
Wood–area	0	0	0	0	0
–point	5,438	959	6,391	1,372	1,529
Liquid Petroleum Gas–point	0	0	0	0	0
Bagasse–point	0	0	0	0	0
Other–point	0	0	0	0	0
Commercial-Institutional Fuel–area	1,119	14,860	2,892	146	211
–point	358	3,809	1,008	41	65
Anthracite Coal–area	33	44	16	0	10
–point	0	0	0	0	0
Bituminous Coal–area	9	6	2	0	2
–point	125	519	189	0	11
Lignite–point	0	0	0	0	0
Residual Oil–area	1,071	14,810	2,794	140	186
–point	219	3,040	568	28	38
Distillate Oil–area	0	0	0	0	0
–point	14	251	249	12	17
Natural Gas–area	7	0	80	5	13
–point	0	0	1	0	0
Wood–area	0	0	0	0	0
–point	0	0	0	0	0
Liquid Petroleum Gas–point	0	0	0	0	0
Miscellaneous–point	0	0	0	0	0
Internal Combustion–point	20	50	432	41	216
Electric Generation	20	50	432	41	216
Distillate Oil	9	49	124	10	28
Natural Gas	0	0	0	0	0
Diesel Fuel	11	1	308	31	187
Industrial Fuel	0	0	0	0	0
Distillate Oil	0	0	0	0	0
Natural Gas	0	0	0	0	0
Gasoline	0	0	0	0	0
Diesel Fuel	0	0	0	0	0

Emission categories	Pollutant, tons per year				
	Particulates	Sulfur oxides	Nitrogen oxides	Hydro-carbons	Carbon monoxide
Other	0	0	0	0	0
Commercial-Institutional	0	0	0	0	0
Diesel Fuel	0	0	0	0	0
Other	0	0	0	0	0
Engine-Testing	0	0	0	0	0
Aircraft	0	0	0	0	0
Other	0	0	0	0	0
Miscellaneous	0	0	0	0	0
INDUSTRIAL PROCESS-POINT	29,139	12,486	1,052	37,292	47,448
Chemical Manufacturing	0	1,703	0	4,673	0
Food/Agriculture	139	0	0	0	0
Primary Metal	0	0	0	0	0
Secondary Metals	13	0	0	0	100
Mineral Products	11,109	5,450	1,012	2	0
Petroleum Industry	0	0	0	0	0
Wood Products	17,863	5,274	12	139	47,346
Evaporation	2	0	0	31,959	0
Metal Fabrication	0	0	0	0	0
Leather Products	2	26	4	468	1
Textile Manufacturing	1	0	0	51	0
Inprocess Fuel	11	34	16	1	2
Other/Not Classified	0	0	9	0	0
SOLID WASTE DISPOSAL-AREA	2,870	218	722	5,910	17,110
-POINT	5,167	330	1,787	9,169	31,741
Government-point	2,153	153	752	3,708	10,451
Municipal Incineration	71	12	9	71	94
Open Burning	1,778	111	667	3,334	9,445
Other	304	30	76	304	912
Residential-area	2,324	97	518	5,324	15,566
On Site Incineration	1,030	16	32	2,897	8,690
Open Burning	1,294	81	485	2,427	6,877
Commercial-Institutional-area	419	104	157	397	1,021
-point	15	7	10	9	23
On Site Incineration-area	311	97	117	195	447
-point	10	7	8	9	22
Open Burning-area	108	7	40	203	574
-point	0	0	0	0	0
Apartment-point	1	0	0	0	0
Other-point	3	0	2	0	0
Industrial-area	126	17	47	189	523
-point	3,000	170	1,025	5,452	21,266
On Site Incineration-area	38	12	14	24	55
-point	424	10	64	652	7,626
Open Burning-area	88	5	33	165	468
-point	2,575	160	961	4,800	13,640
Auto Body Incineration-point	0	0	0	0	0
Other-point	0	0	0	0	0
Miscellaneous-point	0	0	0	0	0
TRANSPORTATION-AREA	5,478	2,457	47,755	66,157	310,108
Land Vehicles	4,776	2,078	46,951	56,162	300,132
Gasoline	4,109	1,125	38,202	55,011	297,151
Light Vehicles	3,666	950	33,130	43,698	228,433
Heavy Vehicles	395	150	4,531	9,789	51,437
Off Highway	47	25	541	1,524	17,281
Diesel Fuel	667	953	8,749	1,151	2,981
Heavy Vehicles	389	545	5,243	520	1,874
Off Highway	162	145	1,799	197	507
Rail	115	263	1,708	434	600
Aircraft	661	137	463	1,845	3,855
Military	569	109	273	1,324	1,421
Civil	84	17	76	372	2,125
Commercial	8	12	114	149	308
Vessels	41	242	341	1,966	6,122
Bituminous Coal	0	0	0	0	0
Diesel Fuel	27	34	256	67	90
Residual Oil	13	194	28	2	1
Gasoline	0	13	56	1,897	6,031
Gas Handling Evaporation Loss	0	0	0	6,183	0
MISCELLANEOUS-AREA	313	0	66	2,947	2,261
Forest Fires	260	0	61	367	2,140
Structural Fires	54	0	5	14	121
Slash Burning	0	0	0	0	0
Frost Control	0	0	0	0	0
Solvent Evaporation Loss	0	0	0	2,566	0

MARYLAND

Emission categories	Pollutant, tons per year				
	Particulates	Sulfur oxides	Nitrogen oxides	Hydro-carbons	Carbon monoxide
GRAND TOTAL	115,444	341,200	291,186	394,150	1,387,658
-AREA	34,360	44,911	180,286	274,041	1,374,332
-POINT	81,084	296,288	110,900	120,109	13,326
FUEL COMBUSTION-AREA	8,463	26,690	18,591	2,250	6,632
-POINT	39,149	237,435	102,946	2,492	5,652
External Combustion-area	8,463	26,690	18,591	2,250	6,632
-point	38,907	236,518	97,886	2,012	4,334
Residential Fuel-area	3,861	11,661	6,321	1,663	5,518
Anthracite Coal	333	857	100	83	2,996
Bituminous Coal	0	0	0	0	0
Distillate Oil	2,486	10,741	2,983	746	1,243
Residual Oil	0	0	0	0	0
Natural Gas	371	22	2,970	297	742
Wood	671	40	269	537	537
Electric Generation-point	32,563	203,785	84,732	1,510	3,470
Anthracite Coal	0	0	0	0	0
Bituminous Coal	30,705	137,550	38,798	647	2,155
Lignite	0	0	0	0	0
Residual Oil	1,762	65,782	44,159	841	1,262
Distillate Oil	84	452	1,098	21	31
Natural Gas	13	1	676	1	22
Process Gas	0	0	0	0	0
Coke	0	0	0	0	0
Solid Waste/Coal	0	0	0	0	0
Other	0	0	0	0	0
Industrial Fuel-area	2,938	6,945	5,711	222	454
-point	4,825	26,967	9,931	333	617
Anthracite Coal-area	0	0	0	0	0
-point	0	0	0	0	0
Bituminous Coal-area	1,709	1,249	246	16	33
-point	3,705	19,854	3,778	74	227
Lignite-point	0	0	0	0	0
Residual Oil-area	740	4,605	1,930	97	129
-point	965	6,745	3,390	169	226
Distillate Oil-area	376	1,085	1,506	75	100
-point	102	326	469	23	31
Natural Gas-area	113	7	2,029	34	192
-point	33	3	2,033	14	80
Process Gas-area	0	0	0	0	0
-point	0	0	0	0	0
Coke-point	0	0	0	0	0
Wood-area	0	0	0	0	0
-point	20	39	260	52	52
Liquid Petroleum Gas-point	0	0	2	0	0
Bagasse-point	0	0	0	0	0
Other-point	0	0	0	0	0
Commercial-Institutional Fuel-area	1,665	8,084	6,559	365	660
-point	1,519	5,766	3,223	169	247
Anthracite Coal-area	0	0	0	0	0
-point	0	0	0	0	0
Bituminous Coal-area	0	0	0	0	0
-point	662	990	180	16	37
Lignite-point	0	0	0	0	0
Residual Oil-area	1,141	7,099	2,976	149	198
-point	666	4,239	2,236	112	149
Distillate Oil-area	338	974	1,353	68	90
-point	186	537	743	37	50
Natural Gas-area	186	11	2,231	149	372
-point	5	0	64	4	11
Wood-area	0	0	0	0	0
-point	0	0	0	0	0
Liquid Petroleum Gas-point	0	0	0	0	0
Miscellaneous-point	0	0	0	0	0
Internal Combustion-point	242	918	5,060	480	1,318
Electric Generation	242	918	5,060	480	1,318
Distillate Oil	130	918	1,764	145	401
Natural Gas	112	0	3,296	335	918
Diesel Fuel	0	0	0	0	0
Industrial Fuel	0	0	0	0	0
Distillate Oil	0	0	0	0	0
Natural Gas	0	0	0	0	0
Gasoline	0	0	0	0	0
Diesel Fuel	0	0	0	0	0

Emission categories	Pollutant, tons per year				
	Particulates	Sulfur oxides	Nitrogen oxides	Hydro- carbons	Carbon monoxide
Other	0	0	0	0	0
Commercial-Institutional	0	0	0	0	0
Diesel Fuel	0	0	0	0	0
Other	0	0	0	0	0
Engine-Testing	0	0	0	0	0
Aircraft	0	0	0	0	0
Other	0	0	0	0	0
Miscellaneous	0	0	0	0	0
INDUSTRIAL PROCESS-POINT	41,156	58,455	7,619	117,316	2,290
Chemical Manufacturing	955	37	956	14,080	0
Food/Agriculture	46	0	0	0	0
Primary Metal	1,542	0	0	0	864
Secondary Metals	41	2	0	0	1,426
Mineral Products	38,264	58,096	6,347	0	0
Petroleum Industry	71	319	316	29	0
Wood Products	0	0	0	1	0
Evaporation	1	0	0	103,206	0
Metal Fabrication	0	0	0	0	0
Leather Products	0	0	0	0	0
Textile Manufacturing	0	0	0	0	0
Inprocess Fuel	237	1	0	0	0
Other/Not Classified	0	0	0	0	0
SOLID WASTE DISPOSAL-AREA	6,083	515	2,259	10,774	30,374
-POINT	779	398	335	301	5,384
Government-point	685	375	311	225	5,251
Municipal Incineration	676	375	300	225	5,251
Open Burning	0	0	0	0	0
Other	9	0	11	0	0
Residential-area	4,650	288	1,721	8,779	24,903
On Site Incineration	65	1	2	182	547
Open Burning	4,585	287	1,719	8,597	24,357
Commercial-Institutional-area	718	106	269	1,041	2,868
-point	0	0	0	0	0
On Site Incineration-area	245	77	92	153	352
-point	0	0	0	0	0
Open Burning-area	474	30	178	888	2,516
-point	0	0	0	0	0
Apartment-point	0	0	0	0	0
Other-point	0	0	0	0	0
Industrial-area	715	122	268	955	2,602
-point	94	23	24	76	133
On Site Incineration-area	308	96	116	193	443
-point	94	23	24	76	133
Open Burning-area	406	25	152	762	2,159
-point	0	0	0	0	0
Auto Body Incineration-point	0	0	0	0	0
Other-point	0	0	0	0	0
Miscellaneous-point	0	0	0	0	0
TRANSPORTATION-AREA	19,814	17,706	159,436	246,646	1,337,327
Land Vehicles	17,008	7,393	155,382	217,236	1,314,348
Gasoline	14,336	3,862	122,738	212,403	1,299,837
Light Vehicles	13,195	3,421	110,635	179,245	1,099,275
Heavy Vehicles	1,078	408	11,389	31,141	177,702
Off Highway	63	33	715	2,016	22,860
Diesel Fuel	2,672	3,531	32,644	4,833	14,511
Heavy Vehicles	1,080	1,512	13,404	1,808	8,647
Off Highway	1,163	1,041	12,887	1,411	3,632
Rail	429	979	6,353	1,614	2,232
Aircraft	2,071	466	1,763	5,778	7,805
Military	1,987	379	955	4,623	4,963
Civil	28	6	26	126	720
Commercial	56	81	783	1,029	2,123
Vessels	734	9,847	2,290	4,968	15,173
Bituminous Coal	0	0	0	0	0
Diesel Fuel	78	98	732	192	256
Residual Oil	656	9,717	1,420	99	48
Gasoline	0	32	138	4,677	14,870
Gas Handling Evaporation Loss	0	0	0	18,665	0
MISCELLANEOUS-AREA	0	0	0	14,370	0
Forest Fires	0	0	0	0	0
Structural Fires	0	0	0	0	0
Slash Burning	0	0	0	0	0
Frost Control	0	0	0	0	0
Solvent Evaporation Loss	0	0	0	14,370	0

MASSACHUSETTS

Emission categories	Pollutant, tons per year				
	Particulates	Sulfur oxides	Nitrogen oxides	Hydro-carbons	Carbon monoxide
GRAND TOTAL	114,230	433,695	405,742	520,930	1,950,351
–AREA	56,952	126,133	267,772	436,665	1,895,927
–POINT	57,278	307,562	137,970	84,265	54,424
FUEL COMBUSTION–AREA	30,539	116,851	85,933	6,183	11,161
–POINT	34,837	304,957	134,973	2,909	4,581
External Combustion–area	30,539	116,851	85,933	6,183	11,161
–point	34,837	304,957	134,973	2,909	4,581
Residential Fuel–area	7,116	18,684	11,242	2,485	5,887
Anthracite Coal	158	407	47	40	1,422
Bituminous Coal	65	184	10	65	291
Distillate Oil	6,267	18,055	7,521	1,880	3,134
Residual Oil	0	0	0	0	0
Natural Gas	449	27	3,593	359	898
Wood	176	11	71	141	141
Electric Generation–point	21,783	222,668	115,108	1,987	3,294
Anthracite Coal	0	0	0	0	0
Bituminous Coal	15,373	37,882	16,352	146	473
Lignite	0	0	0	0	0
Residual Oil	6,360	184,667	96,128	1,831	2,747
Distillate Oil	19	116	283	5	8
Natural Gas	32	2	2,346	4	67
Process Gas	0	0	0	0	0
Coke	0	0	0	0	0
Solid Waste/Coal	0	0	0	0	0
Other	0	0	0	0	0
Industrial Fuel–area	9,144	35,811	28,095	1,331	1,945
–point	10,856	69,719	16,125	734	1,022
Anthracite Coal–area	0	0	0	0	0
–point	0	0	0	0	0
Bituminous Coal–area	986	481	126	8	17
–point	5,567	3,971	1,249	13	45
Lignite–point	0	0	0	0	0
Residual Oil–area	4,623	28,778	12,061	603	804
–point	5,211	65,700	14,181	709	941
Distillate Oil–area	3,408	6,545	13,632	682	909
–point	10	44	42	2	3
Natural Gas–area	126	8	2,275	38	215
–point	17	1	631	5	29
Process Gas–area	0	0	0	0	0
–point	0	0	0	0	0
Coke–point	0	0	0	0	0
Wood–area	0	0	0	0	0
–point	51	3	22	4	4
Liquid Petroleum Gas–point	0	0	0	0	0
Bagasse–point	0	0	0	0	0
Other–point	0	0	0	0	0
Commercial-Institutional Fuel–area	14,279	62,355	46,596	2,367	3,330
–point	2,197	12,570	3,740	188	265
Anthracite Coal–area	0	0	0	0	0
–point	0	0	0	0	0
Bituminous Coal–area	0	0	0	0	0
–point	921	511	142	10	22
Lignite–point	0	0	0	0	0
Residual Oil–area	8,632	51,857	22,518	1,126	1,501
–point	1,240	11,916	3,372	169	225
Distillate Oil–area	5,461	10,487	21,843	1,092	1,456
–point	32	143	126	6	8
Natural Gas–area	186	11	2,236	149	373
–point	4	0	100	4	9
Wood–area	0	0	0	0	0
–point	0	0	0	0	0
Liquid Petroleum Gas–point	0	0	0	0	0
Miscellaneous–point	0	0	0	0	0
Internal Combustion–point	0	0	0	0	0
Electric Generation	0	0	0	0	0
Distillate Oil	0	0	0	0	0
Natural Gas	0	0	0	0	0
Diesel Fuel	0	0	0	0	0
Industrial Fuel	0	0	0	0	0
Distillate Oil	0	0	0	0	0
Natural Gas	0	0	0	0	0
Gasoline	0	0	0	0	0
Diesel Fuel	0	0	0	0	0

Emission categories	Pollutant, tons per year				
	Particulates	Sulfur oxides	Nitrogen oxides	Hydro-carbons	Carbon monoxide
Other	0	0	0	0	0
Commercial-Institutional	0	0	0	0	0
Diesel Fuel	0	0	0	0	0
Other	0	0	0	0	0
Engine-Testing	0	0	0	0	0
Aircraft	0	0	0	0	0
Other	0	0	0	0	0
Miscellaneous	0	0	0	0	0
INDUSTRIAL PROCESS-POINT	11,939	1,301	8	69,996	8,416
Chemical Manufacturing	321	1,294	0	4,644	0
Food/Agriculture	3	0	0	0	0
Primary Metal	0	0	0	0	0
Secondary Metals	7,644	0	0	294	8,415
Mineral Products	3,967	4	0	0	0
Petroleum Industry	0	0	0	0	0
Wood Products	1	0	0	658	0
Evaporation	2	0	8	57,580	1
Metal Fabrication	0	0	0	91	0
Leather Products	0	0	0	13	0
Textile Manufacturing	1	0	0	6,642	0
Inprocess Fuel	0	4	0	0	0
Other/Not Classified	0	0	0	75	0
SOLID WASTE DISPOSAL-AREA	5,020	458	851	10,801	31,628
-POINT	10,502	1,303	2,989	11,181	41,426
Government-point	10,234	1,157	2,806	10,980	40,818
Municipal Incineration	4,603	793	634	476	11,096
Open Burning	5,595	350	2,098	10,490	29,722
Other	36	15	74	15	0
Residential-area	3,694	90	354	9,740	29,002
On Site Incineration	3,001	47	94	8,441	25,322
Open Burning	693	43	260	1,299	3,681
Commercial-Institutional-area	973	290	365	680	1,622
-point	47	12	22	39	70
On Site Incineration-area	915	286	343	572	1,316
-point	43	12	16	37	64
Open Burning-area	58	4	22	108	306
-point	0	0	0	0	0
Apartment-point	4	0	6	2	6
Other-point	0	0	0	0	0
Industrial-area	354	78	133	381	1,004
-point	222	135	161	162	539
On Site Incineration-area	226	71	85	141	324
-point	222	135	161	162	539
Open Burning-area	128	8	48	240	680
-point	0	0	0	0	0
Auto Body Incineration-point	0	0	0	0	0
Other-point	0	0	0	0	0
Miscellaneous-point	0	0	0	0	0
TRANSPORTATION-AREA	21,393	8,824	180,988	325,680	1,853,137
Land Vehicles	20,392	7,698	177,922	290,447	1,824,715
Gasoline	18,568	4,993	155,140	286,740	1,811,507
Light Vehicles	17,101	4,434	139,988	242,181	1,547,447
Heavy Vehicles	1,444	547	14,883	43,801	255,465
Off Highway	24	12	269	758	8,596
Diesel Fuel	1,824	2,705	22,782	3,707	13,208
Heavy Vehicles	1,219	1,706	14,845	2,131	10,631
Off Highway	275	246	3,050	334	860
Rail	330	753	4,888	1,242	1,717
Aircraft	848	286	1,793	3,851	8,883
Military	606	116	291	1,410	1,513
Civil	144	29	130	639	3,651
Commercial	98	142	1,372	1,802	3,718
Vessels	152	839	1,273	6,303	19,539
Bituminous Coal	0	0	0	0	0
Diesel Fuel	107	134	998	262	349
Residual Oil	45	665	97	7	3
Gasoline	0	41	178	6,035	19,187
Gas Handling Evaporation Loss	0	0	0	25,079	0
MISCELLANEOUS-AREA	0	0	0	94,001	0
Forest Fires	0	0	0	0	0
Structural Fires	0	0	0	0	0
Slash Burning	0	0	0	0	0
Frost Control	0	0	0	0	0
Solvent Evaporation Loss	0	0	0	94,001	0

MICHIGAN

Emission categories	Pollutant, tons per year				
	Particulates	Sulfur oxides	Nitrogen oxides	Hydro-carbons	Carbon monoxide
GRAND TOTAL	724,450	1,513,313	1,022,664	824,898	4,535,586
-AREA	171,027	176,091	627,516	764,087	3,745,669
-POINT	553,423	1,337,222	395,148	60,811	789,91*
FUEL COMBUSTION-AREA	105,012	132,334	80,232	8,774	27,640
-POINT	272,980	1,267,934	380,920	7,247	18,267
External Combustion-area	105,012	132,334	80,232	8,774	27,640
-point	272,949	1,267,867	380,731	7,192	18,178
Residential Fuel-area	9,392	33,280	20,620	5,767	20,487
Anthracite Coal	433	3,349	130	108	3,901
Bituminous Coal	2,274	11,233	341	2,274	10,232
Distillate Oil	3,532	15,262	4,238	1,060	1,766
Residual Oil	295	3,265	513	38	51
Natural Gas	1,875	113	15,004	1,500	3,751
Wood	983	59	393	786	786
Electric Generation-point	135,820	1,014,364	272,728	3,564	11,797
Anthracite Coal	0	0	0	0	0
Bituminous Coal	134,724	966,539	219,191	3,027	10,053
Lignite	0	0	0	0	0
Residual Oil	125	39,771	15,342	292	438
Distillate Oil	637	8,022	9,669	184	276
Natural Gas	331	32	24,437	54	914
Process Gas	3	0	4,088	7	116
Coke	0	0	0	0	0
Solid Waste/Coal	0	0	0	0	0
Other	0	0	0	0	0
Industrial Fuel-area	80,859	71,947	38,248	1,495	3,541
-point	131,545	244,671	103,786	3,504	5,868
Anthracite Coal-area	0	0	0	0	0
-point	0	0	0	0	0
Bituminous Coal-area	76,147	52,611	7,987	532	1,065
-point	129,812	232,551	77,054	2,028	4,847
Lignite-point	0	0	0	0	0
Residual Oil-area	1,021	11,291	2,662	133	177
-point	590	8,691	4,000	697	268
Distillate Oil-area	2,774	7,990	11,095	555	740
-point	472	3,310	3,225	161	176
Natural Gas-area	917	55	16,503	275	1,559
-point	667	118	19,474	616	573
Process Gas-area	0	0	0	0	0
-point	0	0	0	0	0
Coke-point	0	0	0	0	0
Wood-area	0	0	0	0	0
-point	0	0	0	0	0
Liquid Petroleum Gas-point	5	0	33	1	4
Bagasse-point	0	0	0	0	0
Other-point	0	0	0	0	0
Commercial-Institutional Fuel-area	14,761	27,107	21,364	1,512	3,612
-point	5,584	8,832	4,218	125	513
Anthracite Coal-area	0	0	0	0	0
-point	0	0	0	0	0
Bituminous Coal-area	11,421	17,687	1,647	358	1,289
-point	5,423	7,991	3,460	83	441
Lignite-point	0	0	0	0	0
Residual Oil-area	265	2,935	692	35	46
-point	42	309	110	5	7
Distillate Oil-area	2,234	6,435	8,935	447	596
-point	104	530	470	23	31
Natural Gas-area	841	50	10,091	673	1,682
-point	15	1	177	13	33
Wood-area	0	0	0	0	0
-point	0	0	0	0	0
Liquid Petroleum Gas-point	0	0	0	0	0
Miscellaneous-point	0	0	0	0	0
Internal Combustion-point	31	68	189	54	89
Electric Generation	31	68	189	54	89
Distillate Oil	9	26	124	10	28
Natural Gas	0	0	0	0	0
Diesel Fuel	22	42	65	44	61
Industrial Fuel	0	0	0	0	0
Distillate Oil	0	0	0	0	0
Natural Gas	0	0	0	0	0
Gasoline	0	0	0	0	0
Diesel Fuel	0	0	0	0	0

Emission categories	Pollutant, tons per year				
	Particulates	Sulfur oxides	Nitrogen oxides	Hydro-carbons	Carbon monoxide
Other.............	0	0	0	0	0
Commercial-Institutional...........	0	0	0	0	0
Diesel Fuel........	0	0	0	0	0
Other........	0	0	0	0	0
Engine-Testing.......	0	0	0	0	0
Aircraft........	0	0	0	0	0
Other........	0	0	0	0	0
Miscellaneous......	0	0	0	0	0
INDUSTRIAL PROCESS-POINT.........	274,992	68,292	13,390	48,721	761,706
Chemical Manufacturing.......	311	4,207	0	8,845	0
Food/Agriculture........	80	1	0	0	0
Primary Metal.......	103,389	15,221	54	5,104	457,000
Secondary Metals........	16,688	130	1	0	304,693
Mineral Products.......	152,722	40,537	5,407	39	14
Petroleum Industry........	442	8,192	7,920	454	0
Wood Products........	22	0	0	0	0
Evaporation........	395	4	7	32,751	0
Metal Fabrication.......	31	0	0	0	0
Leather Products........	0	0	0	0	0
Textile Manufacturing.......	0	0	0	0	0
Inprocess Fuel........	911	0	0	1,528	0
Other/Not Classified........	0	0	0	0	0
SOLID WASTE DISPOSAL-AREA........	8,808	1,163	2,496	15,104	42,932
-POINT.........	5,452	997	838	4,842	9,944
Government-point........	5,327	985	791	4,618	9,315
Municipal Incineration........	5,275	985	788	4,618	9,315
Open Burning........	0	0	0	0	1
Other........	52	0	4	0	0
Residential-area.......	4,840	192	1,008	11,277	33,053
On Site Incineration........	2,348	37	73	6,605	19,814
Open Burning........	2,492	156	934	4,673	13,239
Commercial-Institutional-area........	3,323	834	1,246	3,098	7,942
-point........	1	3	3	3	10
On Site Incineration-area........	2,506	783	940	1,567	3,603
-point........	1	3	3	3	10
Open Burning-area........	817	51	306	1,532	4,339
-point........	0	0	0	0	0
Apartment-point........	0	0	0	0	0
Other-point........	0	0	0	0	0
Industrial-area........	645	136	242	729	1,937
-point........	124	9	44	221	618
On Site Incineration-area........	384	120	144	240	552
-point........	12	2	2	11	23
Open Burning-area........	261	16	98	489	1,386
-point........	112	7	42	210	595
Auto Body Incineration-point........	0	0	0	0	0
Other-point........	0	0	0	0	0
Miscellaneous-point........	0	0	0	0	0
TRANSPORTATION-AREA........	55,326	42,591	544,625	677,631	3,670,847
Land Vehicles........	52,654	40,376	537,457	601,343	3,583,677
Gasoline........	36,215	9,981	313,157	553,863	3,497,884
Light Vehicles........	32,299	8,374	271,032	438,077	2,682,450
Heavy Vehicles........	3,059	1,159	32,354	88,234	503,076
Off Highway........	857	449	9,771	27,552	312,359
Diesel Fuel........	16,439	30,395	224,300	47,480	85,793
Heavy Vehicles........	2,722	3,810	33,874	4,527	21,495
Off Highway........	3,387	3,031	37,529	4,109	10,577
Rail........	10,331	23,554	152,897	38,844	53,721
Aircraft........	2,542	909	5,949	12,262	28,667
Military........	1,749	334	840	4,070	4,369
Civil........	457	91	413	2,025	11,572
Commercial........	335	484	4,695	6,167	12,726
Vessels........	130	1,304	1,219	18,489	58,503
Bituminous Coal........	0	0	0	0	0
Diesel Fuel........	55	69	516	136	181
Residual Oil........	75	1,111	162	11	5
Gasoline........	0	124	540	18,342	58,316
Gas Handling Evaporation Loss........	0	0	0	45,538	0
MISCELLANEOUS-AREA........	1,881	3	164	62,578	4,249
Forest Fires........	0	0	0	0	0
Structural Fires........	1,881	3	164	488	4,249
Slash Burning........	0	0	0	0	0
Frost Control........	0	0	0	0	0
Solvent Evaporation Loss........	0	0	0	62,090	0

MINNESOTA

Emission categories	Pollutant, tons per year				
	Particulates	Sulfur oxides	Nitrogen oxides	Hydro-carbons	Carbon monoxide
GRAND TOTAL	190,669	346,388	353,962	381,938	1,877,531
–AREA	39,066	54,128	217,903	336,153	1,741,492
–POINT	151,603	292,260	136,060	45,785	136,039
FUEL COMBUSTION–AREA	10,366	43,622	30,804	4,920	12,846
–POINT	43,116	260,054	132,489	2,754	7,554
External Combustion-area	10,366	43,622	30,804	4,920	12,846
–point	42,991	258,260	130,243	2,538	6,928
Residential Fuel-area	6,179	17,786	9,135	3,903	10,714
Anthracite Coal	0	0	0	0	0
Bituminous Coal	1,571	5,969	236	1,571	7,068
Distillate Oil	2,708	11,703	3,250	812	1,354
Residual Oil	0	0	0	0	0
Natural Gas	643	39	5,147	515	1,287
Wood	1,256	75	503	1,005	1,005
Electric Generation-point	23,379	215,875	97,591	1,115	3,944
Anthracite Coal	0	0	0	0	0
Bituminous Coal	21,355	185,421	69,920	857	2,658
Lignite	1,547	20,581	9,890	192	761
Residual Oil	104	6,207	1,740	33	50
Distillate Oil	22	216	374	7	11
Natural Gas	64	15	15,039	26	438
Process Gas	0	0	266	0	8
Coke	287	3,435	362	1	20
Solid Waste/Coal	0	0	0	0	0
Other	0	0	0	0	0
Industrial Fuel-area	2,626	21,704	11,873	435	924
–point	18,189	34,895	29,456	1,080	2,294
Anthracite Coal-area	0	0	0	0	0
–point	0	0	0	0	0
Bituminous Coal-area	0	0	0	0	0
–point	6,702	9,557	6,046	122	299
Lignite-point	7,243	9,689	6,399	492	984
Residual Oil-area	1,678	19,719	4,376	219	292
–point	927	13,638	2,488	125	161
Distillate Oil-area	684	1,969	2,734	137	182
–point	91	360	517	26	34
Natural Gas-area	265	16	4,763	79	450
–point	273	74	12,959	107	600
Process Gas-area	0	0	0	0	0
–point	0	1,393	0	0	0
Coke-point	0	29	19	0	3
Wood-area	0	0	0	0	0
–point	2,953	154	1,028	208	212
Liquid Petroleum Gas-point	0	0	0	0	0
Bagasse-point	0	0	0	0	0
Other-point	0	0	0	0	0
Commercial-Institutional Fuel-area	1,561	4,132	9,796	582	1,208
–point	1,423	7,490	3,196	343	689
Anthracite Coal-area	0	0	0	0	0
–point	0	0	0	0	0
Bituminous Coal-area	0	0	0	0	0
–point	809	2,392	773	47	98
Lignite-point	248	332	216	17	33
Residual Oil-area	106	1,242	276	14	18
–point	247	4,702	879	43	57
Distillate Oil-area	993	2,862	3,974	199	265
–point	1	6	5	0	0
Natural Gas-area	462	28	5,546	370	924
–point	58	4	964	57	142
Wood-area	0	0	0	0	0
–point	58	54	359	179	359
Liquid Petroleum Gas-point	0	0	0	0	0
Miscellaneous-point	0	0	0	0	0
Internal Combustion-point	125	1,793	2,246	216	627
Electric Generation	103	1,720	1,774	159	492
Distillate Oil	81	1,708	1,102	91	250
Natural Gas	17	0	505	51	141
Diesel Fuel	5	12	166	17	101
Industrial Fuel	19	70	469	46	127
Distillate Oil	5	70	68	6	15
Natural Gas	14	0	401	41	112
Gasoline	0	0	0	0	0
Diesel Fuel	0	0	0	0	0

Emission categories	Pollutant, tons per year				
	Particulates	Sulfur oxides	Nitrogen oxides	Hydro-carbons	Carbon monoxide
Other	0	0	0	0	0
Commercial-Institutional	0	0	0	0	0
Diesel Fuel	0	0	0	0	0
Other	0	0	0	0	0
Engine-Testing	3	3	3	11	8
Aircraft	3	3	3	11	8
Other	0	0	0	0	0
Miscellaneous	0	0	0	0	0
INDUSTRIAL PROCESS-POINT	106,700	32,139	3,288	42,676	125,898
Chemical Manufacturing	426	2,900	1,238	520	0
Food/Agriculture	49,131	0	0	0	0
Primary Metal	30,069	1,316	17	1,712	500
Secondary Metals	684	709	31	0	15,082
Mineral Products	21,971	2,038	461	2	0
Petroleum Industry	1,039	20,653	1,534	1,990	110,315
Wood Products	3,266	4,517	0	0	0
Evaporation	51	0	0	38,453	1
Metal Fabrication	0	0	0	0	0
Leather Products	0	0	0	0	0
Textile Manufacturing	0	0	0	0	0
Inprocess Fuel	63	5	8	0	0
Other/Not Classified	0	0	0	0	0
SOLID WASTE DISPOSAL-AREA	8,945	559	3,354	16,772	47,519
-POINT	1,787	68	282	354	2,587
Government-point	0	0	0	0	0
Municipal Incineration	0	0	0	0	0
Open Burning	0	0	0	0	0
Other	0	0	0	0	0
Residential-area	8,070	504	3,026	15,132	42,874
On Site Incineration	0	0	0	0	0
Open Burning	8,070	504	3,026	15,132	42,874
Commercial-Institutional-area	874	55	328	1,640	4,645
-point	30	0	4	47	553
On Site Incineration-area	0	0	0	0	0
-point	30	0	4	47	553
Open Burning-area	874	55	328	1,640	4,645
-point	0	0	0	0	0
Apartment-point	0	0	0	0	0
Other-point	0	0	0	0	0
Industrial-area	0	0	0	0	0
-point	1,757	67	278	307	2,035
On Site Incineration-area	0	0	0	0	0
-point	200	18	34	259	2,035
Open Burning-area	0	0	0	0	0
-point	0	0	0	0	0
Auto Body Incineration-point	0	0	0	0	0
Other-point	1,557	49	244	49	0
Miscellaneous-point	0	0	0	0	0
TRANSPORTATION-AREA	19,755	9,946	183,745	292,645	1,681,127
Land Vehicles	19,150	9,282	181,991	258,410	1,649,063
Gasoline	16,020	4,559	141,932	251,932	1,630,423
Light Vehicles	13,597	3,525	115,433	180,540	1,081,012
Heavy Vehicles	1,620	614	17,346	45,585	256,842
Off Highway	803	420	9,152	25,806	292,568
Diesel Fuel	3,130	4,723	40,059	6,478	18,640
Heavy Vehicles	1,646	2,305	20,694	2,673	12,372
Off Highway	696	623	7,712	844	2,174
Rail	787	1,795	11,653	2,961	4,094
Aircraft	559	196	1,273	2,691	6,706
Military	365	70	175	850	912
Civil	123	24	111	546	3,120
Commercial	70	102	987	1,296	2,674
Vessels	47	468	480	8,008	25,358
Bituminous Coal	0	0	0	0	0
Diesel Fuel	20	25	189	50	66
Residual Oil	26	389	57	4	2
Gasoline	0	54	234	7,954	25,290
Gas Handling Evaporation Loss	0	0	0	23,536	0
MISCELLANEOUS-AREA	0	0	0	21,817	0
Forest Fires	0	0	0	0	0
Structural Fires	0	0	0	0	0
Slash Burning	0	0	0	0	0
Frost Control	0	0	0	0	0
Solvent Evaporation Loss	0	0	0	21,817	0

MISSISSIPPI

Emission categories	Pollutant, tons per year				
	Particulates	Sulfur oxides	Nitrogen oxides	Hydro-carbons	Carbon monoxide
GRAND TOTAL	199,401	54,481	216,614	224,298	1,037,166
-AREA	33,358	7,954	135,934	189,714	899,139
-POINT	166,043	46,527	80,680	34,584	138,027
FUEL COMBUSTION-AREA	4,151	1,484	16,247	2,849	4,541
-POINT	21,175	12,191	68,097	1,789	3,160
External Combustion-area	4,151	1,484	16,247	2,849	4,541
-point	21,173	12,190	66,975	1,582	3,124
Residential Fuel-area	3,080	729	3,355	2,479	3,212
Anthracite Coal	0	0	0	0	0
Bituminous Coal	112	532	17	112	504
Distillate Oil	14	20	16	4	7
Residual Oil	0	0	0	0	0
Natural Gas	282	17	2,252	225	563
Wood	2,673	160	1,069	2,138	2,138
Electric Generation-point	1,194	4,807	50,712	202	1,439
Anthracite Coal	0	0	0	0	0
Bituminous Coal	0	0	0	0	0
Lignite	0	0	0	0	0
Residual Oil	167	3,706	2,893	55	83
Distillate Oil	294	1,057	3,853	73	110
Natural Gas	734	44	43,966	73	1,247
Process Gas	0	0	0	0	0
Coke	0	0	0	0	0
Solid Waste/Coal	0	0	0	0	0
Other	0	0	0	0	0
Industrial Fuel-area	631	141	9,767	178	910
-point	19,960	7,380	16,236	1,370	1,664
Anthracite Coal-area	0	0	0	0	0
-point	0	0	0	0	0
Bituminous Coal-area	0	0	0	0	0
-point	227	10	51	3	7
Lignite-point	0	0	0	0	0
Residual Oil-area	0	0	0	0	0
-point	299	4,204	216	11	14
Distillate Oil-area	114	110	456	23	30
-point	227	2,226	1,146	57	76
Natural Gas-area	517	31	9,310	155	879
-point	198	12	8,627	59	327
Process Gas-area	0	0	0	0	0
-point	0	0	0	0	0
Coke-point	0	0	0	0	0
Wood-area	0	0	0	0	0
-point	19,010	928	6,196	1,239	1,240
Liquid Petroleum Gas-point	0	0	0	0	0
Bagasse-point	0	0	0	0	0
Other-point	0	0	0	0	0
Commercial-Institutional Fuel-area	440	615	3,126	191	419
-point	20	3	27	10	20
Anthracite Coal-area	0	0	0	0	0
-point	0	0	0	0	0
Bituminous Coal-area	0	0	0	0	0
-point	0	0	0	0	0
Lignite-point	0	0	0	0	0
Residual Oil-area	29	378	75	4	5
-point	0	0	0	0	0
Distillate Oil-area	236	227	944	47	63
-point	0	0	0	0	0
Natural Gas-area	176	11	2,107	140	351
-point	1	0	8	1	2
Wood-area	0	0	0	0	0
-point	19	3	19	9	19
Liquid Petroleum Gas-point	0	0	0	0	0
Miscellaneous-point	0	0	0	0	0
Internal Combustion-point	1	1	1,121	207	36
Electric Generation	0	0	892	0	0
Distillate Oil	0	0	0	0	0
Natural Gas	0	0	892	0	0
Diesel Fuel	0	0	0	0	0
Industrial Fuel	1	1	229	207	36
Distillate Oil	1	1	14	1	3
Natural Gas	0	0	215	206	33
Gasoline	0	0	0	0	0
Diesel Fuel	0	0	0	0	0

Emission categories	Pollutant, tons per year				
	Particulates	Sulfur oxides	Nitrogen oxides	Hydro-carbons	Carbon monoxide
Other	0	0	0	0	0
Commercial-Institutional	0	0	0	0	0
Diesel Fuel	0	0	0	0	0
Other	0	0	0	0	0
Engine-Testing	0	0	0	0	0
Aircraft	0	0	0	0	0
Other	0	0	0	0	0
Miscellaneous	0	0	0	0	0
INDUSTRIAL PROCESS-POINT	139,970	34,175	11,868	26,633	72,151
Chemical Manufacturing	2,782	10,649	10,289	10,423	2,938
Food/Agriculture	11,306	0	0	144	0
Primary Metal	246	22	0	0	477
Secondary Metals	96	0	0	0	383
Mineral Products	106,866	30	194	0	0
Petroleum Industry	6,131	20,375	1,385	2,046	9,500
Wood Products	11,283	3,090	0	185	58,853
Evaporation	0	0	0	13,596	0
Metal Fabrication	0	0	0	18	0
Leather Products	0	0	0	0	0
Textile Manufacturing	0	0	0	0	0
Inprocess Fuel	1,257	10	0	198	0
Other/Not Classified	3	0	0	23	0
SOLID WASTE DISPOSAL-AREA	4,112	257	1,542	7,710	21,845
-POINT	4,899	161	716	6,162	62,716
Government-point	0	0	0	0	1
Municipal Incineration	0	0	0	0	1
Open Burning	0	0	0	0	0
Other	0	0	0	0	0
Residential-area	3,556	222	1,333	6,668	18,891
On Site Incineration	0	0	0	0	0
Open Burning	3,556	222	1,333	6,668	18,891
Commercial-Institutional-area	362	23	136	680	1,925
-point	70	12	11	66	93
On Site Incineration-area	0	0	0	0	0
-point	69	12	11	66	93
Open Burning-area	362	23	136	680	1,925
-point	0	0	0	0	0
Apartment-point	0	0	0	0	0
Other-point	0	0	0	0	0
Industrial-area	194	12	73	363	1,029
-point	4,829	148	704	6,096	62,622
On Site Incineration-area	0	0	0	0	0
-point	3,961	146	556	5,593	59,675
Open Burning-area	194	12	73	363	1,029
-point	855	3	148	503	2,947
Auto Body Incineration-point	12	0	0	0	0
Other-point	0	0	0	0	0
Miscellaneous-point	0	0	0	0	0
TRANSPORTATION-AREA	13,181	6,213	115,684	156,622	788,330
Land Vehicles	11,642	5,453	111,076	135,389	770,104
Gasoline	9,465	2,553	83,811	131,776	758,710
Light Vehicles	8,698	2,255	75,401	110,948	635,069
Heavy Vehicles	718	272	7,861	19,279	106,074
Off Highway	48	25	550	1,550	17,568
Diesel Fuel	2,177	2,900	27,265	3,613	11,394
Heavy Vehicles	1,236	1,731	15,968	1,870	7,967
Off Highway	704	630	7,797	854	2,198
Rail	237	539	3,500	889	1,230
Aircraft	1,150	246	852	3,088	4,409
Military	1,094	209	526	2,546	2,733
Civil	35	7	31	153	874
Commercial	21	30	295	388	801
Vessels	390	514	3,755	4,901	13,818
Bituminous Coal	0	0	0	0	0
Diesel Fuel	390	487	3,639	955	1,274
Residual Oil	0	0	0	0	0
Gasoline	0	27	116	3,946	12,544
Gas Handling Evaporation Loss	0	0	0	13,245	0
MISCELLANEOUS-AREA	11,913	0	2,461	22,533	84,422
Forest Fires	9,005	0	2,119	12,713	74,158
Structural Fires	0	0	0	0	0
Slash Burning	2,908	0	342	3,421	10,264
Frost Control	0	0	0	0	0
Solvent Evaporation Loss	0	0	0	6,399	0

MISSOURI

Emission categories	Pollutant, tons per year				
	Particulates	Sulfur oxides	Nitrogen oxides	Hydro-carbons	Carbon monoxide
GRAND TOTAL	375,790	1,230,231	564,162	448,299	1,864,069
-AREA	108,176	90,152	255,880	336,158	1,704,200
-POINT	267,615	1,140,079	308,282	112,141	159,869
FUEL COMBUSTION-AREA	80,195	75,032	36,036	5,968	10,742
-POINT	52,300	907,880	278,080	8,974	65,023
External Combustion-area	80,195	75,032	36,036	5,968	10,742
-point	51,255	905,387	263,239	7,808	61,832
Residential Fuel-area	5,868	4,106	9,774	4,470	7,329
Anthracite Coal	0	0	0	0	0
Bituminous Coal	463	2,763	69	463	2,085
Distillate Oil	634	1,058	761	190	317
Residual Oil	0	0	0	0	0
Natural Gas	926	56	7,406	741	1,851
Wood	3,845	231	1,538	3,076	3,076
Electric Generation-point	31,747	868,843	237,461	1,871	5,409
Anthracite Coal	188	1,069	98	2	56
Bituminous Coal	31,184	769,680	140,705	1,720	4,841
Lignite	0	0	0	0	0
Residual Oil	92	55,020	14,477	16	17
Distillate Oil	62	42,993	13,138	4	4
Natural Gas	221	80	69,042	129	491
Process Gas	0	0	0	0	0
Coke	0	0	0	0	0
Solid Waste/Coal	0	0	0	0	0
Other	0	0	0	0	0
Industrial Fuel-area	70,203	61,953	14,585	716	1,579
-point	18,218	32,922	22,963	5,649	56,038
Anthracite Coal-area	0	0	0	0	0
-point	0	0	0	0	0
Bituminous Coal-area	69,100	59,457	6,962	464	928
-point	11,999	25,201	5,137	170	405
Lignite-point	125	433	147	10	20
Residual Oil-area	115	1,590	300	15	20
-point	565	4,750	734	382	72
Distillate Oil-area	715	889	2,862	143	191
-point	59	136	167	38	25
Natural Gas-area	247	15	4,450	74	420
-point	4,918	1,045	16,375	4,996	55,458
Process Gas-area	0	0	0	0	0
-point	54	822	139	7	17
Coke-point	0	0	0	0	0
Wood-area	25	1	10	20	20
-point	359	45	116	25	25
Liquid Petroleum Gas-point	29	480	75	4	9
Bagasse-point	0	0	0	0	0
Other-point	112	10	73	18	7
Commercial-Institutional Fuel-area	4,124	8,973	11,677	782	1,833
-point	1,290	3,623	2,816	287	384
Anthracite Coal-area	0	0	0	0	0
-point	5	23	2	1	3
Bituminous Coal-area	2,436	6,460	460	100	360
-point	994	2,657	533	114	73
Lignite-point	0	0	0	0	0
Residual Oil-area	267	1,477	696	35	46
-point	46	577	86	9	17
Distillate Oil-area	816	1,000	3,265	163	218
-point	37	283	112	15	16
Natural Gas-area	605	36	7,255	484	1,209
-point	207	83	2,080	149	275
Wood-area	0	0	0	0	0
-point	0	0	0	0	0
Liquid Petroleum Gas-point	1	0	3	0	1
Miscellaneous-point	0	0	0	0	0
Internal Combustion-point	1,045	2,492	14,840	1,167	3,192
Electric Generation	14	56	234	13	56
Distillate Oil	8	46	103	2	4
Natural Gas	2	2	44	1	1
Diesel Fuel	3	6	83	10	51
Industrial Fuel	1,030	2,436	14,606	1,153	3,135
Distillate Oil	0	0	0	0	0
Natural Gas	1	2	193	1	0
Gasoline	0	0	0	0	0
Diesel Fuel	1,029	2,434	14,412	1,152	3,134

Emission categories	Pollutant, tons per year				
	Particulates	Sulfur oxides	Nitrogen oxides	Hydro- carbons	Carbon monoxide
Other	1	1	2	1	1
Commercial-Institutional	0	0	0	0	0
Diesel Fuel	0	0	0	0	0
Other	0	0	0	0	0
Engine-Testing	0	0	0	0	0
Aircraft	0	0	0	0	0
Other	0	0	0	0	0
Miscellaneous	0	0	0	0	0
INDUSTRIAL PROCESS–POINT	214,191	231,711	29,714	102,053	79,859
Chemical Manufacturing	66,733	2,381	19,417	41,107	77,682
Food/Agriculture	7,234	38	28	92	5
Primary Metal	52,890	157,092	13	1,322	372
Secondary Metals	611	847	21	10	1,221
Mineral Products	81,083	56,970	8,651	111	123
Petroleum Industry	844	11,426	709	28	9
Wood Products	13	0	1	519	10
Evaporation	52	10	64	54,905	62
Metal Fabrication	0	0	0	0	0
Leather Products	2	0	0	0	0
Textile Manufacturing	0	0	0	0	0
Inprocess Fuel	4,403	2,903	808	767	375
Other/Not Classified	326	45	3	3,192	1
SOLID WASTE DISPOSAL–AREA	5,530	481	2,048	9,747	27,466
–POINT	1,104	488	488	1,114	14,987
Government-point	621	402	312	235	5,405
Municipal Incineration	616	386	310	232	5,403
Open Burning	5	16	2	4	2
Other	0	0	0	0	0
Residential-area	4,515	279	1,667	8,536	24,221
On Site Incineration	75	1	2	211	633
Open Burning	4,440	277	1,665	8,325	23,588
Commercial-Institutional-area	471	82	177	621	1,690
–point	38	14	17	20	62
On Site Incineration-area	209	65	78	131	301
–point	34	14	16	19	50
Open Burning-area	262	16	98	491	1,390
–point	4	0	1	1	12
Apartment-point	0	0	0	0	0
Other-point	0	0	0	0	0
Industrial-area	544	120	204	589	1,554
–point	445	72	160	858	9,520
On Site Incineration-area	345	108	129	216	496
–point	150	44	102	755	8,634
Open Burning-area	199	12	75	374	1,058
–point	295	28	58	104	886
Auto Body Incineration-point	0	0	0	0	0
Other-point	0	0	0	0	0
Miscellaneous-point	0	0	0	0	0
TRANSPORTATION–AREA.	22,450	14,640	217,796	308,879	1,665,992
Land Vehicles	21,302	13,906	213,878	268,163	1,634,256
Gasoline	15,969	4,549	142,162	254,421	1,602,696
Light Vehicles	13,268	3,440	112,798	176,089	1,053,350
Heavy Vehicles	2,111	800	22,639	59,371	334,389
Off Highway	590	309	6,724	18,960	214,956
Diesel Fuel	5,333	9,357	71,716	13,742	31,560
Heavy Vehicles	2,223	3,112	27,960	3,603	16,656
Off Highway	611	546	6,766	741	1,907
Rail	2,499	5,699	36,991	9,398	12,997
Aircraft	916	280	1,578	3,510	5,633
Military	816	156	392	1,898	2,038
Civil	17	3	15	74	422
Commercial	84	121	1,171	1,537	3,173
Vessels	232	454	2,340	8,530	26,104
Bituminous Coal	0	0	0	0	0
Diesel Fuel	224	280	2,088	548	731
Residual Oil	8	120	18	1	1
Gasoline	0	54	235	7,981	25,373
Gas Handling Evaporation Loss	0	0	0	28,677	0
MISCELLANEOUS–AREA	0	0	0	11,564	0
Forest Fires	0	0	0	0	0
Structural Fires	0	0	0	0	0
Slash Burning	0	0	0	0	0
Frost Control	0	0	0	0	0
Solvent Evaporation Loss	0	0	0	11,564	0

MONTANA

Emission categories	Pollutant, tons per year				
	Particulates	Sulfur oxides	Nitrogen oxides	Hydro-carbons	Carbon monoxide
GRAND TOTAL	133,561	132,419	113,400	197,518	960,247
–AREA	90,667	17,377	91,699	177,293	788,430
–POINT	42,894	115,042	21,701	20,225	171,817
FUEL COMBUSTION–AREA	5,219	11,531	7,272	1,353	3,261
–POINT	17,431	18,074	17,483	1,611	2,519
External Combustion–area	5,219	11,531	7,272	1,353	3,261
–point	17,166	17,768	13,766	1,314	1,710
Residential Fuel–area	1,296	1,508	1,592	1,018	2,470
Anthracite Coal	0	0	0	0	0
Bituminous Coal	358	681	54	358	1,613
Distillate Oil	179	774	215	54	90
Residual Oil	1	8	1	0	0
Natural Gas	134	8	1,072	107	268
Wood	624	37	250	499	499
Electric Generation–point	8,249	9,745	8,224	486	761
Anthracite Coal	0	0	0	0	0
Bituminous Coal	1,492	5,119	4,041	67	225
Lignite	6,239	4,270	2,081	48	160
Residual Oil	2	79	29	1	1
Distillate Oil	0	0	0	0	0
Natural Gas	1	0	223	0	6
Process Gas	0	0	0	0	0
Coke	0	0	0	0	0
Solid Waste/Coal	0	0	0	0	0
Other	515	277	1,849	370	370
Industrial Fuel–area	2,854	7,143	3,385	148	295
–point	8,916	8,023	5,538	827	947
Anthracite Coal–area	0	0	0	0	0
–point	0	0	0	0	0
Bituminous Coal–area	2,229	1,629	643	43	86
–point	0	0	0	0	0
Lignite–point	0	0	0	0	0
Residual Oil–area	358	4,892	933	47	62
–point	306	2,982	286	14	7
Distillate Oil–area	215	620	860	43	57
–point	6	45	22	1	1
Natural Gas–area	53	3	949	16	90
–point	40	92	1,453	11	62
Process Gas–area	0	0	0	0	0
–point	266	2,497	0	0	0
Coke–point	0	0	0	0	0
Wood–area	0	0	0	0	0
–point	8,032	567	3,777	801	877
Liquid Petroleum Gas–point	0	0	0	0	0
Bagasse–point	0	0	0	0	0
Other–point	266	1,841	0	0	0
Commercial-Institutional Fuel–area	1,069	2,880	2,295	186	496
–point	1	0	5	0	1
Anthracite Coal–area	0	0	0	0	0
–point	0	0	0	0	0
Bituminous Coal–area	751	1,231	298	65	233
–point	0	0	0	0	0
Lignite–point	0	0	0	0	0
Residual Oil–area	100	1,327	260	13	17
–point	0	0	0	0	0
Distillate Oil–area	110	316	439	22	29
–point	0	0	0	0	0
Natural Gas–area	108	6	1,299	87	216
–point	1	0	5	0	1
Wood–area	0	0	0	0	0
–point	0	0	0	0	0
Liquid Petroleum Gas–point	0	0	0	0	0
Miscellaneous–point	0	0	0	0	0
Internal Combustion–point	266	305	3,716	297	809
Electric Generation	3	22	36	3	8
Distillate Oil	3	22	36	3	8
Natural Gas	0	0	0	0	0
Diesel Fuel	0	0	0	0	0
Industrial Fuel	263	263	3,681	294	800
Distillate Oil	0	0	0	0	0
Natural Gas	0	1	0	0	0
Gasoline	0	0	0	0	0
Diesel Fuel	263	283	3,681	294	800

Emission categories	Pollutant, tons per year				
	Particulates	Sulfur oxides	Nitrogen oxides	Hydro- carbons	Carbon monoxide
Other	0	0	0	0	0
Commercial-Institutional	0	0	0	0	0
Diesel Fuel	0	0	0	0	0
Other	0	0	0	0	0
Engine-Testing	0	0	0	0	0
Aircraft	0	0	0	0	0
Other	0	0	0	0	0
Miscellaneous	0	0	0	0	0
INDUSTRIAL PROCESS-POINT	23,235	96,935	3,881	14,909	125,518
Chemical Manufacturing	141	2,344	0	0	0
Food/Agriculture	180	0	0	0	0
Primary Metal	9,086	71,130	0	0	0
Secondary Metals	14	0	0	0	0
Mineral Products	10,728	4,906	1,003	3	0
Petroleum Industry	1,319	16,854	2,828	11,176	106,724
Wood Products	1,498	1,444	0	19	18,793
Evaporation	0	0	0	3,709	0
Metal Fabrication	0	0	0	0	0
Leather Products	0	0	0	0	0
Textile Manufacturing	0	0	0	0	0
Inprocess Fuel	270	257	50	3	0
Other/Not Classified	0	0	0	0	0
SOLID WASTE DISPOSAL-AREA	3,215	201	1,206	6,029	17,081
-POINT	2,228	34	337	3,705	43,781
Government-point	0	0	0	0	0
Municipal Incineration	0	0	0	0	0
Open Burning	0	0	0	0	0
Other	0	0	0	0	0
Residential-area	2,823	176	1,059	5,294	14,998
On Site Incineration	0	0	0	0	0
Open Burning	2,823	176	1,059	5,294	14,998
Commercial-Institutional-area	290	18	109	543	1,539
-point	0	0	0	0	0
On Site Incineration-area	0	0	0	0	0
-point	0	0	0	0	0
Open Burning-area	290	18	109	543	1,539
-point	0	0	0	0	0
Apartment-point	0	0	0	0	0
Other-point	0	0	0	0	0
Industrial-area	102	6	38	192	544
-point	2,228	34	337	3,705	43,781
On Site Incineration-area	0	0	0	0	0
-point	2,228	34	337	3,704	43,780
Open Burning-area	102	6	38	192	544
-point	0	0	0	0	1
Auto Body Incineration-point	0	0	0	0	0
Other-point	0	0	0	0	0
Miscellaneous-point	0	0	0	0	0
TRANSPORTATION-AREA	6,694	5,644	69,559	61,242	310,462
Land Vehicles	6,215	5,510	68,907	53,122	303,503
Gasoline	3,375	944	30,775	47,058	289,402
Light Vehicles	3,021	783	26,774	36,823	199,316
Heavy Vehicles	170	65	1,906	4,329	23,134
Off Highway	184	96	2,094	5,905	66,951
Diesel Fuel	2,840	4,566	38,132	6,064	14,101
Heavy Vehicles	1,487	2,082	19,719	2,081	7,965
Off Highway	434	388	4,804	526	1,354
Rail	920	2,096	13,609	3,457	4,781
Aircraft	479	126	616	1,635	3,051
Military	413	79	198	961	1,031
Civil	39	8	35	172	983
Commercial	27	39	383	503	1,037
Vessels	0	8	36	1,229	3,909
Bituminous Coal	0	0	0	0	0
Diesel Fuel	0	0	0	0	0
Residual Oil	0	0	0	0	0
Gasoline	0	8	36	1,229	3,909
Gas Handling Evaporation Loss	0	0	0	5,256	0
MISCELLANEOUS-AREA	75,538	0	13,662	108,670	457,626
Forest Fires	40,592	0	9,551	57,306	334,285
Structural Fires	0	0	0	0	0
Slash Burning	34,947	0	4,111	41,114	123,341
Frost Control	0	0	0	0	0
Solvent Evaporation Loss	0	0	0	10,250	0

NEBRASKA

Emission categories	Pollutant, tons per year				
	Particulates	Sulfur oxides	Nitrogen oxides	Hydro-carbons	Carbon monoxide
GRAND TOTAL	300,602	55,386	173,821	378,922	780,087
–AREA	14,086	11,729	113,603	145,889	765,828
–POINT	286,516	43,657	60,218	233,033	14,259
FUEL COMBUSTION–AREA	1,974	4,909	11,471	1,048	2,786
–POINT	10,649	32,705	47,250	438	2,641
External Combustion–area	1,974	4,909	11,471	1,048	2,786
–point	10,610	32,480	46,236	338	2,120
Residential Fuel–area	966	2,286	3,252	681	1,847
Anthracite Coal	0	0	0	0	0
Bituminous Coal	196	1,118	29	196	882
Distillate Oil	263	1,138	316	79	132
Residual Oil	0	0	0	0	0
Natural Gas	356	21	2,846	285	711
Wood	151	9	61	121	121
Electric Generation–point	6,365	30,242	40,769	145	1,663
Anthracite Coal	268	11,651	18,396	31	1,022
Bituminous Coal	5,953	17,497	9,747	82	274
Lignite	0	0	0	0	0
Residual Oil	25	716	350	7	10
Distillate Oil	19	365	271	5	8
Natural Gas	100	12	12,005	21	349
Process Gas	0	0	0	0	0
Coke	0	0	0	0	0
Solid Waste/Coal	0	0	0	0	0
Other	0	0	0	0	0
Industrial Fuel–area	412	1,358	3,790	94	332
–point	4,109	1,532	4,529	144	349
Anthracite Coal–area	0	0	0	0	0
–point	0	0	0	0	0
Bituminous Coal–area	0	0	0	0	0
–point	3,867	308	1,349	90	180
Lignite–point	0	0	0	0	0
Residual Oil–area	57	782	148	7	10
–point	85	767	220	13	14
Distillate Oil–area	196	566	786	39	52
–point	76	452	304	15	20
Natural Gas–area	159	10	2,857	48	270
–point	77	5	2,649	24	131
Process Gas–area	0	0	0	0	0
–point	0	0	0	0	0
Coke–point	0	0	0	0	0
Wood–area	0	0	0	0	0
–point	4	1	4	2	4
Liquid Petroleum Gas–point	0	0	1	0	0
Bagasse–point	0	0	0	0	0
Other–point	0	0	0	0	0
Commercial-Institutional Fuel–area	596	1,264	4,429	273	607
–point	136	706	938	49	108
Anthracite Coal–area	0	0	0	0	0
–point	0	0	0	0	0
Bituminous Coal–area	0	0	0	0	0
–point	12	1	2	0	0
Lignite–point	0	0	0	0	0
Residual Oil–area	26	355	67	3	4
–point	29	343	73	4	5
Distillate Oil–area	310	894	1,241	62	83
–point	48	359	191	10	13
Natural Gas–area	260	16	3,121	208	520
–point	47	3	672	36	90
Wood–area	0	0	0	0	0
–point	0	0	0	0	0
Liquid Petroleum Gas–point	0	0	0	0	0
Miscellaneous–point	0	0	0	0	0
Internal Combustion–point	38	225	1,014	100	521
Electric Generation	38	225	1,005	100	519
Distillate Oil	2	60	24	2	5
Natural Gas	7	0	201	20	56
Diesel Fuel	29	165	780	77	457
Industrial Fuel	1	0	10	1	2
Distillate Oil	1	0	10	1	2
Natural Gas	0	0	0	0	0
Gasoline	0	0	0	0	0
Diesel Fuel	0	0	0	0	0

Emission categories	Pollutant, tons per year				
	Particulates	Sulfur oxides	Nitrogen oxides	Hydro-carbons	Carbon monoxide
Other..	0	0	0	0	0
Commercial-Institutional........................	0	0	0	0	0
Diesel Fuel	0	0	0	0	0
Other..	0	0	0	0	0
Engine-Testing................................	0	0	0	0	0
Aircraft......................................	0	0	0	0	0
Other..	0	0	0	0	0
Miscellaneous.................................	0	0	0	0	0
INDUSTRIAL PROCESS-POINT	275,700	10,929	12,897	232,344	10,905
Chemical Manufacturing	22	0	370	14,202	259
Food/Agriculture	212,402	0	1	2	14
Primary Metal................................	0	0	0	0	0
Secondary Metals.............................	6,554	6,681	14	0	2,127
Mineral Products.............................	56,448	4,056	1,039	1	1
Petroleum Industry...........................	4	163	23	73	4,521
Wood Products...............................	0	0	0	0	0
Evaporation	0	0	0	141,402	0
Metal Fabrication.............................	269	30	11,450	76,666	3,983
Leather Products.............................	0	0	0	0	0
Textile Manufacturing.........................	0	0	0	0	0
Inprocess Fuel................................	0	0	0	0	0
Other/Not Classified	0	0	0	0	0
SOLID WASTE DISPOSAL-AREA..............	890	56	334	1,668	4,726
-POINT...........................	168	22	71	251	713
Government-point.............................	118	7	44	222	628
Municipal Incineration........................	0	0	0	0	0
Open Burning.................................	118	7	44	222	628
Other	0	0	0	0	0
Residential-area..............................	890	56	334	1,668	4,726
On Site Incineration..........................	0	0	0	0	0
Open Burning.................................	890	56	334	1,668	4,726
Commercial-Institutional-area.................	0	0	0	0	0
-point.................	17	5	14	10	21
On Site Incineration-area.....................	0	0	0	0	0
-point....................	12	5	12	10	19
Open Burning-area	0	0	0	0	0
-point...........................	0	0	0	0	1
Apartment-point..............................	0	0	0	0	0
Other-point	4	0	2	0	0
Industrial-area...............................	0	0	0	0	0
-point...............................	32	10	13	19	65
On Site Incineration-area.....................	0	0	0	0	0
-point....................	26	10	11	13	40
Open Burning-area	0	0	0	0	0
-point...........................	7	0	1	6	26
Auto Body Incineration-point	0	0	0	0	0
Other-point	0	0	0	0	0
Miscellaneous-point	0	0	0	0	0
TRANSPORTATION-AREA....................	10,391	6,764	101,700	137,741	755,381
Land Vehicles................................	9,867	6,609	100,933	124,177	746,153
Gasoline	7,118	2,078	64,678	117,591	731,081
Light Vehicles............................	5,520	1,431	47,250	72,158	424,750
Heavy Vehicles	1,313	498	14,183	36,281	202,580
Off Highway..............................	285	149	3,246	9,151	103,752
Diesel Fuel...............................	2,749	4,531	36,255	6,586	15,072
Heavy Vehicles	1,014	1,419	12,842	1,614	7,315
Off Highway..............................	610	546	6,756	740	1,904
Rail......................................	1,126	2,566	16,657	4,232	5,853
Aircraft	515	133	637	1,745	3,441
Military..................................	436	83	209	1,014	1,088
Civil.....................................	52	10	47	231	1,321
Commercial...............................	27	39	381	500	1,031
Vessels...................................	8	22	129	1,832	5,787
Bituminous Coal	0	0	0	0	0
Diesel Fuel...............................	8	10	76	20	27
Residual Oil..............................	0	0	0	0	0
Gasoline	0	12	53	1,812	5,760
Gas Handling Evaporation Loss...............	0	0	0	9,988	0
MISCELLANEOUS-AREA.....................	832	0	98	5,431	2,935
Forest Fires.................................	0	0	0	0	0
Structural Fires..............................	0	0	0	0	0
Slash Burning	832	0	98	978	2,935
Frost Control................................	0	0	0	0	0
Solvent Evaporation Loss.....................	0	0	0	4,453	0

NEVADA

Emission categories	Pollutant, tons per year				
	Particulates	Sulfur oxides	Nitrogen oxides	Hydro-carbons	Carbon monoxide
GRAND TOTAL	119,193	342,314	141,112	53,429	233,651
-AREA	5,777	3,719	35,827	48,267	219,260
-POINT	113,417	338,595	105,285	5,163	14,391
FUEL COMBUSTION-AREA	698	1,319	2,593	311	501
-POINT	6,949	62,472	102,444	1,094	3,591
External Combustion-area	698	1,319	2,593	311	501
-point	6,939	62,472	102,180	1,068	3,518
Residential Fuel-area	320	348	610	198	283
Anthracite Coal	0	0	0	0	0
Bituminous Coal	0	0	0	0	0
Distillate Oil	116	335	140	35	58
Residual Oil	0	0	0	0	0
Natural Gas	51	3	409	41	102
Wood	153	9	61	122	122
Electric Generation-point	6,740	60,780	99,861	949	3,384
Anthracite Coal	0	0	0	0	0
Bituminous Coal	6,558	60,171	88,966	922	3,075
Lignite	0	0	0	0	0
Residual Oil	34	594	444	8	13
Distillate Oil	0	4	13	0	0
Natural Gas	148	10	10,437	17	296
Process Gas	0	0	0	0	0
Coke	0	0	0	0	0
Solid Waste/Coal	0	0	0	0	0
Other	0	0	0	0	0
Industrial Fuel-area	140	458	506	25	34
-point	196	1,673	2,295	118	133
Anthracite Coal-area	0	0	0	0	0
-point	0	0	0	0	0
Bituminous Coal-area	0	0	0	0	0
-point	138	1,399	750	50	100
Lignite-point	0	0	0	0	0
Residual Oil-area	38	262	99	5	7
-point	2	28	0	0	0
Distillate Oil-area	102	195	407	20	27
-point	2	8	10	0	1
Natural Gas-area	0	0	0	0	0
-point	53	238	1,535	67	32
Process Gas-area	0	0	0	0	0
-point	0	0	0	0	0
Coke-point	0	0	0	0	0
Wood-area	0	0	0	0	0
-point	0	0	0	0	0
Liquid Petroleum Gas-point	0	0	0	0	0
Bagasse-point	0	0	0	0	0
Other-point	0	0	0	0	0
Commercial-Institutional Fuel-area	239	513	1,477	88	185
-point	4	20	24	1	2
Anthracite Coal-area	0	0	0	0	0
-point	0	0	0	0	0
Bituminous Coal-area	0	0	0	0	0
-point	0	0	0	0	0
Lignite-point	0	0	0	0	0
Residual Oil-area	38	262	99	5	7
-point	2	15	10	0	1
Distillate Oil-area	129	247	515	26	34
-point	1	5	15	1	1
Natural Gas-area	72	4	863	58	144
-point	0	0	0	0	0
Wood-area	0	0	0	0	0
-point	0	0	0	0	0
Liquid Petroleum Gas-point	0	0	0	0	0
Miscellaneous-point	0	0	0	0	0
Internal Combustion-point	10	0	264	27	73
Electric Generation	10	0	264	27	73
Distillate Oil	1	0	18	1	4
Natural Gas	8	0	247	25	69
Diesel Fuel	0	0	0	0	0
Industrial Fuel	0	0	0	0	0
Distillate Oil	0	0	0	0	0
Natural Gas	0	0	0	0	0
Gasoline	0	0	0	0	0
Diesel Fuel	0	0	0	0	0

Emission categories	Pollutant, tons per year				
	Particulates	Sulfur oxides	Nitrogen oxides	Hydro-carbons	Carbon monoxide
Other	0	0	0	0	0
Commercial-Institutional	0	0	0	0	0
Diesel Fuel	0	0	0	0	0
Other	0	0	0	0	0
Engine-Testing	0	0	0	0	0
Aircraft	0	0	0	0	0
Other	0	0	0	0	0
Miscellaneous	0	0	0	0	0
INDUSTRIAL PROCESS-POINT	106,358	274,173	501	1,728	3,000
Chemical Manufacturing	7	3,567	167	0	0
Food/Agriculture	25	0	0	0	0
Primary Metal	1,562	270,577	334	0	3,000
Secondary Metals	0	0	0	0	0
Mineral Products	104,748	29	0	0	0
Petroleum Industry	0	0	0	0	0
Wood Products	0	0	0	0	0
Evaporation	0	0	0	1,728	0
Metal Fabrication	0	0	0	0	0
Leather Products	0	0	0	0	0
Textile Manufacturing	0	0	0	0	0
Inprocess Fuel	8	0	0	0	0
Other/Not Classified	9	0	0	0	0
SOLID WASTE DISPOSAL-AREA	60	5	22	105	296
-POINT	109	1,950	2,340	2,340	7,800
Government-point	0	0	0	0	0
Municipal Incineration	0	0	0	0	0
Open Burning	0	0	0	0	0
Other	0	0	0	0	0
Residential-area	54	3	20	102	289
On Site Incineration	0	0	0	0	0
Open Burning	54	3	20	102	289
Commercial-Institutional-area	5	2	2	3	7
-point	109	1,950	2,340	2,340	7,800
On Site Incineration-area	5	2	2	3	7
-point	109	1,950	2,340	2,340	7,800
Open Burning-area	0	0	0	0	0
-point	0	0	0	0	0
Apartment-point	0	0	0	0	0
Other-point	0	0	0	0	0
Industrial-area	0	0	0	0	0
-point	0	0	0	0	0
On Site Incineration-area	0	0	0	0	0
-point	0	0	0	0	0
Open Burning-area	0	0	0	0	0
-point	0	0	0	0	0
Auto Body Incineration-point	0	0	0	0	0
Other-point	0	0	0	0	0
Miscellaneous-point	0	0	0	0	0
TRANSPORTATION-AREA	4,697	2,395	33,141	45,689	216,047
Land Vehicles	3,110	1,949	30,914	33,557	199,938
Gasoline	2,360	633	20,734	31,666	195,660
Light Vehicles	2,278	591	19,805	29,048	165,978
Heavy Vehicles	0	0	0	0	0
Off Highway	81	43	929	2,618	29,683
Diesel Fuel	750	1,316	10,180	1,891	4,278
Heavy Vehicles	340	476	4,362	523	2,287
Off Highway	69	62	762	83	215
Rail	342	779	5,056	1,285	1,776
Aircraft	1,587	431	2,163	5,468	9,148
Military	1,416	270	680	3,294	3,536
Civil	70	14	63	308	1,763
Commercial	101	147	1,420	1,865	3,849
Vessels	0	15	64	2,189	6,960
Bituminous Coal	0	0	0	0	0
Diesel Fuel	0	0	0	0	0
Residual Oil	0	0	0	0	0
Gasoline	0	15	64	2,189	6,960
Gas Handling Evaporation Loss	0	0	0	4,475	0
MISCELLANEOUS-AREA	322	0	70	2,161	2,416
Forest Fires	272	0	64	384	2,240
Structural Fires	0	0	0	0	0
Slash Burning	50	0	6	58	175
Frost Control	0	0	0	0	0
Solvent Evaporation Loss	0	0	0	1,718	0

NEW HAMPSHIRE

Emission categories	Pollutant, tons per year				
	Particulates	Sulfur oxides	Nitrogen oxides	Hydro-carbons	Carbon monoxide
GRAND TOTAL	17,536	93,436	79,289	88,366	271,969
-AREA	9,584	18,698	41,482	55,946	248,379
-POINT	7,952	74,738	37,807	32,420	23,590
FUEL COMBUSTION-AREA	3,628	17,267	8,293	959	1,567
-POINT	2,386	73,885	36,749	490	1,034
External Combustion-area	3,628	17,267	8,293	959	1,567
-point	2,369	73,856	36,523	471	983
Residential Fuel-area	1,429	3,118	1,638	604	981
Anthracite Coal	15	38	4	4	134
Bituminous Coal	0	0	0	0	0
Distillate Oil	1,062	3,059	1,274	319	531
Residual Oil	0	0	0	0	0
Natural Gas	29	2	230	23	57
Wood	324	19	130	259	259
Electric Generation-point	942	60,653	33,553	298	698
Anthracite Coal	0	0	0	0	0
Bituminous Coal	302	34,716	25,123	137	457
Lignite	0	0	0	0	0
Residual Oil	640	25,936	8,429	161	241
Distillate Oil	0	0	1	0	0
Natural Gas	0	0	0	0	0
Process Gas	0	0	0	0	0
Coke	0	0	0	0	0
Solid Waste/Coal	0	0	0	0	0
Other	0	0	0	0	0
Industrial Fuel-area	1,090	7,640	2,731	135	187
-point	1,230	10,678	2,439	147	249
Anthracite Coal-area	17	23	13	0	2
-point	0	1	0	0	1
Bituminous Coal-area	230	67	44	3	6
-point	22	33	5	17	76
Lignite-point	0	0	0	0	0
Residual Oil-area	529	6,953	1,381	69	92
-point	758	10,397	1,992	100	133
Distillate Oil-area	310	596	1,240	62	83
-point	28	230	113	6	8
Natural Gas-area	3	0	52	1	5
-point	5	0	213	1	8
Process Gas-area	0	0	0	0	0
-point	0	0	0	0	0
Coke-point	0	0	0	0	0
Wood-area	0	0	0	0	0
-point	418	17	116	23	23
Liquid Petroleum Gas-point	0	0	1	0	0
Bagasse-point	0	0	0	0	0
Other-point	0	0	0	0	0
Commercial-Institutional Fuel-area	1,109	6,509	3,924	220	399
-point	197	2,525	531	27	36
Anthracite Coal-area	22	30	11	0	7
-point	0	0	0	0	0
Bituminous Coal-area	145	95	38	8	30
-point	0	0	0	0	0
Lignite-point	0	0	0	0	0
Residual Oil-area	422	5,546	1,101	55	73
-point	185	2,397	483	24	32
Distillate Oil-area	433	832	1,733	87	116
-point	12	128	47	2	3
Natural Gas-area	87	5	1,040	69	173
-point	0	0	2	0	1
Wood-area	0	0	0	0	0
-point	0	0	0	0	0
Liquid Petroleum Gas-point	0	0	0	0	0
Miscellaneous-point	0	0	0	0	0
Internal Combustion-point	16	29	225	19	51
Electric Generation	16	29	225	19	51
Distillate Oil	16	29	222	18	50
Natural Gas	0	0	4	0	1
Diesel Fuel	0	0	0	0	0
Industrial Fuel	0	0	0	0	0
Distillate Oil	0	0	0	0	0
Natural Gas	0	0	0	0	0
Gasoline	0	0	0	0	0
Diesel Fuel	0	0	0	0	0

Emission categories	Pollutant, tons per year				
	Particulates	Sulfur oxides	Nitrogen oxides	Hydro-carbons	Carbon monoxide
Other	0	0	0	0	0
Commercial-Institutional	0	0	0	0	0
Diesel Fuel	0	0	0	0	0
Other	0	0	0	0	0
Engine-Testing	0	0	0	0	0
Aircraft	0	0	0	0	0
Other	0	0	0	0	0
Miscellaneous	0	0	0	0	0
INDUSTRIAL PROCESS-POINT	2,287	631	10	26,877	7,560
Chemical Manufacturing	0	0	0	6	0
Food/Agriculture	212	0	0	0	0
Primary Metal	0	0	0	0	0
Secondary Metals	0	0	0	0	0
Mineral Products	511	0	10	24	0
Petroleum Industry	0	0	0	0	0
Wood Products	1,517	630	0	0	7,560
Evaporation	1	0	0	26,702	0
Metal Fabrication	0	0	0	0	0
Leather Products	46	1	0	38	0
Textile Manufacturing	0	0	0	79	0
Inprocess Fuel	1	0	0	23	0
Other/Not Classified	0	0	0	5	0
SOLID WASTE DISPOSAL-AREA	2,080	161	512	4,292	12,436
-POINT	3,279	222	1,048	5,053	14,996
Government-point	3,279	222	1,048	5,053	14,996
Municipal Incineration	601	55	44	33	771
Open Burning	2,678	167	1,004	5,020	14,225
Other	0	0	0	0	0
Residential-area	1,731	72	381	3,976	11,630
On Site Incineration	780	12	24	2,192	6,577
Open Burning	951	59	357	1,784	5,053
Commercial-Institutional-area	318	80	119	297	761
-point	0	0	0	0	0
On Site Incineration-area	240	75	90	150	344
-point	0	0	0	0	0
Open Burning-area	78	5	29	147	417
-point	0	0	0	0	0
Apartment-point	0	0	0	0	0
Other-point	0	0	0	0	0
Industrial-area	31	10	12	20	45
-point	0	0	0	0	0
On Site Incineration-area	31	10	12	20	45
-point	0	0	0	0	0
Open Burning-area	0	0	0	0	0
-point	0	0	0	0	0
Auto Body Incineration-point	0	0	0	0	0
Other-point	0	0	0	0	0
Miscellaneous-point	0	0	0	0	0
TRANSPORTATION-AREA	3,725	1,270	32,648	48,528	233,400
Land Vehicles	3,387	1,191	32,341	42,242	228,328
Gasoline	3,127	853	28,997	41,880	227,164
Light Vehicles	2,809	728	25,362	33,719	177,739
Heavy Vehicles	285	108	3,263	7,114	37,554
Off Highway	33	17	371	1,047	11,872
Diesel Fuel	260	338	3,344	362	1,164
Heavy Vehicles	186	260	2,492	250	915
Off Highway	65	58	721	79	203
Rail	9	20	131	33	46
Aircraft	338	74	285	1,045	2,699
Military	261	50	125	607	651
Civil	71	14	64	313	1,789
Commercial	7	10	96	126	259
Vessels	0	5	22	746	2,372
Bituminous Coal	0	0	0	0	0
Diesel Fuel	0	0	0	0	0
Residual Oil	0	0	0	0	0
Gasoline	0	5	22	746	2,372
Gas Handling Evaporation Loss	0	0	0	4,493	0
MISCELLANEOUS-AREA	152	0	29	2,167	976
Forest Fires	106	0	25	150	872
Structural Fires	46	0	4	12	103
Slash Burning	0	0	0	0	0
Frost Control	0	0	0	0	0
Solvent Evaporation Loss	0	0	0	2,006	0

NEW JERSEY

Emission categories	Pollutant, tons per year				
	Particulates	Sulfur oxides	Nitrogen oxides	Hydro-carbons	Carbon monoxide
GRAND TOTAL	129,306	486,975	568,424	639,325	2,411,999
-AREA	73,057	111,368	346,996	446.152	2,269,396
-POINT	56,249	375,607	221,428	193,173	142,603
FUEL COMBUSTION-AREA	24,044	90,162	75,519	5,469	13,111
-POINT	27,217	303,266	192,747	3,697	7,452
External Combustion-area	24,044	90,162	75,519	5,469	13,111
-point	27,062	301,930	190,109	3,461	6,802
Residential Fuel-area	6,879	17,195	12,955	2,482	8,413
Anthracite Coal	446	1,149	134	112	4,015
Bituminous Coal	0	0	0	0	0
Distillate Oil	5,551	15,992	6,662	1,665	2,776
Residual Oil	0	0	0	0	0
Natural Gas	764	46	6,112	611	1,528
Wood	118	7	47	94	94
Electric Generation-point	16,642	272,358	165,048	2,356	4,862
Anthracite Coal	0	0	0	0	0
Bituminous Coal	13,727	147,324	60,529	564	1,879
Lignite	0	0	0	0	0
Residual Oil	2,847	123,866	90,291	1,720	2,580
Distillate Oil	24	1,156	2,839	54	81
Natural Gas	45	11	11,388	19	323
Process Gas	0	0	0	0	0
Coke	0	0	0	0	0
Solid Waste/Coal	0	0	0	0	0
Other	0	0	0	0	0
Industrial Fuel-area	6,973	21,179	26,604	1,130	1,951
-point	9,588	27,249	23,043	992	1,744
Anthracite Coal-area	0	0	0	0	0
-point	1,439	1,875	1,093	12	349
Bituminous Coal-area	989	321	127	8	17
-point	977	733	736	8	26
Lignite-point	0	0	0	0	0
Residual Oil-area	1,567	13,000	4,087	204	272
-point	6,877	23,874	18,508	923	1,226
Distillate Oil-area	4,081	7,838	16,325	816	1,088
-point	155	762	634	32	42
Natural Gas-area	337	20	6,066	101	573
-point	97	4	2,069	18	100
Process Gas-area	0	0	0	0	0
-point	0	0	0	0	0
Coke-point	0	0	0	0	0
Wood-area	0	0	0	0	0
-point	4	0	1	0	0
Liquid Petroleum Gas-point	0	0	1	0	0
Bagasse-point	0	0	0	0	0
Other-point	39	0	0	0	0
Commercial-Institutional Fuel-area	10,192	51,789	35,960	1,856	2,748
-point	832	2,323	2,018	112	195
Anthracite Coal-area	0	0	0	0	0
-point	90	22	11	0	4
Bituminous Coal-area	0	0	0	0	0
-point	266	560	311	21	41
Lignite-point	0	0	0	0	0
Residual Oil-area	5,137	42,625	13,401	670	893
-point	324	1,200	844	42	56
Distillate Oil-area	4,762	9,146	19,050	952	1,270
-point	122	540	490	24	33
Natural Gas-area	292	18	3,509	234	585
-point	31	2	362	24	61
Wood-area	0	0	0	0	0
-point	0	0	0	0	0
Liquid Petroleum Gas-point	0	0	0	0	0
Miscellaneous-point	0	0	0	0	0
Internal Combustion-point	155	1,335	2,638	236	651
Electric Generation	155	1,335	2,638	236	651
Distillate Oil	121	1,335	1,635	134	371
Natural Gas	34	0	1,003	102	279
Diesel Fuel	0	0	0	0	0
Industrial Fuel	0	0	0	0	0
Distillate Oil	0	0	0	0	0
Natural Gas	0	0	0	0	0
Gasoline	0	0	0	0	0
Diesel Fuel	0	0	0	0	0

Emission categories	Pollutant, tons per year				
	Particulates	Sulfur oxides	Nitrogen oxides	Hydro-carbons	Carbon monoxide
Other	0	0	0	0	0
Commercial-Institutional	0	0	0	0	0
Diesel Fuel	0	0	0	0	0
Other	0	0	0	0	0
Engine-Testing	0	0	0	0	0
Aircraft	0	0	0	0	0
Other	0	0	0	0	0
Miscellaneous	0	0	0	0	0
INDUSTRIAL PROCESS-POINT	28,414	72,069	28,503	188,792	133,652
Chemical Manufacturing	3,079	27,944	11,297	6,005	19,804
Food/Agriculture	223	0	5	2	0
Primary Metal	247	2	1	0	0
Secondary Metals	3,343	2,077	50	166	30,307
Mineral Products	12,659	3,505	402	124	0
Petroleum Industry	8,084	35,843	16,200	19,444	83,541
Wood Products	38	0	0	0	0
Evaporation	7	0	0	162,940	0
Metal Fabrication	20	0	0	1	0
Leather Products	0	0	0	0	0
Textile Manufacturing	0	0	0	0	0
Inprocess Fuel	685	2,696	548	100	0
Other/Not Classified	29	2	0	10	0
SOLID WASTE DISPOSAL-AREA	18,268	3,934	4,795	24,496	68,112
-POINT	619	272	179	684	1,499
Government-point	393	56	93	558	1,161
Municipal Incineration	245	47	37	281	375
Open Burning	148	9	56	278	786
Other	0	0	0	0	0
Residential-area	5,979	93	187	16,815	50,445
On Site Incineration	5,979	93	187	16,815	50,445
Open Burning	0	0	0	0	0
Commercial-Institutional-area	11,663	3,645	4,374	7,289	16,765
-point	29	4	4	27	43
On Site Incineration-area	11,663	3,645	4,374	7,289	16,765
-point	26	4	4	26	35
Open Burning-area	0	0	0	0	0
-point	3	0	0	1	8
Apartment-point	0	0	0	0	0
Other-point	0	0	0	0	0
Industrial-area	627	196	235	392	901
-point	197	212	82	99	295
On Site Incineration-area	627	196	235	392	901
-point	195	212	81	95	286
Open Burning-area	0	0	0	0	0
-point	2	0	1	3	9
Auto Body Incineration-point	0	0	0	0	0
Other-point	1	0	0	0	0
Miscellaneous-point	0	0	0	0	0
TRANSPORTATION-AREA	30,745	17,272	266,682	406,508	2,188,173
Land Vehicles	26,252	11,367	235,017	342,464	2,137,853
Gasoline	22,784	6,060	190,929	335,226	2,113,512
Light Vehicles	21,663	5,616	179,120	301,566	1,895,406
Heavy Vehicles	990	375	10,309	29,430	170,144
Off Highway	132	69	1,500	4,231	47,962
Diesel Fuel	3,468	5,307	44,088	7,238	24,341
Heavy Vehicles	2,323	3,252	28,634	3,954	19,220
Off Highway	401	359	4,443	486	1,252
Rail	744	1,696	11,011	2,797	3,869
Aircraft	1,243	345	1,798	4,484	8,502
Military	1,054	201	506	2,452	2,632
Civil	104	21	94	459	2,624
Commercial	86	124	1,198	1,574	3,247
Vessels	3,250	5,559	29,866	17,639	41,818
Bituminous Coal	0	0	0	0	0
Diesel Fuel	3,144	3,930	29,346	7,703	10,271
Residual Oil	105	1,562	228	16	8
Gasoline	0	67	292	9,920	31,539
Gas Handling Evaporation Loss	0	0	0	41,920	0
MISCELLANEOUS-AREA	0	0	0	9,679	0
Forest Fires	0	0	0	0	0
Structural Fires	0	0	0	0	0
Slash Burning	0	0	0	0	0
Frost Control	0	0	0	0	0
Solvent Evaporation Loss	0	0	0	9,679	0

NEW MEXICO

Emission categories	Pollutant, tons per year				
	Particulates	Sulfur oxides	Nitrogen oxides	Hydro-carbons	Carbon monoxide
GRAND TOTAL	132,114	426,227	219,869	143,116	503,918
-AREA	15,369	8,292	90,070	100,533	478,963
-POINT	116,745	417,935	129,799	42,583	24,955
FUEL COMBUSTION-AREA	2,124	2,429	8,077	1,367	2,026
-POINT	22,732	138,975	127,246	14,571	7,739
External Combustion-area	2,124	2,429	8,077	1,367	2,026
-point	22,210	136,494	118,260	1,530	5,315
Residential Fuel-area	1,390	161	2,025	1,103	1,336
Anthracite Coal	0	0	0	0	0
Bituminous Coal	0	0	0	0	0
Distillate Oil	18	79	22	6	9
Residual Oil	0	0	0	0	0
Natural Gas	191	11	1,531	153	383
Wood	1,180	71	472	944	944
Electric Generation-point	22,053	129,043	113,590	1,460	5,091
Anthracite Coal	0	0	0	0	0
Bituminous Coal	21,713	126,492	99,130	1,408	4,680
Lignite	0	0	0	0	0
Residual Oil	109	2,318	1,437	27	41
Distillate Oil	16	220	205	4	6
Natural Gas	214	13	12,819	21	364
Process Gas	0	0	0	0	0
Coke	0	0	0	0	0
Solid Waste/Coal	0	0	0	0	0
Other	0	0	0	0	0
Industrial Fuel-area	352	1,603	3,046	77	266
-point	147	7,436	4,572	50	205
Anthracite Coal-area	0	0	0	0	0
-point	0	0	0	0	0
Bituminous Coal-area	0	0	0	0	0
-point	0	0	0	0	0
Lignite-point	0	0	0	0	0
Residual Oil-area	86	1,191	225	11	15
-point	0	0	0	0	0
Distillate Oil-area	141	404	564	28	38
-point	17	150	68	2	2
Natural Gas-area	125	8	2,257	38	213
-point	119	7,175	4,361	35	203
Process Gas-area	0	0	0	0	0
-point	9	111	133	13	0
Coke-point	0	0	0	0	0
Wood-area	0	0	0	0	0
-point	0	0	0	0	0
Liquid Petroleum Gas-point	2	0	10	0	0
Bagasse-point	0	0	0	0	0
Other-point	0	0	0	0	0
Commercial-Institutional Fuel-area	381	665	3,006	188	424
-point	11	15	98	20	20
Anthracite Coal-area	0	0	0	0	0
-point	0	0	0	0	0
Bituminous Coal-area	0	0	0	0	0
-point	0	0	0	0	0
Lignite-point	0	0	0	0	0
Residual Oil-area	9	122	23	1	2
-point	0	0	0	0	0
Distillate Oil-area	186	532	744	37	50
-point	0	0	0	0	0
Natural Gas-area	187	11	2,239	149	373
-point	0	0	0	0	0
Wood-area	0	0	0	0	0
-point	11	15	98	20	20
Liquid Petroleum Gas-point	0	0	0	0	0
Miscellaneous-point	0	0	0	0	0
Internal Combustion-point	521	2,481	8,986	13,041	2,424
Electric Generation	34	41	1,757	720	193
Distillate Oil	7	20	54	11	11
Natural Gas	4	0	69	18	17
Diesel Fuel	9	10	157	224	73
Industrial Fuel	487	2,440	7,229	12,321	2,231
Distillate Oil	60	98	1,182	119	179
Natural Gas	380	2,340	5,379	12,121	525
Gasoline	1	1	19	30	729
Diesel Fuel	46	1	648	52	141

Emission categories	Pollutant, tons per year				
	Particulates	Sulfur oxides	Nitrogen oxides	Hydro-carbons	Carbon monoxide
Other..	0	0	0	0	657
Commercial-Institutional..........................	0	0	0	0	0
Diesel Fuel	0	0	0	0	0
Other..	0	0	0	0	0
Engine-Testing..................................	0	0	0	0	0
Aircraft......................................	0	0	0	0	0
Other..	0	0	0	0	0
Miscellaneous.....................................	0	0	0	0	0
INDUSTRIAL PROCESS-POINT..................	93,338	278,882	2,454	26,947	4,780
Chemical Manufacturing	131	45,322	0	0	0
Food/Agriculture.................................	21	0	0	0	0
Primary Metal....................................	1,344	145,000	0	0	0
Secondary Metals.................................	0	0	0	0	0
Mineral Products.................................	91,551	2,009	513	0	0
Petroleum Industry...............................	270	86,550	1,940	1,945	4,780
Wood Products...................................	0	0	0	0	0
Evaporation	0	0	0	25,002	0
Metal Fabrication................................	0	0	0	0	0
Leather Products.................................	0	0	0	0	0
Textile Manufacturing............................	0	0	0	0	0
Inprocess Fuel...................................	21	0	1	0	0
Other/Not Classified	0	0	0	0	0
SOLID WASTE DISPOSAL-AREA..............	2,665	206	870	5,065	14,451
-POINT..............	676	79	99	1,065	12,436
Government-point.................................	9	1	3	17	48
Municipal Incineration...........................	0	0	0	0	0
Open Burning....................................	9	1	3	17	48
Other...	0	0	0	0	0
Residential-area..................................	1,091	51	280	2,398	6,972
On Site Incineration.............................	376	6	12	1,057	3,172
Open Burning....................................	715	45	268	1,341	3,800
Commercial-Institutional-area.....................	1,444	127	541	2,522	7,097
-point	0	0	0	0	0
On Site Incineration-area........................	148	46	55	92	212
-point...............	0	0	0	0	0
Open Burning-area	1,296	81	486	2,430	6,885
-point...............	0	0	0	0	0
Apartment-point	0	0	0	0	0
Other-point......................................	0	0	0	0	0
Industrial-area...................................	130	28	49	144	382
-point....................................	667	78	95	1,048	12,387
On Site Incineration-area........................	80	25	30	50	114
-point.......................	667	78	95	1,048	12,387
Open Burning-area	50	3	19	95	268
-point.............................	0	0	0	0	0
Auto Body Incineration-point	0	0	0	0	0
Other-point	0	0	0	0	0
Miscellaneous-point	0	0	0	0	0
TRANSPORTATION-AREA......................	9,151	5,656	80,819	89,009	452,020
Land Vehicles....................................	7,830	5,356	79,725	76,482	441,220
Gasoline......................................	5,338	1,419	46,998	71,016	428,013
Light Vehicles...............................	5,193	1,346	45,328	66,546	381,414
Heavy Vehicles	27	10	319	661	3,416
Off Highway................................	118	62	1,351	3,809	43,183
Diesel Fuel	2,492	3,937	32,727	5,466	13,207
Heavy Vehicles	1,104	1,546	14,260	1,669	7,148
Off Highway................................	558	500	6,188	678	1,744
Rail...	830	1,892	12,278	3,119	4,314
Aircraft	1,320	289	1,042	3,617	5,195
Military......................................	1,253	239	602	2,915	3,129
Civil...	38	8	34	169	966
Commercial...................................	29	42	406	533	1,100
Vessels..	0	12	52	1,763	5,606
Bituminous Coal	0	0	0	0	0
Diesel Fuel	0	0	0	0	0
Residual Oil..................................	0	0	0	0	0
Gasoline	0	12	52	1,763	5,606
Gas Handling Evaporation Loss	0	0	0	7,148	0
MISCELLANEOUS-AREA	1,430	0	304	5,091	10,465
Forest Fires.....................................	1,211	0	285	1,709	9,970
Structural Fires..................................	219	0	19	57	496
Slash Burning	0	0	0	0	0
Frost Control....................................	0	0	0	0	0
Solvent Evaporation Loss.........................	0	0	0	3,325	0

NEW YORK

Emission categories	Pollutant, tons per year				
	Particulates	Sulfur oxides	Nitrogen oxides	Hydro-carbons	Carbon monoxide
GRAND TOTAL	280,825	1,033,251	996,740	1,116,330	4,949,33
-AREA	155,248	277,775	692,545	1,109,156	4,936,51
-POINT	125,577	755,476	304,195	7,174	12,81
FUEL COMBUSTION-AREA	75,601	243,299	196,406	15,105	41,92
-POINT	106,871	474,196	270,962	5,768	12,56
External Combustion-area	75,601	243,299	196,406	15,105	41,92
-point	105,750	472,406	253,153	4,211	8,27
Residential Fuel-area	25,274	64,169	45,117	7,472	30,51
Anthracite Coal	2,051	5,284	615	513	18,46
Bituminous Coal	52	249	8	52	23
Distillate Oil	11,378	32,779	13,654	3,414	5,68
Residual Oil	8,871	25,681	15,428	1,157	1,54
Natural Gas	1,874	112	14,993	1,499	3,74
Wood	1,046	63	419	837	83
Electric Generation-point	96,204	447,799	245,779	3,889	7,75
Anthracite Coal	0	0	0	0	
Bituminous Coal	88,148	155,214	57,053	709	2,36
Lignite	0	0	0	0	
Residual Oil	7,802	292,550	164,808	3,139	4,70
Distillate Oil	0	12	30	1	
Natural Gas	254	24	23,887	40	67
Process Gas	0	0	0	0	
Coke	0	0	0	0	(
Solid Waste/Coal	0	0	0	0	(
Other	0	0	0	0	(
Industrial Fuel-area	18,733	88,196	55,829	2,782	3,73
-point	4,586	5,943	1,484	37	8
Anthracite Coal-area	5	18	10	0	(
-point	0	0	0	0	(
Bituminous Coal-area	0	0	0	0	(
-point	4,417	4,249	794	13	4
Lignite-point	0	0	0	0	
Residual Oil-area	13,868	78,873	36,178	1,809	2,41
-point	155	1,608	405	20	2
Distillate Oil-area	4,844	9,304	19,378	969	1,29
-point	10	85	39	2	
Natural Gas-area	15	1	264	4	2
-point	4	0	246	1	
Process Gas-area	0	0	0	0	(
-point	0	0	0	0	(
Coke-point	0	0	0	0	(
Wood-area	0	0	0	0	(
-point	0	0	0	0	(
Liquid Petroleum Gas-point	0	0	0	0	(
Bagasse-point	0	0	0	0	(
Other-point	0	0	0	0	(
Commercial-Institutional Fuel-area	31,595	90,934	95,460	4,851	7,684
-point	4,961	18,664	5,891	285	44
Anthracite Coal-area	994	3,350	1,243	25	746
-point	2	3	1	0	
Bituminous Coal-area	1,062	1,159	112	24	88
-point	3,008	1,741	469	13	74
Lignite-point	0	0	0	0	
Residual Oil-area	20,046	69,087	52,293	2,615	3,48
-point	1,720	15,891	4,488	224	299
Distillate Oil-area	9,013	17,309	36,051	1,803	2,403
-point	228	1,028	908	45	6
Natural Gas-area	480	29	5,761	384	960
-point	3	0	26	2	
Wood-area	0	0	0	0	(
-point	0	0	0	0	(
Liquid Petroleum Gas-point	0	0	0	0	(
Miscellaneous-point	0	0	0	0	(
Internal Combustion-point	1,120	1,790	17,808	1,558	4,29
Electric Generation	1,120	1,790	17,808	1,558	4,29
Distillate Oil	956	1,720	12,966	1,065	2,945
Natural Gas	164	69	4,842	492	1,348
Diesel Fuel	0	0	0	0	0
Industrial Fuel	0	0	0	0	0
Distillate Oil	0	0	0	0	0
Natural Gas	0	0	0	0	0
Gasoline	0	0	0	0	C
Diesel Fuel	0	0	0	0	C

Emission categories	Pollutant, tons per year				
	Particulates	Sulfur oxides	Nitrogen oxides	Hydro- carbons	Carbon monoxide
Other..	0	0	0	0	0
Commercial-Institutional.................................	0	0	0	0	0
Diesel Fuel	0	0	0	0	0
Other..	0	0	0	0	0
Engine-Testing...	0	0	0	0	0
Aircraft..	0	0	0	0	0
Other..	0	0	0	0	0
Miscellaneous...	0	0	0	0	0
INDUSTRIAL PROCESS-POINT	18,596	281,265	33,221	1,333	109
Chemical Manufacturing....................................	289	0	0	90	106
Food/Agriculture..	78	0	0	116	3
Primary Metal..	0	0	0	0	0
Secondary Metals...	143	0	0	0	0
Mineral Products..	18,071	281,265	33,221	0	0
Petroleum Industry...	0	0	0	0	0
Wood Products...	6	0	0	0	0
Evaporation...	8	0	0	1,090	0
Metal Fabrication...	0	0	0	0	0
Leather Products..	0	0	0	0	0
Textile Manufacturing.......................................	0	0	0	37	0
Inprocess Fuel...	2	0	0	0	0
Other/Not Classified	0	0	0	0	0
SOLID WASTE DISPOSAL-AREA	23,874	2,777	7,894	40,506	114,305
-POINT	110	15	12	74	141
Government-point..	110	15	12	74	141
Municipal Incineration.......................................	110	15	12	73	141
Open Burning...	0	0	0	0	0
Other...	0	0	0	0	0
Residential-area..	15,817	844	4,873	32,545	93,656
On Site Incineration...	3,080	48	96	8,664	25,992
Open Burning...	12,737	796	4,776	23,882	67,664
Commercial-Institutional-area..............................	5,702	1,512	2,138	4,915	12,385
-point	0	0	0	0	0
On Site Incineration-area...................................	4,621	1,444	1,733	2,888	6,643
-point.............................	0	0	0	0	0
Open Burning-area..	1,081	68	405	2,027	5,742
-point..........................	0	0	0	0	0
Apartment-point...	0	0	0	0	0
Other-point..	0	0	0	0	0
Industrial-area..	2,355	421	883	3,046	8,264
-point..	0	0	0	0	0
On Site Incineration-area...................................	1,096	342	411	685	1,575
-point.............................	0	0	0	0	0
Open Burning-area..	1,259	79	472	2,361	6,690
-point..........................	0	0	0	0	0
Auto Body Incineration-point	0	0	0	0	0
Other-point..	0	0	0	0	0
Miscellaneous-point..	0	0	0	0	0
TRANSPORTATION-AREA...............................	55,773	31,698	488,244	838,943	4,780,283
Land Vehicles...	53,360	20,750	477,562	737,544	4,678,481
Gasoline...	48,272	13,181	413,394	727,113	4,645,304
Light Vehicles...	44,137	11,443	368,817	603,169	3,721,879
Heavy Vehicles	2,950	1,118	31,063	85,840	491,433
Off Highway...	1,185	620	13,514	38,104	431,991
Diesel Fuel...	5,088	7,569	64,168	10,431	33,177
Heavy Vehicles	2,916	4,083	35,959	4,959	24,081
Off Highway...	1,058	947	11,723	1,284	3,304
Rail..	1,114	2,540	16,485	4,188	5,792
Aircraft...	1,550	832	6,600	10,924	24,119
Military..	898	172	432	2,090	2,244
Civil..	226	45	204	999	5,708
Commercial...	426	615	5,965	7,835	16,167
Vessels...	863	10,116	4,082	24,815	77,684
Bituminous Coal	0	0	0	0	0
Diesel Fuel...	209	262	1,953	513	684
Residual Oil..	654	9,691	1,416	98	47
Gasoline...	0	164	712	24,204	76,953
Gas Handling Evaporation Loss	0	0	0	65,660	0
MISCELLANEOUS-AREA	0	0	0	214,602	0
Forest Fires...	0	0	0	0	0
Structural Fires..	0	0	0	0	0
Slash Burning..	0	0	0	0	0
Frost Control...	0	0	0	0	0
Solvent Evaporation Loss...................................	0	0	0	214,602	0

NORTH CAROLINA

Emission categories	Pollutant, tons per year				
	Particulates	Sulfur oxides	Nitrogen oxides	Hydro-carbons	Carbon monoxide
GRAND TOTAL	513,714	582,959	565,923	548,584	2,341,955
-AREA	118,582	68,117	325,723	466,139	2,195,558
-POINT	395,132	514,842	240,200	82,446	146,397
FUEL COMBUSTION-AREA	36,851	47,895	35,169	9,067	18,816
-POINT	155,731	492,618	232,733	6,407	14,723
External Combustion-area	36,851	47,895	35,169	9,067	18,816
-point	155,731	492,618	232,733	6,407	14,723
Residential Fuel-area	10,326	16,603	7,081	7,271	15,639
Anthracite Coal	0	0	0	0	0
Bituminous Coal	2,173	4,129	326	2,173	9,780
Distillate Oil	2,849	12,155	3,419	855	1,425
Residual Oil	0	0	0	0	0
Natural Gas	160	10	1,278	128	320
Wood	5,144	309	2,058	4,115	4,115
Electric Generation-point	120,309	401,600	192,677	3,136	10,327
Anthracite Coal	0	0	0	0	0
Bituminous Coal	120,141	400,630	187,723	3,056	10,185
Lignite	0	0	0	0	0
Residual Oil	1	8	75	1	2
Distillate Oil	154	962	4,104	78	117
Natural Gas	13	1	774	1	22
Process Gas	0	0	0	0	0
Coke	0	0	0	0	0
Solid Waste/Coal	0	0	0	0	0
Other	0	0	0	0	0
Industrial Fuel-area	20,462	10,399	10,385	780	1,514
-point	34,849	87,649	38,935	3,228	4,302
Anthracite Coal-area	0	0	0	0	0
-point	5	0	11	0	6
Bituminous Coal-area	19,519	9,525	3,760	251	501
-point	14,497	28,959	11,831	403	1,109
Lignite-point	4	3	1	0	• 1
Residual Oil-area	53	735	137	7	9
-point	3,350	55,338	10,579	525	698
Distillate Oil-area	30	88	122	6	8
-point	218	1,582	908	45	59
Natural Gas-area	342	21	6,160	103	582
-point	113	9	4,538	35	190
Process Gas-area	0	0	0	0	0
-point	0	0	0	0	0
Coke-point	3	96	13	0	2
Wood-area	518	31	207	414	414
-point	16,641	1,656	11,038	2,218	2,235
Liquid Petroleum Gas-point	1	4	8	0	1
Bagasse-point	0	0	0	0	0
Other-point	18	2	8	2	2
Commercial-Institutional Fuel-area	6,063	20,893	17,702	1,016	1,662
-point	573	3,369	1,121	42	94
Anthracite Coal-area	0	0	0	0	0
-point	0	0	0	0	0
Bituminous Coal-area	1,703	1,859	450	98	352
-point	400	1,285	518	13	47
Lignite-point	0	0	0	0	0
Residual Oil-area	626	8,720	1,633	82	109
-point	151	1,803	394	20	26
Distillate Oil-area	3,585	10,305	14,341	717	956
-point	16	281	64	3	4
Natural Gas-area	105	6	1,260	84	210
-point	6	0	145	7	17
Wood-area	44	3	18	35	35
-point	0	0	0	0	0
Liquid Petroleum Gas-point	0	0	0	0	0
Miscellaneous-point	0	0	0	0	0
Internal Combustion-point	0	0	0	0	0
Electric Generation	0	0	0	0	0
Distillate Oil	0	0	0	0	0
Natural Gas	0	0	0	0	0
Diesel Fuel	0	0	0	0	0
Industrial Fuel	0	0	0	0	0
Distillate Oil	0	0	0	0	0
Natural Gas	0	0	0	0	0
Gasoline	0	0	0	0	0
Diesel Fuel	0	0	0	0	0

Emission categories	Pollutant, tons per year				
	Particulates	Sulfur oxides	Nitrogen oxides	Hydro-carbons	Carbon monoxide
Other	0	0	0	0	0
Commercial-Institutional	0	0	0	0	0
Diesel Fuel	0	0	0	0	0
Other	0	0	0	0	0
Engine-Testing	0	0	0	0	0
Aircraft	0	0	0	0	0
Other	0	0	0	0	0
Miscellaneous	0	0	0	0	0
INDUSTRIAL PROCESS-POINT	236,834	21,978	6,806	73,030	113,307
Chemical Manufacturing	1,594	9,022	5,450	13,368	4
Food/Agriculture	5,323	0	1	3	5
Primary Metal	86	1,296	1	0	12,621
Secondary Metals	464	11	0	20	2,364
Mineral Products	179,921	3,976	1,114	66	156
Petroleum Industry	0	0	0	0	0
Wood Products	47,154	7,474	59	79	98,146
Evaporation	17	0	50	58,550	0
Metal Fabrication	8	0	18	28	0
Leather Products	2	0	0	0	0
Textile Manufacturing	107	0	18	552	1
Inprocess Fuel	2,152	199	96	257	10
Other/Not Classified	7	0	0	108	0
SOLID WASTE DISPOSAL-AREA	7,654	1,151	2,450	11,847	33,165
-POINT	2,567	246	661	3,009	18,368
Government-point	24	8	6	47	63
Municipal Incineration	24	8	6	47	63
Open Burning	0	0	0	0	0
Other	0	0	0	0	0
Residential-area	3,127	138	752	7,009	20,432
On Site Incineration	1,223	19	38	3,439	10,317
Open Burning	1,904	119	714	3,570	10,115
Commercial-Institutional-area	1,919	472	720	1,838	4,737
-point	38	4	8	16	83
On Site Incineration-area	1,409	440	528	881	2,025
-point	15	4	4	11	21
Open Burning-area	510	32	191	957	2,712
-point	21	0	3	5	63
Apartment-point	0	0	0	0	0
Other-point	2	0	1	0	0
Industrial-area	2,608	541	978	3,000	7,997
-point	2,505	234	647	2,946	18,221
On Site Incineration-area	1,512	473	567	945	2,174
-point	2,301	221	571	2,569	17,152
Open Burning-area	1,096	68	411	2,055	5,823
-point	203	13	75	377	1,069
Auto Body Incineration-point	0	0	0	0	0
Other-point	0	0	0	0	0
Miscellaneous-point	0	0	0	0	0
TRANSPORTATION-AREA	30,358	19,069	282,124	375,808	1,955,843
Land Vehicles	25,157	14,854	256,033	325,216	1,907,141
Gasoline	20,027	5,846	186,357	311,800	1,882,169
Light Vehicles	15,687	4,067	137,828	193,741	1,067,518
Heavy Vehicles	3,409	1,292	37,906	88,106	475,067
Off Highway	932	488	10,623	29,953	339,585
Diesel Fuel	5,130	9,008	69,676	13,416	24,972
Heavy Vehicles	1,305	1,827	17,204	1,866	7,392
Off Highway	1,111	995	12,315	1,348	3,471
Rail	2,713	6,186	40,156	10,202	14,109
Aircraft	2,708	648	2,811	8,566	17,121
Military	2,310	441	1,110	5,375	5,770
Civil	295	59	266	1,306	7,461
Commercial	103	148	1,435	1,885	3,890
Vessels	2,494	3,566	23,280	13,442	31,581
Bituminous Coal	0	0	0	0	0
Diesel Fuel	2,464	3,080	22,998	6,037	8,049
Residual Oil	29	436	64	4	2
Gasoline	0	50	218	7,401	23,529
Gas Handling Evaporation Loss	0	0	0	28,583	0
MISCELLANEOUS-AREA	43,718	2	5,980	69,417	187,735
Forest Fires	7,398	0	1,741	10,444	60,922
Structural Fires	1,084	2	94	281	2,450
Slash Burning	35,236	0	4,145	41,454	124,363
Frost Control	0	0	0	0	0
Solvent Evaporation Loss	0	0	0	17,238	0

NORTH DAKOTA

Emission categories	Pollutant, tons per year				
	Particulates	Sulfur oxides	Nitrogen oxides	Hydro-carbons	Carbon monoxide
GRAND TOTAL	85,067	79,696	98,284	71,522	411,208
–AREA	12,016	12,488	54,918	66,861	393,753
–POINT	73,051	67,209	43,365	4,660	17,455
FUEL COMBUSTION–AREA	6,571	9,248	4,430	2,335	9,361
–POINT	39,556	62,056	42,948	933	3,078
External Combustion–area	6,571	9,248	4,430	2,335	9,361
–point	39,556	62,056	42,948	933	3,078
Residential Fuel–area	2,629	4,874	1,537	2,171	9,028
Anthracite Coal	0	0	0	0	0
Bituminous Coal	1,902	2,169	285	1,902	8,561
Distillate Oil	625	2,699	750	187	312
Residual Oil	0	0	0	0	0
Natural Gas	61	4	486	49	121
Wood	41	2	17	33	33
Electric Generation–point	34,132	56,438	40,585	801	2,804
Anthracite Coal	0	0	0	0	0
Bituminous Coal	0	0	0	0	0
Lignite	34,092	56,418	39,635	796	2,735
Residual Oil	0	0	0	0	0
Distillate Oil	1	18	38	1	1
Natural Gas	40	2	912	4	67
Process Gas	0	0	0	0	0
Coke	0	0	0	0	0
Solid Waste/Coal	0	0	0	0	0
Other	0	0	0	0	0
Industrial Fuel–area	3,749	3,416	1,654	86	159
–point	2,210	4,245	1,723	84	177
Anthracite Coal–area	0	0	0	0	0
–point	0	0	0	0	0
Bituminous Coal–area	3,446	975	641	43	86
–point	0	0	0	0	0
Lignite–point	1,979	908	437	37	88
Residual Oil–area	263	2,361	685	34	46
–point	17	131	45	2	3
Distillate Oil–area	28	80	110	6	7
–point	193	3,204	772	39	51
Natural Gas–area	12	1	217	4	20
–point	20	1	468	6	35
Process Gas–area	0	0	0	0	0
–point	0	0	0	0	0
Coke–point	0	0	0	0	0
Wood–area	0	0	0	0	0
–point	0	0	0	0	0
Liquid Petroleum Gas–point	0	0	0	0	0
Bagasse–point	0	0	0	0	0
Other–point	0	0	0	0	0
Commercial-Institutional Fuel–area	193	957	1,239	77	174
–point	3,214	1,374	640	48	98
Anthracite Coal–area	0	0	0	0	0
–point	0	0	0	0	0
Bituminous Coal–area	0	0	0	0	0
–point	212	41	33	2	4
Lignite–point	2,982	1,274	587	45	92
Residual Oil–area	101	905	262	13	17
–point	4	48	10	1	1
Distillate Oil–area	17	48	67	3	4
–point	1	7	5	0	0
Natural Gas–area	76	5	910	61	152
–point	0	0	2	0	0
Wood–area	0	0	0	0	0
–point	0	0	0	0	0
Liquid Petroleum Gas–point	0	0	0	0	0
Miscellaneous–point	0	0	0	0	0
Internal Combustion–point	0	0	0	0	0
Electric Generation	0	0	0	0	0
Distillate Oil	0	0	0	0	0
Natural Gas	0	0	0	0	0
Diesel Fuel	0	0	0	0	0
Industrial Fuel	0	0	0	0	0
Distillate Oil	0	0	0	0	0
Natural Gas	0	0	0	0	0
Gasoline	0	0	0	0	0
Diesel Fuel	0	0	0	0	0

Emission categories	Pollutant, tons per year				
	Particulates	Sulfur oxides	Nitrogen oxides	Hydro-carbons	Carbon monoxide
Other	0	0	0	0	0
Commercial-Institutional	0	0	0	0	0
Diesel Fuel	0	0	0	0	0
Other	0	0	0	0	0
Engine-Testing	0	0	0	0	0
Aircraft	0	0	0	0	0
Other	0	0	0	0	0
Miscellaneous	0	0	0	0	0
INDUSTRIAL PROCESS-POINT	33,496	5,152	418	3,727	14,377
Chemical Manufacturing	62	1	0	0	0
Food/Agriculture	12,576	3	6	8	16
Primary Metal	0	0	0	0	0
Secondary Metals	18	0	0	0	151
Mineral Products	19,979	1	1	1	1
Petroleum Industry	1	5,144	405	3,710	14,193
Wood Products	0	0	0	0	0
Evaporation	0	0	0	0	0
Metal Fabrication	0	0	0	0	0
Leather Products	0	0	0	0	0
Textile Manufacturing	0	0	0	0	0
Inprocess Fuel	859	4	7	9	17
Other/Not Classified	0	0	0	0	0
SOLID WASTE DISPOSAL-AREA	207	65	78	129	297
-POINT	0	0	0	0	0
Government-point	0	0	0	0	0
Municipal Incineration	0	0	0	0	0
Open Burning	0	0	0	0	0
Other	0	0	0	0	0
Residential-area	0	0	0	0	0
On Site Incineration	0	0	0	0	0
Open Burning	0	0	0	0	0
Commercial-Institutional-area	183	57	69	114	263
-point	0	0	0	0	0
On Site Incineration-area	183	57	69	114	263
-point	0	0	0	0	0
Open Burning-area	0	0	0	0	0
-point	0	0	0	0	0
Apartment-point	0	0	0	0	0
Other-point	0	0	0	0	0
Industrial-area	24	8	9	15	34
-point	0	0	0	0	0
On Site Incineration-area	24	8	9	15	34
-point	0	0	0	0	0
Open Burning-area	0	0	0	0	0
-point	0	0	0	0	0
Auto Body Incineration-point	0	0	0	0	0
Other-point	0	0	0	0	0
Miscellaneous-point	0	0	0	0	0
TRANSPORTATION-AREA	5,095	3,175	50,397	62,517	383,732
Land Vehicles	4,696	3,065	49,838	56,339	377,098
Gasoline	2,996	964	29,055	53,599	369,888
Light Vehicles	1,935	502	17,112	23,714	129,214
Heavy Vehicles	642	243	7,170	16,424	88,065
Off Highway	419	219	4,774	13,461	152,609
Diesel Fuel	1,700	2,101	20,783	2,740	7,210
Heavy Vehicles	552	773	7,256	795	3,174
Off Highway	931	834	10,321	1,130	2,909
Rail	217	494	3,206	815	1,126
Aircraft	399	105	536	1,498	4,084
Military	276	53	132	641	688
Civil	101	20	91	446	2,548
Commercial	22	32	312	410	847
Vessels	0	5	24	802	2,550
Bituminous Coal	0	0	0	0	0
Diesel Fuel	0	0	0	0	0
Residual Oil	0	0	0	0	0
Gasoline	0	5	24	802	2,550
Gas Handling Evaporation Loss	0	0	0	3,879	0
MISCELLANEOUS-AREA	143	0	13	1,881	363
Forest Fires	7	0	2	10	56
Structural Fires	136	0	12	35	307
Slash Burning	0	0	0	0	0
Frost Control	0	0	0	0	0
Solvent Evaporation Loss	0	0	0	1,836	0

OHIO

Emission categories	Particulates	Sulfur oxides	Nitrogen oxides	Hydro-carbons	Carbon monoxide
GRAND TOTAL	2,028,090	3,347,838	1,186,261	1,117,174	5,624,951
–AREA	499,458	375,370	590,295	933,474	4,237,389
–POINT	1,528,632	2,972,468	595,966	183,700	1,387,562
FUEL COMBUSTION–AREA	411,538	344,508	118,851	12,567	37,705
–POINT	729,115	2,819,799	542,729	10,145	30,000
External Combustion–area	411,538	344,508	118,851	12,567	37,705
–point	729,100	2,819,777	542,502	10,039	29,960
Residential Fuel–area	9,019	22,063	23,637	6,403	23,258
Anthracite Coal	284	124	85	71	2,556
Bituminous Coal	3,112	14,388	467	3,112	14,004
Distillate Oil	2,557	7,367	3,069	767	1,279
Residual Oil	0	0	0	0	0
Natural Gas	2,472	148	19,779	1,978	4,945
Wood	594	36	238	475	475
Electric Generation–point	426,775	2,085,954	404,392	5,752	19,025
Anthracite Coal	657	6,353	855	13	488
Bituminous Coal	426,013	2,078,777	397,888	5,706	18,392
Lignite	0	0	0	0	0
Residual Oil	18	426	369	7	9
Distillate Oil	26	394	955	18	25
Natural Gas	60	3	3,723	6	98
Process Gas	0	0	601	1	17
Coke	0	0	0	0	0
Solid Waste/Coal	0	0	0	0	0
Other	0	0	0	0	0
Industrial Fuel–area	364,050	260,102	64,275	3,573	7,816
–point	290,018	709,628	133,262	4,003	10,023
Anthracite Coal–area	0	0	0	0	0
–point	8	739	63	1	36
Bituminous Coal–area	362,393	258,263	47,549	3,170	6,340
–point	278,297	648,675	103,730	3,586	9,033
Lignite–point	289	478	74	6	11
Residual Oil–area	0	0	0	0	0
–point	1,176	13,237	3,178	157	190
Distillate Oil–area	935	1,796	3,741	187	249
–point	104	314	1,087	54	69
Natural Gas–area	721	43	12,984	216	1,226
–point	912	1,185	23,213	186	657
Process Gas–area	0	0	0	0	0
–point	8,255	43,674	1,799	0	0
Coke–point	872	1,319	74	1	10
Wood–area	0	0	0	0	0
–point	105	7	44	12	17
Liquid Petroleum Gas–point	0	0	0	0	0
Bagasse–point	0	0	0	0	0
Other–point	0	0	0	0	0
Commercial-Institutional Fuel–area	38,469	62,343	30,939	2,590	6,631
–point	12,307	24,195	4,848	284	909
Anthracite Coal–area	0	0	0	0	0
–point	32	1,295	65	2	108
Bituminous Coal–area	32,816	52,059	5,866	1,275	4,591
–point	12,092	21,979	4,257	250	743
Lignite–point	39	111	13	3	10
Residual Oil–area	0	0	0	0	0
–point	100	690	261	13	17
Distillate Oil–area	5,345	10,266	21,381	1,069	1,425
–point	32	119	135	6	9
Natural Gas–area	308	18	3,692	246	615
–point	11	1	118	9	22
Wood–area	0	0	0	0	0
–point	0	0	0	0	0
Liquid Petroleum Gas–point	0	0	0	0	0
Miscellaneous–point	0	0	0	0	0
Internal Combustion–point	15	22	226	106	39
Electric Generation	1	13	23	2	8
Distillate Oil	1	13	15	1	3
Natural Gas	0	0	0	0	0
Diesel Fuel	0	1	7	1	4
Industrial Fuel	14	9	204	104	32
Distillate Oil	0	0	0	0	0
Natural Gas	0	0	0	0	0
Gasoline	4	0	59	92	0
Diesel Fuel	10	9	145	12	32

Emission categories	Pollutant, tons per year				
	Particulates	Sulfur oxides	Nitrogen oxides	Hydro-carbons	Carbon monoxide
Other	0	0	0	0	0
Commercial–Institutional	0	0	0	0	0
Diesel Fuel	0	0	0	0	0
Other	0	0	0	0	0
Engine–Testing	0	0	0	0	0
Aircraft	0	0	0	0	0
Other	0	0	0	0	0
Miscellaneous	0	0	0	0	0
INDUSTRIAL PROCESS–POINT	793,844	147,937	52,319	169,230	1,344,472
Chemical Manufacturing	11,168	11,950	2,346	61,368	27,011
Food/Agriculture	6,114	0	0	119	18
Primary Metal	375,263	35,164	1,747	26,624	148,449
Secondary Metals	14,690	4,699	13	189	218,707
Mineral Products	368,596	11,922	1,111	26	37
Petroleum Industry	10,033	56,794	37,226	18,790	938,662
Wood Products	1,581	465	0	0	6,510
Evaporation	0	0	0	51,836	0
Metal Fabrication	13	1,068	22	5	0
Leather Products	0	0	0	0	0
Textile Manufacturing	11	0	0	2,858	0
Inprocess Fuel	3,273	9,976	2,621	6,198	5,019
Other/Not Classified	3,105	15,899	7,233	1,217	58
SOLID WASTE DISPOSAL–AREA	32,651	3,006	8,648	63,749	183,585
–POINT	5,672	4,731	918	4,325	13,090
Government–point	4,246	647	699	3,367	9,326
Municipal Incineration	3,767	618	519	2,469	6,781
Open Burning	479	30	180	898	2,545
Other	0	0	0	0	0
Residential–area	23,247	962	5,121	53,396	156,193
On Site Incineration	10,463	163	327	29,426	88,278
Open Burning	12,784	799	4,794	23,970	67,915
Commercial–Institutional–area	5,099	1,245	1,912	4,928	12,727
–point	187	23	32	210	1,147
On Site Incineration–area	3,706	1,158	1,390	2,316	5,327
–point	154	23	29	202	1,052
Open Burning–area	1,393	87	522	2,612	7,399
–point	32	0	4	8	95
Apartment–point	0	0	0	0	0
Other–point	0	0	0	0	0
Industrial–area	4,306	799	1,615	5,425	14,665
–point	1,240	4,061	186	749	2,617
On Site Incineration–area	2,119	662	795	1,324	3,046
–point	252	4,048	73	208	524
Open Burning–area	2,187	137	820	4,101	11,620
–point	975	13	113	537	2,078
Auto Body Incineration–point	13	0	1	3	16
Other–point	0	0	0	0	0
Miscellaneous–point	0	0	0	0	0
TRANSPORTATION–AREA	52,832	27,851	462,584	697,540	4,010,593
Land Vehicles	48,157	21,540	443,026	613,744	3,936,876
Gasoline	39,857	10,937	342,309	600,603	3,883,917
Light Vehicles	36,378	9,431	304,503	495,633	3,048,883
Heavy Vehicles	2,178	825	22,977	63,156	360,970
Off Highway	1,301	681	14,830	41,815	474,064
Diesel Fuel	8,300	10,603	100,717	13,141	52,959
Heavy Vehicles	5,670	7,939	70,739	9,379	44,279
Off Highway	2,406	2,153	26,657	2,918	7,513
Rail	224	512	3,321	844	1,167
Aircraft	1,750	517	3,019	7,646	23,442
Military	993	190	477	2,310	2,480
Civil	616	122	556	2,726	15,579
Commercial	142	205	1,986	2,609	5,383
Vessels	2,924	5,794	16,539	17,754	50,275
Bituminous Coal	1,177	2,942	177	1,177	5,296
Diesel Fuel	1,704	2,130	15,904	4,175	5,566
Residual Oil	43	638	93	6	3
Gasoline	0	84	365	12,395	39,409
Gas Handling Evaporation Loss	0	0	0	58,397	0
MISCELLANEOUS–AREA	2,437	5	212	159,619	5,505
Forest Fires	0	0	0	0	0
Structural Fires	2,437	5	212	632	5,505
Slash Burning	0	0	0	0	0
Frost Control	0	0	0	0	0
Solvent Evaporation Loss	0	0	0	158,987	0

OKLAHOMA

Emission categories	Pollutant, tons per year				
	Particulates	Sulfur oxides	Nitrogen oxides	Hydro-carbons	Carbon monoxide
GRAND TOTAL	140,967	109,699	244,764	391,672	1,708,984
–AREA	35,484	19,149	171,806	303,445	1,480,750
–POINT	105,484	90,550	72,957	88,228	228,233
FUEL COMBUSTION–AREA	4,006	10,235	18,895	2,064	3,516
–POINT	4,386	2,174	64,268	330	17,605
External Combustion–area	4,006	10,235	18,895	2,064	3,516
–point	4,363	2,062	63,756	170	2,013
Residential Fuel–area	1,857	141	4,397	1,482	2,060
Anthracite Coal	0	0	0	0	0
Bituminous Coal	0	0	0	0	0
Distillate Oil	7	30	8	2	3
Residual Oil	0	0	0	0	0
Natural Gas	480	29	3,841	384	960
Wood	1,370	82	548	1,096	1,096
Electric Generation–point	1,165	97	61,064	109	1,848
Anthracite Coal	0	0	0	0	0
Bituminous Coal	78	31	8	0	0
Lignite	0	0	0	0	0
Residual Oil	0	0	0	0	0
Distillate Oil	0	0	0	0	0
Natural Gas	1,087	65	61,056	108	1,847
Process Gas	0	0	0	0	0
Coke	0	0	0	0	0
Solid Waste/Coal	0	0	0	0	0
Other	0	0	0	0	0
Industrial Fuel–area	1,279	6,800	9,095	257	771
–point	131	1,966	2,684	61	163
Anthracite Coal–area	0	0	0	0	0
–point	0	0	0	0	0
Bituminous Coal–area	0	0	0	0	0
–point	0	0	0	0	0
Lignite–point	0	0	0	0	0
Residual Oil–area	456	5,357	1,189	59	79
–point	1	0	2	0	0
Distillate Oil–area	494	1,423	1,976	99	132
–point	12	114	65	2	1
Natural Gas–area	329	20	5,930	99	560
–point	109	1,852	2,616	58	161
Process Gas–area	0	0	0	0	0
–point	0	0	0	0	0
Coke–point	0	0	0	0	0
Wood–area	9	0	1	0	0
–point	0	0	0	0	0
Liquid Petroleum Gas–point	0	0	0	0	0
Bagasse–point	0	0	0	0	0
Other–point	0	0	0	0	0
Commercial-Institutional Fuel–area	870	3,293	5,403	324	685
–point	3,068	0	8	1	2
Anthracite Coal–area	0	0	0	0	0
–point	0	0	0	0	0
Bituminous Coal–area	0	0	0	0	0
–point	0	0	0	0	0
Lignite–point	0	0	0	0	0
Residual Oil–area	175	2,056	456	23	30
–point	0	0	0	0	0
Distillate Oil–area	424	1,221	1,695	85	113
–point	0	0	0	0	0
Natural Gas–area	271	16	3,251	217	542
–point	3,068	0	8	1	2
Wood–area	0	0	0	0	0
–point	0	0	0	0	0
Liquid Petroleum Gas–point	0	0	0	0	0
Miscellaneous–point	0	0	0	0	0
Internal Combustion–point	23	112	513	160	15,593
Electric Generation	15	72	436	44	134
Distillate Oil	0	0	1	0	0
Natural Gas	13	71	397	40	111
Diesel Fuel	1	1	37	4	23
Industrial Fuel	8	40	77	116	15,459
Distillate Oil	3	1	39	3	8
Natural Gas	5	38	38	113	15,451
Gasoline	0	0	0	0	0
Diesel Fuel	0	0	0	0	0

Emission categories	Pollutant, tons per year				
	Particulates	Sulfur oxides	Nitrogen oxides	Hydro-carbons	Carbon monoxide
Other	0	0	0	0	0
Commercial-Institutional	0	0	0	0	0
Diesel Fuel	0	0	0	0	0
Other	0	0	0	0	0
Engine-Testing	0	0	0	0	0
Aircraft	0	0	0	0	0
Other	0	0	0	0	0
Miscellaneous	0	0	0	0	0
INDUSTRIAL PROCESS-POINT	101,091	88,375	8,687	87,886	210,597
Chemical Manufacturing	2,018	25	0	2,538	27,414
Food/Agriculture	136	0	1	0	0
Primary Metal	2,174	54,419	120	0	0
Secondary Metals	205	965	0	0	457
Mineral Products	81,652	2,560	1,036	1	3
Petroleum Industry	4,979	27,673	6,966	20,518	156,834
Wood Products	3,018	0	0	0	0
Evaporation	0	0	151	56,788	0
Metal Fabrication	0	0	0	0	0
Leather Products	0	0	0	0	0
Textile Manufacturing	0	0	0	0	0
Inprocess Fuel	6,852	2,733	413	2,064	25,890
Other/Not Classified	58	0	0	5,977	0
SOLID WASTE DISPOSAL-AREA	9,807	613	3,678	18,389	52,101
-POINT	6	0	2	11	31
Government-point	6	0	2	11	31
Municipal Incineration	0	0	0	0	0
Open Burning	6	0	2	11	31
Other	0	0	0	0	0
Residential-area	9,807	613	3,678	18,389	52,101
On Site Incineration	0	0	0	0	0
Open Burning	9,807	613	3,678	18,389	52,101
Commercial-Institutional-area	0	0	0	0	0
-point	0	0	0	0	0
On Site Incineration-area	0	0	0	0	0
-point	0	0	0	0	0
Open Burning-area	0	0	0	0	0
-point	0	0	0	0	0
Apartment-point	0	0	0	0	0
Other-point	0	0	0	0	0
Industrial-area	0	0	0	0	0
-point	0	0	0	0	0
On Site Incineration-area	0	0	0	0	0
-point	0	0	0	0	0
Open Burning-area	0	0	0	0	0
-point	0	0	0	0	0
Auto Body Incineration-point	0	0	0	0	0
Other-point	0	0	0	0	0
Miscellaneous-point	0	0	0	0	0
TRANSPORTATION-AREA	20,987	8,300	149,174	265,278	1,423,588
Land Vehicles	15,177	7,103	145,611	228,691	1,389,402
Gasoline	12,484	3,703	112,958	224,395	1,373,646
Light Vehicles	8,894	2,306	74,696	120,435	736,249
Heavy Vehicles	3,337	1,265	35,378	95,827	545,199
Off Highway	253	132	2,884	8,132	92,198
Diesel Fuel	2,693	3,400	32,653	4,296	15,756
Heavy Vehicles	1,563	2,188	19,586	2,556	11,924
Off Highway	986	882	10,922	1,196	3,078
Rail	145	330	2,144	545	753
Aircraft	5,809	1,164	3,419	14,442	18,584
Military	5,655	1,080	2,716	13,156	14,122
Civil	112	22	101	496	2,832
Commercial	43	62	601	790	1,630
Vessels	0	33	144	4,907	15,602
Bituminous Coal	0	0	0	0	0
Diesel Fuel	0	0	0	0	0
Residual Oil	0	0	0	0	0
Gasoline	0	33	144	4,907	15,602
Gas Handling Evaporation Loss	0	0	0	17,238	0
MISCELLANEOUS-AREA	684	1	60	17,714	1,545
Forest Fires	0	0	0	0	0
Structural Fires	684	1	60	177	1,545
Slash Burning	0	0	0	0	0
Frost Control	0	0	0	0	0
Solvent Evaporation Loss	0	0	0	17,537	0

OREGON

Emission categories	Pollutant, tons per year				
	Particulates	Sulfur oxides	Nitrogen oxides	Hydro-carbons	Carbon monoxide
GRAND TOTAL	**147,909**	**41,532**	**198,111**	**290,495**	**1,188,700**
–AREA	**62,480**	**22,976**	**147,521**	**246,327**	**1,157,951**
–POINT	**85,428**	**18,555**	**50,590**	**44,168**	**30,749**
FUEL COMBUSTION–AREA	7,660	13,626	12,368	4,606	5,770
–POINT	26,439	10,184	33,320	8,867	7,391
External Combustion–area	7,660	13,626	12,368	4,606	5,770
–point	26,323	9,920	30,892	8,867	7,283
Residential Fuel–area	4,680	3,888	3,799	3,157	3,901
Anthracite Coal	0	0	0	0	0
Bituminous Coal	99	188	15	99	446
Distillate Oil	1,214	3,498	1,457	364	607
Residual Oil	0	0	0	0	0
Natural Gas	129	8	1,032	103	258
Wood	3,238	194	1,295	2,590	2,590
Electric Generation–point	29	381	675	6	19
Anthracite Coal	0	0	0	0	0
Bituminous Coal	0	0	0	0	0
Lignite	0	0	0	0	0
Residual Oil	8	154	103	2	3
Distillate Oil	13	227	166	3	5
Natural Gas	8	1	407	1	12
Process Gas	0	0	0	0	0
Coke	0	0	0	0	0
Solid Waste/Coal	0	0	0	0	0
Other	0	0	0	0	0
Industrial Fuel–area	2,294	8,092	5,957	1,292	1,600
–point	26,295	9,539	30,216	8,861	7,264
Anthracite Coal–area	0	0	0	0	0
–point	1	0	5	0	0
Bituminous Coal–area	0	0	0	0	0
–point	422	621	422	28	56
Lignite–point	0	0	0	0	0
Residual Oil–area	638	7,938	1,664	83	111
–point	725	6,634	3,087	242	80
Distillate Oil–area	29	56	116	6	8
–point	101	117	513	36	123
Natural Gas–area	200	12	3,605	60	341
–point	413	1,418	3,885	415	138
Process Gas–area	1	0	1	2	0
–point	3	0	39	9	0
Coke–point	0	0	0	0	0
Wood–area	1,426	86	571	1,141	1,141
–point	24,626	749	22,223	8,124	6,862
Liquid Petroleum Gas–point	3	0	43	7	4
Bagasse–point	0	0	0	0	0
Other–point	0	0	0	0	0
Commercial-Institutional Fuel–area	686	1,646	2,612	157	269
–point	0	0	0	0	0
Anthracite Coal–area	0	0	0	0	0
–point	0	0	0	0	0
Bituminous Coal–area	113	114	28	6	22
–point	0	0	0	0	0
Lignite–point	0	0	0	0	0
Residual Oil–area	53	660	138	7	9
–point	0	0	0	0	0
Distillate Oil–area	452	868	1,808	90	121
–point	0	0	0	0	0
Natural Gas–area	53	3	632	42	105
–point	0	0	0	0	0
Wood–area	15	1	6	12	12
–point	0	0	0	0	0
Liquid Petroleum Gas–point	0	0	0	0	0
Miscellaneous–point	0	0	0	0	0
Internal Combustion–point	116	264	2,428	0	108
Electric Generation	116	264	2,428	0	108
Distillate Oil	116	264	2,428	0	108
Natural Gas	0	0	0	0	0
Diesel Fuel	0	0	0	0	0
Industrial Fuel	0	0	0	0	0
Distillate Oil	0	0	0	0	0
Natural Gas	0	0	0	0	0
Gasoline	0	0	0	0	0
Diesel Fuel	0	0	0	0	0

Emission categories	Pollutant, tons per year				
	Particulates	Sulfur oxides	Nitrogen oxides	Hydro-carbons	Carbon monoxide
Other	0	0	0	0	0
Commercial-Institutional	0	0	0	0	0
Diesel Fuel	0	0	0	0	0
Other	0	0	0	0	0
Engine-Testing	0	0	0	0	0
Aircraft	0	0	0	0	0
Other	0	0	0	0	0
Miscellaneous	0	0	0	0	0
INDUSTRIAL PROCESS-POINT	54,446	8,305	16,615	34,105	2,204
Chemical Manufacturing	211	46	24	3,354	476
Food/Agriculture	3,228	0	0	0	0
Primary Metal	0	0	0	0	0
Secondary Metals	8,522	1,178	48	10	337
Mineral Products	5,755	377	869	42	9
Petroleum Industry	11	0	0	7	3
Wood Products	32,125	6,282	14,860	6,409	1,373
Evaporation	10	0	0	24,115	0
Metal Fabrication	0	0	0	0	0
Leather Products	0	0	0	0	0
Textile Manufacturing	0	0	0	0	0
Inprocess Fuel	3,608	397	814	68	6
Other/Not Classified	977	25	0	100	0
SOLID WASTE DISPOSAL-AREA	2,924	190	1,047	5,548	15,768
-POINT	4,543	66	655	1,196	21,154
Government-point	203	19	131	324	879
Municipal Incineration	52	9	74	41	79
Open Burning	151	10	57	283	800
Other	0	0	0	0	0
Residential-area	2,453	147	871	4,734	13,480
On Site Incineration	143	2	4	402	1,206
Open Burning	2,310	144	866	4,332	12,274
Commercial-Institutional-area	304	28	114	525	1,475
-point	89	4	141	46	167
On Site Incineration-area	36	11	13	22	51
-point	89	4	141	46	167
Open Burning-area	268	17	100	503	1,424
-point	0	0	0	0	0
Apartment-point	0	0	0	0	0
Other-point	0	0	0	0	0
Industrial-area	167	15	63	289	813
-point	4,251	43	383	826	20,108
On Site Incineration-area	19	6	7	12	27
-point	4,250	36	381	826	20,108
Open Burning-area	148	9	55	278	786
-point	0	0	0	0	0
Auto Body Incineration-point	0	0	0	0	0
Other-point	1	7	2	0	0
Miscellaneous-point	0	0	0	0	0
TRANSPORTATION-AREA	13,692	9,160	128,570	177,637	959,961
Land Vehicles	12,702	7,841	125,485	156,617	933,802
Gasoline	9,506	2,659	83,658	149,207	915,098
Light Vehicles	8,077	2,094	68,302	108,038	651,970
Heavy Vehicles	1,263	479	13,470	35,851	202,832
Off Highway	165	87	1,886	5,318	60,296
Diesel Fuel	3,196	5,182	41,827	7,410	18,704
Heavy Vehicles	1,430	2,003	17,966	2,326	10,791
Off Highway	611	547	6,771	741	1,908
Rail	1,155	2,633	17,090	4,342	6,005
Aircraft	814	271	1,738	3,985	12,240
Military	416	79	200	968	1,039
Civil	308	61	278	1,363	7,786
Commercial	90	130	1,260	1,655	3,415
Vessels	176	1,048	1,347	4,552	13,919
Bituminous Coal	0	0	0	0	0
Diesel Fuel	117	147	1,094	287	383
Residual Oil	59	872	127	9	4
Gasoline	0	29	125	4,256	13,532
Gas Handling Evaporation Loss	0	0	0	12,483	0
MISCELLANEOUS-AREA	38,205	1	5,535	58,537	176,452
Forest Fires	8,965	0	2,109	12,656	73,825
Structural Fires	451	0	39	117	1,020
Slash Burning	28,789	1	3,387	33,869	101,607
Frost Control	0	0	0	0	0
Solvent Evaporation Loss	0	0	0	11,895	0

PENNSYLVANIA

Emission categories	Pollutant, tons per year				
	Particulates	Sulfur oxides	Nitrogen oxides	Hydro-carbons	Carbon monoxide
GRAND TOTAL	876,861	3,017,782	1,227,190	811,992	4,360,272
–AREA	115,671	213,139	551,288	717,435	3,962,123
–POINT	761,190	2,804,642	675,902	94,556	398,150
FUEL COMBUSTION–AREA	64,777	170,947	102,086	13,247	120,808
–POINT	486,563	2,623,955	662,621	14,128	41,408
External Combustion–area	64,777	170,947	102,086	13,247	120,808
–point	486,277	2,620,505	658,598	13,831	40,518
Residential Fuel–area	23,056	60,189	24,926	9,994	114,323
Anthracite Coal	10,142	26,125	3,043	2,535	91,277
Bituminous Coal	3,509	13,335	526	3,509	15,792
Distillate Oil	7,148	20,593	8,578	2,144	3,574
Residual Oil	0	0	0	0	0
Natural Gas	1,563	94	12,502	1,250	3,125
Wood	694	42	278	555	555
Electric Generation–point	279,860	2,260,154	557,219	9,195	30,444
Anthracite Coal	20,494	27,187	11,507	129	2,644
Bituminous Coal	257,427	2,180,256	488,743	7,971	26,248
Lignite	0	0	0	0	0
Residual Oil	1,652	51,051	51,327	980	1,393
Distillate Oil	280	1,659	5,501	114	148
Natural Gas	6	0	141	1	10
Process Gas	0	0	0	0	0
Coke	0	0	0	0	0
Solid Waste/Coal	0	0	0	0	0
Other	0	0	0	0	0
Industrial Fuel–area	33,394	72,221	52,959	1,941	4,328
–point	199,880	353,976	98,207	4,413	9,558
Anthracite Coal–area	0	0	0	0	0
–point	4,664	4,066	2,032	32	952
Bituminous Coal–area	22,464	13,133	2,592	173	346
–point	185,841	279,725	57,068	2,543	5,587
Lignite–point	0	0	0	0	0
Residual Oil–area	7,800	55,401	20,347	1,017	1,356
–point	5,960	63,705	19,014	948	1,212
Distillate Oil–area	1,881	3,612	7,523	376	502
–point	358	2,870	2,330	116	154
Natural Gas–area	1,250	75	22,497	375	2,125
–point	1,090	151	14,948	146	821
Process Gas–area	0	0	0	0	0
–point	1,207	3,215	1,696	188	0
Coke–point	85	89	79	1	10
Wood–area	0	0	0	0	0
–point	675	156	1,041	438	822
Liquid Petroleum Gas–point	0	0	0	0	0
Bagasse–point	0	0	0	0	0
Other–point	0	0	0	0	0
Commercial–Institutional Fuel–area	8,327	38,537	24,200	1,311	2,157
–point	6,537	6,375	3,172	223	516
Anthracite Coal–area	0	0	0	0	0
–point	4,965	802	494	30	108
Bituminous Coal–area	1,363	1,786	216	47	169
–point	771	1,297	294	35	110
Lignite–point	0	0	0	0	0
Residual Oil–area	4,646	32,901	12,119	606	808
–point	665	4,056	1,384	69	86
Distillate Oil–area	1,994	3,830	7,978	399	532
–point	34	214	137	7	9
Natural Gas–area	324	19	3,887	259	648
–point	101	6	863	81	203
Wood–area	0	0	0	0	0
–point	0	0	0	0	0
Liquid Petroleum Gas–point	0	0	0	0	0
Miscellaneous–point	0	0	0	0	0
Internal Combustion–point	286	3,450	4,023	298	890
Electric Generation	263	2,927	3,813	276	735
Distillate Oil	250	2,898	3,592	256	614
Natural Gas	6	0	23	0	0
Diesel Fuel	7	29	199	20	121
Industrial Fuel	23	523	210	21	155
Distillate Oil	23	523	207	17	47
Natural Gas	0	0	0	0	0
Gasoline	0	0	3	4	108
Diesel Fuel	0	0	0	0	0

Emission categories	Pollutant, tons per year				
	Particulates	Sulfur oxides	Nitrogen oxides	Hydro- carbons	Carbon monoxide
Other..	0	0	0	0	0
Commercial-Institutional................................	0	0	0	0	0
Diesel Fuel..	0	0	0	0	0
Other...	0	0	0	0	0
Engine-Testing...	0	0	0	0	0
Aircraft..	0	0	0	0	0
Other...	0	0	0	0	0
Miscellaneous..	0	0	0	0	0
INDUSTRIAL PROCESS-POINT..................	265,669	179,272	12,124	79,265	337,180
Chemical Manufacturing.................................	2,925	2,666	1,687	8,913	14,612
Food/Agriculture..	3,722	624	0	11	94
Primary Metal...	49,147	146,801	707	7,221	86,483
Secondary Metals..	13,624	5,398	1,106	725	71,330
Mineral Products...	188,889	8,963	552	880	127
Petroleum Industry..	3,022	14,502	8,015	15,934	160,832
Wood Products..	3,661	263	0	· 0	3,702
Evaporation..	20	0	10	44,601	0
Metal Fabrication...	5	0	11	100	0
Leather Products...	0	0	0	0	0
Textile Manufacturing.....................................	542	38	0	875	0
Inprocess 'Fuel..	111	17	35	6	0
Other/Not Classified.......................................	2	0	0	0	0
SOLID WASTE DISPOSAL-AREA..............	1,115	312	376	966	2,465
-POINT.............	8,959	1,415	1,157	1,162	19,562
Government-point..	8,476	1,326	1,064	823	18,527
Municipal Incineration.................................	8,407	1,325	1,060	820	18,519
Open Burning..	2	0	1	3	8
Other...	68	1	3	1	0
Residential-area..	123	2	4	346	1,039
On Site Incineration.....................................	123	2	4	346	1,039
Open Burning..	0	0	0	0	0
Commercial-Institutional-area.........................	466	146	175	292	670
-point......................	7	6	7	8	26
On Site Incineration-area..............................	466	146	175	292	670
-point.............................	7	6	7	8	26
Open Burning-area.......................................	0	0	0	0	0
-point......................................	0	0	0	0	0
Apartment-point..	0	0	0	0	0
Other-point..	1	0	0	0	0
Industrial-area..	526	164	197	329	756
-point..	476	84	86	332	1,009
On Site Incineration-area..............................	526	164	197	329	756
-point.............................	345	77	64	222	659
Open Burning-area.......................................	0	0	0	0	0
-point......................................	107	3	22	109	350
Auto Body Incineration-point........................	0	0	0	0	0
Other-point..	24	4	1	1	0
Miscellaneous-point...	0	0	0	0	0
TRANSPORTATION-AREA..........................	49,779	41,881	448,827	687,696	3,838,849
Land Vehicles...	47,315	22,536	441,102	616,271	3,797,672
Gasoline..	39,930	10,938	345,600	600,654	3,747,332
Light Vehicles..	35,973	9,326	302,976	484,659	2,947,206
Heavy Vehicles......................................	3,181	1,205	33,772	91,034	517,135
Off Highway..	776	406	8,853	24,961	282,990
Diesel Fuel...	7,385	11,598	95,502	15,617	50,340
Heavy Vehicles......................................	5,103	7,144	63,740	8,414	39,597
Off Highway..	540	484	5,987	655	1,687
Rail...	1,742	3,971	25,774	6,548	9,056
Aircraft...	1,035	438	3,141	5,795	12,853
Military...	691	132	332	1,607	1,725
Civil..	154	31	139	681	3,892
Commercial..	191	275	2,670	3,507	7,237
Vessels..	1,429	18,907	4,584	9,314	28,325
Bituminous Coal..	0	0	0	0	0
Diesel Fuel..	172	215	1,605	421	562
Residual Oil..	1,257	18,633	2,723	189	91
Gasoline..	0	59	256	8,703	27,672
Gas Handling Evaporation Loss......................	0	0	0	56,317	'0
MISCELLANEOUS-AREA.............................	0	0	0	15,526	0
Forest Fires..	0	0	0	0	0
Structural Fires...	0	0	0	0	0
Slash Burning...	0	0	0	0	0
Frost Control..	0	0	0	0	0
Solvent Evaporation Loss................................	0	0	0	15,526	0

PUERTO RICO

Emission categories	Pollutant, tons per year				
	Particulates	Sulfur oxides	Nitrogen oxides	Hydro-carbons	Carbon monoxide
GRAND TOTAL	117,681	172,551	93,224	109,317	406,637
–AREA	25,065	20,068	46,137	83,495	369,497
–POINT	92,616	152,484	47,087	25,822	37,140
FUEL COMBUSTION–AREA	1,197	13,521	4,312	226	350
–POINT	27,732	114,145	36,733	2,188	2,882
External Combustion–area	1,197	13,521	4,312	226	350
–point	27,563	112,537	34,410	1,997	2,356
Residential Fuel–area	0	0	0	0	0
Anthracite Coal	0	0	0	0	0
Bituminous Coal	0	0	0	0	0
Distillate Oil	0	0	0	0	0
Residual Oil	0	0	0	0	0
Natural Gas	0	0	0	0	0
Wood	0	0	0	0	0
Electric Generation–point	2,023	88,462	26,988	510	773
Anthracite Coal	0	0	0	0	0
Bituminous Coal	0	1,091	431	4	14
Lignite	0	0	0	0	0
Residual Oil	1,970	87,110	25,859	493	739
Distillate Oil	53	261	699	13	20
Natural Gas	0	0	0	0	0
Process Gas	0	0	0	0	0
Coke	0	0	0	0	0
Solid Waste/Coal	0	0	0	0	0
Other	0	0	0	0	0
Industrial Fuel–area	820	11,574	2,430	121	162
–point	25,536	24,013	7,410	1,486	1,582
Anthracite Coal–area	0	0	0	0	0
–point	0	0	0	0	0
Bituminous Coal–area	0	0	0	0	0
–point	0	0	0	0	0
Lignite–point	0	0	0	0	0
Residual Oil–area	611	10,564	1,594	80	106
–point	1,911	21,679	5,006	250	334
Distillate Oil–area	209	1,009	836	42	56
–point	181	646	726	36	48
Natural Gas–area	0	0	0	0	0
–point	0	0	1	0	0
Process Gas–area	0	0	0	0	0
–point	0	1,688	0	0	0
Coke–point	0	0	0	0	0
Wood–area	0	0	0	0	0
–point	0	0	0	0	0
Liquid Petroleum Gas–point	0	0	0	0	0
Bagasse–point	23,443	0	1,200	1,200	1,200
Other–point	0	0	477	0	0
Commercial–Institutional Fuel–area	377	1,947	1,882	105	188
–point	4	62	11	1	1
Anthracite Coal–area	0	0	0	0	0
–point	0	0	0	0	0
Bituminous Coal–area	0	0	0	0	0
–point	0	0	0	0	0
Lignite–point	0	0	0	0	0
Residual Oil–area	30	517	78	4	5
–point	3	57	9	1	1
Distillate Oil–area	295	1,427	1,182	59	79
–point	1	5	2	0	0
Natural Gas–area	52	3	623	42	104
–point	0	0	0	0	0
Wood–area	0	0	0	0	0
–point	0	0	0	0	0
Liquid Petroleum Gas–point	0	0	0	0	0
Miscellaneous–point	0	0	0	0	0
Internal Combustion–point	169	1,608	2,323	191	526
Electric Generation	118	1,543	1,605	132	364
Distillate Oil	118	1,543	1,605	132	364
Natural Gas	0	0	0	0	0
Diesel Fuel	0	0	0	0	0
Industrial Fuel	51	65	718	59	162
Distillate Oil	24	33	323	27	73
Natural Gas	1	0	36	4	10
Gasoline	0	0	0	0	0
Diesel Fuel	26	32	359	29	78

Emission categories	Pollutant, tons per year				
	Particulates	Sulfur oxides	Nitrogen oxides	Hydro-carbons	Carbon monoxide
Other	0	0	0	0	0
Commercial-Institutional	0	0	0	0	0
Diesel Fuel	0	0	0	0	0
Other	0	0	0	0	0
Engine-Testing	0	0	0	0	0
Aircraft	0	0	0	0	0
Other	0	0	0	0	0
Miscellaneous	0	0	0	0	0
INDUSTRIAL PROCESS-POINT	64,708	38,328	10,288	23,306	33,327
Chemical Manufacturing	108	201	0	4,702	0
Food/Agriculture	816	0	0	0	0
Primary Metal	0	0	0	0	0
Secondary Metals	299	0	0	0	0
Mineral Products	59,438	15,899	2,871	0	0
Petroleum Industry	1,764	22,228	7,417	1,865	33,288
Wood Products	0	0	0	0	0
Evaporation	9	0	0	16,739	39
Metal Fabrication	0	0	0	0	0
Leather Products	0	0	0	0	0
Textile Manufacturing	0	0	0	0	0
Inprocess Fuel	2,274	0	0	0	0
Other/Not Classified	0	0	0	0	0
SOLID WASTE DISPOSAL-AREA	0	0	0	0	0
-POINT	175	11	66	329	931
Government-point	0	0	0	0	0
Municipal Incineration	0	0	0	0	0
Open Burning	0	0	0	0	0
Other	0	0	0	0	0
Residential-area	0	0	0	0	0
On Site Incineration	0	0	0	0	0
Open Burning	0	0	0	0	0
Commercial-Institutional-area	0	0	0	0	0
-point	0	0	0	0	0
On Site Incineration-area	0	0	0	0	0
-point	0	0	0	0	0
Open Burning-area	0	0	0	0	0
-point	0	0	0	0	0
Apartment-point	0	0	0	0	0
Other-point	0	0	0	0	0
Industrial-area	0	0	0	0	0
-point	175	11	66	329	931
On Site Incineration-area	0	0	0	0	0
-point	0	0	0	0	0
Open Burning-area	0	0	0	0	0
-point	175	11	66	329	931
Auto Body Incineration-point	0	0	0	0	0
Other-point	0	0	0	0	0
Miscellaneous-point	0	0	0	0	0
TRANSPORTATION-AREA	5,635	6,547	39,680	59,041	304,796
Land Vehicles	4,170	1,563	37,239	50,263	298,246
Gasoline	3,749	973	31,931	49,584	295,125
Light Vehicles	3,743	970	31,866	49,442	294,383
Heavy Vehicles	6	2	65	141	742
Off Highway	0	0	0	0	0
Diesel Fuel	421	590	5,308	679	3,121
Heavy Vehicles	421	590	5,308	679	3,121
Off Highway	0	0	0	0	0
Rail	0	0	0	0	0
Aircraft	1,151	331	1,761	4,149	6,527
Military	1,040	199	500	2,419	2,597
Civil	22	4	20	99	566
Commercial	89	128	1,241	1,630	3,364
Vessels	314	4,653	680	47	23
Bituminous Coal	0	0	0	0	0
Diesel Fuel	0	0	0	0	0
Residual Oil	314	4,653	680	47	23
Gasoline	0	0	0	0	0
Gas Handling Evaporation Loss	0	0	0	4,583	0
MISCELLANEOUS-AREA	18,233	0	2,145	24,227	64,351
Forest Fires	0	0	0	0	0
Structural Fires	0	0	0	0	0
Slash Burning	18,233	0	2,145	21,450	64,351
Frost Control	0	0	0	0	0
Solvent Evaporation Loss	0	0	0	2,777	0

RHODE ISLAND

Emission categories	Pollutant, tons per year				
	Particulates	Sulfur oxides	Nitrogen oxides	Hydro-carbons	Carbon monoxide
GRAND TOTAL	14,827	46,470	56,205	85,283	328,142
-AREA	10,560	19,035	43,559	67,570	321,861
-POINT	4,268	27,435	12,646	17,713	6,281
FUEL COMBUSTION-AREA	5,070	17,315	12,875	955	1,616
-POINT	1,662	26,994	12,335	312	476
External Combustion-area	5,070	17,315	12,875	955	1,616
-point	1,662	26,994	12,335	312	476
Residential Fuel-area	1,203	3,189	1,881	409	839
Anthracite Coal	15	38	4	4	132
Bituminous Coal	0	0	0	0	0
Distillate Oil	1,092	3,145	1,310	328	546
Residual Oil	0	0	0	0	0
Natural Gas	69	4	556	56	139
Wood	28	2	11	22	22
Electric Generation-point	514	15,682	8,961	150	256
Anthracite Coal	0	0	0	0	0
Bituminous Coal	0	0	0	0	0
Lignite	0	0	0	0	0
Residual Oil	494	15,681	7,781	148	222
Distillate Oil	0	0	0	0	0
Natural Gas	19	1	1,180	2	33
Process Gas	0	0	0	0	0
Coke	0	0	0	0	0
Solid Waste/Coal	0	0	0	0	0
Other	0	0	0	0	0
Industrial Fuel-area	1,559	4,667	4,079	195	284
-point	892	8,876	2,597	123	168
Anthracite Coal-area	0	0	0	0	0
-point	0	0	0	0	0
Bituminous Coal-area	357	261	51	3	7
-point	0	0	0	0	0
Lignite-point	0	0	0	0	0
Residual Oil-area	729	3,526	1,900	95	127
-point	889	8,876	2,442	122	163
Distillate Oil-area	458	879	1,831	92	122
-point	0	0	0	0	0
Natural Gas-area	16	1	296	5	28
-point	3	0	154	1	5
Process Gas-area	0	0	0	0	0
-point	0	0	0	0	0
Coke-point	0	0	0	0	0
Wood-area	0	0	0	0	0
-point	0	0	0	0	0
Liquid Petroleum Gas-point	0	0	0	0	0
Bagasse-point	0	0	0	0	0
Other-point	0	0	0	0	0
Commercial-Institutional Fuel-area	2,307	9,459	6,915	351	494
-point	257	2,435	777	39	53
Anthracite Coal-area	10	12	4	0	3
-point	0	0	0	0	0
Bituminous Coal-area	13	22	3	1	2
-point	0	0	0	0	0
Lignite-point	0	0	0	0	0
Residual Oil-area	1,741	8,427	4,542	227	303
-point	217	2,085	616	31	41
Distillate Oil-area	519	997	2,076	104	138
-point	39	350	155	8	10
Natural Gas-area	24	1	290	19	48
-point	1	0	6	1	1
Wood-area	0	0	0	0	0
-point	0	0	0	0	0
Liquid Petroleum Gas-point	0	0	0	0	0
Miscellaneous-point	0	0	0	0	0
Internal Combustion-point	0	0	0	0	0
Electric Generation	0	0	0	0	0
Distillate Oil	0	0	0	0	0
Natural Gas	0	0	0	0	0
Diesel Fuel	0	0	0	0	0
Industrial Fuel	0	0	0	0	0
Distillate Oil	0	0	0	0	0
Natural Gas	0	0	0	0	0
Gasoline	0	0	0	0	0
Diesel Fuel	0	0	0	0	0

Emission categories	Pollutant, tons per year				
	Particulates	Sulfur oxides	Nitrogen oxides	Hydro-carbons	Carbon monoxide
Other...	0	0	0	0	0
Commercial-Institutional...	0	0	0	0	0
Diesel Fuel	0	0	0	0	0
Other...	0	0	0	0	0
Engine-Testing...	0	0	0	0	0
Aircraft...	0	0	0	0	0
Other...	0	0	0	0	0
Miscellaneous...	0	0	0	0	0
INDUSTRIAL PROCESS-POINT	648	251	108	16,997	2,449
Chemical Manufacturing	35	0	0	726	0
Food/Agriculture	0	0	0	0	0
Primary Metal	0	0	0	0	0
Secondary Metals	125	0	0	0	2,449
Mineral Products	451	0	0	0	0
Petroleum Industry	31	251	108	5	0
Wood Products	0	0	0	0	0
Evaporation	5	0	0	16,087	0
Metal Fabrication	0	0	0	0	0
Leather Products	0	0	0	0	0
Textile Manufacturing	0	0	0	180	0
Inprocess Fuel	0	0	0	0	0
Other/Not Classified	0	0	0	0	0
SOLID WASTE DISPOSAL-AREA	1,605	105	556	3,079	8,771
-POINT	1,957	190	203	403	3,356
Government-point	1,957	190	203	403	3,356
Municipal Incineration	1,800	180	144	108	2,520
Open Burning	157	10	59	295	836
Other	0	0	0	0	0
Residential-area	1,354	78	462	2,665	7,614
On Site Incineration	134	2	4	378	1,133
Open Burning	1,220	76	457	2,288	6,481
Commercial-Institutional-area	144	19	54	219	607
-point	0	0	0	0	0
On Site Incineration-area	41	13	15	26	59
-point	0	0	0	0	0
Open Burning-area	103	6	39	194	548
-point	0	0	0	0	0
Apartment-point	0	0	0	0	0
Other-point	0	0	0	0	0
Industrial-area	107	8	40	195	550
-point	0	0	0	0	0
On Site Incineration-area	4	1	2	3	6
-point	0	0	0	0	0
Open Burning-area	102	6	38	192	544
-point	0	0	0	0	0
Auto Body Incineration-point	0	0	0	0	0
Other-point	0	0	0	0	0
Miscellaneous-point	0	0	0	0	0
TRANSPORTATION-AREA	3,885	1,614	30,128	56,453	311,473
Land Vehicles	3,321	1,276	29,222	47,923	300,025
Gasoline	2,950	805	24,809	47,314	297,453
Light Vehicles	2,617	678	21,384	37,177	238,237
Heavy Vehicles	333	126	3,426	10,137	59,216
Off Highway	0	0	0	0	0
Diesel Fuel	371	471	4,413	609	2,572
Heavy Vehicles	247	345	3,001	433	2,164
Off Highway	114	102	1,258	138	355
Rail	10	24	154	39	54
Aircraft	535	136	629	1,718	2,748
Military	488	93	234	1,134	1,218
Civil	20	4	18	89	510
Commercial	27	39	376	494	1,020
Vessels	30	203	277	2,764	8,700
Bituminous Coal	0	0	0	0	0
Diesel Fuel	19	23	174	46	61
Residual Oil	11	162	24	2	1
Gasoline	0	18	80	2,717	8,639
Gas Handling Evaporation Loss	0	0	0	4,047	0
MISCELLANEOUS-AREA	0	0	0	7,084	0
Forest Fires	0	0	0	0	0
Structural Fires	0	0	0	0	0
Slash Burning	0	0	0	0	0
Frost Control	0	0	0	0	0
Solvent Evaporation Loss	0	0	0	7,084	0

SOUTH CAROLINA

Emission categories	Pollutant, tons per year				
	Particulates	Sulfur oxides	Nitrogen oxides	Hydro-carbons	Carbon monoxide
GRAND TOTAL	213,308	301,083	288,282	360,971	1,319,415
-AREA	75,072	28,600	155,631	323,185	1,187,484
-POINT	138,235	272,483	132,651	37,785	131,931
FUEL COMBUSTION-AREA	21,840	19,962	17,743	3,749	6,942
-POINT	45,542	255,711	130,236	3,090	6,461
External Combustion-area	21,840	19,962	17,743	3,749	6,942
-point	45,523	255,705	129,975	3,070	6,404
Residential Fuel-area	3,989	1,150	3,035	2,941	5,053
Anthracite Coal	0	0	0	0	0
Bituminous Coal	518	984	78	518	2,330
Distillate Oil	706	0	848	212	353
Residual Oil	0	0	0	0	0
Natural Gas	132	8	1,056	106	264
Wood	2,633	158	1,053	2,106	2,106
Electric Generation-point	20,847	179,985	93,285	1,122	3,265
Anthracite Coal	0	0	0	0	0
Bituminous Coal	20,563	122,342	66,515	751	2,502
Lignite	0	0	0	0	0
Residual Oil	261	57,616	18,584	354	531
Distillate Oil	1	19	211	4	6
Natural Gas	23	8	7,974	13	226
Process Gas	0	0	0	0	0
Coke	0	0	0	0	0
Solid Waste/Coal	0	0	0	0	0
Other	0	0	0	0	0
Industrial Fuel-area	12,480	5,578	5,917	218	637
-point	23,447	73,681	36,139	1,913	3,075
Anthracite Coal-area	0	0	0	0	0
-point	0	0	0	0	0
Bituminous Coal-area	12,220	5,567	2,197	146	293
-point	15,273	26,561	14,280	479	1,171
Lignite-point	0	0	0	0	0
Residual Oil-area	0	0	0	0	0
-point	3,184	44,948	9,190	457	609
Distillate Oil-area	69	0	276	14	18
-point	340	1,535	1,355	67	90
Natural Gas-area	191	11	3,444	57	325
-point	164	12	7,099	60	342
Process Gas-area	0	0	0	0	0
-point	0	0	0	0	0
Coke-point	0	0	0	0	0
Wood-area	0	0	0	0	0
-point	4,304	623	4,212	850	862
Liquid Petroleum Gas-point	0	0	3	0	0
Bagasse-point	0	0	0	0	0
Other-point	181	0	0	0	0
Commercial-Institutional Fuel-area	5,371	13,234	8,790	590	1,252
-point	1,229	2,039	551	34	64
Anthracite Coal-area	0	0	0	0	0
-point	307	142	59	4	8
Bituminous Coal-area	3,261	3,392	821	179	643
-point	866	1,197	338	23	45
Lignite-point	0	0	0	0	0
Residual Oil-area	711	9,838	1,856	93	124
-point	52	692	135	7	9
Distillate Oil-area	1,334	0	5,335	267	356
-point	3	7	13	1	1
Natural Gas-area	65	4	778	52	130
-point	1	0	6	0	1
Wood-area	0	0	0	0	0
-point	0	0	0	0	0
Liquid Petroleum Gas-point	0	0	0	0	0
Miscellaneous-point	0	0	0	0	0
Internal Combustion-point	19	6	262	21	57
Electric Generation	0	0	0	0	0
Distillate Oil	0	0	0	0	0
Natural Gas	0	0	0	0	0
Diesel Fuel	0	0	0	0	0
Industrial Fuel	19	6	262	21	57
Distillate Oil	0	0	0	0	0
Natural Gas	0	0	0	0	0
Gasoline	0	0	0	0	0
Diesel Fuel	19	6	262	21	57

Emission categories	Pollutant, tons per year				
	Particulates	Sulfur oxides	Nitrogen oxides	Hydro- carbons	Carbon monoxide
Other	0	0	0	0	0
Commercial-Institutional	0	0	0	0	0
Diesel Fuel	0	0	0	0	0
Other	0	0	0	0	0
Engine-Testing	0	0	0	0	0
Aircraft	0	0	0	0	0
Other	0	0	0	0	0
Miscellaneous	0	0	0	0	0
INDUSTRIAL PROCESS-POINT	91,761	16,752	2,282	33,282	109,004
Chemical Manufacturing	502	1,410	443	6,415	6,228
Food/Agriculture	176	0	0	73	0
Primary Metal	187	0	0	0	0
Secondary Metals	948	163	186	1	836
Mineral Products	58,362	7,717	1,654	120	111
Petroleum Industry	0	0	0	0	0
Wood Products	30,954	7,463	0	519	101,725
Evaporation	0	0	0	21,846	0
Metal Fabrication	2	0	0	0	0
Leather Products	0	0	0	0	0
Textile Manufacturing	1	0	0	2,126	0
Inprocess Fuel	626	0	0	2,178	52
Other/Not Classified	3	0	0	5	52
SOLID WASTE DISPOSAL-AREA	21,106	1,319	7,915	39,573	112,124
-POINT	932	20	132	1,413	16,466
Government-point	16	3	1	0	0
Municipal Incineration	0	0	0	0	0
Open Burning	0	0	0	0	0
Other	16	3	1	0	0
Residential-area	18,911	1,182	7,092	35,459	100,466
On Site Incineration	0	0	0	0	0
Open Burning	18,911	1,182	7,092	35,459	100,466
Commercial-Institutional-area	1,958	122	734	3,672	10,404
-point	1	0	0	1	4
On Site Incineration-area	0	0	0	0	0
-point	1	0	0	1	4
Open Burning-area	1,958	122	734	3,672	10,404
-point	0	0	0	0	0
Apartment-point	0	0	0	0	0
Other-point	0	0	0	0	0
Industrial-area	236	15	88	443	1,254
-point	915	16	131	1,412	16,462
On Site Incineration-area	0	0	0	0	0
-point	863	16	131	1,412	16,462
Open Burning-area	236	15	88	443	1,254
-point	0	0	0	0	0
Auto Body Incineration-point	0	0	0	0	0
Other-point	52	0	0	0	0
Miscellaneous-point	0	0	0	0	0
TRANSPORTATION-AREA	14,982	7,319	125,940	250,163	927,225
Land Vehicles	13,269	5,811	124,186	156,708	900,786
Gasoline	11,249	2,995	98,528	153,219	889,361
Light Vehicles	10,655	2,762	92,026	136,889	790,144
Heavy Vehicles	546	207	5,955	14,787	81,717
Off Highway	48	25	547	1,544	17,499
Diesel Fuel	2,020	2,816	25,658	3,489	11,425
Heavy Vehicles	1,328	1,859	17,086	2,029	8,759
Off Highway	448	401	4,969	544	1,400
Rail	244	555	3,604	916	1,266
Aircraft	1,613	343	1,168	4,307	6,240
Military	1,531	292	736	3,563	3,824
Civil	54	11	49	241	1,377
Commercial	27	40	383	504	1,039
Vessels	99	1,166	585	6,399	20,198
Bituminous Coal	0	0	0	0	0
Diesel Fuel	26	32	240	63	84
Residual Oil	74	1,091	159	11	5
Gasoline	0	43	186	6,325	20,109
Gas Handling Evaporation Loss	0	0	0	82,749	0
MISCELLANEOUS-AREA	17,145	0	4,034	29,701	141,194
Forest Fires	17,145	0	4,034	24,205	141,194
Structural Fires	0	0	0	0	0
Slash Burning	0	0	0	0	0
Frost Control	0	0	0	0	0
Solvent Evaporation Loss	0	0	0	5,496	0

SOUTH DAKOTA

Emission categories	Pollutant, tons per year				
	Particulates	Sulfur oxides	Nitrogen oxides	Hydro-carbons	Carbon monoxide
GRAND TOTAL	**59,767**	**14,663**	**52,649**	**85,161**	**463,404**
–AREA	**8,936**	**5,342**	**46,552**	**77,482**	**449,474**
–POINT	**50,831**	**9,321**	**6,097**	**7,679**	**13,930**
FUEL COMBUSTION–AREA	1,423	2,897	2,662	933	2,796
–POINT	3,697	5,413	4,632	199	518
External Combustion–area	1,423	2,897	2,662	933	2,796
–point	3,690	5,359	4,466	189	456
Residential Fuel–area	1,296	2,713	1,443	873	2,640
Anthracite Coal	0	0	0	0	0
Bituminous Coal	447	510	67	447	2,013
Distillate Oil	505	2,183	606	152	253
Residual Oil	0	0	0	0	0
Natural Gas	83	5	666	67	166
Wood	260	16	104	208	208
Electric Generation–point	3,015	3,584	3,402	137	316
Anthracite Coal	0	0	0	0	0
Bituminous Coal	725	613	654	44	87
Lignite	2,241	2,806	1,299	81	188
Residual Oil	42	165	652	11	16
Distillate Oil	0	0	0	0	0
Natural Gas	6	1	750	1	21
Process Gas	1	0	48	0	4
Coke	0	0	0	0	0
Solid Waste/Coal	0	0	0	0	0
Other	0	0	0	0	0
Industrial Fuel–area	30	29	403	8	37
–point	127	489	368	13	23
Anthracite Coal–area	0	0	0	0	0
–point	0	0	0	0	0
Bituminous Coal–area	0	0	0	0	0
–point	0	0	0	0	0
Lignite–point	0	0	0	0	0
Residual Oil–area	0	0	0	0	0
–point	38	425	100	5	7
Distillate Oil–area	10	28	39	2	3
–point	9	60	36	2	2
Natural Gas–area	20	1	364	6	34
–point	6	0	212	2	10
Process Gas–area	0	0	0	0	0
–point	0	0	0	0	0
Coke–point	0	0	0	0	0
Wood–area	0	0	0	0	0
–point	73	3	20	4	4
Liquid Petroleum Gas–point	0	0	0	0	0
Bagasse–point	0	0	0	0	0
Other–point	0	0	0	0	0
Commercial-Institutional Fuel–area	97	154	816	52	119
–point	549	1,286	696	40	117
Anthracite Coal–area	0	0	0	0	0
–point	0	0	0	0	0
Bituminous Coal–area	0	0	0	0	0
–point	0	0	0	0	0
Lignite–point	461	846	237	18	82
Residual Oil–area	3	32	7	0	0
–point	0	0	0	0	0
Distillate Oil–area	41	118	164	8	11
–point	83	439	330	17	22
Natural Gas–area	54	3	644	43	107
–point	6	0	128	5	12
Wood–area	0	0	0	0	0
–point	0	0	0	0	0
Liquid Petroleum Gas–point	0	0	0	0	0
Miscellaneous–point	0	0	0	0	0
Internal Combustion–point	7	54	166	10	62
Electric Generation	7	54	166	10	62
Distillate Oil	2	35	32	0	0
Natural Gas	1	0	32	0	0
Diesel Fuel	4	19	102	10	62
Industrial Fuel	0	0	0	0	0
Distillate Oil	0	0	0	0	0
Natural Gas	0	0	0	0	0
Gasoline	0	0	0	0	0
Diesel Fuel	0	0	0	0	0

Emission categories	Pollutant, tons per year				
	Particulates	Sulfur oxides	Nitrogen oxides	Hydro-carbons	Carbon monoxide
Other	0	0	0	0	0
Commercial-Institutional	0	0	0	0	0
Diesel Fuel	0	0	0	0	0
Other	0	0	0	0	0
Engine-Testing	0	0	0	0	0
Aircraft	0	0	0	0	0
Other	0	0	0	0	0
Miscellaneous	0	0	0	0	0
INDUSTRIAL PROCESS-POINT	45,591	3,832	983	4,719	8
Chemical Manufacturing	0	0	0	51	0
Food/Agriculture	16,410	3	3	3	3
Primary Metal	3,692	0	0	0	0
Secondary Metals	0	0	0	0	0
Mineral Products	25,489	3,826	976	1	1
Petroleum Industry	0	0	0	0	0
Wood Products	0	0	0	0	0
Evaporation	0	0	0	4,661	0
Metal Fabrication	0	0	0	0	0
Leather Products	0	0	0	0	0
Textile Manufacturing	0	0	0	0	0
Inprocess Fuel	0	4	4	4	4
Other/Not Classified	0	0	0	0	0
SOLID WASTE DISPOSAL-AREA	1,736	111	332	3,894	11,408
-POINT	1,542	76	483	2,760	13,404
Government-point	1,147	71	426	2,139	6,064
Municipal Incineration	0	0	0	0	0
Open Burning	1,147	71	426	2,139	6,064
Other	0	0	0	0	0
Residential-area	1,551	53	262	3,779	11,143
On Site Incineration	929	15	29	2,612	7,837
Open Burning	622	39	233	1,167	3,307
Commercial-Institutional-area	128	40	48	80	183
-point	0	0	0	0	0
On Site Incineration-area	128	40	48	80	183
-point	0	0	0	0	0
Open Burning-area	0	0	0	0	0
-point	0	0	0	0	0
Apartment-point	0	0	0	0	0
Other-point	0	0	0	0	0
Industrial-area	57	18	21	36	82
-point	396	6	57	621	7,340
On Site Incineration-area	57	18	21	36	82
-point	395	6	56	621	7,339
Open Burning-area	0	0	0	0	0
-point	0	0	0	0	1
Auto Body Incineration-point	0	0	0	0	0
Other-point	0	0	0	0	0
Miscellaneous-point	0	0	0	0	0
TRANSPORTATION-AREA	5,137	2,3?	43,429	70,018	430,852
Land Vehicles	4,292	2,125	42,559	60,932	421,628
Gasoline	3,534	1,088	33,007	59,603	417,708
Light Vehicles	2,641	685	23,001	33,360	188,793
Heavy Vehicles	441	167	4,846	11,692	63,949
Off Highway	453	237	5,160	14,551	164,966
Diesel Fuel	758	1,037	9,552	1,329	3,920
Heavy Vehicles	398	557	5,136	601	2,557
Off Highway	246	220	2,721	298	767
Rail	115	261	1,695	431	595
Aircraft	845	198	828	2,579	4,729
Military	746	142	358	1,736	1,864
Civil	70	14	63	309	1,764
Commercial	29	42	407	534	1,102
Vessels	0	10	42	1,414	4,495
Bituminous Coal	0	0	0	0	0
Diesel Fuel	0	0	0	0	0
Residual Oil	0	0	0	0	0
Gasoline	0	10	42	1,414	4,495
Gas Handling Evaporation Loss	0	0	0	5,093	0
MISCELLANEOUS-AREA	641	0	129	2,637	4,418
Forest Fires	497	0	117	702	4,094
Structural Fires	144	0	13	37	325
Slash Burning	0	0	0	0	0
Frost Control	0	0	0	0	0
Solvent Evaporation Loss	0	0	0	1,898	0

TENNESSEE

Emission categories	Pollutant, tons per year				
	Particulates	Sulfur oxides	Nitrogen oxides	Hydro-carbons	Carbon monoxide
GRAND TOTAL	417,905	1,304,896	536,918	391,719	1,936,094
–AREA	41,061	40,339	243,768	318,887	1,608,799
–POINT	376,845	1,264,557	293,151	72,831	327,295
FUEL COMBUSTION–AREA	13,555	26,583	19,793	6,031	22,419
–POINT	238,020	1,149,484	271,733	5,327	115,291
External Combustion–area	13,555	26,583	19,793	6,031	22,419
–point	237,971	1,148,680	270,930	5,257	115,096
Residential Fuel–area	5,712	15,544	3,798	5,250	20,314
Anthracite Coal	0	0	0	0	0
Bituminous Coal	4,182	15,021	627	4,182	18,819
Distillate Oil	313	451	375	94	156
Residual Oil	0	0	0	0	0
Natural Gas	304	18	2,430	243	607
Wood	914	55	366	731	731
Electric Generation–point	167,793	1,082,841	224,018	3,048	10,284
Anthracite Coal	0	0	0	0	0
Bituminous Coal	167,781	1,082,765	218,554	3,038	10,126
Lignite	0	0	0	0	0
Residual Oil	5	70	26	1	1
Distillate Oil	0	1	3	0	0
Natural Gas	7	6	5,434	9	158
Process Gas	0	0	0	0	0
Coke	0	0	0	0	0
Solid Waste/Coal	0	0	0	0	0
Other	0	0	0	0	0
Industrial Fuel–area	643	1,450	7,654	180	697
–point	69,209	64,227	41,976	2,005	104,304
Anthracite Coal–area	0	0	0	0	0
–point	0	0	0	0	0
Bituminous Coal–area	0	0	0	0	0
–point	65,080	54,346	25,791	967	2,263
Lignite–point	0	0	0	0	0
Residual Oil–area	97	1,278	254	13	17
–point	234	2,961	689	36	46
Distillate Oil–area	154	148	616	31	41
–point	140	893	821	100	42
Natural Gas–area	376	23	6,766	113	639
–point	393	3,745	10,851	112	422
Process Gas–area	16	2	18	24	0
–point	41	703	0	0	0
Coke–point	0	0	0	0	0
Wood–area	0	0	0	0	0
–point	3,258	311	3,824	791	101,531
Liquid Petroleum Gas–point	0	0	0	0	0
Bagasse–point	0	0	0	0	0
Other–point	64	1,268	0	0	0
Commercial-Institutional Fuel–area	7,200	9,589	8,340	600	1,408
–point	969	1,611	4,936	203	508
Anthracite Coal–area	0	0	0	0	0
–point	0	0	0	0	0
Bituminous Coal–area	5,720	8,257	861	187	674
–point	734	1,502	489	43	107
Lignite–point	31	44	9	2	7
Residual Oil–area	7	95	19	1	1
–point	3	19	8	0	0
Distillate Oil–area	1,276	1,225	5,103	255	340
–point	5	36	22	1	1
Natural Gas–area	196	12	2,358	157	393
–point	196	12	4,400	157	392
Wood–area	0	0	0	0	0
–point	0	0	0	0	0
Liquid Petroleum Gas–point	0	0	0	0	0
Miscellaneous–point	0	0	7	0	0
Internal Combustion–point	49	804	803	71	195
Electric Generation	49	804	803	71	195
Distillate Oil	41	804	556	46	126
Natural Gas	8	0	247	25	69
Diesel Fuel	0	0	0	0	0
Industrial Fuel	0	0	0	0	0
Distillate Oil	0	0	0	0	0
Natural Gas	0	0	0	0	0
Gasoline	0	0	0	0	0
Diesel Fuel	0	0	0	0	0

Emission categories	Pollutant, tons per year				
	Particulates	Sulfur oxides	Nitrogen oxides	Hydro-carbons	Carbon monoxide
Other	0	0	0	0	0
Commercial-Institutional	0	0	0	0	0
Diesel Fuel	0	0	0	0	0
Other	0	0	0	0	0
Engine-Testing	0	0	0	0	0
Aircraft	0	0	0	0	0
Other	0	0	0	0	0
Miscellaneous	0	0	0	0	0
INDUSTRIAL PROCESS-POINT	134,797	114,185	20,636	63,236	202,727
Chemical Manufacturing	9,112	77,842	16,019	42,505	51,430
Food/Agriculture	3,605	0	0	4	878
Primary Metal	21,072	1,861	8	656	13,140
Secondary Metals	2,663	371	19	0	96,892
Mineral Products	77,780	21,968	3,694	2,373	3,110
Petroleum Industry	175	5,459	282	29	0
Wood Products	12,999	976	0	1,379	36,195
Evaporation	229	0	152	16,214	146
Metal Fabrication	5	0	0	0	0
Leather Products	0	0	0	0	0
Textile Manufacturing	0	0	0	0	0
Inprocess Fuel	7,084	5,707	463	77	937
Other/Not Classified	73	0	0	0	0
SOLID WASTE DISPOSAL-AREA	3,474	217	1,303	6,513	18,454
-POINT	4,027	888	782	4,268	9,276
Government-point	3,458	744	595	3,412	7,119
Municipal Incineration	3,458	744	595	3,412	7,119
Open Burning	0	0	0	0	0
Other	0	0	0	0	0
Residential-area	2,038	127	764	3,822	10,829
On Site Incineration	0	0	0	0	0
Open Burning	2,038	127	764	3,822	10,829
Commercial-Institutional-area	1,281	80	480	2,402	6,804
-point	15	5	6	17	51
On Site Incineration-area	0	0	0	0	0
-point	14	5	6	17	51
Open Burning-area	1,281	80	480	2,402	6,804
-point	0	0	0	0	0
Apartment-point	0	0	0	0	0
Other-point	0	0	0	0	0
Industrial-area	154	10	58	290	820
-point	555	140	180	839	2,106
On Site Incineration-area	0	0	0	0	0
-point	525	139	175	812	2,027
Open Burning-area	154	10	58	290	820
-point	16	1	5	27	79
Auto Body Incineration-point	0	0	0	0	0
Other-point	15	0	0	0	0
Miscellaneous-point	0	0	0	0	0
TRANSPORTATION-AREA	23,189	13,537	222,599	292,900	1,566,023
Land Vehicles	22,054	12,438	214,463	255,486	1,528,574
Gasoline	16,817	4,597	147,371	244,699	1,499,340
Light Vehicles	15,276	3,960	130,534	200,352	1,183,693
Heavy Vehicles	1,175	445	12,666	32,586	182,304
Off Highway	366	191	4,171	11,762	133,343
Diesel Fuel	5,237	7,841	67,092	10,787	29,234
Heavy Vehicles	2,470	3,458	31,316	3,924	17,735
Off Highway	1,390	1,244	15,400	1,686	4,340
Rail	1,377	3,139	20,376	5,177	7,159
Aircraft	483	231	1,818	3,414	10,864
Military	120	23	58	280	301
Civil	253	50	229	1,122	6,412
Commercial	109	158	1,531	2,011	4,151
Vessels	653	868	6,318	9,290	26,585
Bituminous Coal	0	0	0	0	0
Diesel Fuel	653	816	6,092	1,599	2,132
Residual Oil	0	0	0	0	0
Gasoline	0	52	226	7,691	24,453
Gas Handling Evaporation Loss	0	0	0	24,710	0
MISCELLANEOUS-AREA	842	2	73	13,443	1,903
Forest Fires	0	0	0	0	0
Structural Fires	842	2	73	218	1,903
Slash Burning	0	0	0	0	0
Frost Control	0	0	0	0	0
Solvent Evaporation Loss	0	0	0	13,225	0

TEXAS

Emission categories	Pollutant, tons per year				
	Particulates	Sulfur oxides	Nitrogen oxides	Hydro-carbons	Carbon monoxide
GRAND TOTAL	608,297	800,689	1,587,862	2,211,509	7,215,631
-AREA	167,110	86,863	831,477	1,043,837	4,223,930
-POINT	441,188	713,825	756,385	1,167,671	2,991,700
FUEL COMBUSTION-AREA	13,359	32,159	143,299	4,454	15,450
-POINT	33,177	80,657	625,978	33,907	26,240
External Combustion-area	13,359	32,159	143,299	4,454	15,450
-point	31,756	73,354	461,243	6,258	15,148
Residential Fuel-area	1,480	250	11,587	1,166	2,904
Anthracite Coal	0	0	0	0	0
Bituminous Coal	0	0	0	0	0
Distillate Oil	38	163	45	11	19
Residual Oil	0	0	0	0	0
Natural Gas	1,443	87	11,542	1,154	2,885
Wood	0	0	0	0	0
Electric Generation-point	19,982	53,831	372,386	724	10,764
Anthracite Coal	0	0	0	0	0
Bituminous Coal	0	0	0	0	0
Lignite	13,523	42,670	8,784	1	5
Residual Oil	527	6,170	6,916	130	195
Distillate Oil	0	0	0	0	0
Natural Gas	5,931	4,991	356,686	592	10,564
Process Gas	0	0	0	0	0
Coke	0	0	0	0	0
Solid Waste/Coal	0	0	0	0	0
Other	0	0	0	0	0
Industrial Fuel-area	9,190	23,114	115,429	2,325	10,567
-point	10,359	17,171	85,021	5,193	4,281
Anthracite Coal-area	0	0	0	0	0
-point	0	0	0	0	0
Bituminous Coal-area	0	0	0	0	0
-point	0	0	0	0	0
Lignite-point	0	0	0	0	0
Residual Oil-area	1,252	16,449	3,266	163	218
-point	0	0	0	0	0
Distillate Oil-area	2,194	6,320	8,776	439	585
-point	4	0	1,459	1	1
Natural Gas-area	5,744	345	103,387	1,723	9,764
-point	3,595	8,395	76,678	4,895	3,983
Process Gas-area	0	0	0	0	0
-point	1	8,505	5,307	0	0
Coke-point	0	0	0	0	0
Wood-area	0	0	0	0	0
-point	6,758	271	1,560	296	296
Liquid Petroleum Gas-point	2	0	17	0	1
Bagasse-point	0	0	0	0	0
Other-point	0	0	0	0	0
Commercial-Institutional Fuel-area	2,688	8,795	16,282	963	1,979
-point	1,414	2,353	3,836	341	103
Anthracite Coal-area	0	0	0	0	0
-point	0	0	0	0	0
Bituminous Coal-area	0	0	0	0	0
-point	0	0	0	0	0
Lignite-point	0	0	0	0	0
Residual Oil-area	307	4,036	801	40	53
-point	0	0	1	0	0
Distillate Oil-area	1,637	4,715	6,547	327	436
-point	0	0	1	0	0
Natural Gas-area	745	45	8,935	596	1,489
-point	1,413	2,353	3,833	341	103
Wood-area	0	0	0	0	0
-point	0	0	0	0	0
Liquid Petroleum Gas-point	0	0	0	0	0
Miscellaneous-point	0	0	0	0	0
Internal Combustion-point	1,421	7,303	164,735	27,650	11,093
Electric Generation	7	0	189	0	0
Distillate Oil	0	0	0	0	0
Natural Gas	7	0	189	0	0
Diesel Fuel	0	0	0	0	0
Industrial Fuel	1,293	7,303	164,464	27,614	10,968
Distillate Oil	0	0	0	0	0
Natural Gas	1,284	7,300	164,389	27,557	10,424
Gasoline	3	3	27	49	543
Diesel Fuel	6	0	48	8	1

Emission categories	Pollutant, tons per year				
	Particulates	Sulfur oxides	Nitrogen oxides	Hydro-carbons	Carbon monoxide
Other	0	0	0	0	0
Commercial-Institutional	0	0	0	0	0
Diesel Fuel	0	0	0	0	0
Other	0	0	0	0	0
Engine-Testing	121	0	82	36	125
Aircraft	121	0	82	36	125
Other	0	0	0	0	0
Miscellaneous	0	0	0	0	0
INDUSTRIAL PROCESS-POINT	406,829	620,296	130,018	1,109,202	2,959,670
Chemical Manufacturing	55,520	153,774	12,767	498,814	1,535,832
Food/Agriculture	5,233	56	172	37	35
Primary Metal	156,469	133,049	6,950	2,672	50,709
Secondary Metals	18,718	59,867	443	296	22,023
Mineral Products	119,831	12,614	3,415	2,134	644
Petroleum Industry	40,548	253,309	92,484	330,450	1,309,422
Wood Products	8,906	5,177	678	355	35,484
Evaporation	0	1,606	390	268,249	1,964
Metal Fabrication	0	0	0	6	0
Leather Products	0	0	0	0	0
Textile Manufacturing	0	0	0	0	0
Inprocess Fuel	1,583	843	12,698	5,947	3,557
Other/Not Classified	21	0	20	243	0
SOLID WASTE DISPOSAL-AREA	15,873	1,414	4,528	30,566	87,724
-POINT	1,182	12,873	389	24,562	5,790
Government-point	0	0	0	0	0
Municipal Incineration	0	0	0	0	0
Open Burning	0	0	0	0	0
Other	0	0	0	0	0
Residential-area	12,020	557	3,083	26,423	76,808
On Site Incineration	4,144	65	130	11,655	34,966
Open Burning	7,876	492	2,953	14,768	41,841
Commercial-Institutional-area	2,194	502	823	2,289	5,997
-point	176	3	25	275	3,255
On Site Incineration-area	1,461	457	548	913	2,100
-point	175	3	25	275	3,252
Open Burning-area	734	46	275	1,376	3,897
-point	1	0	0	0	3
Apartment-point	0	0	0	0	0
Other-point	0	0	0	0	0
Industrial-area	1,658	355	622	1,854	4,919
-point	1,006	12,870	364	24,286	2,535
On Site Incineration-area	1,004	314	376	627	1,443
-point	504	9,712	256	499	1,929
Open Burning-area	654	41	245	1,227	3,477
-point	463	8	40	23,708	584
Auto Body Incineration-point	0	0	0	0	0
Other-point	38	3,150	68	79	22
Miscellaneous-point	0	0	0	0	0
TRANSPORTATION-AREA	125,199	53,286	681,022	910,399	4,030,677
Land Vehicles	61,333	35,231	624,088	648,354	3,718,437
Gasoline	44,563	12,362	412,964	617,211	3,647,622
Light Vehicles	39,909	10,347	359,825	487,034	2,616,598
Heavy Vehicles	2,910	1,103	33,253	74,106	395,336
Off Highway	1,744	913	19,886	56,071	635,688
Diesel Fuel	16,770	22,869	211,124	31,143	70,815
Heavy Vehicles	4,813	6,738	64,050	6,653	25,330
Off Highway	8,036	7,192	89,053	9,750	25,099
Rail	3,920	8,938	58,022	14,741	20,386
Aircraft	61,857	12,599	38,838	157,746	218,955
Military	59,373	11,337	28,523	138,138	148,282
Civil	1,869	371	1,688	8,276	47,284
Commercial	616	890	8,628	11,332	23,384
Vessels	2,008	5,457	18,095	31,934	93,284
Bituminous Coal	0	0	0	0	0
Diesel Fuel	1,805	2,256	16,846	4,422	5,896
Residual Oil	203	3,014	441	31	15
Gasoline	0	186	809	27,481	87,373
Gas Handling Evaporation Loss	0	0	0	72,365	0
MISCELLANEOUS-AREA	12,680	4	2,628	98,419	90,079
Forest Fires	10,280	0	2,419	14,513	84,657
Structural Fires	2,400	4	209	622	5,422
Slash Burning	0	0	0	0	0
Frost Control	0	0	0	0	0
Solvent Evaporation Loss	0	0	0	83,284	0

UTAH

Emission categories	Pollutant, tons per year				
	Particulates	Sulfur oxides	Nitrogen oxides	Hydro-carbons	Carbon monoxide
GRAND TOTAL	80,580	183,007	107,592	103,047	503,995
-AREA	35,046	30,763	81,777	95,466	442,436
-POINT	45,534	152,244	25,814	7,582	61,559
FUEL COMBUSTION-AREA	22,476	25,780	13,374	2,197	7,672
-POINT	11,007	22,044	20,054	339	1,132
External Combustion-area	22,476	25,780	13,374	2,197	7,672
-point	10,838	22,036	19,894	325	920
Residential Fuel-area	1,821	2,107	2,594	1,678	6,600
Anthracite Coal	0	0	0	0	0
Bituminous Coal	1,306	1,736	196	1,306	5,875
Distillate Oil	80	344	96	24	40
Residual Oil	0	0	0	0	0
Natural Gas	280	17	2,240	224	560
Wood	156	9	63	125	125
Electric Generation-point	3,382	12,582	10,799	180	511
Anthracite Coal	0	0	0	0	0
Bituminous Coal	3,283	7,395	6,870	125	398
Lignite	0	0	0	0	0
Residual Oil	92	5,162	2,749	52	79
Distillate Oil	3	24	35	1	1
Natural Gas	5	1	1,145	2	33
Process Gas	0	0	0	0	0
Coke	0	0	0	0	0
Solid Waste/Coal	0	0	0	0	0
Other	0	0	0	0	0
Industrial Fuel-area	19,218	19,680	8,570	377	779
-point	6,913	8,197	8,124	95	291
Anthracite Coal-area	0	0	0	0	0
-point	0	0	0	0	0
Bituminous Coal-area	17,702	3,622	2,043	136	272
-point	6,445	2,857	2,648	29	94
Lignite-point	0	0	0	0	0
Residual Oil-area	1,104	15,274	2,881	144	192
-point	207	2,436	814	41	54
Distillate Oil-area	269	775	1,076	54	72
-point	5	33	20	1	1
Natural Gas-area	143	9	2,570	43	243
-point	90	621	4,641	25	142
Process Gas-area	0	0	0	0	0
-point	166	2,250	0	0	0
Coke-point	0	0	0	0	0
Wood-area	0	0	0	0	0
-point	0	0	0	0	0
Liquid Petroleum Gas-point	0	0	0	0	0
Bagasse-point	0	0	0	0	0
Other-point	0	0	0	0	0
Commercial-Institutional Fuel-area	1,437	3,994	2,211	142	293
-point	542	1,256	972	50	118
Anthracite Coal-area	0	0	0	0	0
-point	0	0	0	0	0
Bituminous Coal-area	920	422	146	32	114
-point	459	911	547	26	78
Lignite-point	0	0	0	0	0
Residual Oil-area	199	2,756	520	26	35
-point	1	0	4	0	0
Distillate Oil-area	282	814	1,130	56	75
-point	78	345	311	16	21
Natural Gas-area	35	2	415	28	69
-point	3	1	109	7	19
Wood-area	0	0	0	0	0
-point	0	0	0	0	0
Liquid Petroleum Gas-point	0	0	0	0	0
Miscellaneous-point	0	0	0	0	0
Internal Combustion-point	169	8	159	14	212
Electric Generation	5	8	137	14	47
Distillate Oil	1	2	11	1	3
Natural Gas	3	0	99	10	28
Diesel Fuel	1	6	27	3	16
Industrial Fuel	0	0	0	0	0
Distillate Oil	0	0	0	0	0
Natural Gas	0	0	0	0	0
Gasoline	0	0	0	0	0
Diesel Fuel	0	0	0	0	0

Emission categories	Pollutant, tons per year				
	Particulates	Sulfur oxides	Nitrogen oxides	Hydro-carbons	Carbon monoxide
Other	0	0	0	0	0
Commercial-Institutional	0	0	0	0	0
Diesel Fuel	0	0	0	0	0
Other	0	0	0	0	0
Engine-Testing	164	0	22	0	165
Aircraft	0	0	0	0	0
Other	164	0	22	0	165
Miscellaneous	0	0	0	0	0
INDUSTRIAL PROCESS-POINT	33,913	130,123	5,681	6,980	56,806
Chemical Manufacturing	65	26,470	166	256	0
Food/Agriculture	0	0	0	0	0
Primary Metal	8,561	83,148	36	3,753	21,410
Secondary Metals	161	7	0	0	5,675
Mineral Products	23,930	4,181	698	608	365
Petroleum Industry	1,195	16,317	4,780	1,654	29,355
Wood Products	0	0	0	0	0
Evaporation	0	0	0	709	0
Metal Fabrication	0	0	0	0	0
Leather Products	0	0	0	0	0
Textile Manufacturing	0	0	0	0	0
Inprocess Fuel	0	0	1	1	1
Other/Not Classified	0	0	0	0	0
SOLID WASTE DISPOSAL-AREA	978	124	244	1,773	5,086
-POINT	614	77	80	263	3,621
Government-point	475	75	60	45	1,047
Municipal Incineration	475	75	60	45	1,047
Open Burning	0	0	0	0	0
Other	0	0	0	0	0
Residential-area	662	25	126	1,576	4,631
On Site Incineration	356	6	11	1,003	3,008
Open Burning	306	19	115	573	1,624
Commercial-Institutional-area	220	69	83	138	317
-point	0	0	0	0	0
On Site Incineration-area	220	69	83	138	317
-point	0	0	0	0	0
Open Burning-area	0	0	0	0	0
-point	0	0	0	0	0
Apartment-point	0	0	0	0	0
Other-point	0	0	0	0	0
Industrial-area	96	30	36	60	138
-point	139	2	20	218	2,574
On Site Incineration-area	96	30	36	60	138
-point	139	2	20	218	2,574
Open Burning-area	0	0	0	0	0
-point	0	0	0	0	0
Auto Body Incineration-point	0	0	0	0	0
Other-point	0	0	0	0	0
Miscellaneous-point	0	0	0	0	0
TRANSPORTATION-AREA	8,402	4,859	67,527	82,101	408,170
Land Vehicles	6,251	4,376	65,646	69,196	396,645
Gasoline	4,374	1,247	40,522	64,679	387,495
Light Vehicles	3,657	948	32,438	45,027	246,184
Heavy Vehicles	531	201	5,962	13,669	73,474
Off Highway	186	97	2,122	5,984	67,837
Diesel Fuel	1,877	3,129	25,124	4,517	9,150
Heavy Vehicles	601	841	7,901	862	3,445
Off Highway	450	403	4,987	546	1,406
Rail	827	1,885	12,236	3,109	4,299
Aircraft	2,151	484	1,881	6,301	11,525
Military	1,912	365	919	4,449	4,776
Civil	181	36	164	802	4,584
Commercial	57	82	799	1,049	2,165
Vessels	0	0	0	0	0
Bituminous Coal	0	0	0	0	0
Diesel Fuel	0	0	0	0	0
Residual Oil	0	0	0	0	0
Gasoline	0	0	0	0	0
Gas Handling Evaporation Loss	0	0	0	6,604	0
MISCELLANEOUS-AREA	3,189	0	632	9,394	21,508
Forest Fires	2,245	0	528	3,169	18,484
Structural Fires	244	0	21	63	·550
Slash Burning	701	0	82	825	2,474
Frost Control	0	0	0	0	0
Solvent Evaporation Loss	0	0	0	5,338	0

VERMONT

Emission categories	Pollutant, tons per year				
	Particulates	Sulfur oxides	Nitrogen oxides	Hydro-carbons	Carbon monoxide
GRAND TOTAL	16,922	11,443	29,200	41,372	163,365
–AREA	6,166	5,207	26,482	37,507	162,712
–POINT	10,756	6,236	2,718	3,866	653
FUEL COMBUSTION–AREA	1,879	4,007	3,195	622	1,140
–POINT	2,688	6,216	2,713	184	362
External Combustion–area	1,879	4,007	3,195	622	1,140
–point	2,663	6,103	2,294	147	213
Residential Fuel–area	1,128	2,214	1,135	518	965
Anthracite Coal	32	84	10	8	292
Bituminous Coal	0	0	0	0	0
Distillate Oil	732	2,109	878	220	366
Residual Oil	0	0	0	0	0
Natural Gas	13	1	107	11	27
Wood	350	21	140	280	280
Electric Generation–point	1,146	698	470	18	39
Anthracite Coal	0	0	0	0	0
Bituminous Coal	1,140	616	248	17	33
Lignite	0	0	0	0	0
Residual Oil	3	79	36	1	1
Distillate Oil	1	2	9	0	0
Natural Gas	2	0	177	0	5
Process Gas	0	0	0	0	0
Coke	0	0	0	0	0
Solid Waste/Coal	0	0	0	0	0
Other	0	0	0	0	0
Industrial Fuel–area	236	309	541	25	40
–point	1,378	3,894	1,405	108	145
Anthracite Coal–area	33	45	25	0	3
–point	0	0	0	0	0
Bituminous Coal–area	86	25	16	1	2
–point	154	74	15	1	3
Lignite–point	0	0	0	0	0
Residual Oil–area	2	21	5	0	0
–point	301	3,307	786	39	52
Distillate Oil–area	113	217	453	23	30
–point	53	475	211	11	14
Natural Gas–area	2	0	41	1	4
–point	7	0	143	2	11
Process Gas–area	0	0	0	0	0
–point	0	0	0	0	0
Coke–point	0	0	0	0	0
Wood–area	0	0	0	0	0
–point	862	37	246	55	65
Liquid Petroleum Gas–point	1	0	4	0	1
Bagasse–point	0	0	0	0	0
Other–point	0	0	0	0	0
Commercial-Institutional Fuel–area	514	1,484	1,519	79	135
–point	139	1,511	420	21	29
Anthracite Coal–area	59	80	30	1	18
–point	0	0	0	0	0
Bituminous Coal–area	70	46	18	4	14
–point	4	19	4	0	0
Lignite–point	0	0	0	0	0
Residual Oil–area	74	768	193	10	13
–point	118	1,359	341	17	23
Distillate Oil–area	307	590	1,229	61	82
–point	18	133	70	4	5
Natural Gas–area	4	0	49	3	8
–point	0	0	5	0	1
Wood–area	0	0	0	0	0
–point	0	0	0	0	0
Liquid Petroleum Gas–point	0	0	0	0	0
Miscellaneous–point	0	0	0	0	0
Internal Combustion–point	25	112	419	37	149
Electric Generation	16	97	295	27	120
Distillate Oil	11	92	154	13	35
Natural Gas	0	0	0	0	0
Diesel Fuel	5	5	140	14	85
Industrial Fuel	9	15	124	10	28
Distillate Oil	9	15	124	10	28
Natural Gas	0	0	0	0	0
Gasoline	0	0	0	0	0
Diesel Fuel	0	0	0	0	0

Emission categories	Pollutant, tons per year				
	Particulates	Sulfur oxides	Nitrogen oxides	Hydro- carbons	Carbon monoxide
Other	0	0	0	0	0
Commercial-Institutional	0	0	0	0	0
Diesel Fuel	0	0	0	0	0
Other	0	0	0	0	0
Engine-Testing	0	0	0	0	0
Aircraft	0	0	0	0	0
Other	0	0	0	0	0
Miscellaneous	0	0	0	0	0
INDUSTRIAL PROCESS-POINT	8,049	19	0	3,674	277
Chemical Manufacturing	3	0	0	0	0
Food/Agriculture	581	0	0	0	0
Primary Metal	0	0	0	0	0
Secondary Metals	36	19	0	0	277
Mineral Products	7,424	0	0	0	0
Petroleum Industry	0	0	0	0	0
Wood Products	0	0	0	15	0
Evaporation	1	0	0	3,659	0
Metal Fabrication	2	0	0	0	0
Leather Products	0	0	0	0	0
Textile Manufacturing	0	0	0	0	0
Inprocess Fuel	3	0	0	0	0
Other/Not Classified	0	0	0	0	0
SOLID WASTE DISPOSAL-AREA	1,148	87	282	2,380	6,897
-POINT	18	1	5	8	14
Government-point	0	0	0	0	0
Municipal Incineration	0	0	0	0	0
Open Burning	0	0	0	0	0
Other	0	0	0	0	0
Residential-area	962	40	212	2,209	6,460
On Site Incineration	432	7	13	1,214	3,642
Open Burning	530	33	199	995	2,818
Commercial-Institutional-area	175	44	66	165	422
-point	6	1	1	7	10
On Site Incineration-area	131	41	49	82	189
-point	6	1	1	7	10
Open Burning-area	44	3	16	83	234
-point	0	0	0	0	0
Apartment-point	0	0	0	0	0
Other-point	0	0	0	0	0
Industrial-area	10	3	4	7	15
-point	12	0	4	0	3
On Site Incineration-area	10	3	4	7	15
-point	11	0	3	0	0
Open Burning-area	0	0	0	0	0
-point	1	0	0	0	3
Auto Body Incineration-point	0	0	0	0	0
Other-point	0	0	0	0	0
Miscellaneous-point	0	0	0	0	0
TRANSPORTATION-AREA	3,045	1,113	22,994	33,783	154,348
Land Vehicles	2,256	921	22,203	27,749	148,131
Gasoline	1,990	552	18,714	27,332	146,946
Light Vehicles	1,719	446	15,593	20,461	106,578
Heavy Vehicles	249	94	2,870	6,163	32,336
Off Highway	22	12	251	708	8,032
Diesel Fuel	266	369	3,489	417	1,185
Heavy Vehicles	181	253	2,436	240	858
Off Highway	56	51	625	68	176
Rail	29	66	427	109	150
Aircraft	784	181	722	2,276	3,424
Military	733	140	352	1,706	1,831
Civil	26	5	23	114	653
Commercial	25	36	347	455	940
Vessels	5	12	69	885	2,793
Bituminous Coal	0	0	0	0	0
Diesel Fuel	5	6	44	11	15
Residual Oil	0	0	0	0	0
Gasoline	0	6	26	874	2,778
Gas Handling Evaporation Loss	0	0	0	2,873	0
MISCELLANEOUS-AREA	95	0	11	722	327
Forest Fires	17	0	4	24	140
Structural Fires	71	0	6	18	160
Slash Burning	8	0	1	9	27
Frost Control	0	0	0	0	0
Solvent Evaporation Loss	0	0	0	670	0

VIRGINIA

Emission categories	Pollutant, tons per year				
	Particulates	Sulfur oxides	Nitrogen oxides	Hydro- carbons	Carbon monoxide
GRAND TOTAL	444,529	575,054	434,569	483,501	1,881,071
-AREA	49,441	85,294	252,924	353,760	1,694,394
-POINT	395,088	489,760	181,645	129,742	186,677
FUEL COMBUSTION-AREA	18,087	70,398	29,461	7,863	18,302
-POINT	170,512	421,252	150,354	4,976	21,426
External Combustion-area	18,087	70,398	29,461	7,863	18,302
-point	170,508	421,235	150,335	4,916	21,383
Residential Fuel-area	9,395	4,086	7,298	6,846	16,457
Anthracite Coal	0	0	0	0	0
Bituminous Coal	2,509	3,814	376	2,509	11,290
Distillate Oil	2,345	0	2,814	703	1,172
Residual Oil	0	0	0	0	0
Natural Gas	301	18	2,412	241	603
Wood	4,240	254	1,696	3,392	3,392
Electric Generation-point	92,182	255,249	95,964	1,695	3,769
Anthracite Coal	0	0	0	0	0
Bituminous Coal	90,750	65,111	40,337	654	2,180
Lignite	0	0	0	0	0
Residual Oil	1,311	189,840	53,088	1,011	1,517
Distillate Oil	111	296	1,474	28	42
Natural Gas	10	1	1,065	2	30
Process Gas	0	0	0	0	0
Coke	0	0	0	0	0
Solid Waste/Coal	0	0	0	0	0
Other	0	0	0	0	0
Industrial Fuel-area	4,374	12,883	8,703	309	732
-point	75,635	158,070	51,290	2,956	17,088
Anthracite Coal-area	0	0	0	0	0
-point	0	0	0	0	0
Bituminous Coal-area	2,855	1,171	578	39	77
-point	60,606	84,108	29,401	756	2,134
Lignite-point	0	0	0	0	0
Residual Oil-area	811	11,698	2,116	106	141
-point	3,823	70,363	12,094	644	13,307
Distillate Oil-area	481	0	1,924	96	128
-point	1,219	1,286	586	27	36
Natural Gas-area	227	14	4,085	68	386
-point	96	8	2,620	182	185
Process Gas-area	0	0	0	0	0
-point	0	3	59	0	0
Coke-point	0	0	0	0	0
Wood-area	0	0	0	0	0
-point	8,741	970	6,461	1,342	1,424
Liquid Petroleum Gas-point	2	6	12	0	2
Bagasse-point	0	0	0	0	0
Other-point	1,149	1,326	57	5	1
Commercial-Institutional Fuel-area	4,318	53,429	13,460	709	1,113
-point	2,691	7,916	3,080	264	527
Anthracite Coal-area	0	0	0	0	0
-point	0	0	0	0	0
Bituminous Coal-area	0	0	0	0	0
-point	2,104	3,757	1,575	128	295
Lignite-point	0	0	0	0	0
Residual Oil-area	3,770	53,418	9,835	492	656
-point	358	3,607	935	47	62
Distillate Oil-area	368	0	1,471	74	98
-point	89	532	355	17	23
Natural Gas-area	179	11	2,153	144	359
-point	6	0	76	5	13
Wood-area	0	0	0	0	0
-point	132	20	132	66	132
Liquid Petroleum Gas-point	1	0	7	1	1
Miscellaneous-point	0	0	0	0	0
Internal Combustion-point	5	17	19	60	43
Electric Generation	0	0	0	0	0
Distillate Oil	0	0	0	0	0
Natural Gas	0	0	0	0	0
Diesel Fuel	0	0	0	0	0
Industrial Fuel	0	0	0	0	0
Distillate Oil	0	0	0	0	0
Natural Gas	0	0	0	0	0
Gasoline	0	0	0	0	0
Diesel Fuel	0	0	0	0	0

Emission categories	Pollutant, tons per year				
	Particulates	Sulfur oxides	Nitrogen oxides	Hydro-carbons	Carbon monoxide
Other	0	0	0	0	0
Commercial-Institutional	0	0	0	0	0
Diesel Fuel	0	0	0	0	0
Other	0	0	0	0	0
Engine-Testing	5	17	19	60	43
Aircraft	5	17	19	60	43
Other	0	0	0	0	0
Miscellaneous	0	0	0	0	0
INDUSTRIAL PROCESS-POINT	222,822	68,239	30,937	123,610	157,418
Chemical Manufacturing	5,273	12,161	21,173	30,819	302
Food/Agriculture	1,880	0	0	6	51
Primary Metal	2,590	1,437	25	2,465	689
Secondary Metals	4,637	1,711	37	45	27,733
Mineral Products	193,730	608	99	302	1,507
Petroleum Industry	2,049	46,433	6,389	1,218	57,506
Wood Products	10,076	5,325	22	3,947	68,915
Evaporation	668	4	2,890	75,320	1
Metal Fabrication	705	0	282	197	0
Leather Products	0	0	0	0	0
Textile Manufacturing	15	0	0	569	0
Inprocess Fuel	426	58	4	769	221
Other/Not Classified	774	502	16	7,955	492
SOLID WASTE DISPOSAL-AREA	4,940	605	1,796	7,896	22,042
-POINT	1,753	269	354	1,156	7,834
Government-point	829	212	179	432	2,008
Municipal Incineration	774	150	120	341	1,819
Open Burning	35	2	13	66	188
Other	20	60	46	25	1
Residential-area	3,470	209	1,245	6,660	18,946
On Site Incineration	164	3	5	460	1,381
Open Burning	3,306	207	1,240	6,200	17,565
Commercial-Institutional-area	803	213	301	689	1,734
-point	14	4	3	2	3
On Site Incineration-area	653	204	245	408	939
-point	14	4	3	2	3
Open Burning-area	150	9	56	281	795
-point	0	0	0	0	0
Apartment-point	0	0	0	0	0
Other-point	0	0	0	0	0
Industrial-area	667	182	250	547	1,362
-point	910	54	172	722	5,822
On Site Incineration-area	563	176	211	352	810
-point	701	46	116	521	4,998
Open Burning-area	104	6	39	195	553
-point	206	6	48	199	824
Auto Body Incineration-point	0	0	0	0	0
Other-point	3	2	8	2	0
Miscellaneous-point	0	0	0	0	0
TRANSPORTATION-AREA	26,414	14,291	221,667	317,747	1,654,049
Land Vehicles	22,851	11,420	215,433	275,543	1,616,843
Gasoline	18,920	5,056	163,784	266,639	1,593,573
Light Vehicles	17,787	4,612	151,547	234,587	1,394,424
Heavy Vehicles	1,028	389	11,045	28,688	161,017
Off Highway	105	55	1,193	3,363	38,132
Diesel Fuel	3,931	6,364	51,649	8,904	23,270
Heavy Vehicles	2,006	2,808	25,393	3,198	14,509
Off Highway	602	538	6,668	730	1,879
Rail	1,324	3,018	19,588	4,976	6,882
Aircraft	3,262	853	4,089	10,751	16,993
Military	2,976	568	1,430	6,924	7,433
Civil	103	20	93	456	2,606
Commercial	183	265	2,566	3,370	6,954
Vessels	301	2,018	2,145	6,633	20,213
Bituminous Coal	0	0	0	0	0
Diesel Fuel	183	229	1,708	448	598
Residual Oil	118	1,747	255	18	9
Gasoline	0	42	181	6,167	19,607
Gas Handling Evaporation Loss	0	0	0	24,820	0
MISCELLANEOUS-AREA	0	0	0	20,254	0
Forest Fires	0	0	0	0	0
Structural Fires	0	0	0	0	0
Slash Burning	0	0	0	0	0
Frost Control	0	0	0	0	0
Solvent Evaporation Loss	0	0	0	20,254	0

WASHINGTON

Emission categories	Pollutant, tons per year				
	Particulates	Sulfur oxides	Nitrogen oxides	Hydro-carbons	Carbon monoxide
GRAND TOTAL	183,904	350,342	348,836	336,944	1,586,480
-AREA	46,665	36,076	201,138	294,860	1,320,802
-POINT	137,239	314,266	147,698	42,084	265,678
FUEL COMBUSTION-AREA	6,942	23,245	15,706	3,032	4,337
-POINT	43,610	67,189	69,288	4,620	18,031
External Combustion-area	6,942	23,245	15,706	3,032	4,337
-point	43,609	67,184	69,279	4,619	18,029
Residential Fuel-area	4,438	7,959	4,936	2,555	3,443
Anthracite Coal	0	0	0	0	0
Bituminous Coal	87	383	13	87	393
Distillate Oil	1,677	4,913	2,013	503	839
Residual Oil	260	2,518	452	34	45
Natural Gas	196	12	1,571	157	393
Wood	2,218	133	887	1,774	1,774
Electric Generation-point	12,217	22,037	34,959	602	1,899
Anthracite Coal	0	0	0	0	0
Bituminous Coal	12,108	19,000	33,750	563	1,875
Lignite	0	0	0	0	0
Residual Oil	69	2,919	280	29	3
Distillate Oil	8	115	243	5	7
Natural Gas	33	3	686	5	14
Process Gas	0	0	0	0	0
Coke	0	0	0	0	0
Solid Waste/Coal	0	0	0	0	0
Other	0	0	0	0	0
Industrial Fuel-area	1,168	7,622	5,566	198	438
-point	29,308	42,039	32,730	3,927	15,965
Anthracite Coal-area	0	0	0	0	0
-point	0	0	0	0	0
Bituminous Coal-area	0	0	^0	0	0
-point	852	1,737	696	43	88
Lignite-point	0	0	0	0	0
Residual Oil-area	697	6,869	1,819	91	121
-point	2,729	29,344	5,462	431	1,592
Distillate Oil-area	337	745	1,349	67	90
-point	42	180	167	8	11
Natural Gas-area	133	8	2,398	40	226
-point	503	2,997	10,309	235	394
Process Gas-area	0	0	0	0	0
-point	565	5,699	1,172	110	8,366
Coke-point	0	0	0	0	0
Wood-area	0	0	0	0	0
-point	24,163	1,747	14,825	3,089	4,475
Liquid Petroleum Gas-point	3	0	17	0	2
Bagasse-point	0	0	0	0	0
Other-point	450	335	82	10	1,037
Commercial-Institutional Fuel-area	1,335	7,664	5,203	278	456
-point	2,084	3,108	1,591	90	165
Anthracite Coal-area	0	0	0	0	0
-point	0	0	0	0	0
Bituminous Coal-area	0	0	0	0	0
-point	1,724	477	287	27	66
Lignite-point	0	0	0	0	0
Residual Oil-area	622	6,447	1,622	81	108
-point	250	2,388	642	32	43
Distillate Oil-area	623	1,212	2,490	125	166
-point	94	241	378	19	25
Natural Gas-area	91	5	1,091	73	182
-point	15	1	284	12	31
Wood-area	0	0	0	0	0
-point	0	0	0	0	0
Liquid Petroleum Gas-point	0	0	0	0	0
Miscellaneous-point	1	0	0	0	2
Internal Combustion-point	1	5	8	1	2
Electric Generation	1	5	8	1	2
Distillate Oil	1	5	8	1	2
Natural Gas	0	0	0	0	0
Diesel Fuel	0	0	0	0	0
Industrial Fuel	0	0	0	0	0
Distillate Oil	0	0	0	0	0
Natural Gas	0	0	0	0	0
Gasoline	0	0	0	0	0
Diesel Fuel	0	0	0	0	0

Emission categories	Pollutant, tons per year				
	Particulates	Sulfur oxides	Nitrogen oxides	Hydro-carbons	Carbon monoxide
Other	0	0	0	0	0
Commercial-Institutional	0	0	0	0	0
Diesel Fuel	0	0	0	0	0
Other	0	0	0	0	0
Engine-Testing	0	0	0	0	0
Aircraft	0	0	0	0	0
Other	0	0	0	0	0
Miscellaneous	0	0	0	0	0
INDUSTRIAL PROCESS-POINT	87,797	246,855	77,780	33,235	196,530
Chemical Manufacturing	119	1,427	2,316	679	679
Food/Agriculture	5,831	0	0	57	5
Primary Metal	29,647	206,230	473	1,798	122,748
Secondary Metals	1,183	1,422	47	34	944
Mineral Products	23,022	8,759	1,694	543	8,104
Petroleum Industry	9,374	11,479	73,203	4,250	565
Wood Products	17,677	16,341	25	2,595	60,735
Evaporation	0	0	0	20,331	0
Metal Fabrication	50	0	0	0	0
Leather Products	0	0	0	0	0
Textile Manufacturing	0	0	0	0	0
Inprocess Fuel	895	1,196	21	2,947	2,750
Other/Not Classified	0	0	0	0	0
SOLID WASTE DISPOSAL-AREA	3,911	205	788	8,917	26,119
-POINT	5,832	222	630	4,229	51,118
Government-point	209	13	69	363	1,035
Municipal Incineration	0	0	0	0	0
Open Burning	184	11	66	338	960
Other	25	3	3	25	75
Residential-area	3,198	107	520	7,849	23,164
On Site Incineration	1,975	31	62	5,555	16,666
Open Burning	1,223	76	459	2,294	6,498
Commercial-Institutional-area	426	68	160	590	1,617
-point	7	0	1	2	20
On Site Incineration-area	167	52	63	104	240
-point	0	0	0	0	0
Open Burning-area	259	16	97	486	1,377
-point	7	0	1	2	20
Apartment-point	0	0	0	0	0
Other-point	0	0	0	0	0
Industrial-area	286	30	107	478	1,339
-point	5,617	209	560	3,865	50,064
On Site Incineration-area	47	15	18	30	68
-point	5,589	41	557	3,854	49,991
Open Burning-area	239	15	90	449	1,271
-point	25	168	3	11	61
Auto Body Incineration-point	2	0	0	1	3
Other-point	0	0	0	0	10
Miscellaneous-point	0	0	0	0	0
TRANSPORTATION-AREA	19,870	12,624	182,609	236,944	1,227,707
Land Vehicles	17,730	8,924	174,912	204,451	1,188,683
Gasoline	13,888	3,847	127,035	197,728	1,171,454
Light Vehicles	12,326	3,196	109,419	154,313	857,933
Heavy Vehicles	1,152	437	12,943	30,238	164,127
Off Highway	410	215	4,673	13,177	149,393
Diesel Fuel	3,842	5,077	47,877	6,723	17,229
Heavy Vehicles	1,374	1,923	17,994	1,992	8,106
Off Highway	1,786	1,598	19,789	2,167	5,578
Rail	682	1,555	10,094	2,564	3,546
Aircraft	1,396	359	1,795	5,211	14,926
Military	934	178	449	2,174	2,333
Civil	391	78	353	1,733	9,903
Commercial	71	102	993	1,304	2,690
Vessels	744	3,342	5,902	8,412	24,098
Bituminous Coal	0	0	0	0	0
Diesel Fuel	570	712	5,319	1,396	1,862
Residual Oil	174	2,583	377	26	13
Gasoline	0	47	206	6,990	22,224
Gas Handling Evaporation Loss	0	0	0	18,870	0
MISCELLANEOUS-AREA	15,943	1	2,036	45,966	62,638
Forest Fires	1,553	0	365	2,192	12,786
Structural Fires	737	1	64	191	1,665
Slash Burning	13,653	0	1,606	16,063	48,188
Frost Control	0	0	0	0	0
Solvent Evaporation Loss	0	0	0	27,521	0

WEST VIRGINIA

Emission categories	Pollutant, tons per year				
	Particulates	Sulfur oxides	Nitrogen oxides	Hydro- carbons	Carbon monoxide
GRAND TOTAL	305,146	913,153	355,233	113,711	1,117,761
-AREA	16,965	20,475	91,687	107,335	509,578
-POINT	288,182	892,678	263,546	6,376	608,183
FUEL COMBUSTION-AREA	5,325	16,121	16,025	3,920	14,689
-POINT	263,322	882,819	262,239	3,035	9,588
External Combustion-area	5,325	16,121	16,025	3,920	14,689
-point	263,320	882,818	262,218	3,033	9,583
Residential Fuel-area	3,926	11,133	3,414	3,549	13,447
Anthracite Coal	0	0	0	0	0
Bituminous Coal	2,709	10,293	406	2,709	12,190
Distillate Oil	267	783	321	80	134
Residual Oil	0	0	0	0	0
Natural Gas	304	18	2,428	243	607
Wood	646	39	259	517	517
Electric Generation-point	258,796	868,174	257,417	2,856	9,192
Anthracite Coal	201	1,847	1,215	2	68
Bituminous Coal	258,589	866,185	255,683	2,844	9,110
Lignite	0	0	0	0	0
Residual Oil	0	0	0	0	0
Distillate Oil	6	142	519	10	15
Natural Gas	0	0	0	0	0
Process Gas	0	0	0	0	0
Coke	0	0	0	0	0
Solid Waste/Coal	0	0	0	0	0
Other	0	0	0	0	0
Industrial Fuel-area	1,074	3,438	10,477	238	937
-point	4,524	14,639	4,799	176	391
Anthracite Coal-area	0	0	0	0	0
-point	0	0	0	0	0
Bituminous Coal-area	0	0	0	0	0
-point	4,252	9,101	3,868	153	351
Lignite-point	0	0	0	0	0
Residual Oil-area	355	2,943	925	46	62
-point	19	807	156	8	10
Distillate Oil-area	243	466	970	49	65
-point	125	2,918	733	15	26
Natural Gas-area	477	29	8,581	143	810
-point	2	0	42	1	3
Process Gas-area	0	0	0	0	0
-point	0	0	0	0	0
Coke-point	0	0	0	0	0
Wood-area	0	0	0	0	0
-point	0	0	0	0	0
Liquid Petroleum Gas-point	0	0	0	0	0
Bagasse-point	0	0	0	0	0
Other-point	126	1,813	0	0	0
Commercial-Institutional Fuel-area	325	1,550	2,134	134	305
-point	0	5	2	0	0
Anthracite Coal-area	0	0	0	0	0
-point	0	0	0	0	0
Bituminous Coal-area	0	0	0	0	0
-point	0	0	0	0	0
Lignite-point	0	0	0	0	0
Residual Oil-area	182	1,527	474	24	32
-point	0	0	0	0	0
Distillate Oil-area	7	14	30	1	2
-point	0	5	1	0	0
Natural Gas-area	136	8	1,630	109	272
-point	0	0	1	0	0
Wood-area	0	0	0	0	0
-point	0	0	0	0	0
Liquid Petroleum Gas-point	0	0	0	0	0
Miscellaneous-point	0	0	0	0	0
Internal Combustion-point	2	1	21	2	5
Electric Generation	2	1	21	2	5
Distillate Oil	2	1	21	2	5
Natural Gas	0	0	0	0	0
Diesel Fuel	0	0	0	0	0
Industrial Fuel	0	0	0	0	0
Distillate Oil	0	0	0	0	0
Natural Gas	0	0	0	0	0
Gasoline	0	0	0	0	0
Diesel Fuel	0	0	0	0	0

Emission categories	Pollutant, tons per year				
	Particulates	Sulfur oxides	Nitrogen oxides	Hydro-carbons	Carbon monoxide
Other	0	0	0	0	0
Commercial-Institutional	0	0	0	0	0
Diesel Fuel	0	0	0	0	0
Other	0	0	0	0	0
Engine-Testing	0	0	0	0	0
Aircraft	0	0	0	0	0
Other	0	0	0	0	0
Miscellaneous	0	0	0	0	0
INDUSTRIAL PROCESS-POINT	24,751	9,826	1,242	3,297	598,533
Chemical Manufacturing	263	3,685	0	218	0
Food/Agriculture	0	0	0	0	0
Primary Metal	21,688	4,798	1,242	2,064	304,000
Secondary Metals	0	0	0	0	0
Mineral Products	2,730	1,343	0	0	0
Petroleum Industry	0	0	0	0	0
Wood Products	0	0	0	0	0
Evaporation	0	0	0	1,015	0
Metal Fabrication	0	0	0	0	0
Leather Products	0	0	0	0	0
Textile Manufacturing	0	0	0	0	0
Inprocess Fuel	70	0	0	0	294,533
Other/Not Classified	0	0	0	0	0
SOLID WASTE DISPOSAL-AREA	1,556	97	583	2,918	8,266
-POINT	109	33	65	44	62
Government-point	0	0	0	0	0
Municipal Incineration	0	0	0	0	0
Open Burning	0	0	0	0	0
Other	0	0	0	0	0
Residential-area	1,366	85	512	2,561	7,255
On Site Incineration	0	0	0	0	0
Open Burning	1,366	85	512	2,561	7,255
Commercial-Institutional-area	139	9	52	261	740
-point	0	0	0	0	0
On Site Incineration-area	0	0	0	0	0
-point	0	0	0	0	0
Open Burning-area	139	9	52	261	740
-point	0	0	0	0	0
Apartment-point	0	0	0	0	0
Other-point	0	0	0	0	0
Industrial-area	51	3	19	96	272
-point	109	33	65	44	62
On Site Incineration-area	0	0	0	0	0
-point	93	33	65	44	62
Open Burning-area	51	3	19	96	272
-point	0	0	0	0	0
Auto Body Incineration-point	0	0	0	0	0
Other-point	16	0	0	0	0
Miscellaneous-point	0	0	0	0	0
TRANSPORTATION-AREA	7,911	4,256	74,623	92,661	470,968
Land Vehicles	7,528	3,990	72,853	81,947	464,407
Gasoline	5,931	1,572	52,075	78,708	456,051
Light Vehicles	5,704	1,479	49,569	72,411	412,137
Heavy Vehicles	176	67	1,936	4,689	25,684
Off Highway	50	26	570	1,608	18,231
Diesel Fuel	1,597	2,418	20,778	3,239	8,356
Heavy Vehicles	796	1,114	10,328	1,188	4,975
Off Highway	377	337	4,173	457	1,176
Rail	424	967	6,277	1,595	2,205
Aircraft	242	73	427	1,064	3,194
Military	140	27	67	326	350
Civil	82	16	74	362	2,069
Commercial	20	29	286	376	775
Vessels	142	194	1,342	1,259	3,367
Bituminous Coal	0	0	0	0	0
Diesel Fuel	141	176	1,314	345	460
Residual Oil	1	11	2	0	0
Gasoline	0	6	27	914	2,907
Gas Handling Evaporation Loss	0	0	0	8,391	0
MISCELLANEOUS-AREA	2,173	1	456	7,836	15,654
Forest Fires	1,798	0	423	2,539	14,808
Structural Fires	374	1	33	97	846
Slash Burning	0	0	0	0	0
Frost Control	0	0	0	0	0
Solvent Evaporation Loss	0	0	0	5,200	0

WISCONSIN

Emission categories	Pollutant, tons per year				
	Particulates	Sulfur oxides	Nitrogen oxides	Hydro-carbons	Carbon monoxide
GRAND TOTAL	380,064	745,998	465,065	574,454	1,886,15:
-AREA	110,466	85,359	229,109	378,307	1,815,03(
-POINT	269,597	660,638	235,956	196,147	71,11;
FUEL COMBUSTION-AREA	73,929	74,116	36,702	5,525	14,544
-POINT	211,186	620,165	189,246	3,218	15,96!
External Combustion-area	73,929	74,116	36,702	5,525	14,544
-point	211,186	620,165	188,960	3,218	15,96
Residential Fuel-area	6,398	18,341	9,739	3,701	9,70
Anthracite Coal	0	0	0	0	
Bituminous Coal	1,307	3,724	196	1,307	5,88
Distillate Oil	3,359	14,513	4,030	1,008	1,67!
Residual Oil	0	0	0	0	
Natural Gas	634	38	5,073	507	1,26
Wood	1,099	66	440	879	87
Electric Generation-point	158,015	518,898	147,101	1,739	5,57!
Anthracite Coal	0	0	0	0	(
Bituminous Coal	157,833	518,092	137,722	1,694	5,31:
Lignite	0	0	0	0	
Residual Oil	96	676	1,269	26	3(
Distillate Oil	5	122	297	6	;
Natural Gas	81	8	7,813	13	22:
Process Gas	0	0	0	0	(
Coke	0	0	0	0	
Solid Waste/Coal	0	0	0	0	
Other	0	0	0	0	
Industrial Fuel-area	52,595	34,091	16,705	781	1,79(
-point	51,007	98,063	40,065	1,388	10,18:
Anthracite Coal-area	0	0	0	0	
-point	0	0	0	0	
Bituminous Coal-area	51,361	30,026	7,902	527	1,05<
-point	40,987	92,001	26,499	827	1,95:
Lignite-point	0	0	0	0	
Residual Oil-area	343	2,370	894	45	6(
-point	985	3,618	742	38	52:
Distillate Oil-area	582	1,677	2,328	116	15:
-point	300	308	1,216	61	8:
Natural Gas-area	310	19	5,582	93	52
-point	465	17	9,570	83	46!
Process Gas-area	0	0	0	0	(
-point	4	0	0	0	(
Coke-point	0	0	0	0	
Wood-area	0	0	0	0	
-point	4,606	754	1,869	366	84(
Liquid Petroleum Gas-point	8	30	54	1	
Bagasse-point	0	0	0	0	
Other-point	3,651	1,335	115	13	6,30
Commercial-Institutional Fuel-area	14,935	21,683	10,258	1,044	3,04
-point	2,165	3,204	1,794	91	20
Anthracite Coal-area	0	0	0	0	
-point	0	0	0	0	!
Bituminous Coal-area	13,544	17,747	2,864	623	2,24.
-point	2,059	2,985	604	30	6
Lignite-point	0	0	0	0	!
Residual Oil-area	161	1,114	420	21	2:
-point	13	96	35	2	
Distillate Oil-area	974	2,807	3,897	195	26(
-point	17	117	74	4	
Natural Gas-area	256	15	3,076	205	51:
-point	47	3	1,053	42	10:
Wood-area	0	0	0	0	
-point	27	4	27	14	2;
Liquid Petroleum Gas-point	0	0	0	0	
Miscellaneous-point	0	0	0	0	
Internal Combustion-point	0	0	286	0	
Electric Generation	0	0	286	0	
Distillate Oil	0	0	0	0	
Natural Gas	0	0	286	0	
Diesel Fuel	0	0	0	0	
Industrial Fuel	0	0	0	0	
Distillate Oil	0	0	0	0	
Natural Gas	0	0	0	0	
Gasoline	0	0	0	0	
Diesel Fuel	0	0	0	0	

Emission categories	Pollutant, tons per year				
	Particulates	Sulfur oxides	Nitrogen oxides	Hydro-carbons	Carbon monoxide
Other...............	0	0	0	0	0
Commercial-Institutional........	0	0	0	0	0
Diesel Fuel........	0	0	0	0	0
Other........	0	0	0	0	0
Engine-Testing........	0	0	0	0	0
Aircraft........	0	0	0	0	0
Other........	0	0	0	0	0
Miscellaneous........	0	0	0	0	0
INDUSTRIAL PROCESS-POINT........	54,802	40,066	45,908	192,254	50,302
Chemical Manufacturing........	1,035	0	0	596	144
Food/Agriculture........	2,932	0	0	145	11
Primary Metal........	1,292	661	5	444	110
Secondary Metals........	3,036	0	0	24	32,089
Mineral Products........	36,115	22,991	42,252	3,533	13,314
Petroleum Industry........	30	259	97	5	0
Wood Products........	9,592	15,006	1,470	185	4,002
Evaporation........	1	0	0	108,143	0
Metal Fabrication........	0	0	0	89	0
Leather Products........	0	0	0	0	0
Textile Manufacturing........	0	0	0	0	0
Inprocess Fuel........	762	1,133	2,054	111	632
Other/Not Classified........	10	17	31	78,980	0
SOLID WASTE DISPOSAL-AREA........	16,093	1,678	4,231	30,503	87,662
-POINT........	3,609	407	803	676	4,846
Government-point........	3,172	279	224	414	3,638
Municipal Incineration........	3,172	279	224	414	3,638
Open Burning........	0	0	0	0	0
Other........	0	0	0	0	0
Residential-area........	10,198	391	2,020	24,040	70,572
On Site Incineration........	5,247	82	164	14,758	44,273
Open Burning........	4,950	309	1,856	9,282	26,299
Commercial-Institutional-area........	5,158	1,164	1,934	5,464	14,359
-point........	26	3	6	32	234
On Site Incineration-area........	3,366	1,052	1,262	2,104	4,839
-point........	25	2	3	31	232
Open Burning-area........	1,792	112	672	3,360	9,520
-point........	0	0	0	0	0
Apartment-point........	1	0	2	1	2
Other-point........	0	0	0	0	0
Industrial-area........	737	123	276	1,000	2,731
-point........	411	125	574	230	974
On Site Incineration-area........	306	96	115	191	440
-point........	224	125	552	186	423
Open Burning-area........	431	27	162	809	2,291
-point........	187	0	22	44	551
Auto Body Incineration-point........	0	0	0	0	0
Other-point........	0	0	0	0	0
Miscellaneous-point........	0	0	0	0	0
TRANSPORTATION-AREA........	20,444	9,566	188,176	304,307	1,712,830
Land Vehicles........	19,858	8,968	186,759	271,094	1,680,505
Gasoline........	16,939	4,780	149,926	265,585	1,662,642
Light Vehicles........	14,346	3,719	121,790	190,468	1,140,397
Heavy Vehicles........	2,053	778	21,978	57,753	325,389
Off Highway........	540	283	6,158	17,364	196,856
Diesel Fuel........	2,919	4,188	36,833	5,509	17,863
Heavy Vehicles........	1,777	2,488	22,358	2,877	13,280
Off Highway........	653	584	7,231	792	2,038
Rail........	490	1,116	7,245	1,841	2,545
Aircraft........	475	166	1,072	2,270	5,609
Military........	313	60	151	729	783
Civil........	102	20	92	451	2,577
Commercial........	59	86	830	1,090	2,249
Vessels........	112	433	344	8,374	26,716
Bituminous Coal........	96	241	14	96	433
Diesel Fuel........	7	9	68	18	24
Residual Oil........	9	127	19	1	1
Gasoline........	0	56	243	8,259	26,258
Gas Handling Evaporation Loss........	0	0	0	22,569	0
MISCELLANEOUS-AREA........	0	0	0	37,971	0
Forest Fires........	0	0	0	0	0
Structural Fires........	0	0	0	0	0
Slash Burning........	0	0	0	0	0
Frost Control........	0	0	0	0	0
Solvent Evaporation Loss........	0	0	0	37,971	0

WYOMING

Emission categories	Pollutant, tons per year				
	Particulates	Sulfur oxides	Nitrogen oxides	Hydro-carbons	Carbon monoxide
GRAND TOTAL	87,051	70,191	102,238	67,654	381,753
-AREA	13,646	6,023	52,900	47,473	195,490
-POINT	73,405	64,168	49,338	20,181	186,264
FUEL COMBUSTION-AREA	1,269	1,359	6,155	721	2,354
-POINT	38,492	44,781	45,165	1,079	2,521
External Combustion-area	1,269	1,359	6,155	721	2,354
-point	38,492	44,781	45,165	1,079	2,521
Residential Fuel-area	576	423	827	518	1,820
Anthracite Coal	0	0	0	0	0
Bituminous Coal	341	410	51	341	1,534
Distillate Oil	22	0	26	6	11
Residual Oil	0	0	0	0	0
Natural Gas	87	5	700	70	175
Wood	126	8	51	101	101
Electric Generation-point	37,718	40,151	37,076	676	2,150
Anthracite Coal	0	0	0	0	0
Bituminous Coal	36,848	39,683	36,844	660	2,119
Lignite	870	426	196	15	30
Residual Oil	0	35	9	0	0
Distillate Oil	0	7	14	0	0
Natural Gas	0	0	13	0	0
Process Gas	0	0	0	0	0
Coke	0	0	0	0	0
Solid Waste/Coal	0	0	0	0	0
Other	0	0	0	0	0
Industrial Fuel-area	422	8	3,603	98	309
-point	774	4,630	8,084	403	370
Anthracite Coal-area	0	0	0	0	0
-point	0	0	0	0	0
Bituminous Coal-area	0	0	0	0	0
-point	22	46	12	6	20
Lignite-point	0	0	0	0	0
Residual Oil-area	0	0	0	0	0
-point	525	4,199	1,316	218	84
Distillate Oil-area	285	0	1,141	57	76
-point	55	173	219	11	15
Natural Gas-area	137	8	2,462	41	233
-point	172	48	6,416	168	251
Process Gas-area	0	0	0	0	0
-point	0	165	120	0	0
Coke-point	0	0	0	0	0
Wood-area	0	0	0	0	0
-point	0	0	0	0	0
Liquid Petroleum Gas-point	0	0	2	0	0
Bagasse-point	0	0	0	0	0
Other-point	0	0	0	0	0
Commercial-Institutional Fuel-area	271	928	1,724	105	225
-point	0	0	6	0	1
Anthracite Coal-area	0	0	0	0	0
-point	0	0	0	0	0
Bituminous Coal-area	0	0	0	0	0
-point	0	0	0	0	0
Lignite-point	0	0	0	0	0
Residual Oil-area	67	922	174	9	12
-point	0	0	0	0	0
Distillate Oil-area	112	0	449	22	30
-point	0	0	0	0	0
Natural Gas-area	92	6	1,101	73	183
-point	0	0	6	0	1
Wood-area	0	0	0	0	0
-point	0	0	0	0	0
Liquid Petroleum Gas-point	0	0	0	0	0
Miscellaneous-point	0	0	0	0	0
Internal Combustion-point	0	0	0	0	0
Electric Generation	0	0	0	0	0
Distillate Oil	0	0	0	0	0
Natural Gas	0	0	0	0	0
Diesel Fuel	0	0	0	0	0
Industrial Fuel	0	0	0	0	0
Distillate Oil	0	0	0	0	0
Natural Gas	0	0	0	0	0
Gasoline	0	0	0	0	0
Diesel Fuel	0	0	0	0	0

Emission categories	Pollutant, tons per year				
	Particulates	Sulfur oxides	Nitrogen oxides	Hydro-carbons	Carbon monoxide
Other............	0	0	0	0	0
Commercial-Institutional...........	0	0	0	0	0
Diesel Fuel	0	0	0	0	0
Other.........	0	0	0	0	0
Engine-Testing..........	0	0	0	0	0
Aircraft.........	0	0	0	0	0
Other.........	0	0	0	0	0
Miscellaneous..........	0	0	0	0	0
INDUSTRIAL PROCESS-POINT	33,515	19,367	3,974	16,906	157,790
Chemical Manufacturing	14,180	1,530	275	0	0
Food/Agriculture	517	0	0	0	0
Primary Metal.........	356	761	1,866	221	5,557
Secondary Metals.........	0	0	0	0	0
Mineral Products	17,267	2,142	235	0	0
Petroleum Industry.........	1,195	14,934	1,597	4,707	152,233
Wood Products	0	0	0	0	0
Evaporation	0	0	0	11,979	0
Metal Fabrication	0	0	0	0	0
Leather Products.........	0	0	0	0	0
Textile Manufacturing.........	0	0	0	0	0
Inprocess Fuel.........	0	0	0	0	0
Other/Not Classified	0	0	0	0	0
SOLID WASTE DISPOSAL-AREA	1,659	94	131	4,163	12,387
-POINT	1,397	20	200	2,196	25,952
Government-point.........	0	0	0	0	0
Municipal Incineration.........	0	0	0	0	0
Open Burning.........	0	0	0	0	0
Other	0	0	0	0	0
Residential-area.........	1,427	22	45	4,014	12,042
On Site Incineration.........	1,427	22	45	4,014	12,042
Open Burning.........	0	0	0	0	0
Commercial-Institutional-area.........	206	64	77	132	306
-point	0	0	0	0	0
On Site Incineration-area.........	204	64	76	128	293
-point.........	0	0	0	0	0
Open Burning-area	2	0	1	5	13
-point.........	0	0	0	0	0
Apartment-point.........	0	0	0	0	0
Other-point.........	0	0	0	0	0
Industrial-area.........	25	8	9	17	39
-point.........	1,397	20	200	2,196	25,952
On Site Incineration-area.........	24	8	9	15	35
-point.........	1,397	20	200	2,196	25,952
Open Burning-area	1	0	0	2	4
-point.........	0	0	0	0	0
Auto Body Incineration-point	0	0	0	0	0
Other-point	0	0	0	0	0
Miscellaneous-point.........	0	0	0	0	0
TRANSPORTATION-AREA.........	4,162	4,570	45,120	32,546	128,751
Land Vehicles.........	3,735	4,464	44,645	27,673	122,801
Gasoline	1,626	441	15,148	21,502	112,613
Light Vehicles	1,465	380	13,299	17,513	91,628
Heavy Vehicles	161	61	1,849	3,989	20,985
Off Highway.........	0	0	0	0	0
Diesel Fuel.........	2,109	4,023	29,497	6,171	10,188
Heavy Vehicles	394	552	5,299	530	1,929
Off Highway.........	316	283	3,502	383	987
Rail	1,398	3,188	20,696	5,258	7,272
Aircraft	427	102	458	1,470	4,106
Military.........	302	58	145	704	755
Civil.........	109	22	99	485	2,770
Commercial.........	15	22	214	281	581
Vessels.........	0	4	17	580	1,844
Bituminous Coal	0	0	0	0	0
Diesel Fuel.........	0	0	0	0	0
Residual Oil.........	0	0	0	0	0
Gasoline	0	4	17	580	1,844
Gas Handling Evaporation Loss	0	0	0	2,823	0
MISCELLANEOUS-AREA	6,556	0	1,493	10,043	51,997
Forest Fires.........	6,153	0	1,448	8,687	50,675
Structural Fires.........	79	0	7	20	·178
Slash Burning.........	324	0	38	381	1,144
Frost Control.........	0	0	0	0	0
Solvent Evaporation Loss.........	0	0	0	954	0

AMERICAN SAMOA

Emission categories	Pollutant, tons per year				
	Particulates	Sulfur oxides	Nitrogen oxides	Hydro-carbons	Carbon monoxide
GRAND TOTAL..	27	20	258	237	930
-AREA....................................	27	20	258	237	930
-POINT...................................	0	0	0	0	0
FUEL COMBUSTION–AREA............................	0	0	0	0	0
-POINT.............................	0	0	0	0	0
External Combustion–area............................	0	0	0	0	0
-point............................	0	0	0	0	0
Residential Fuel–area....................................	0	0	0	0	0
Anthracite Coal	0	0	0	0	0
Bituminous Coal......................................	0	0	0	0	0
Distillate Oil	0	0	0	0	0
Residual Oil...	0	0	0	0	0
Natural Gas	0	0	0	0	0
Wood	0	0	0	0	0
Electric Generation–point............................	0	0	0	0	0
Anthracite Coal	0	0	0	0	0
Bituminous Coal......................................	0	0	0	0	0
Lignite	0	0	0	0	0
Residual Oil...	0	0	0	0	0
Distillate Oil	0	0	0	0	0
Natural Gas	0	0	0	0	0
Process Gas..	0	0	0	0	0
Coke...	0	0	0	0	0
Solid Waste/Coal......................................	0	0	0	0	0
Other...	0	0	0	0	0
Industrial Fuel–area....................................	0	0	0	0	0
-point....................................	0	0	0	0	0
Anthracite Coal–area.................................	0	0	0	0	0
-point.....................	0	0	0	0	0
Bituminous Coal–area	0	0	0	0	0
-point...................	0	0	0	0	0
Lignite–point	0	0	0	0	0
Residual Oil–area	0	0	0	0	0
-point..............................	0	0	0	-0	0
Distillate Oil–area....................................	0	0	0	0	0
-point.............................	0	0	0	0	0
Natural Gas–area......................................	0	0	0	0	0
-point............................	0	0	0	0	0
Process Gas–area	0	0	0	0	0
-point...........................	0	0	0	0	0
Coke–point..	0	0	0	0	0
Wood–area...	0	0	0	0	0
-point	0	0	0	0	0
Liquid Petroleum Gas–point	0	0	0	0	0
Bagasse–point..	0	0	0	0	0
Other–point...	0	0	0	0	0
Commercial-Institutional Fuel–area................	0	0	0	0	0
-point................	0	0	0	0	0
Anthracite Coal–area.................................	0	0	0	0	0
-point.....................	0	0	0	0	0
Bituminous Coal–area	0	0	0	0	0
-point...................	0	0	0	0	0
Lignite–point	0	0	0	0	0
Residual Oil–area	0	0	0	0	0
-point..............................	0	0	0	0	0
Distillate Oil–area....................................	0	0	0	0	0
-point.............................	0	0	0	0	0
Natural Gas–area......................................	0	0	0	0	0
-point............................	0	0	0	0	0
Wood–area...	0	0	0	0	0
-point	0	0	0	0	0
Liquid Petroleum Gas–point	0	0	0	0	0
Miscellaneous–point...................................	0	0	0	0	0
Internal Combustion–point...........................	0	0	0	0	0
Electric Generation....................................	0	0	0	0	0
Distillate Oil	0	0	0	0	0
Natural Gas	0	0	0	0	0
Diesel Fuel	0	0	0	0	0
Industrial Fuel...	0	0	0	0	0
Distillate Oil	0	0	0	0	0
Natural Gas	0	0	0	0	0
Gasoline...	0	0	0	0	0
Diesel Fuel	0	0	0	0	0

Emission categories	Pollutant, tons per year				
	Particulates	Sulfur oxides	Nitrogen oxides	Hydro-carbons	Carbon monoxide
Other	0	0	0	0	0
Commercial-Institutional	0	0	0	0	0
Diesel Fuel	0	0	0	0	0
Other	0	0	0	0	0
Engine-Testing	0	0	0	0	0
Aircraft	0	0	0	0	0
Other	0	0	0	0	0
Miscellaneous	0	0	0	0	0
INDUSTRIAL PROCESS-POINT	0	0	0	0	0
Chemical Manufacturing	0	0	0	0	0
Food/Agriculture	0	0	0	0	0
Primary Metal	0	0	0	0	0
Secondary Metals	0	0	0	0	0
Mineral Products	0	0	0	0	0
Petroleum Industry	0	0	0	0	0
Wood Products	0	0	0	0	0
Evaporation	0	0	0	0	0
Metal Fabrication	0	0	0	0	0
Leather Products	0	0	0	0	0
Textile Manufacturing	0	0	0	0	0
Inprocess Fuel	0	0	0	0	0
Other/Not Classified	0	0	0	0	0
SOLID WASTE DISPOSAL-AREA	0	0	0	0	0
-POINT	0	0	0	0	0
Government-point	0	0	0	0	0
Municipal Incineration	0	0	0	0	0
Open Burning	0	0	0	0	0
Other	0	0	0	0	0
Residential-area	0	0	0	0	0
On Site Incineration	0	0	0	0	0
Open Burning	0	0	0	0	0
Commercial-Institutional-area	0	0	0	0	0
-point	0	0	0	0	0
On Site Incineration-area	0	0	0	0	0
-point	0	0	0	0	0
Open Burning-area	0	0	0	0	0
-point	0	0	0	0	0
Apartment-point	0	0	0	0	0
Other-point	0	0	0	0	0
Industrial-area	0	0	0	0	0
-point	0	0	0	0	0
On Site Incineration-area	0	0	0	0	0
-point	0	0	0	0	0
Open Burning-area	0	0	0	0	0
-point	0	0	0	0	0
Auto Body Incineration-point	0	0	0	0	0
Other-point	0	0	0	0	0
Miscellaneous-point	0	0	0	0	0
TRANSPORTATION-AREA	27	20	258	237	930
Land Vehicles	15	4	135	169	851
Gasoline	15	4	132	169	850
Light Vehicles	15	4	132	169	850
Heavy Vehicles	0	0	0	0	0
Off Highway	0	0	0	0	0
Diesel Fuel	0	0	3	0	1
Heavy Vehicles	0	0	3	0	1
Off Highway	0	0	0	0	0
Rail	0	0	0	0	0
Aircraft	1	2	15	20	41
Military	0	0	0	0	0
Civil	0	0	0	0	0
Commercial	1	2	15	20	41
Vessels	12	14	108	28	38
Bituminous Coal	0	0	0	0	0
Diesel Fuel	12	14	108	28	38
Residual Oil	0	0	0	0	0
Gasoline	0	0	0	0	0
Gas Handling Evaporation Loss	0	0	0	20	0
MISCELLANEOUS-AREA	0	0	0	0	0
Forest Fires	0	0	0	0	0
Structural Fires	0	0	0	0	0
Slash Burning	0	0	0	0	0
Frost Control	0	0	0	0	0
Solvent Evaporation Loss	0	0	0	0	0

GUAM

Emission categories	Pollutant, tons per year				
	Particulates	Sulfur oxides	Nitrogen oxides	Hydro-carbons	Carbon monoxide
GRAND TOTAL	2,197	13,654	7,290	7,037	25,695
-AREA	689	246	3,283	4,550	18,523
-POINT	1,508	13,408	4,007	2,487	7,172
FUEL COMBUSTION-AREA	0	1	2	0	0
-POINT	244	13,329	3,533	117	456
External Combustion-area	0	1	2	0	0
-point	222	13,097	2,920	56	83
Residential Fuel-area	0	0	0	0	0
Anthracite Coal	0	0	0	0	0
Bituminous Coal	0	0	0	0	0
Distillate Oil	0	0	0	0	0
Residual Oil	0	0	0	0	0
Natural Gas	0	0	0	0	0
Wood	0	0	0	0	0
Electric Generation-point	222	13,097	2,920	56	83
Anthracite Coal	0	0	0	0	0
Bituminous Coal	0	0	0	0	0
Lignite	0	0	0	0	0
Residual Oil	222	13,097	2,920	56	83
Distillate Oil	0	0	0	0	0
Natural Gas	0	0	0	0	0
Process Gas	0	0	0	0	0
Coke	0	0	0	0	0
Solid Waste/Coal	0	0	0	0	0
Other	0	0	0	0	0
Industrial Fuel-area	0	0	2	0	0
-point	0	0	0	0	0
Anthracite Coal-area	0	0	0	0	0
-point	0	0	0	0	0
Bituminous Coal-area	0	0	0	0	0
-point	0	0	0	0	0
Lignite-point	0	0	0	0	0
Residual Oil-area	0	0	0	0	0
-point	0	0	0	0	0
Distillate Oil-area	0	0	0	0	0
-point	0	0	0	0	0
Natural Gas-area	0	0	2	0	0
-point	0	0	0	0	0
Process Gas-area	0	0	0	0	0
-point	0	0	0	0	0
Coke-point	0	0	0	0	0
Wood-area	0	0	0	0	0
-point	0	0	0	0	0
Liquid Petroleum Gas-point	0	0	0	0	0
Bagasse-point	0	0	0	0	0
Other-point	0	0	0	0	0
Commercial-Institutional Fuel-area	0	1	0	0	0
-point	0	0	0	0	0
Anthracite Coal-area	0	0	0	0	0
-point	0	0	0	0	0
Bituminous Coal-area	0	0	0	0	0
-point	0	0	0	0	0
Lignite-point	0	0	0	0	0
Residual Oil-area	0	0	0	0	0
-point	0	0	0	0	0
Distillate Oil-area	0	1	0	0	0
-point	0	0	0	0	0
Natural Gas-area	0	0	0	0	0
-point	0	0	0	0	0
Wood-area	0	0	0	0	0
-point	0	0	0	0	0
Liquid Petroleum Gas-point	0	0	0	0	0
Miscellaneous-point	0	0	0	0	0
Internal Combustion-point	22	232	613	61	373
Electric Generation	22	232	613	61	373
Distillate Oil	0	0	0	0	0
Natural Gas	0	0	0	0	0
Diesel Fuel	22	232	613	61	373
Industrial Fuel	0	0	0	0	0
Distillate Oil	0	0	0	0	0
Natural Gas	0	0	0	0	0
Gasoline	0	0	0	0	0
Diesel Fuel	0	0	0	0	0

Emission categories	Pollutant, tons per year				
	Particulates	Sulfur oxides	Nitrogen oxides	Hydro-carbons	Carbon monoxide
Other	0	0	0	0	0
Commercial-Institutional	0	0	0	0	0
Diesel Fuel	0	0	0	0	0
Other	0	0	0	0	0
Engine-Testing	0	0	0	0	0
Aircraft	0	0	0	0	0
Other	0	0	0	0	0
Miscellaneous	0	0	0	0	0
INDUSTRIAL PROCESS-POINT	0	0	0	0	0
Chemical Manufacturing	0	0	0	0	0
Food/Agriculture	0	0	0	0	0
Primary Metal	0	0	0	0	0
Secondary Metals	0	0	0	0	0
Mineral Products	0	0	0	0	0
Petroleum Industry	0	0	0	0	0
Wood Products	0	0	0	0	0
Evaporation	0	0	0	0	0
Metal Fabrication	0	0	0	0	0
Leather Products	0	0	0	0	0
Textile Manufacturing	0	0	0	0	0
Inprocess Fuel	0	0	0	0	0
Other/Not Classified	0	0	0	0	0
SOLID WASTE DISPOSAL-AREA	0	0	0	0	0
-POINT	1,264	79	474	2,370	6,716
Government-point	1,264	79	474	2,370	6,716
Municipal Incineration	0	0	0	0	0
Open Burning	1,264	79	474	2,370	6,716
Other	0	0	0	0	0
Residential-area	0	0	0	0	0
On Site Incineration	0	0	0	0	0
Open Burning	0	0	0	0	0
Commercial-Institutional-area	0	0	0	0	0
-point	0	0	0	0	0
On Site Incineration-area	0	0	0	0	0
-point	0	0	0	0	0
Open Burning-area	0	0	0	0	0
-point	0	0	0	0	0
Apartment-point	0	0	0	0	0
Other-point	0	0	0	0	0
Industrial-area	0	0	0	0	0
-point	0	0	0	0	0
On Site Incineration-area	0	0	0	0	0
-point	0	0	0	0	0
Open Burning-area	0	0	0	0	0
-point	0	0	0	0	0
Auto Body Incineration-point	0	0	0	0	0
Other-point	0	0	0	0	0
Miscellaneous-point	0	0	0	0	0
TRANSPORTATION-AREA	689	246	3,281	4,550	18,523
Land Vehicles	313	144	3,013	3,228	17,365
Gasoline	258	67	2,288	3,151	17,072
Light Vehicles	258	67	2,288	3,151	17,072
Heavy Vehicles	0	0	0	0	0
Off Highway	0	0	0	0	0
Diesel Fuel	55	77	725	77	293
Heavy Vehicles	55	77	725	77	293
Off Highway	0	0	0	0	0
Rail	0	0	0	0	0
Aircraft	374	79	265	972	1,157
Military	368	70	177	857	919
Civil	0	0	0	0	0
Commercial	6	9	88	115	238
Vessels	2	23	3	0	0
Bituminous Coal	0	0	0	0	0
Diesel Fuel	0	0	0	0	0
Residual Oil	2	23	3	0	0
Gasoline	0	0	0	0	0
Gas Handling Evaporation Loss	0	0	0	351	0
MISCELLANEOUS-AREA	0	0	0	0	0
Forest Fires	0	0	0	0	0
Structural Fires	0	0	0	0	0
Slash Burning	0	0	0	0	0
Frost Control	0	0	0	0	0
Solvent Evaporation Loss	0	0	0	0	0

VIRGIN ISLANDS

Emission categories	Pollutant, tons per year				
	Particulates	Sulfur oxides	Nitrogen oxides	Hydro-carbons	Carbon monoxide
GRAND TOTAL	5,059	7,483	5,744	7,439	32,086
-AREA	465	269	4,635	7,370	31,995
-POINT	4,595	7,213	1,109	69	91
FUEL COMBUSTION-AREA	1	4	3	0	0
-POINT	422	5,907	1,105	55	74
External Combustion-area	1	4	3	0	0
-point	422	5,907	1,105	55	74
Residential Fuel-area	0	0	0	0	0
Anthracite Coal	0	0	0	0	0
Bituminous Coal	0	0	0	0	0
Distillate Oil	0	0	0	0	0
Residual Oil	0	0	0	0	0
Natural Gas	0	0	0	0	0
Wood	0	0	0	0	0
Electric Generation-point	0	0	0	0	0
Anthracite Coal	0	0	0	0	0
Bituminous Coal	0	0	0	0	0
Lignite	0	0	0	0	0
Residual Oil	0	0	0	0	0
Distillate Oil	0	0	0	0	0
Natural Gas	0	0	0	0	0
Process Gas	0	0	0	0	0
Coke	0	0	0	0	0
Solid Waste/Coal	0	0	0	0	0
Other	0	0	0	0	0
Industrial Fuel-area	1	4	3	0	0
-point	420	5,887	1,097	55	73
Anthracite Coal-area	0	0	0	0	0
-point	0	0	0	0	0
Bituminous Coal-area	0	0	0	0	0
-point	0	0	0	0	0
Lignite-point	0	0	0	0	0
Residual Oil-area	0	0	0	0	0
-point	419	5,880	1,092	55	73
Distillate Oil-area	1	4	3	0	0
-point	1	7	5	0	0
Natural Gas-area	0	0	0	0	0
-point	0	0	0	0	0
Process Gas-area	0	0	0	0	0
-point	0	0	0	0	0
Coke-point	0	0	0	0	0
Wood-area	0	0	0	0	0
-point	0	0	0	0	0
Liquid Petroleum Gas-point	0	0	0	0	0
Bagasse-point	0	0	0	0	0
Other-point	0	0	0	0	0
Commercial-Institutional Fuel-area	0	0	0	0	0
-point	2	20	9	0	1
Anthracite Coal-area	0	0	0	0	0
-point	0	0	0	0	0
Bituminous Coal-area	0	0	0	0	0
-point	0	0	0	0	0
Lignite-point	0	0	0	0	0
Residual Oil-area	0	0	0	0	0
-point	0	0	0	0	0
Distillate Oil-area	0	0	0	0	0
-point	2	20	9	0	1
Natural Gas-area	0	0	0	0	0
-point	0	0	0	0	0
Wood-area	0	0	0	0	0
-point	0	0	0	0	0
Liquid Petroleum Gas-point	0	0	0	0	0
Miscellaneous-point	0	0	0	0	0
Internal Combustion-point	0	0	0	0	0
Electric Generation	0	0	0	0	0
Distillate Oil	0	0	0	0	0
Natural Gas	0	0	0	0	0
Diesel Fuel	0	0	0	0	0
Industrial Fuel	0	0	0	0	0
Distillate Oil	0	0	0	0	0
Natural Gas	0	0	0	0	0
Gasoline	0	0	0	0	0
Diesel Fuel	0	0	0	0	0

Emission categories	Pollutant, tons per year				
	Particulates	Sulfur oxides	Nitrogen oxides	Hydro- carbons	Carbon monoxide
Other	0	0	0	0	0
Commercial-Institutional	0	0	0	0	0
Diesel Fuel	0	0	0	0	0
Other	0	0	0	0	0
Engine-Testing	0	0	0	0	0
Aircraft	0	0	0	0	0
Other	0	0	0	0	0
Miscellaneous	0	0	0	0	0
INDUSTRIAL PROCESS-POINT	4,162	1,304	2	0	0
Chemical Manufacturing	70	652	1	0	0
Food/Agriculture	0	0	0	0	0
Primary Metal	0	0	0	0	0
Secondary Metals	0	0	0	0	0
Mineral Products	4,022	0	0	0	0
Petroleum Industry	0	0	0	0	0
Wood Products	0	0	0	0	0
Evaporation	0	0	0	0	0
Metal Fabrication	0	0	0	0	0
Leather Products	0	0	0	0	0
Textile Manufacturing	0	0	0	0	0
Inprocess Fuel	70	652	1	0	0
Other/Not Classified	0	0	0	0	0
SOLID WASTE DISPOSAL-AREA	0	0	0	0	0
-POINT	11	2	2	13	18
Government-point	11	2	2	13	18
Municipal Incineration	11	2	2	13	18
Open Burning	0	0	0	0	0
Other	0	0	0	0	0
Residential-area	0	0	0	0	0
On Site Incineration	0	0	0	0	0
Open Burning	0	0	0	0	0
Commercial-Institutional-area	0	0	0	0	0
-point	0	0	0	0	0
On Site Incineration-area	0	0	0	0	0
-point	0	0	0	0	0
Open Burning-area	0	0	0	0	0
-point	0	0	0	0	0
Apartment-point	0	0	0	0	0
Other-point	0	0	0	0	0
Industrial-area	0	0	0	0	0
-point	0	0	0	0	0
On Site Incineration-area	0	0	0	0	0
-point	0	0	0	0	0
Open Burning-area	0	0	0	0	0
-point	0	0	0	0	0
Auto Body Incineration-point	0	0	0	0	0
Other-point	0	0	0	0	0
Miscellaneous-point	0	0	0	0	0
TRANSPORTATION-AREA	464	266	4,632	7,337	31,995
Land Vehicles	376	105	3,440	5,274	28,780
Gasoline	375	103	3,425	5,272	28,773
Light Vehicles	327	85	2,885	4,026	22,067
Heavy Vehicles	48	18	540	1,247	6,705
Off Highway	0	0	0	0	0
Diesel Fuel	1	2	15	2	7
Heavy Vehicles	1	2	15	2	7
Off Highway	0	0	0	0	0
Rail	0	0	0	0	0
Aircraft	85	122	1,186	1,558	3,214
Military	0	0	0	0	0
Civil	0	0	0	0	0
Commercial	85	122	1,186	1,558	3,214
Vessels	3	39	6	0	0
Bituminous Coal	0	0	0	0	0
Diesel Fuel	0	0	0	0	0
Residual Oil	3	39	6	0	0
Gasoline	0	0	0	0	0
Gas Handling Evaporation Loss	0	0	0	505	0
MISCELLANEOUS-AREA	0	0	0	33	0
Forest Fires	0	0	0	0	0
Structural Fires	0	0	0	0	0
Slash Burning	0	0	0	0	0
Frost Control	0	0	0	0	0
Solvent Evaporation Loss	0	0	0	33	0

REFERENCES

Chaput, L. S. "Federal Standards of Performance for New Stationary Sources of Air Pollution," *J. Air Poll. Control Assoc.* (November 1976).

Environmental Protection Agency, U.S. 40CFR 51.3 (July 1, 1975).

Environmental Protection Agency, U.S. "Compilation of Air Pollution Factors," AP-42 (1976a).

Environmental Protection Agency, U.S. "National Emission Report (1972)," EPA-451/2-76-007 (1976b).

Gerstle, R. W. and D. A. Kemnitz. "Atmospheric Emissions from Open Burning," *J. Air Poll. Control Assoc.* 12:324-327 (1967).

Holzworth, G. W. "Mixing Heights, Wind Speeds, and Potential for Urban Air Pollution Throughout the Contiguous United States," Environmental Protection Agency (January 1972).

Resources Research, Inc. "Air Pollution Emission Factors," Final Report, prepared for National Air Pollution Control Administration, Durham, NC, CPA-22-69-119 (April 1970).

CHAPTER 7

WATER RESOURCES

Data collection is the first task of the water assessment process. This task need not be by means of bottles and equipment in the field, since EPA's STORET system has water quality data on almost all major streams of the U.S. STORET data is recorded from 200,000 water quality stations, measuring up to 3,000 parameters. Table 7-1 gives typical water quality data available from the STORET computer printout of EPA. Table 7-2 gives state codes. Table 7-3 shows other federal agencies that collect and store both water quality and quantity data.

Table 7-4 lists data gathering techniques and methods for stream analysis, should field work be dictated by the project. The table summarizes data and equipment needs, as well as applicable stream types and agencies involved in these measurements. Table 7-5 summarizes other techniques used for assessment of fishery habitat and stream flow requirements. The first column includes the author and original year published; the second contains the general limits of application of technique. The middle column refers to type of data acquired, while the fourth column gives data needed. Table 7-6 gives a summary of urban pollution sources. The pollutant is listed in the first column, while other columns quantify runoff and waste in pounds per acre. Figures 7-1 and 7-2 quantify nutrient pollution in mg/l, for phosphorus and nitrogen, respectively. Both figures show nutrient concentrations in streams increasing with land use changes from forest cover, to urban, to agricultural use, the largest contributor to nutrient enrichment of streams. Table 7-7 summarizes sources of oil pollution at sea. More than one third of oil in the oceans is from transportation sources.

Tables 7-8 through 7-14 summarize water quality standards and criteria. Table 7-8 lists federal water quality criteria for public water supply for

Table 7-1. Water Quality Data, From STORET Computer Printout of EPA

Code	Parameter			Number	Mean	Variance	Standard Deviation	Maximum	Minimum	Beginning Date	Ending Date
00010	Water	Temperature	Cent	3	22.3666	.013550	.116404	22.5000	22.3000	66/08/16	66/08/18
00070	Turbidity	Jackson	JTU	3	17.8333	5.083620	2.25469	20.0000	15.5000	66/08/16	66/08/18
00081	AP Color	PT-CO	Units	3	30.0000	.000000	.00000	30.0000	30.0000	66/08/16	66/08/18
00300	DO		mg/l	3	7.03333	.003456	.058789	7.10000	7.00000	66/08/16	66 08/18
00301	DO	Saturday	%	3	80.3666	.406250	.637377	81.1000	80.0000	66/08/16	66/08/18
00310	BOD	5-day	mg/l	5	1.84000	.923000	.960729	3.00000	.80000	66/08/16	72/08/25
00400	PH		SU	3	8.1000	.190140	.436050	8.40000	7.60000	66/08/16	66/08/18
00500	Residue	Total	mg/l	5	365.400	23196.9	152.302	460.000	95.0000	66/08/16	66/08/18
00501	Invalid			5	365.400	23195.9	152.302	460.000	95.0000	66/08/16	72/08/25
00510	Residue	Total fix	mg/l	5	278.000	13219.5	114.976	352.000	77.0000	66/08/16	72/08/25
00515	Residue	DISS-105	100 mg/l	2	13.50000	.000000	.000000	13.5000	13.5000	72/08/25	72/08/25
00525	Residue	Fix FLT	mg/l	2	2.50000	.000000	.000000	2.50000	2.50000	72/08/25	72/08/25
00940	Chloride	CL	mg/l	3	5.73333	.203384	.450982	6.20000	5.30000	66/08/16	66/08/18
31501	Total Coliforms	MFIMENDO	/100 ml	4	87 0000	20091.7	141.745	300.000	10.0000	66/08/16	72/08/24
31616	Fecal Coliforms	MFM-FCBR	/100 ml	1	15.0000			15.0000	15.0000	72/08/24	72/08/24

Table 7-2. State Codes

State	STORET[a] Code	State	STORET[a] Code
Alabama	01	Missouri	29
Alaska	02	Montana	30
Arizona	04	Nebraska	31
Arkansas	05	Nevada	32
California	06	New Hampshire	33
Colorado	08	New Jersey	34
Connecticut	09	New Mexico	35
Delaware	10	New York	36
District of Columbia	11	North Carolina	37
Florida	12	North Dakota	38
Georgia	13	Ohio	39
Guam	14	Oklahoma	40
Hawaii	15	Oregon	41
Idaho	16	Pennsylvania	42
Illinois	17	Puerto Rico	43
Indiana	18	Rhode Island	44
Iowa	19	South Carolina	45
Kansas	20	South Dakota	46
Kentucky	21	Tennessee	47
Louisiana	22	Texas	48
Maine	23	Utah	49
Maryland	24	Vermont	50
Massachusetts	25	Virginia	51
Michigan	26	Washington	53
Minnesota	27	West Virginia	54
Mississippi	28	Wisconsin	55
		Wyoming	56

[a]Federal Code (FIPS)

Table 7-3. Background Data Sources on Water Resources

Agency	Hydraulic Data	Water Quality Data
U.S. Geological Survey topographical maps and data for each state are available in USGS Regional Offices by State	1. Gaging stations (a) Flow records (b) Stage-discharge curves (c) Channel cross sections 2. Topographical maps (a) River distances (travel times) (b) Channel slopes (c) Location of tributaries, point loads and point diversions	1. Water quality stations (a) Cation and anion balances (b) Chemical analysis (c) Temperature (d) Pesticide analysis (e) Suspended and sediment discharge (f) Specific conductance (g) Phytoplankton
Environmental Protection Agency	n/a	1. STORET data: Water quality raw data and statistics 2. Specific water quality reports are available from Region Offices.
U.S. Fish and Wildlife Service	Regional Offices, National Reservoir Inventory, Ecological Services	Regional Offices, Research reports
U.S. Bureau of Reclamation	Usually uses USGS data but reservoir releases, etc. and research reports are important	Research reports
U.S. Bureau of Land Management	Environmental Impact Statements and specific research projects	Environmental Impact Statements and specific research projects
U.S. Forest Service	Watershed Resources Inventory System	USFS River Basin Planning Studies, Resource Capability System
Universities	Applied and basic research projects	Water Resources Research Centers
U.S. Army Corps of Engineers, District Offices	Water Supply Studies, flood records, reservoir volumes	Wastewater Management Studies, Tulsa District Environmental Workroom; Vicksburg Waterways Experiment Station

U.S. Coast Guard	Coastal cruise data, oceanography, bathymetry, currents	n/a

State Agencies	Limited	1. State Engineers Office
		  (a) Water use data
		  (b) Irrigation district
		2. State Environmental Regulatory Agency
		  (a) 303e studies
		  (b) 208 studies
		3. State Wildlife Fisheries Resources and State Parks
		4. Water Resources Control Board

Table 7-4. Data and Methods for Stream Analysis (Stalnaker and Arnette, 1976).

Method	Types of Streams	Techniques Involved
USGS stream gages, USBR, TVA, Corps of Engineers, River Authorities, Power Companies, and Federal Power Commission	Small (jumpable), wadable, and large streams, reservoir releases	Staff gage, rating curve establishing relation between flow and stage (elevation of water surface). Releases from reservoirs would be a good source of downstream flow data.
Weirs or measuring flumes	Small and some wadable streams	Construction of a weir with known hydraulic capacities so that stream flow as a function of stage can be determined. Need to measure stage height.
Tracer studies used primarily to measure mixing rates or changes in flow. With precise additions can measure flow by dilution.	Small, wadable and large streams	Fluorescent dyes, salt, radioactive tracers, manmade or natural conservative pollutants (e.g., point source discharges).
Three-point method	Wadable and large streams (for small streams only a single measurement is usually made)	Measured at a particular time. Stream depth and velocity are determined at quartile points on the stream. Velocity is estimated at 0.6 depth with a current meter.
Flow assessment	Small, wadable and large streams	Estimate (actually measure when possible) depth and width (1) based on experience estimate on velocity, or (2) use an orange or similar object which barely floats and time the passage past two measured points.

Table 7-4, continued

How to Obtain Data	Time Lag in Getting Data	Data Requirements and Functional Relationships
Stations are marked on quadrangle maps, listed by river basin in USGS publications (published annually by state) or obtained in river basin office. USBR where reservoir releases occur.	Available to public annually in reports or within 2-3 months from river basin office. Occasionally, arrangements may be made with local office to accompany engineer on his calibration trips to obtain data immediately.	Stage height with time, $Q = f$ (stage height, time) usually calculated from graphs
Usually constructed for a specific purpose: US Forest Service, Fish & Game agencies, irrigation companies, and USGS use these.	Usually immediate if relationships are known.	$Q - VA$, A is a function of stage, V is a function of stage.
Field analysis: Fluorometer; conductivity meter; other measurement devices as appropriate. Sampling devices: Sample bottles, timer. A boat is needed for larger streams.	Time to measure and calculate Q.	Flow changes between points 1, 2. $Q_2 = Q_1 (C_1/C_2)$. Flow rate $Q = Q_t (C_1 - C_2/(C_2 - C_0))$ where Q_t is the steady dosing rate of tracer, C_0 is background concentration of tracer, C_1 is concentration in feed, C_2 is concentration in the stream.
Sometimes agencies responsible for water resources have equipment and reaches defined for such measurements. Tape, depth and current meters are needed. A boat is needed for larger streams. Timer.	None	Calculate mean depth, mean velocity, and measure width. $Q = V \cdot W \cdot D$
Field analysis. Should have at least a tape, timer.	None	$Q = V \cdot W \cdot D$

Table 7-5. A Summary of Methods to Assess Fishery and Stream Habitat Flow Requirements (Stalnaker and Arnette, 1976)

Author	Application	Analysis	Data Needs	Remarks
Tennant, 1975	Reconnaissance All size streams Widely applied to warm and cold water streams in the mid-West, Northern Great Plains	General habitat, fish, wildlife and recreation	Type: Flow records Input: Mean annual flow records over several years Output: Preservation and survival flows biannually	Moderate data needs Low time and cost requirements Best used when prior data exists Low to moderate resolution Characterizes entire stream
Anonymous, 1974	Reconnaissance All size streams Applied to Northern Great Plains streams	General habitat, fish, wildlife and recreation	Type: Flow records Input: Mean daily discharge records Output: Preservation flows, monthly	Moderate data, time and cost requirements Best used when prior data exists Low to moderate resolution Needs field testing in different regions
Hoppe & Finnell, 1970	Reconnaissance Small streams and wadable rivers Applied to Frying Pan River, CO	Spawning, fish food production, and sediment flushing	Type: Flow duration curves Input: Flow records Output: Minimum flows for spawning, flushing and food production	Moderate data, time and cost requirements Requires prior data Low to moderate resolution Needs verification on other streams Characterizes only critical areas of stream
Robinson, 1969	Reconnaissance All size streams Applied to streams in CT River Basin	Fishery flows	Type: Flow records Input: Average monthly, median and lowest flows Output: Preservation and optimum flows for fisheries	Moderate data needs Low time and cost requirements Best used when prior data exists Low to moderate resolution Characterizes entire stream Needs testing in different regions
Herrington & Dunham, 1967 Chrostowski, 1972 Dunham & Collotzi, 1975	Intensive field measures Small streams and wadable rivers Applied to many trout streams in intermountain area	General habitat, fish and riparian vegetation	Type: Transects Input: Hydraulic parameters Output: Preservation flows for fish, wildlife and recreation	High data needs Moderate ease, high time and cost requirements Best measured at low flows Moderate to high resolution Characterizes the entire stream Needs followup analyses after flow reductions applied Would be applicable for evaluat-

Reference	Application	Type/Input/Output	Remarks
Anonymous, 1973 (Critical Area Method)	Limited field measures / Small streams and wadable rivers / Applied trout streams on USFS lands in CO	General habitat, riparian vegetation, recreation and aesthetics	Type: Transects / Input: Visual examination of entire stream by team approach / Output: Preservation flows and optimum for fish, wildlife and recreation	Minimal data needs / Moderate time and cost requirements / Requires team of experts / Moderate resolution / Characterizes critical area of the stream / Needs followup analyses for validation
Hoppe, 1975	Reconnaissance and limited field measures / Small streams and wadable rivers / Applied to Frying Pan River, CO	Spawning, cover, riffle (food production) for trout	Type: Transects / Input: Hydraulic parameters / Output: Preservation flows for fish	Moderate data, time and cost requirements. / Requires judgment of experienced biologist / Resolution dependent on experience of biologist / Characterizes only the most critical section of stream
Thompson, 1972, 1974 Oregon State Game Commission, 1972	Intensive field measures / Small streams, wadable rivers, larger rivers with wadable spawning bars / Applied to several OR streams and the Snake River, ID	Passage, spawning of salmonids	Type: Transects / Input: Hydraulic parameters / Output: Minimum passage minimum and optimum spawning flows	Moderately high data, time and cost requirements / High resolution / Characterizes only the riffle areas / Assumes reproduction is the limiting or overriding consideration / Criteria needs to be developed for additional species
Rantz, 1964	Reconnaissance / Regional or basinwide / All size streams / Applied to Mad and Eel Rivers, CA	Spawning, production of young of Chinook salmon	Type: Predicting formulae / Input: Average annual flow, drainage area average stream width / Output: Optimum spawning discharge	Minimal data, time and cost requirements / Low resolution / Characterizes spawning bars by computing a discharge at one downstream point only: assumed optimum for spawning and incubation / Must be developed for each major watershed and needs considerable field data for development
Collings, 1974	Reconnaissance, regional or basinwide / All size streams / Applied to western WA streams	Spawning flows for five salmon species	Type: Predicting formulae / Input: Drainage area, mean basin altitude, reach altitude, width, slope, hydraulic radius / Output: Optimum spawning flow	Minimal data, time and cost requirements / Low resolution / Must be developed for each physiographic region / Needs considerable field data for development / Could provide information for future regional assessment studies

Table 7-5, continued

Author	Application	Analysis	Data Needs	Remarks
Sams & Pearson, 1963 (weighted usable width, average velocity analyses)	Intensive field measures; Small streams and wadable rivers; Applied to four streams in Williamette River Basin, OR	Spawning, incubation flows for Chinook, Coho and Steelhead	Type: Transect; Input: Hydraulic parameters, substrate-permeability data, intra-gravel DO, velocity distribution curves; Output: Optimum spawning and incubation flows	Considerable data, time and cost requirements; High resolution; Requires accurate depth-velocity criteria for each species; Characterizes spawning areas only; Need development of criteria for additional riffle spawning species
Sams & Pearson, 1963 (average stream width)	Limited field measures; All size streams; Applied to four Western OR streams	Spawning flows	Type: Transects; Input: Average pool and stream width; Output: Optimum spawning flows	Moderate data, time and cost requirements; Low resolution; Requires velocity criteria for each species; Could be used for interpretation from aerial photos on larger streams and rivers; Limited to streams with average pool width $\cong$ to average stream width; Applicable to gravel spawning species for which velocity criteria is known
Bishop & Scott, 1973; Collings, 1974	Intensive field measures; Small streams and wadable rivers; Applied to coastal streams in western WA	Spawning of salmon	Type: Transects with additional random point measurements; Input: Hydraulic parameters, plainimetric maps; Output: Optimum (preferred) and "sustaining" spawning flows	High data, time and cost requirements; Resolution high; Characterizes spawning reach only; Needs additional criteria; Could be applicable to large rivers by using sounding devices, etc., and to reaches other than spawning, and to evaluation of augmented flows
Wickett, 1954; Terhune, 1958	Intensive field measure; Small streams and wadable rivers	Incubation	Type: Standpipe technique; Input: Permeability rates, dissolved oxygen levels; Output: Incubation flows, percolation flows, percolation rates	Moderate to high data, time and cost requirements; Resolution high; Characterizes intragravel flow and percolation rates; Could be applied to augmented, as well as reduced flow, but requires measurement at actual flow
Hoppe & Finnell, 1970	Limited field measures; All flowing water; Applied to Frying Pan River, trout-streams in southern CO	Incubation	Type: Predictive formula; Input: Stream gradient, velocity measurement; Output: incubation flows	Low to moderate data, time and cost requirements; Low to moderate resolution; Characterization and application same as Wickett et al., 1954; Could be applied to evaluation of aug...

Reference	Application	Category	Method	Requirements
Thompson, 1974	Intensive field measures Small streams and wadable rivers Applied to Snake River, ID	Incubation	Type: Standpipe and egg basket Input: Permeability rates, dissolved oxygen levels, introduced incubating eggs Output: Percolation rates, incubation flows	Moderate to high data, time and cost requirements High Resolution Characterization and application same as Wickett et al., 1954
Banks et al., 1974	Intensive field measures Small streams and wadable rivers Applied to Green River, WY	Food production, resting microhabitat, total usable habitat	Type: Transects, aerial photographs Input: Hydraulic parameters, area estimates from planimetered aerial photographs Output: Maximum surface acreage for food production, resting microhabitat and total usable habitat	Moderate to high data, time and cost requirements Low to moderate resolution Characterizes entire stream Requires measurement at varying flows Could be applied to evaluation of augmented flow
Collings, 1974	Limited or intensive field measures Small streams and wadable rivers Applied to coastal streams in western WA	Food production (rearing)	Type: Transects Input: Hydraulic parameters, wetted perimeter-discharge curve Output: Minimum (preservation) food production (rearing) flow	Moderate data, time and cost requirements. Low resolution Characterizes riffle areas only Could be applied to evaluation of augmented flow
Wesche, 1973	Intensive field measures Small streams and wadable rivers Applied to brown trout streams in southeastern WY	Cover	Type: Transects Input: Substrate size, hydraulic parameters, surface area, size of undercut banks, mapping of stream reaches Output: Cover rating	High time, data and cost requirements Moderate to high resolution Characterize the entire stream Could be applied to evaluation of augmented flows
Bovee, 1974	Intensive field measures Small streams and wadable rivers Tested in Yellowstone River drainage in southeastern MT	Passage, spawning riffle productivity	Type: Transects Input: Hydraulic Parameters planimetric mapping Output: Identification of optimum flows for passage, spawning, riffle productivity	High data, time and cost requirements Moderate to high resolution Key indicator species and their depth velocity criteria need to be established Characterizes spawning reaches and riffle areas

Table 7-6. Annual Yield of Pollutants from Urban Runoff and Municipal Waste (Colston, 1975).

Pollutant	Urban Runoff (lb/ac)	Raw Municipal Waste (lb/ac)	Total Annual Yield (lb/ac)
COD	938	1027	1965
Suspended Solids	.6690	335	7025
Kjeldahl Nitrogen	6.1		6.1
Nitrate Nitrogen		7.2	7.2
Total Phosphorus	4.7	11	15.7
Chromium	1.6	0.1	1.7
Copper	1.6	0.2	1.8
Lead	2.9	<0.8	3.7
Nickel	1.2	0.16	1.3
Zinc	2.0	1.5	3.5
Aluminum[a]	64		64
Calcium[a]	52		52
Cobalt[a]	1.9		1.9
Iron[a]	102		102
Magnesium[a]	71		71
Manganese[a]	4.9		4.9
TOTAL	7944 (85%)	1283 (15%)	9327 (100%)
Fecal Coliform	230/ml		

[a]Estimated.

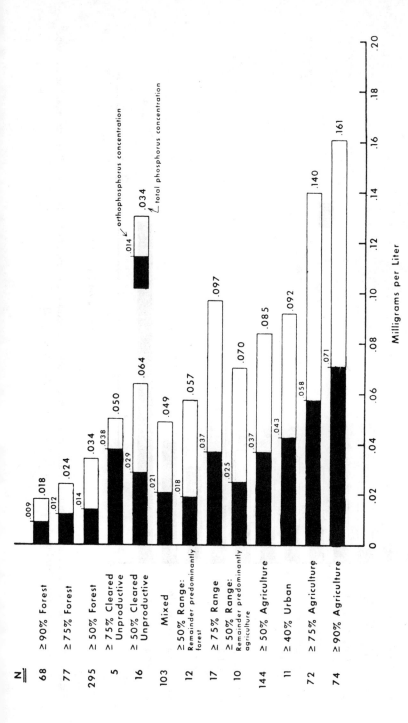

Figure 7-1. Land use vs mean total phosphorus and mean orthophosphorus stream concentrations—data from 904 "nonpoint source-type" watersheds distributed throughout the United States (Omernik, 1977).

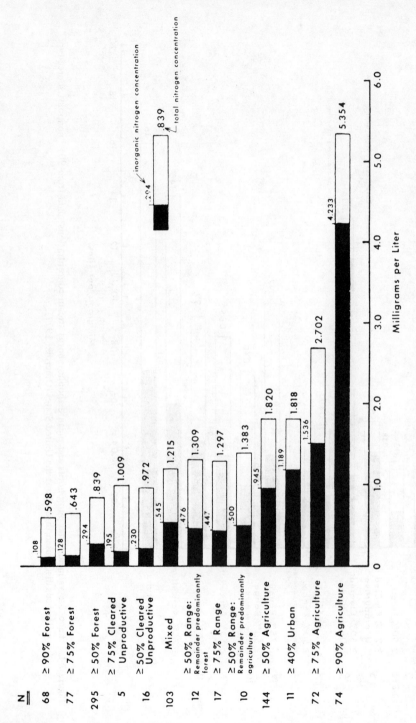

Figure 7-2. Land use vs mean total nitrogen and mean inorganic nitrogen stream concentrations—data from 904 "nonpoint source-type" watersheds distributed throughout the United States (Omernik, 1977).

Table 7-7. Contributions of Various Sources to Oil in the Oceans (NAS, 1973).

Source	Estimated Contribution (tons/yr)	%
Transportation		
Tankers, dry docking, terminal operation, bilges, accidents	2,350,000	34.9
Coastal Refineries, Municipal and Industrial Waste	875,000	13.0
Offshore Oil Productions	87,500	1.3
River and Urban Runoff	2,100,000	31.2
Atmospheric Fallout	660,000	9.8
Natural Seeps	660,000	9.8
Total	6,732,500	100.0

Table 7-8. EPA Numerical Water Quality Criteria for
Public Water Supply Intake (EPA, 1976a)

Parameter	μg/l (unless otherwise specified)	Crop Irrigation
Arsenic	50	100
Barium	1 mg/l	
Beryllium		100 μg/l: or 500 μg/l for neutral to alkaline fine-textured soils
Boron		750 μg/l - sensitive crops
Cadmium	10	
Chromium	50	
Copper	1,000	
2, 4-D chlorophenoxy herbicides	100	
Endrin	0.2	
Iron	0.3 mg/l	
Lead	50	
Lindane	4	
Mangenese	50	
Mercury	2	
Methoxychlor	100	
Nitrate nitrogen (N)	10 mg/l	
pH	5-9	
Phenols	1.0	
Selenium	10	
Silver	50	
Solids (dissolved), salinity	250 mg/l for chlorides & sulfates	
2, 4, 5-TP chlorophenoxy herbicides	10	
Toxaphene	5	
Zinc	5,000	

Table 7-9. EPA Numerical Water Quality Criteria for Marine Aquatic Life (EPA 1976a)

Parameter	$\mu g/l$ (unless otherwise specified)
Aldrin-Dieldrin	0.003
Cadmium	5
Chlorine (total residual)	10
Chlorodane	0.004
Copper	0.1 LC50 (96 hr)
Cyanides	5
DDT	0.001
Demeton	0.1
Endosulfan	0.001
Endrin	0.004
Guthion	0.01
Heptachlor	0.001
Hydrogen Sulfide	2
Lindane	0.004
Malathion	0.1
Manganese	100 for Marine mollusks
Mercury	0.1
Methoxychlor	0.03
Mirex	0.001
Nickel	0.01 LC 50 (96 hr)
Oil and Grease	Not detectable as a visible film, sheen, discoloration of the surface, or by odor. Does not cause tainting of fish or invertebrates or damage to biota. Does not form an oil deposit on the shores or bottom of the receiving body of water.
pH	6.5-8.5 (but not more than 0.2 ± normally occurring range
PCB	0.001
Parathion	0.04
Phosphorus	0.1 (P)
Selenium	0.01 LC50 (96 hr)
Silver	0.01 LC50 (96 hr)
Toxaphene	0.005

Table 7-10. EPA Numerical Water Quality Criteria
for Freshwater Aquatic Life (EPA, 1976a)

Parameter	$\mu g/l$ (unless otherwise specified)
Aldrin-Dieldrin	.003
Alkalinity	$\geqslant 20$ mg/l as $CaCO_3$
Ammonia	20 as un-ionized
Beryllium	11-soft water; 1,100-hard water
Cadmium	0.4 (soft); 1.2 (hard) - cladocerams and salmonid
	4.0 (soft); 12.0 (hard) - other
Chlorine (total residual)	2-salmonid; 10-other
Chlorodane	0.01
Chromium	100
Color	10% change in compensation point
Copper	0.01 LC50 (96 hr)
Cyanides	.005 mg/l
DDT	0.001
Demeton	0.1
DO	5.0 mg/l
Endosulfan	0.003
Endrin	0.004
Fecal Coliform	$\geqslant 14$ MPN/100 ml; no more than 10%
	$\geqslant 43$ MPN/100 ml - shell fish harvesting
Guthion	0.01
Heptachlor	0.001
Iron	1.0 mg/l
Lead	0.01 LC50 (96 hr)
Lindane	0.01
Malathion	0.1
Mercury	0.05
Methoxychlor	0.03
Mirex	0.001
Nickel	0.01 LC50 (96 hr)
Oils	None visible on surface - 0.01 LC50
Parathion	0.04
PCB	0.001
pH	6.5 - 9
Phthalate esters	3
Selenium	0.01 LC50 (96 hr)
Silver	0.01 LC50 (96 hr)
Sulfides	2 as undissociated H_2S
Suspended and Settleable Solids ⎫ ⎬ Turbidity and Light Penetration ⎭	Should not reduce depth of compensation point for photosynthetic activity by more than 10% from seasonally estimated norms
Toxaphene	0.005
Zinc	0.01 LC50 (96 hr)

Table 7-11. Summary of Specific Quality Characteristics of Surface Waters that Have Been Used as Sources for Industrial Water Supplies[a]

Characteristic	Boiler Makeup Water		Cooling Water			
			Fresh		Brackish	
	Industrial 0-1,500 psig	Utility 700-5,000 psig	Once Through	Makeup Recycle	Once Through	Makeup Recycle
Silica (SiO$_2$)	150	150	50	150	25	25
Aluminum	3	3	3	3	–	–
Iron (Fe)	80	80	14	80	1.0	1.0
Manganese (Mn)	10	10	2.5	10	0.02	0.01
Copper (Cu)	–	–	–	–	–	–
Calcium (Ca)	–	–	500	500	1,200	1,200
Magnesium (Mg)	–	–	–	–	–	–
Sodium and potassium (Na + K)	–	–	–	–	–	–
Ammonia (NH$_3$)	–	–	–	–	–	–
Bicarbonate (HCO$_3$)	600	600	600	600	180	180
Sulfate (SO$_4$)	1,400	1,400	680	680	2,700	2,700
Chloride (Cl)	19,000	19,000	600	500	22,000	22,000
Fluoride (F)	–	–	–	–	–	–
Nitrate (NO$_3$)	–	–	30	30	–	–
Phosphate (PO$_4$)	–	50	4	4	5	5
Dissolved Solids	35,000	35,000	1,000	1,000	35,000	35,000
Suspended Solids	15,000	15,000	5,000	15,000	250	250
Hardness (CaCO$_3$)	5,000	5,000	850	850	7,000	7,000
Alkalinity (CaCO$_3$)	500	500	500	500	150 ~	150
Acidity (CaCO$_3$)	1,000	1,000	0	200	0	0
pH, Units	–	–	5.0-8.9	3.5-9.1	5.0-8.4	5.0-8.4
Color, Units	1,200	1,000	–	1,200	–	–
Organics:						
Methylene blue active substances	2[d]	10	1.3	1.3	–	1.3
Carbon tetrachloride extract	100	100	e	100	e	100
Chemical oxygen demand (O$_2$)	100	500	–	100	–	200
Hydrogen sulfide (H$_2$S)	–	–	–	–	4	4
Temperature, °F	120	120	100	120	100	12

[a]Unless otherwise indicated, units are mg/l and values are maximums; no one water will have all the maximum values shown (Hann, 1972).
[b]Water containing in excess of 1,000 mg/l dissolved solids
[c]May be ≤ 1,000 for mechanical pulping operations.
[d]No large particles ≤ 3 mm diameter.
[e]1 mg/l for pressures up to 700 psig.
[f]No floating oil.
[g]Applied to bleached chemical pulp and paper only.

Table 7-11, continued

			Process Water				
Textile Industry SIC-22	Lumber Industry SIC-24	Pulp and Paper Industry SIC-26	Chemical Industry SIC-28	Petroleum Industry SIC-29	Primary Metals Industry SIC-33	Food and Kindred Products, SIC-20	Leather Industry SIC-31
–	–	50	–	50	–	For the above 2 cate-	
–	–	–	–	–	–	gories, the quality of	
0.3	–	2.6	5	15	–	raw surface supply	
1.0	–	–	2	–	–	should be that pre-	
0.5	–	–	–	–	–	scribed by the MTS	
–	–	–	200	220	–	subcommittee on	
–	–	–	100	85	–	Water Quality Require-	
–	–	–	–	230	–	ments for Public Water	
						Supplies	
–	–	–	600	480	–		
–	–	–	850	570	–		
–	–	200^b	500	1,600	500		
–	–	–	–	1.2	–		
–	–	–	–	8	–		
150	–	1,080	2,500	3,500	1,500		
1,000	c	–	10,000	5,000	3,000		
120	–	475	1,000	900	1,000		
–	–	–	500	–	200		
–	–	–	–	–	75		
6.0-8.0	5-9	4.6-9.4	5.5-9.0	6.0-9.0	3-9		
–	–	360	500	25	–		
–	–	–	–	–	–		
–	–	–	–	–	30		
–	–	–	–	–	–		
–	–	94^f	–	–	100		

Table 7-12. Ranges of Promulgated Standards for Raw Water Sources of Domestic Water Supply (Hann, 1972).

Constituent	Excellent Source of Water Supply Requiring Disinfection Only, as Treatment	Good Source of Water Supply, Requiring Usual Treatment such as Filtration and Disinfection	Poor Source of Water Supply, Requiring Special or Auxiliary Treatment and Disinfection
BOD (5-day), mg/l			
Monthly average	0.75-1.5	1.5-2.5	Over 2.5
Maximum day, or sample	1.0-3.0	3.0-4.0	Over 4.0
Coliform MPN per 100 ml			
Monthly average	50-100	50-5,000	Over 5,000
Maximum day, or sample	Less than 5% over 100	Less than 20% over 5,000	Less than 5% over 20,000
Dissolved Oxygen			
mg/l average	4.0-7.5	4.0-6.5	4.0
% saturation	75% or better	60% or better	—
pH			
Average	6.0-8.5	5.0-9.0	3.8-10.5
Chlorides, max. mg/l	50 or less	50-250	Over 250
Fluorides, mg/l	Less than 1.5	1.5-3.0	Over 3.0
Phenolic compounds, max. mg/l.	None	0.005	Over 0.005
Color, units	0-20	20-150	Over 150
Turbidity, units	0-10	10-250	Over 250

Table 7-13. Summary of Categories for which Effluent Guidelines and Federal Standards Have Been Promulgated (as of January 1977) (EPA, 1977)

Part	Subpart
Dairy Products	Receiving stations
	Fluid products
	Cultured products
	Butter
	Cottage cheese and cultured cream cheese
	Natural and processed cheese
	Fluid mix for ice cream and other frozen desserts
	Ice cream, frozen desserts, novelties and other dairy desserts
	Condensed milk
	Dry milk
	Condensed whey
	Dry whey
Grain Mills	Corn wet milling
	Corn dry milling
	Normal wheat flour milling
	Bulgur wheat flour milling
	Normal rice milling
	Parboiled rice processing
	Animal feed
	Hot cereal
	Ready-to-eat cereal
	Wheat starch and gluten
Canned and Preserved Fruits and Vegetables	Apple juice
	Apple products
	Citrus products
	Frozen potato products
	Dehydrated potato products
	Canned and preserved fruits
	Canned and preserved vegetables
	Canned and misc. specialties
Canned and Preserved Seafood	Farm-raised catfish processing
	Conventional blue crab processing
	Mechanized blue crab processing
	Nonremote Alaskan crab meat processing
	Remote Alaskan crab meat processing
	Nonremote Alaskan whole crab and crab section processing
	Remote Alaskan whole crab and crab section processing
	Dungeness and tanner crab processing in the contiguous state
	Nonremote Alaskan shrimp processing

Table 7-13, continued

Part	Subpart
Seafood (continued)	Remote Alaskan shrimp processing
	Northern shrimp processing in the contiguous states
	Southern nonbreaded shrimp processing in the contiguous states
	Breaded shrimp processing in the contiguous states
	Tuna processing
	Fish meal processing
	Alaskan hand-butchered salmon processing
	Alaskan mechanized salmon processing
	West Coast hand-butchered salmon
	West Coast mechanized salmon processing
	Alaskan bottom fish processing
	Non-Alaskan conventional bottom fish processing
	Non-Alaskan mechanized bottom fish processing
	Hand-shucked clam processing
	Mechanized clam processing
	Pacific Coast hand-shucked oyster processing
	Atlantic and Gulf Coast hand-shucked oyster processing
	Steamed and canned oyster processing
	Sardine processing
	Alaskan scallop processing
	Non-Alaskan scallop processing
	Alaskan herring fillet processing
	Non-Alaskan herring fillet processing
	Abalone processing
Sugar Processing Industries	Beet Sugar Processing
	Crystalline cane sugar refining
	Liquid cane sugar refining
	Louisiana raw cane sugar processing
	Florida and Texas raw cane sugar
	Hilo-Hamakua Coast of the island of Hawaii raw cane sugar processing
	Hawaiian raw cane sugar processing
	Puerto Rican raw cane sugar processing
Textile Industry	Wool scouring
	Wool finishing
	Dry processing
	Woven fabric finishing
	Knit fabric finishing
	Carpet mills
	Stock and yarn dyeing and finishing

Table 7-13, continued

Part	Subpart
Cement Manufacturing	Nonleaching Leaching Materials storage piles runoff
Feedlots	All subcategories except duck Ducks
Electroplating	Electroplating of copper, nickel, chromium, and zinc on ferrous and nonferrous materials Electroplating of precious metals Electroplating of specialty metals Anodizing Coatings Chemical etching and milling
Organic Chemicals	Nonaqueous processes Processes with process water contact as steam diluent or absorbent Aqueous liquid phase reaction systems
Inorganic Chemicals	Aluminum chloride production Aluminum sulfate production Calcium carbide production Calcium chloride production Calcium oxide and calcium hydroxide production Chlorine and sodium or potassium hydroxide production Hydrochloric acid production Hydrofluoric acid production Hydrogen peroxide production Nitric acid production Potassium metal production Potassium dichromate production Potassium sulfate production Sodium bicarbonate production Sodium carbonate production Sodium chloride production Sodium dichromate and sodium sulfate production Sodium metal production Sodium silicate production Sodium sulfite production Sulfuric acid production Titanium dioxide production Aluminun fluoride production Ammonium chloride production Ammonium hydroxide production

Table 7-13, continued

Part	Subpart
	Boric acid production
	Bromine production
	Calcium carbonate production
	Calcium hydroxide production
	Carbon dioxide production
	Carbon monoxide and byproduct hydrogen production
	Chrome pigments production
	Chromic acid production
	Copper sulfate production
	Cuprous oxide production
	Ferric chloride producdtion
	Ferrous sulfate production
	Fluorine production
	Hydrogen production
	Hydrogen cyanide production
	Iodine production
	Lead monoxide production
	Lithium carbonate production
	Manganese sulfate production
	Nickel sulfate production
	Strong nitric acid production
	Oxygen and nitrogen production
	Potassium chloride production
	Potassium iodide production
	Potassium permanganate production
	Silver nitrate production
	Sodium bisulfite production
	Sodium fluoride production
	Sodium hydrosulfide production
	Sodium hydrosulfite production
	Sodium silicofluoride production
	Sodium thiosulfate production
	Stannic oxide production
	Sulfur dioxide production
	Zinc oxide production
	Zinc sulfate production
Plastics and Synthetics	Ethylene-vinyl acetate copolymers
	Polytetrafluoroethylene
	Polypropylene fiber
	Alkyds and unsaturated polyester resins
	Cellulose nitrate
	Polyamide (nylon 6/12)
	Polyester resins (thermoplastic)
	Silicones

Table 7-13, continued

Part	Subpart
Soap and Detergent	Soap manufacturing by batch kettle
	Fatty acid manufacturing by fat splitting
	Soap manufacturing by fatty acid neutralization
	Glycerine concentration
	Glycerine distillation
	Manufacture of soap flakes and powders
	Manufacture of bar soaps
	Manufacture of liquid soaps
	Oleum sulfonation and sulfation
	Air-SO_3 sulfation and sulfonation
	SO_3 solvent and vacuum sulfonation
	Sulfamic acid sulfation
	Chlorosulfonic acid sulfation
	Neutralization of sulfuric acid esters and sulfonic acids
	Manufacture of spray dried detergents
	Manufacture of liquid detergents
	Manufacture of detergents by dry blending
	Manufacture of drum-dried detergents
	Manufacture of detergent bars and cakes
Fertilizer Manufacturing	Phosphate
	Ammonia
	Urea
	Ammonium nitrate
	Nitric acid
	Ammonium sulfate production
	Mixed and blended fertilizer production
Petroleum Refining	Topping subcategory
	Cracking
	Petrochemical
	Lube
	Integrated
Iron and Steel Manufacturing	By-product coke
	Beehive coke
	Sintering
	Blast furnace (iron)
	Blast furnace (ferromanganese)
	Basic oxygen furnace (wet air pollution control methods)
	Open hearth furnace
	Electric arc furnace (wet air pollution control methods)
	Vacuum degassing
	Continuous casting

Table 7-13, continued

Part	Subpart
Iron (continued)	Hot forming–primary
	Hot forming–section
	Hot forming–flat
	Pipe and tube
	Pickling-sulfuric acid-batch and continuous
	Pickling-hydrochloric acid-batch and continuous
	Cold rolling
	Hot coatings–galvanizing
	Hot coatings–terne
	Mixcellaneous runoffs–storage piles, casting and slagging
	Combination acid pickling (batch and continuous)
	Scale removal (kolene and hydride)
	Wire pickling and coating
	Continuous alkaline cleaning
Nonferrous Metals	Bauxite refining
	Primary aluminum smelting
	Secondary aluminum smelting
	Primary copper smelting (apply to BPT and BAT)
	Primary copper refining (apply to BPT and BAT)
	Primary lead (apply to BPT and BAT)
	Primary zinc
Phosphate Manufacturing	Phosphorus production
	Phosphorus consuming
	Phosphate
	Defluorinated phosphate rock (apply to BPT and BAT)
	Defluorinated phosphoric acid (apply to BPT and BAT)
	Sodium phosphates
Steam Electric Power Generation	Generating unit
	Small unit
	Old unit (apply to BPT and BAT)
	Area runoff–material storage runoff and construction runoff
Ferroalloy Manufacturing	Open electric furnaces with wet air pollution control devices
	Covered electric furnaces and other smelting operations with wet air pollution control devices
	Slag processing

Table 7-13, continued

Part	Subpart
Ferroalloy (continued)	Covered calcium carbide furnaces with wet air pollution control devices Other calcium carbide furnaces Electrolytic manganese products Electrolytic chromium
Leather Tanning and Finishing	Hair pulp unhairing with chrome tanning and finishing Hair save unhairing with chrome Unhairing with vegetable or alum tanning and finishing Finishing of tanned hides Vegetable or chrome tanning of unhaired hides Unhairing with chrome tanning and no finishing
Glass Manufacturing	Insulation fiberglass Sheet glass manufacturing Rolled glass manufacturing Plate glass manufacturing Float glass manufacturing Automotive glass tempering Automotive glass Laminating Glass container manufacturing Machine-pressed and -blown glass manufacturing Glass tubing (danner) manufacturing Television picture tube envelope manufacturing Incandescent lamp envelope manufacturing Hand-pressed and blown-glass manufacturing
Asbestos Manufacturing	Asbestos-cement pipe Asbestos-cement sheet Asbestos paper (starch binder) Asbestos paper (elastomeric binder) Asbestos millboard Asbestos roofing Asbestos floor tile Coating or finishing of asbestos textiles Solvent recovery Vapor absorption Wet dust collection
Rubber Processing	Tire and inner tube plants Emulsion crumb rubber Solution crumb rubber Latex rubber

Table 7-13, continued

Part	Subpart
Rubber (continued)	Small-sized general molded, extruded and fabricated rubber plants
	Medium-sized general molded, extruded, and fabricated rubber plants
	Large-sized general molded, extruded, and fabricated rubber plants
	Wet digestion reclaimed rubber
	Pan, dry digestion, and mechanical reclaimed rubber
	Latex-dipped, latex-extruded, and latex-molded rubber
	Latex foam
Timber Products	Barking
	Veneer
	Plywood
	Hardboard—dry process
	Hardboard—wet process
	Wood preserving
	Wood preserving—steam
	Wood preserving—boultonizing
	Wet storage
	Log washing
	Sawmills and planning mills
	Finishing
	Particle board
	N-P reserved
	Wood furniture and fixture production without water wash spray booth(s) or laundry facilities
	Wood furniture and fixture production with water wash spray booth(s) or with laundry facilities
Pulp, Paper, and Paperboard	Unbleached kraft
	Sodium-based neutral sulfite semichemical
	Ammonia base neutral sulfite semichemical
	Unbleached kraft—neutral sulfite semichemical (cross recovery)
	Paperboard from wastepaper
	Dissolving kraft
	Market-bleached kraft
	BCT-bleached kraft
	Fine-bleached kraft
	Papergrade sulfite
	Low alpha dissolving sulfite pulp
	Groundwood chemi-mechanical
	Groundwood-thermo-mechanical

Table 7-13, continued

Part	Subpart
Pulp (continued)	Groundwood-CMN papers Groundwood-fine papers Soda Deink NI fine papers NI tissue papers NI tissue (FWP) High alpha dissolving sulfite pulp Papergrade sulfite market pulp
Builders Paper and Board	Builders paper and roofing felt
Meat Products	Simple slaughterhouse Complex slaughterhouse Low-processing packinghouse High-processing packinghouse Small processor Meat cutter Sausage and luncheon meats processor Ham processor Canned meats processor Renderer
Coal Preparation	Coal preparation plant Coal storage, refuse storage, and coal preparation plant ancillary area Acid or ferruginous mine drainage Alkaline mine drainage
Oil and Gas Extraction	Offshore segment of the oil and gas extraction Far-offshore Onshore Coastal Beneficial use Stripper
Mineral Mining and Processing	Dimension stone Crushed stone Construction sand and gravel Industrial sand Gypsum Asphaltic mineral Asbestos and wollastonite Lightweight aggregates Mica and sericite Barite Fluorspar Saline from brine lakes

Table 7-13, continued

Part	Subpart
Minerals (continued)	Borax
	Potash
	Sodium sulfate
	Trona
	Rock salt
	Phosphate rock
	Frasch sulfur
	Mineral pigments
	Lithium
	Bentonite
	Magnesite
	Diatomite
	Jade
	Novaculite
	Fire clay
	Attapulgite and montmorillonite
	Kyanite
	Shale and common clay
	Aplite
	Tripoli
	Kaolin
	Ball clay
	Feldspar
	Talc, steatite, soapstone and pyrophyllite
	Garnet
	Graphite
Pharmaceutical Manufacturing	Fermentation products (apply to BPT only)
	Extraction products
	Chemical synthesis products
	Mixing/compounding and formulation
	Research
Ore Mining and Dressing	Iron ore
	Base and **precious metals**
	Bauxite
	Ferroalloy ores
	Uranium, radium and vanadium ores
	Mercury ore
	Titanium ore
Paving and Roofing Materials (Tars and Asphalt)	Asphalt emulsion
	Asphalt concrete
	Asphalt roofing
	Linoleum and printed asphalt felt
Paint Formulating	Oil-base solvent wash paint
Ink Formulating	Oil-base solvent wash ink

Table 7-13, continued

Part	Subpart
Gum and Wood Chemicals Manufacturing	Char and charcoal briquets Gum rosin and turpentine Wood rosin, turpentine, and pine oil Tall oil rosin, pitch and fatty acids Essential oils Rosin-based derivatives
Pesticide Chemicals	Halogenated organic pesticides Organophosphorus pesticides Organonitrogen pesticides Metalloorganic pesticides Pesticide formulators and packagers
Explosives Manufacturing	Manufacture of explosives B—Reserved Explosives load, assemble, and pack plants
Carbon Black Manufacturing	Carbon black furnace process Carbon black thermal process Carbon black channel process Carbon black lamp process
Photographic	Photographic processing
Hospital Point Source	Hospital

Table 7-14. State Numerical[a] Water Quality Standards (Patterson, 1976)

Parameter	Standard
ALABAMA	
Bacteria—Fecal #/100 ml	200
Dissolved Oxygen, mg/1	5
pH	6.0-8.5
Temperature, °F	Max. of 90° or 5°F increase
Turbidity, JTU	50
ALASKA	
Alkyl Benzene Sulfonate, mg/1	0.05
Arsenic, mg/1	0.01
Bacteria—Total Coliform, #/100 ml	1000
Chloride, mg/1	250
Color, color units	15
Copper, mg/1	1.0
Carbon Chloroform Extract, mg/1	0.2
Cyanide, mg/1	0.01
Fluoride, mg/1	0.7-1.2
Iron, mg/1	0.3
Manganese, mg/1	0.05
Nitrate mg/1	45
Odor, odor units	3
Oxygen (dissolved), mg/1	60% saturation or 5 mg/1
pH	6.5-8.5
Phenols	0.0001
Radioactivity	
Radium-226 pCi/1	3
Strontium-90 pCi/1	10 ·
Gross Beta pCi/1	1000
Sulfate	250
Temperature (maximum), °F	60
Total Dissolved Solids	500
Turbidity, JTU	5
Zinc, mg/1	5
ARIZONA	
Arsenic, mg/1	0.05
Bacteria—Fecal, #/100 ml	1000
Barium, mg/1	1.0
Cadmium, mg/1	0.01
Chromium (hexavalent), mg/1	0.05
Copper, mg/1	1.0
Cyanide, mg/1	0.2
Mercury, mg/1	0.005
Lead, mg/1	0.05
Phenol, mg/1	0.001
Selenium, mg/1	0.01

[a]A variety of non-numerical standards also have been specified for a number of states. These non-numerical standards and criteria are not given here.

Table 7-14, continued

Parameter	Standard
Silver, mg/1	0.05
Zinc, mg/l	5.0
ARKANSAS	
Bacteria—Fecal Coliform, #/100 mg	1000
Chlorides, mg/1	250
Oxygen (dissolved), mg/1	5
pH	6.0-9.0
Phosphorus, μg/1	100-stream
	50-lake
Solids—Total Dissolved, mg/1	500
Sulfates, mg/1	250
Radioactivity	
Radium-226 pCi/1	3
Strontium-90 pCi/1	10
Gross Beta pCi/1	1000
Temperature, $^\circ$F	5° increase streams
	3° increase lakes
CALIFORNIA	
Bacteria	
Total, #/100 ml	100
Fecal, #/100 ml	50-200
Biostimulatory Substances	
Total nitrogen, mg/1	0.5-2.0
Total phosphorus, mg/1	0.05-0.2
Chemical Constituents	
Aluminum, mg/1	0.11
Arsenic, mg/1	0.10
Barium, mg/1	1.0
Boron, mg/1	0.5
Cadmium, mg/1	0.01
Chromium, mg/1	0.05
Cobalt, mg/1	0.2
Copper, mg/1	0.02-0.06
Cyanide, mg/1	0.2
Fluoride, mg/1	0.7-1.2
Iron, mg/1	0.22
Lead, mg/1	0.05
Manganese, mg/1	0.06
Mercury, mg/1	0.005
Nitrate + Nitrite, mg/1	10.0
Silver, mg/1	0.06
Selenium, mg/1	0.01
Zinc, mg/1	0.01
Color, color units	free of coloration
Dissolved Oxygen, mg/1	5.0-9.0
Floating Materials	free of floating materials
Oil and Grease, mg/1	no visible oil or grease

Table 7-14, continued

Parameter	Standard
Organic Chemicals	
Carbon-alcohol extract, mg/l	3.0
Carbon-chloroform extract, mg/l	0.7
MBAS, mg/l	0.2-0.5
Phenols, mg/l	0.1
PCB, μg/l	0.3
Phthalate esters, μg/l	0.002
Pesticides, mg/l	
Aldrin	0.017
Chlordan	0.003
DDT	0.042
Dieldrin	0.017
Endrin	0.001
Heptachlor	0.018
Heptachlor epoxide	0.018
Lindane	0.056
Methoxychlor	1.0
Organophosphorus and carba-	
mate compounds	0.1
Toxophene	0.005
Herbicides	
2,4-D plus, mg/l	0.1
2,2,5-T plus, mg/l	0.1
2,4,5-TP, mg/l	0.1
pH	6.5-8.5
Radioactivity	
Radium-226, pCi/l	3
Strontium-90, pCi/l	10
Gross Beta, pCi/l	1000
Sediment	No adverse effects
Settleable Materials	No adverse effects
Suspended Materials	No adverse effects
Taste and Odor	No adverse effects
Temperature, °F	No adverse effects
Turbidity, JTU	5°F increase

1. Where natural turbidity is between 0 and 50 JTU, increases shall not exceed 20%.
2. Where natural turbidity is between 50 and 100 JTU, increases shall not exceed 10 JTU.
3. Where natural turbidity is greater than 100 JTU, increases shall not exceed 10%.

COLORADO

Parameter	Standard
Bacteria—Fecal, #/100 ml	200
Fecal Streptococcus, #/100 ml	20
Dissolved Oxygen, mg/l	5
Oil and Grease	Cause a film or other discoloration

Table 7-14, continued

Parameter	Standard
pH	6.5-8.5
Radioactivity	
Radium-226, pCi/1	3
Strontium-90, pCi/1	10
Gross Beta, pCi/1	1000
Solids	
Settleable	Free from
Floating	Free from
Taste, Odor, Color	Free from
Temperature, °F	Max. of 90°F or 3-5°F
Toxic Materials	Free from
Turbidity, JTU	10
CONNECTICUT	
Bacteria−Total Coliform, #/100 ml	100
Color	None other than natural
Dissolved Oxygen, mg/1	5 or 75% or saturation
pH	As naturally occurs
Silt	As naturally occurs
Sludge Deposits	As naturally occurs
Taste and Odor	As naturally occurs
Temperature	As naturally occurs
DELAWARE	
Acidity (total as $CaCO_3$), mg/1	20
Alkalinity (total as $CaCO_3$), mg/1	20
Ammonia (as N), mg/1	0.4
Actinomycetes, colonies/100 ml	None
Bacteria−Fecal Coliform, #/100 ml	200
Dissolved Oxygen, mg/1	6.0
Fluorides, mg/1	0.2
Nitrogen (Total), mg/1	3.0
pH	6.5-8.5
Phenols, mg/1	0.01
Radioactivity	
Alpha Emitters, pCi/1	3
Beta Emitters, pCi/1	1000
Synthetic Detergents (MBAS), mg/1	0.5
Temperature, °F	Max. of 85°F or 5° increase
Total dissolved Solids, mg/1	250
Toxic Substances	None
Turbidity, JTU	10
FLORIDA	
Bacteria−Total, #/100 ml	1000
Chlorides, mg/1	250
Detergents, mg/1	0.5
Dissolved Oxygen, mg/1	5.0
Dissolved Solids, mg/1	500

Table 7-14, continued

Parameter	Standard
Fluorides, mg/1	1.4-1.6
Metals	
Arsenic, mg/1	0.05
Chromium, mg/1 (hex)	0.5
Copper, mg/1	0.5
Cyanide, mg/1	None detectable
Iron, mg/1	0.3
Lead, mg/1	0.05
Mercury, mg/1	None detectable
Zinc, mg/1	1.0
Oils and Grease, mg/1	15
Odor	24 @ 60°C
pH	6.0-8.5
Phenols, mg/1	0.001
Radioactivity	
Gross Beta pCi/1	1000
Specific Conductance, micromhos/cm	Max. of 100% increase over 500
Turbidity, JTU	50

GEORGIA

Parameter	Standard
Bacteria–Fecal, #/100 ml	1000
Dissolved Oxygen, mg/1	5
pH	6.0-8.5
Temperature, °F	Max. of 90°F or 5°F increase

HAWAII

Parameter	Standard
Bacteria, Fecal, #/100 ml	400
Dissolved Oxygen, mg/1	4.5
Total Nitrogen, mg/1	0.20
pH	6.5-8.5
Total Phosphorus, mg/1	0.30
Radionuclides	
Radium-226, $\mu\mu$c/1	3
Strontium-90, $\mu\mu$c/1	10
Gross Beta, $\mu\mu$c/1	1000

IDAHO

Parameter	Standard
Bacteria	
Total, #/100 ml	240
Fecal, #/100 ml	50
Dissolved Oxygen, mg/1	6.0 or 90% of saturation
pH	6.5-9.0
Temperature, °F	2°F increase
Turbidity, JTU	5
Total Dissolved Gases	110% of saturation

ILLINOIS

Parameter	Standard
Ammonia Nitrogen (as N), mg/1	1.5
Arsenic, mg/1	1.0

Table 7-14, continued

Parameter	Standard
Bacteria−Fecal, #/100 ml	200
Barium−Total, mg/1	5.0
Boron−Total, mg/1	1.0
Cadmium−Total, mg/1	0.05
Chloride, mg/1	500
Chromium−Total hexavalent, mg/1	0.05
Chromium−Total trivalent, mg/1	1.0
Copper−Total, mg/1	0.02
Cyanide, mg/1	0.025
Dissolved Oxygen, mg/1	6.0
Fluoride, mg/1	5.0
Iron−Total mg/1	1.0
Lead-Total mg/1	0.1
Manganese−Total, mg/1	1.0
Mercury−Total, mg/1	0.0005
Nickel−Total, mg/1	1.0
pH	6.5-9.0
Phenols, mg/l	0.1
Phosphorus, mg/1	0.05
Radioactivity	
Radium-226, pCi/1	1
Strontium-90, pCi/1	2
Gross Beta, pCi/1	100
Selenium−Total, mg/1	1.0
Silver−Total, mg/1	0.005
Sulfate, mg/1	500
Temperature °F	5°F increase
Total Dissolved Solids	1000
Toxic Substances	1/10 the 48-hr TLm
Zinc, mg/1	1.0

INDIANA

Bacteria−Total, #/100 ml	5000
Odor	3
Dissolved Solids, mg/1	500
Radioactivity	
Radium-226, pCi/1	3
Strontium-90, pCi/1	10
Gross Beta, pCi/1	1000

IOWA

Arsenic, mg/1	0.05
Barium, mg/1	1.0
Cadmium, mg/1 [2]	0.01
Chlorides, mg/1	250.0
Chromium−hexavalent, mg/1	0.05
Copper, mg/1	1.0

Table 7-14, continued

Parameter	Standard
Cyanide, mg/1	0.025
Fluoride, mg/1	1.5
Lead, mg/1	0.05
pH	6.5-9.0
Phenols, mg/1	0.001
Mercury, mg/1	0.005
Nitrate (NO_3), mg/1	45.0
Radioactivity	
Radium-226, pCi/1	3
Strontium-90, pCi/1	10
Gross Beta, pCi/1	1000
Selenium, mg/l	sum of lead, cadmium, hexavalent chromium, mercury and selenium shall not exceed 1.5 mg/l
Total Dissolved Solids, mg/1	750.0
Zinc, mg/1	1.0
KANSAS	
Ammonia (as N), mg/1	0.15
Bacteria–Fecal, #/100 ml	200
Dissolved Oxygen, mg/1	5
pH	6.5-8.5
Temperature, °F	Max. of 90°F or 5°F increase
KENTUCKY	
Arsenic, mg/1	0.05
Bacteria–Coliform #/100 ml	5000
Cadmium, mg/1	0.01
Chromium–Hexavalent, mg/1	0.05
Cyanide, mg/1	0.025
Fluoride, mg/1	1.0
Lead, mg/1	0.05
Odor	3
Radioactivity	
Radium-226, pCi/1	3
Strontium-90, pCi/1	10
Gross Beta, pCi/1	1000
Selenium, mg/1	0.01
Silver, mg/1	0.05
Total Dissolved Solids, mg/1	750
LOUISIANA	
Bacteria–Fecal, #/100 ml	200
Chlorides, mg/1	10-250
Dissolved Oxygen	5
pH	6.0-9.0
Sulfate, mg/1	5-50
Temperature	Max. of 90°F or 5°F increase
Total Dissolved Solids, mg/1	100-500

Table 7-14, continued

Parameter	Standard

MAINE
    Bacteria
        Total, #/100 ml — 1000
        Fecal, #/100 ml — 200
    Dissolved Oxygen, mg/1 — 5 or 60% of saturation
    pH — 6.0-8.5

MARYLAND
    Bacteria–Fecal, #/100 ml — 200
    Dissolved Oxygen — 5
    pH — 6.5-8.5
    Temperature — Max. of $90°F$ or $5°F$ increase
    Turbidity, JTU — 50

MASSACHUSETTS
    Bacterial–Total #/100 ml — 1000
    Color and Turbidity — None other than natural in origin
    Chemical Constituents — None detrimental to life forms
    Dissolved Oxygen, mg/1 — 5 or 75% of saturation
    pH — 6.5-8.0
    Radioactivity
        Radium-226, pCi/1 — 3
        Strontium-90, pCi/1 — 10
        Gross Beta, pCi/1 — 1000
    Sludge Deposits — None allowable
    Taste and Odor — None other than natural origin
    Temperature — $4°F$ increase

MICHIGAN
    Bacteria–Fecal, #/100 ml — 200
    Dissolved Oxygen, mg/1 — 6
    pH — 6.5-8.8
    Temperature, $°F$ — $3°F$ increase

MINNESOTA
    Alkyl Benzene Sulfonate, mg/1 — 0.05
    Arsenic — 0.01
    Barium, mg/1 — 1.0
    Bacteria
        Total, #/100 ml — 4
        Fecal, #/100 ml — 200
    Cadmium, mg/1 — 0.01
    Carbon Chloroform Extract, mg/1 — 0.2
    Chlorides, mg/1 — 250
    Chromium–hexavelent, mg/1 — 0.05
    Color, color units — 15
    Copper, mg/1 — 1.0
    Cyanides, mg/1 — 0.01
    Fluorides, mg/1 — 1.5

Table 7-14, continued

Parameter	Standard
Iron, mg/1	0.3
Lead, mg/1	0.05
Manganese, mg/1	0.05
MBAS, mg/1	0.5
Nitrate, mg/1	45
Odor	3
Phenols, mg/1	0.001
Radioactivity	
Radium-226, pCi/1	3
Strontium-90, pCi/1	10
Gross Beta, pCi/1	1000
Selenium, mg/1	0.01
Silver, mg/1	0.05
Sulfate, mg/1	250
Total Dissolved Solids, mg/1	500
Turbidity, JTU	25
Zinc, mg/1	5
MINNESOTA	
Arsenic, mg/1	0.05
Barium, mg/1	1.0
Bacteria−Fecal, #/100 ml	2000
Cadmium, mg/1	0.01
Chlorides, mg/1	250
Chromium−hexavalent, mg/1	0.05
Cyanide, mg/1	0.2
Dissolved Oxygen, mg/1	4.0
Fluoride, mg/1	1.2
Lead, mg/1	0.05
Odor	24 @ 60°C
pH	6.0-8.5
Phenol, mg/1	0.001
Radioactivity	
Gross Beta pCi/1	1000
Selenium, mg/1	0.01
Specific Conductance, μmhos/cm	500
Silver, mg/1	0.05
Temperature, °F	90°F or 5°F increase
Total Dissolved Solids, mg/1	500
MISSOURI	
Bacteria−Fecal, #/100 ml	200
Dissolved Oxygen, mg/1	5
Fluoride, mg/1	1.2
pH	6.5-8.5

Table 7-14, continued

Parameter	Standard
Radioactivity	
Radium-226, pCi/1	3
Strontium-90, pCi/1	10
Gross Beta, pCi/1	1000
Temperature, °F	90°F or 5°F increase
MONTANA	
Bacteria	
Fecal, #/100 ml	200
Total, #/100 ml	1000
Color, color units	5
Dissolved Oxygen, mg/1	7
pH	6.5-8.5
Radioactivity	
Iodine-131, pCi/1	5
Radium-226, pCi/1	1
Strontium-89, pCi/1	100
Strontium-90, pCi/1	10
Tritium, pCi/1	3000
Gross Beta, pCi/1	100
Temperature, °F	67°F or 0.5°F increase
Turbidity, JTU	5
NEBRASKA	
Ammonia (as N), mg/1	1.4
Bacteria–Fecal, #/100 ml	200
Dissolved Oxygen, mg/1	5.0
Oils and Grease, mg/1	10
pH	6.5-8.5
Phenols, mg/1	0.001
Temperature, °F	90°F or 5°F increase
Total Dissolved Solids, mg/1	600
NEVADA	
Bacteria–Fecal, #/100 ml	200-1000
BOD, mg/1	3-15
Boron, mg/1	0.5
Chlorides, mg/1	20-40
Color, color units	3-10
Dissolved Oxygen, mg/1	5-7
MBAS, mg/1	1.0
Nitrates, mg/1	2.5-5.0
pH	6.5-8.5
Phosphates, mg/1	0.04-1.0
Suspended Solids, mg/1	5.0
Temperature, °F	3°F increase
Total Dissolved Solids, mg/1	125-500
Turbidity, JTU	5-10

Table 7-14, continued

Parameter	Standard
NEW HAMPSHIRE	
Bacteria—Total, #/100 ml	240
Color	Not in objectionable amounts
Dissolved Oxygen	75% of saturation
Odor	None
Oil and Grease	None
Sludge Deposits	Not objectionable kinds or amounts
Toxic Substances	Not in toxic concentrations or combinations
Turbidity, JTU	10-25
NEW JERSEY	
Arsenic, mg/1	0.05
Bacteria—Fecal, #/100 ml	200
Barium, mg/1	1.0
Cadmium, mg/1	0.01
Chromium—Hexavalent, mg/1	0.05
Dissolved Oxygen, mg/1	4.0-7.0
Lead, mg/1	0.05
Mercury, mg/1	0.005
pH	6.5-8.5
Phosphorus (as P) μg/1	50
Radioactivity	
Radium-226, pCi/1	3
Strontium-90, pCi/1	10
Gross Beta, pCi/1	1000
Selenium, mg/1	0.01
Silver, mg/1	0.05
Temperature, °F	Max. of 82° or 3°F increase
Total Dissolved Solids, mg/1	133% of background or 500
Toxic Substances	1/20 of the TL_{50} at 96 hr
Turbidity, JTU	20
NEW MEXICO	
Bacteria—Fecal, #/100 ml	100-1000
Chlorides, mg/1	25-10,000
Dissolved Oxygen, mg/1	5.0-6.0 or 85% of saturation
pH	6.0-9.0
Phosphorus, mg/1	0.1
Specific Conductance, μmhos	300
Sulfate, mg/1	150-3000
Temperature, °F	Max. of 77-93.2°F
Total Dissolved Solids, mg/1	1500-20,000
Total Organic Carbons, mg/1	7
Turibidity, JTU	10-50

Table 7-14, continued

Parameter	Standard
NEW YORK	
Ammonia, mg/1	2.0
Bacteria	
Fecal, #/100 ml	200
Total, #/100 ml	5000
Cadmium, mg/1	0.3
Copper, mg/1	0.2
Cyanide, mg/1	0.1
Dissolved Oxygen, mg/1	7
Ferro-Ferricyanide (as $Fe(CN)_6$),	
mg/1	0.4
pH	6.5-8.5
Phenol, mg/1	0.005
Radioactivity	
Radium-226, pCi/1	3
Strontium-90, pCi/1	10
Gross Beta, pCi/1	1000
Total Dissolved Solids, mg/1	500
Zinc, mg/1	0.3
NORTH CAROLINA	
Bacteria	
Fecal #/100 ml	1000
Total #/100 ml	5000
Dissolved Oxygen, mg/1	4.0-6.0
pH	6.0-8.5
Radioactivity	
Gross Beta, pCi/1	1000
Temperature, °F	Max. of 84°F or 5°F increase
Total Hardness, mg/1	100
NORTH DAKOTA	
Ammonia, mg/1	1.0
Arsenic, mg/1	0.05
Bacteria	
Total Coliform, #/100 ml	1000
Fecal Coliform, #100 ml	200
Barium, mg/1	1.0
Boron, mg/1	0.5
Cadmium, mg/1	0.01
Chlorides, mg/1	100
Chromium–Hexavalent, mg/1	0.05
Color	15
Copper, mg/1	0.05
Cyanides, mg/1	0.01
Lead, mg/1	0.05
Nitrates, mg/1	4.0
pH	7-8.5

Table 7-14, continued

Parameter	Standard
Phenols, mg/1	0.01
Phosphate (as P), mg/1	0.1
Radioactivity	
Radium-226, pCi/1	5
Strontium-89, pCi/1	1
Strontium-90, pCi/1	100
Tritium, pCi/1	3000
Selenium, mg/1	0.01
Sodium	50% of total cations as meq/1
Temperature, $^\circ$F	Max. of 85°F or 5°F increase
Total Dissolved Solids, mg/1	500
Turbidity, JTU	10
Zinc, mg/1	0.5
OHIO	
Ammonia, mg/1	1.5
Arsenic, μg/1	50
Bacteria, Fecal, #/100 ml	200
Barium, μg/1	800
Cadmium, μg/1	5
Chloride, mg/1	250
Chromium, μg/1	300
Chromium–Hexavalent, μg/1	50
Chromium–Hexavalent, μg/1^2	10
Copper, μg/1	5-75
Cyanide (free), mg/1	0.005
Cyanide, mg/1	0.2
Cyanide, mg/1	0.005
Dissolved Oxygen, mg/1	5
Fluoride, mg/1	1.3
MBAS, mg/1	0.5
Iron (dissolved), μg/1	1000
Iron (dissolved), μg/1	300
Lead, μg/1	40
Nitrate (as N), mg/1	8
Manganese (dissolved), μg/1	1000
Manganese (dissolved), μg/1^2	50
Mercury, μg/1	0.5
Odor	24 @ 40°C
Oil and Grease, mg/1	5
pH	6.0-9.0
Phosphorus, mg/1	1.0
Phenols, μg/1	10
Phenols, μg/1	1.0
Radioactivity	
Alpha Emitters, pCi/1	3
Strontium-90, pCi/1	10
Gross Beta, pCi/1	100

Table 7-14, continued

Parameter	Standard
Selenium, μg/1	5
Silver, μg/1	1
Temperature, $^\circ$F	3-5°F increase
Total Dissolved Solids, mg/1	1500
Total Dissolved Solids, mg/1	500
Zinc, μg/1	75-500
OKLAHOMA	
Bacteria–Fecal, #/100 ml	200
Dissolved Oxygen, mg/1	5
pH	6.5-8.5
Temperature	Max. of 68-90° or 3-5°F increase
Turbidity, JTU	10-50
OREGON	
Arsenic, mg/1	0.1
Bacteria–Total, #/100 ml	240-1000
Barium, mg/1	1.0
Boron, mg/1	0.5
Cadmium, mg/1	0.003-0.01
Chloride, mg/1	25
Chromium, mg/1	0.02-0.05
Copper, mg/1	0.005
Cyanide, mg/1	0.005-0.01
Dissolved Oxygen, mg/1	6
Fluoride, mg/1	1.0
Iron, mg/1	0.1
Lead, mg/1	0.05
Manganese, mg/1	0.05
pH	6.5-9.0
Phenols, mg/1	0.001
Temperature, $^\circ$F	0.5-20°F increase
Total Dissolved Solids, mg/1	100-750
Turbidity, JTU	5-JTU increase
Zinc, mg/1	0.1
PENNSYLVANIA	
Alkalinity, mg/1	20-100
Ammonia (as N), mg/1	0.5-1.5
Bacteria	
Fecal, #/100 ml	200
Total, #/100 ml	5000
Chlorides, mg/1	50-250
Color, color units	20-50
Copper, mg/1	0.02-0.10
Cyanide, mg/1	0.025
Dissolved Oxygen, mg/1	4.0-7.0
Fluoride, mg/1	1.0
Hardness, mg/1	95-150

Table 7-14, continued

Parameter	Standard
Iron (Dissolved), mg/1	0.3
Iron (Total), mg/1	1.5
Manganese, mg/1	1.0
MBAS, mg/1	0.5-1.0
Odor	24 @ 60°C
pH	6.0-9.0
Phenols, mg/1	0.005-0.02
Phosphate, mg/1	0.03-0.40
Radioactivity	
Alpha Emitters, pCi/1	3
Beta Emitters, pCi/1	1000
Sulfate, mg/1	250
Temperature, °F	85°F max or 2-5°F increase
Total Dissolved Solids, mg/1	500-750 or 133% of background
Turbidity, JTU	10-150
Zinc, mg/1	0.05
RHODE ISLAND	
Bacteria	
Fecal, #/100 ml	200
Total, #/100 ml	1000
Dissolved Oxygen, mg/1	5 or 75% of saturation
pH	6.5-8.0
Temperature, °F	Max. of 83°F or 4°F increase
Turbidity, JTU	10
SOUTH CAROLINA	
Fecal coliform, #/100 ml	1000
pH	6.0-8.5
Dissolved Oxygen, mg/1	5
Phenolic compounds, mg/1	0.001
SOUTH DAKOTA	
Ammonia (as N), mg/1	0.6-1.0
Bacteria−Total, #/100 ml	5000
Chlorides, mg/1	100
Chlorine Residue, mg/1	0.02
Cyanide−Total, mg/1	0.02
Cyanide−Free, mg/1	0.005
Dissolved Oxygen, mg/1	5.0-7.0
Hydrogen, Sulfide, mg/1	0.0002
Iron−Total, mg/l	0.02-0.2
Nitrogen (as N), mg/1	10
Nitrogen (as NO_3), mg/1	45
pH	6.0-9.0
Radioactivity	
Iodine-131, pCi/1	5
Radium-226, pCi/1	1

Table 7-14, continued

Parameter	Standard
Strontium-89, pCi/1	100
Strontium-90, pCi/1	10
Tritium, pCi/1	300
Suspended Solids, mg/1	30-950
Temperature $^\circ$F	Max. 65°F-90°F
Total Dissolved Solids, mg/1	1000
Turibidity, JTU	10-50

TENNESSEE

ABS, mg/1	0.5
Arsenic, mg/1	0.01
Bacteria–Fecal #/100 ml	1000
Chlorides, mg/1	250
Color, color units	15
Copper, mg/1	1.0
CCE, mg/1	0.2
Cyanide, mg/1	0.01
Fluorides, mg/1	1.3
Hardness, mg/1	150
Iron, mg/1	0.3
Manganese, mg/1	0.05
Nitrate, mg/1	35
pH	6.0-9.0
Phenols, mg/1	0.001
Sulfates, mg/1	250
Temperature, $^\circ$C	Max. of 30.5°C or 3°C increase
Total Dissolved Solids, mg/1	500
Turibidity, TJU	12

TEXAS

Bacteria–Fecal, #/100 ml	200-1000
Chloride, mg/1	40-700
Dissolved Oxygen, mg/1	5.0-6.0
pH	6.5-9.0
Sulfate, mg/1	40-700
Temperature, $^\circ$F	Max. 95°F or 1.5-4.0°F increase
Total Dissolved Solids, mg/1	200-400

VIRGINIA

Bacteria–Fecal, #/100 ml	200
Dissolved Oxygen, mg/1	4
pH	6.0-8.5
Temperature, $^\circ$F	Max. of 90°F or 5°F increase

In addition to other standards established for the protection of public or municipal water supplies, the following standards will apply at the raw water intake point:

    Physical
        Color, color units   75

Table 7-14, continued

Parameter	Standard
Inorganic Chemicals	
Alkalinity, mg/l	30-500
Arsenic, mg/l	0.05
Barium, mg/l	1.0
Boron, mg/l	1.0
Cadmium, mg/l	0.01
Chloride, mg/l	250
Chromium, hexavalent, mg/l	0.05
Copper, mg/l	1.0
Fluoride, mg/l	1.7
Iron (filterable), mg/l	0.3
Lead, mg/l	0.05
Manganese (filterable), mg/l	0.05
Nitrate plus nitrites, mg/l	10 (as N)
Selenium, mg/l	0.01
Silver, mg/l	0.05
Sulfate, mg/l	250
Total Dissolved Solids, mg/l	
(filterable residue)	500
Uranyl Ion, mg/l	5
Organic Chemicals	
Carbon Chloroform Extract	
(CCE) mg/l	0.15
Cyanide, mg/l	0.20
Methylene Blue Active Sub-	
stances, mg/l	0.5
Pesticides	
Aldrin, mg/l	0.017
Chlordane, mg/l	0.003
DDT, mg/l	0.042
Dieldrin, mg/l	0.017
Endrin, mg/l	0.001
Heptachlor, mg/l	0.018
Heptachlor epoxide, mg/l	0.018
Lindane, mg/l	0.056
Methoxychlor, mg/l	0.035
Organic phosphates plus	
Carbamates, mg/l	0.1
Toxaphene, mg/l	0.005
Herbicides	
2,4-D plus 2,4,5-T plus	
2,4,5-TP	
mg/l	0.1
Phenols, mg/l	0.001

Table 7-14, continued

Parameter	Standard
Radioactivity	
Gross Beta, pCi/1	1000
Radium-226, pCi/1	3
Strontium-90, pCi/1	10
Arsenic, mg/1	0.01
Bacteria	
Total, #/100 ml	1000
Fecal, #/100 ml	200
Barium, mg/1	0.50
Cadmium, mg/1	0.01
Chloride, mg/1	100
Chromium, mg/1	0.05
Cyanide, mg/1	0.025
Dissolved Oxygen, mg/1	5
Fluoride, mg/1	1.0
Lead, mg/1	0.05
Nitrates, mg/1	45
Odor	8 at $40^\circ C$
pH	6.0-8.5
Phenols, mg/1	0.001
Radioactivity	
Alpha Emitters pCi/1	3
Strontium-90, pCi/1	10
Gross Beta, pCi/1	1000
Selenium, mg/1	0.01
Silver, mg/1	0.05
Temperature, $^\circ F$	Max. of $87^\circ F$ or $5^\circ F$ increase
Toxic Substances	1/10 of 96-hr TLW
UTAH	
Bacteria	
Total Coliform, #/100 ml	5000
Fecal Coliform, #/100 ml	2000
BOD, mg/1	5
Dissolved Oxygen, mg/1	5.5
pH	6.5-8.5
VERMONT	
Bacteria	
Total Coliform, #/100 ml	500
Fecal Coliform, #/100 ml	200
Color, color units	25
Dissolved Oxygen, mg/1	6
pH	6.5-8.0
Sludge Deposits (solids, oil and grease	None
Taste and Odor	None that impair usage

Table 7-14, continued

Parameter	Standard
Temperature, °F	1°F increase
Turbidity, JTU	25
WASHINGTON	
Bacteria–Total #/100 ml	240
Dissolved Oxygen, mg/1	8.0
pH	6.5-8.5
Temperature, °F	Max. 65°F
Turibidity, JTU	5 JTU increase
WISCONSIN	
Bacteria–Fecal, #/100 ml	200
Dissolved Oxygen, mg/1	5
pH	6.0-9.0
Temperature, °F	Max. of 89°F or 5°F increase
Total Dissolved Solids, mg/1	500
WYOMING	
Bacteria–Fecal, #/100 ml	200
Dissolved Oxygen, mg/1	6
Odor	3
Oil, mg/1	10
pH	6.5-8.5
Temperature, °F	Max. of 68°F or 2°F increase
Turbidity, JTU	10

Table 7-15. Recommended Maximum Concentrations of Biocides in Whole Unfiltered Water in Coastal Waters (Clark, 1974)

Organochlorine Pesticides		Organophosphate Insecticides		Herbicides, Fungicides and Defoliants		Botanicals	
Name	µg/l	Name	µg/l	Name	µg/l	Name	µg/l
Aldrin[a]	0.01	Asinphosmethyl	0.001	Aminotriazole	300.0	Allethrin	0.002
DDT[b]	0.002	Ciodrin	0.10	Dalapon	110.0	Pyrethrum	0.01
DDE[b]	0.006	Coumaphos	0.001	Dicamba	200.0	Rotenone	10.0
Dieldrin[a]	0.005	Diazinon	0.009	Dichlobenil	37.0		
Chlordane[b]	0.04	Dichlorvos	0.001	Dichlone	0.2		
Endosulfon[b]	0.003	Dioxathion	0.09	Diquat	0.5		
Endrin[a]	0.002	Disulfonton	0.05	Diuron	1.6		
Heptachlor[a]	0.01	Dursban	0.001	2·4, D (BEE)	4.0		
Lindane[b]	0.02	Ethion	0.02	Fenac (Sodium Salt)	45.0		
Methoxychlor[b]	0.005	EPN	0.06	Silvex (BEE)	2.5		
Toxaphene[b]	0.01	Fenthion	0.006	Silvex (PGBE)	2.0		
		Malathion	0.008	Simazine	10.0		
		Mevinphos	0.002				
		Naled	0.004				
		Oxydemeton Methyl	0.40				
		Parathion	0.0004				
		Phosphamidon	0.03				
		TEPP	0.40				
		Trichlorophon	0.002				

a, bMaximum acceptable concentration in any sample consisting of a homogenate of 25 or more whole fish of any species that is consumed by fish-eating birds and mammals, within the size consumed on a net weight basis, expressed as µg/kg (EPA data available only for organo-chlorine pesticides). Note a: 5 µg/kg; Note b: 50 µg/kg.

Table 7-16. Hazardous and Minimal Risk Concentrations of Selected Inorganic Chemicals (Including Heavy Metals) Which Should be Considered for Protection of Marine Biota (NAS, 1973)

Elements	Natural Concentration in Sea Water (μg/l)	Hazardous Concentrations (μg/l)	Minimal Risk Concentrations (μg/l)	Hazardous/Natural
Aluminum	10	>1500	<200	150
Ammonia	NA[a]	>400 (nonionized)	<10 (nonionized)	–
Antimony	0.45	>200	NA	444
Arsenic	2.6	>50	10	19.2
Barium	20	>1000	<500	50.0
Beryllium	0.0006	>1500	<100	25×10^5
Bismuth	0.2	NA	NA	–
Boron	4.5×10^3	>5000	<5000	1.1
Bromine	6.7×10^4	NA	$<10 \times 10^4$ (ionic bromine in the form of bromate) >100 (molecular)	–
Cadmium[b]	0.02	>10	0.2	500.0
Chlorine	NA	>10 (free residual chlorine)	NA	–
Chromium[c]	0.04	>100	<50	2500.0
Copper	1	>50	<10	50.0
Cyanides	NA	>10	<5	–
Fluorides	1340	>1500	<500	1.1
Iron	10	>300	<50	30.0
Lead	0.02	>50	<10	2500.0
Manganese	2	>100	<20	50.0
Mercury	0.1	>0.1	2[d]	1.0
Nickel	7	>100	<2	14.3
Nitrate	6.7×10^2	NA	NA	–
Phosphorus	NA	>1 (elemental phosphorus)	NA	–
Selenium	0.45	>10	<5	22.2
Silver	0.3	>5	<1	16.7
Sulfides	NA	>10	<5	–
Thallium	2	>100	<50	50.0
Uranium	3	>500	<100	167.0
Zinc[e]	2	>100	<20	50.0

[a] NA: Not available.
[b] The application factor should be lower by at least one order of magnitude in the presence of copper and/or zinc at 1 mg/l or more.
[c] Concentrations should be maintained at less than 0.01 mg/l in oyster areas.
[d] This level is the level in the water supply sources.
[e] The application factor may have to be lowered by an order of magnitude when zinc is present with other heavy metals—e.g., copper and cadmium.

Table 7-17. Estimated Effects of Underwater Explosion Tests on
Marine Life in the Patuxent River and Chesapeake Bay (Young, 1973)

Degree of Damage to Fish[a]	Types of Fish in Designated Areas	
	Chesapeake Bay Depths Greater Than 40 ft	Tributary Rivers Depths Greater Than 40 ft
Maximum probable damage, December, January, February	Maximal concentration of bass occurs near the bottom in deep water. There is a high probability that large kills of striped bass will result. Some white perch and juveniles of other species will be killed.	Maximal concentration of white perch occurs near the bottom in deep water. There is a high probability that large kills of white perch will result. Some striped bass will be killed.
Heavy, probable damage, November and March	Since striped bass and large white perch are migrating into deep, oxygen-rich water in late fall and early spring, large kills may result among striped bass. Few white perch will be killed.	Some striped bass concentrate in deep water of lower estuaries and most white perch concentrate in the same areas. Large numbers of white perch and some striped bass will be killed.
Moderate probable damage, April May, September, October.	Migratory fishes, including striped bass, shad, river herrings, white perch, etc., will appear in kills. Schooling surface fish may be killed.	Same as open bay.
Least probable damage, June, July, August	Since most fish do not frequent deep oxygen-poor waters, few marketable fish will be killed. Menhaden will be killed in large numbers. Schooling near-surface striped bass and other species may be killed at times.	Same as open bay.

[a]Assuming no efforts are made to avoid fish-kill.

Table 7-18. Effects of Underwater Explosions on Aquatic Organisms

Weight of Explosives Used (lb)	Type of Explosives Used	Distance from Blast and Pressure (psi)		Major Aquatic Life Involved in the Experiment	Findings at Distances Indicated	Source
		Distance	Pressure[a]			
10	60% petrogel	50	560	Fish	Fish with swim bladders were largely injured.	Alpin, 1947
		55	509	Fish	Fish without swim bladders were largely uninjured.	
40	60% petrogel	250	178	Fish	A few fish were injured up to the indicated distance.	
20	60% petrogel	50	706	Spiny lobsters (Panulirus interruptus)	Lobsters were not injured.	
200	60% gelatine dynamite	50	1520	Shrimp	Shrimp were not injured.	Gowanloch, J. N. and J. E. McDougall, 1945.
200	60% gelatine dynamite	200	380	Croakers (Micropogon undulatus)	Croakers were not injured	
800	60% gelatin dynamite	50	2414	Shrimp	Shrimp were not injured.	
30	TNT	100	404	Oysters	5% of oysters sustained fatal injury within indicated distance.	Chesapeake Biological Laboratory, 1948.
300	TNT	200	435	Oysters	5% of oysters sustained fatal injury within indicated distance.	

				Species	Remarks	Reference
30	TNT	200	202	Trout (*Cynoscion regalis*) Striped bass (*Roccus Saxatilis*)	Injured at 200 feet. Subsequent deaths due to injury occurred in generally decreasing proportions up to a radius of 500 feet (80 psi).	
3 x 30 (successive)	TNT	250	162	Striped bass	Increased the range of initial mortality from 200 to 350 ft.	
3 x 30 (successive)	TNT	350	115	Trout	Increased the range of initial mortality from 200 to 350 ft.	
300	TNT	150	580	Crabs	Lethal damage was limited to the indicated distance.	Thompson, 1958
2,750,000	Unknown	2640	690	Fish	Fish lethality was confined to an area less than half a mile.	
10	High explosive	160	175	Fish (Arctic cisco and small *Coregonedes*)	Lethal damage to all fish within the indicated distance (equivalent to 25,450 ft^2)	Folk and Lawrence, 1973.

aThe method used to calculate pressure is similar to that described in Table 7-7.

both drinking and for crop irrigation. Table 7-9 summarizes federal
marine water quality standards, while Table 7-10 shows criteria for freshwater aquatic life.

Table 7-11 is a summary of maximum levels of industrial water characteristics that have been used for industrial water supplies. These parameters cover uses for boiler makeup, cooling and industrial process water.
Table 7-12 is a summary of recommended water quality standards for
domestic water supply. Table 7-13 lists industrial categories for which
EPA has federal regulations. The exact standards and numerical ranges
for each can be found in EPA's *Summary of Final Effluent Guidelines
and Standards*.

Table 7-14 is a 1976 summary of state water quality standards. The
states (listed alphabetically) and parameters controlled are on the left,
while numerical standards are on the right.

Tables 7-15 through 7-21 are used for determining impacts of actions
on fish and other biota in aquatic ecosystems. Table 7-15 lists recommended limits for biocides in coastal waters. The first set of standards
are for pesticides, such as the chlorinated hydrocarbons. The second set
of standards are for organophosphate insecticides. The third list of bio-
cide standards are for chemicals used to kill plants. The final list are
botanicals, with the latter rotenone, used to kill fish. Table 7-16 lists
limits of pollutants in coastal waters for protection of marine biota. One
column lists the element or heavy metal; the second column gives natural
concentrations of that substance; the third column lists high hazard levels;
and the fourth minimum risk levels.

Figure 7-3 shows normal summer water temperature isotherms. These
would be used to compare impacts of actions, such as cooling, which
would warm surface waters. Since summer temperatures are usually the
critical factor, changes in water temperature during July and August would
have the greatest influence on fisheries.

Tables 7-19 through 7-20 specifically refer to underwater explosions
and predicting impacts on fish. Table 7-17 estimates effects of explosions
on fish. Table 7-18 compares weights of explosives to potential underwater effects on fish and invertebrates. Table 7-19 gives noise ranges from
underwater sources in terms of charge weight. Table 7-20 and Figure 7-4
show relationships between force and distance from explosion, which are
used to calculate area of explosion influence.

Figure 7-5 and Tables 7-21 and 7-22 deal with estimation of quantities
of water, and low flow impacts on fishery resources. Figure 7-5 shows
normal low stream flow seasons. Consumption, which lowers flow during
these critical times, would have more severe impacts. Table 7-21 shows
specific spawning needs for certain sport fish (column 1). Water depth

Table 7-19. Maximum Range of Noise Audibility (R_a) Generated
by Different Charges of Underwater Explosions[a] (Young, 1973)

Charge Weight (W) (lb)	$W^{1/3}$	Maximum Range of Audibility (R_a) in Nautical Miles
1	1.00	7.9
2	1.26	10.0
5	1.71	13.5
10	2.15	17.0
20	2.71	21.4
50	3.68	29.1
100	4.64	36.7
150	5.31	42.0
200	5.85	46.2

[a]Calculation of R_a values is based on the following relationship:

$$R_a = 7.9 \times W^{1/3}$$

where R_a =   maximum range of audibility (nautical miles)
W =   charge weight (lb)
$W^{1/3}$ =   cube root of charge weight

and velocity are listed as spawning requirements, along with primary
source of original data. Table 7-22 gives a low flow matrix which
compares water quantity with impacts on fish, recreation and water
quality.

Tables 7-22 through 7-27 and Figures 7-6, 7-7 present quantifiable
data for evaluation of human uses of water. Table 7-23 gives typical
per capita uses of water in houses, public buildings, schools and camps,
to estimate consumption of freshwater in urban areas. Tables 7-24
and 7-25 present water consumption data for power plants. Table
7-24 compares three types of power plants, fossil, nuclear [high-tempera-
ture gas reactor (HGTR)] and nuclear [(light water reactor (LWR)].
Table 7-25 estimates water consumption for cooling and evaporation for
six selected locations in the U.S. Figure 7-6 shows water consumption
for energy conversion processes and refining. Energy industries are on
the vertical line, and are compared in terms of gallons of water used
per Btu output (horizontal). Table 7-26 summarizes water uses of
various energy conversion processes.

Table 7-27 gives a quantifiable methodology used for measuring
aesthetics of rivers. The Leopold (1973) method allows for rating
values of aquatic resources. Figure 7-9 illustrates the locations of current federally designated scenic rivers, and gives miles designated officially

Table 7-20. Force in Pounds per Square Inch (psi) Expected at Different Distances (ft) As a Result of Detonating Different Charges (lb) of Explosives[a] (U.S. Navy, 1970)

Radius (R) from Explosion (ft)	πR²		Force (psi) Resulting from the Following Weights of Explosives (lb)								
	(ft²)	(ac)	1	2	5	10	20	50	100	150	200
5	79	0.0018	2,600	3,276	4,446	5,600	7,056	9,578	12,069	13,814	15,205
10	314	0.0072	1,300	1,638	2,223	2,800	3,528	4,789	6,035	6,907	7,602
20	1,256	0.029	650	819	1,112	1,400	1,764	2,395	3,017	3,453	3,801
50	7,850	0.18	260	328	445	560	706	958	1,207	1,381	1,520
80	20,096	0.46	163	205	278	350	441	599	754	863	950
100	31,400	0.72	130	164	223	280	353	479	603	691	760
150	70,650	1.62	87[b]	109	148	187	235	319	402	460	507
200	125,600	2.88	65	82	111	140	176	239	302	345	380
250	196,250	4.51	52	66	89	112	141	192	241	276	304
300	282,600	6.49	43[c]	55	74	93	118	160	201	230	253
350	384,650	8.83	37	47	64	80	101	137	172	197	217
400	502,400	11.53	33	41	56	70	88	120	151	173	190
450	635,850	14.60	29	36	49	62	78	106	134	153	169
500	785,000	18.02	26	33	44	56	71	96	121	138	152

[a] Values based on the following formula:

$$P = \frac{13,000\sqrt[3]{W}}{d},$$

where P = force, psi.

W = weight of explosive, in pounds (tetryl or TNT).

d = distance of explosion from receptor (ft).

[b] 40 psi threshold.
[c] 70 psi threshold.

Table 7-21. Spawning Requirements of Fish (Stalnaker and Arnette, 1976)

Species	Depth (ft)	Velocity (ft/sec)	Reference
Coho	1.0-1.25	1.2-1.8[a]	Chambers et al., 1955
Coho	0.3-1.90	0.5-3.0	Sams and Pearson, 1963
Coho	0.6	1.0-3.0	Thompson, 1972
Coho	0.5[b]	0.7-2.3	Smith, 1973
Pink	0.5-1.75	0.7-3.3[a]	Collings, 1974
Chum	0.5-1.75	0.7-3.3[a]	Collings, 1974
Chum	0.6[b]	1.5-3.3	Smith, 1973
Chum	0.6	1.5-3.2	Thompson, 1972
Fall Chinook	1.0-1.5	1.0-2.3[a]	Chambers et al., 1955
Fall Chinook	0.3-1.5	0.9-3.1	Sam and Pearson, 1963
Fall Chinook	0.8	1.0-3.0	Thompson, 1972
Fall Chinook	0.8[b]	1.0-2.5	Smith, 1973
Spring Chinook	1.5-1.75	1.8-2.3[c]	Chambers et al., 1955
Spring Chinook	0.3-2.0	<0.4-2.8	Sams and Pearson, 1963
Spring Chinook	0.8	1.0-3.0	Thompson, 1972
Spring Chinook	0.6[b]	0.7-2.1	Smith, 1973
Sockeye	1.0-1.5	1.8[a]	Chambers et al., 1955
Sockeye	–	1.8[a]	Clay, 1961
Kokanee	0.4-0.6	0.8-2.1	Thompson, 1972
Kokanee	0.2[b]	0.5-2.4	Smith, 1973
Kokanee	> 0.2	0.4-2.4	Hunter, 1973
Kokanee	0.4-0.6	0.8-2.1	Thompson, 1972
Steelhead	0.6	1.0-3.0	Thompson, 1972
Steelhead	1.27	1.2-3.4	Hooper, 1973
Steelhead	0.8[b]	1.3-3.0	Smith, 1973
Steelhead	> 0.5	1.3-3.2	Hunter, 1973
Steelhead	0.4-2.3	1.2-3.6	Hunter, 1973
Rainbow Trout	0.7-1.1	1.4-2.7[c]	Hooper, 1973
Rainbow Trout	0.5	1.4-2.7	Bovee, 1974
Rainbow Trout	.29-3.0	0.7-3.0	Waters[d]
Rainbow Trout	0.6-1.1	1.4-3.0	Hunter, 1973
Cutthroat Trout	–	1.0-3.0	Hooper, 1973
Cutthroat Trout	0.2-1.5	0.4-2.4	Hunter, 1973
Brown Trout	> 0.8	0.7-2.5	Hunter, 1973
Brown Trout	–	> 1.5[e]	Hoppe and Finnell, 1972
Brown Trout	0.8	0.7-2.1	Thompson, 1972
Brown Trout	–	1.0-3.0[f]	Hooper, 1973
Brown Trout	0.5	1.3-1.7	Bovee, 1974
Brown Trout	0.8[b]	0.7-2.3	Smith, 1973
Brook Trout	29.7[b]	0.03-0.8	Smith, 1973
Brook Trout	–	0.2-3.0	Hooper, 1973
Brook Trout	0.5	0.5-3.0	Bovee, 1974
Brook Trout	0.3-2.0	0.03-2.1	Hunter, 1973
Dolly Varden	0.7-1.4	1.1-2.2	Hunter, 1973
Grayling	> 0.4	–	Hunter, 1973
Whitefish	> 0.4	–	Hunter, 1973

Table 7-21, continued

Species	Depth (ft)	Velocity (ft/sec)	Reference
Paddlefish	Variable	1.6-3.0	Bovee, 1974
Shovelnose Sturgeon	1.0-3.0	2.5-4.9	Bovee, 1974
Lake Sturgeon	2.0-15.0	–	Carlander, 1969
Lake Sturgeon	2.0-15.2	–	Scott and Crossman, 1973
Sturgeon, Russian sp.	5.0-16.4	2.3-3.6	White[g]
Creek Club	–	1.6-3.0	Bovee, 1974
Longnose Dace	0.1-1.0	0.5-1.5	Bovee, 1974
Longnose Sucker	0.7-1.0	1.0-1.5	Bovee, 1974
White Sucker	0.7-1.0	1.0-1.5	Bovee, 1974
Shorthead Redhorse	1.0-3.0	1.0-2.0	Bovee, 1974
Smallmouth Bass	3.0-6.0	0.4	Bovee, 1974
Smallmouth Bass	2.0-20.0	–	Scott and Crossman, 1973
Largemouth Bass	1.0-0.6	Still	Bovee, 1974
Walleye	4.0-5.0	0-1.6	Bovee, 1974
Sauger	4.0-5.0	0-1.6	Bovee, 1974

[a]Measured at 0.4 ft above streambed.
[b]Minimum.
[c]Measured at 0.20 ft above streambed.
[d]Unpublished data (1975). Brian Waters, Pacific Gas and Electric Co.
[e]Measured at 0.6 water depth from flow surface.
[f]Measured at 0.25 ft above streambed.
[g]Draft proposal (1975). Robert White, FWS.

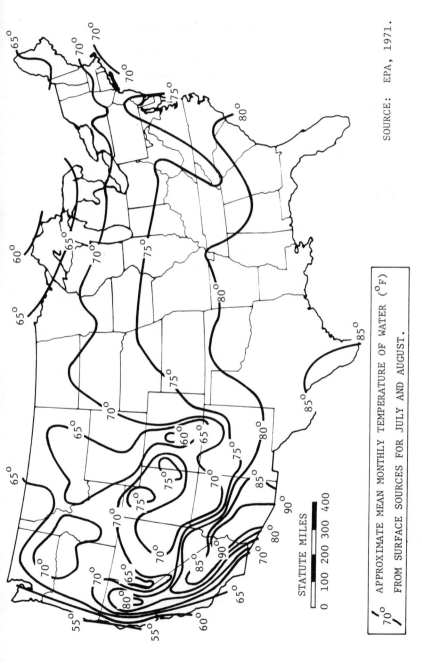

SOURCE: EPA, 1971.

Figure 7-3. Typical U.S. surface water temperature isotherms—July and August.

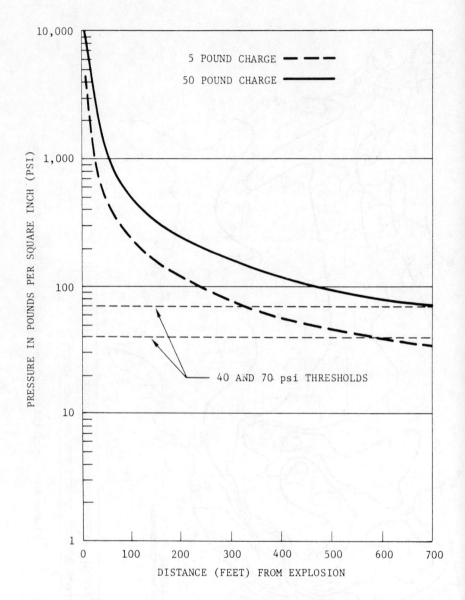

Figure 7-4. Relationship between pressure and distance from explosion for two charge weights.

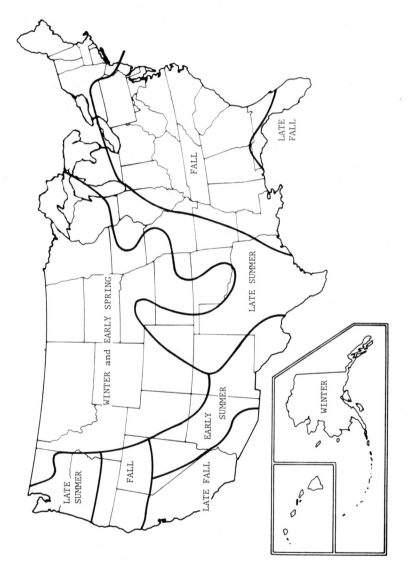

Figure 7-5. Seasons of lowest stream flow.

Table 7-22. Low Flow Evaluation Matrix (Stalnaker and Arnette, 1976)

Flow (cfs)	Fish			Recreation			Water Quality
	Salmon	Steelhead	Trout	Swimming	Canoeing and Kayaking	Fishing	Class
300	Adult migration and spawning capacity reduced by 80%. Egg incubation reduced by 60%. Rearing capacity reduced by 30%. Smolt migration reduced by 75%.	Adult migration and spawning reduced by 80%. Egg incubation reduced by 50%. Rearing reduced by 30%. Smolt migration reduced by 60%.	Spawning reduced by 60%. Adult migration, egg incubation and rearing reduced by 20%.	Acceptable wading marginal for swimming.	Too little water.	Fishing is often poor at this flow.	Water would be reduced to Class B with existing development and discharge.
600	Adult migration and spawning capacity reduced by 30%. Egg incubation reduced by 20%. Optimum flow for rearing. Smolt migration reduced by 25%.	Adult migration and spawning reduced by 30%. Egg incubation reduced by 20%. Optimum for rearing. Smolt migration reduced by 20%.	Optimum for adult migration, egg incubation, and rearing. Spawning reduced by 20%.	Flow satisfactory for swimming.	Danger of damaging canoes	"Best" fishing conditions generally occur at this flow and above.	Minimum flow to maintain Class AA water with existing development and discharge
1000	Optimum for adult migration, spawning, egg incubation and smolt migration.	Optimum for adult migration, spawning, egg incubation and smolt migration	Optimum for spawning.	Too much flow for wading, approaching upper limit for satisfactory swimming.	Minimum flow for canoeing and kayaking.	Fishing is usually good at this flow.	This flow has dilution capacity for additional development and discharge at Class AA standards.

Table 7-23. Water Requirements for Domestic Service, Public Buildings,
Schools and Camps (Todd, 1970)

Domestic Fixtures	
Fill lavatory	2 gal
Fill bathtub	30 gal
Shower bath	30-60 gal
Flush toilet	6 gal
Dishwasher	3 gal/load
Automatic laundry machine	30-50 gal/load
Lawn sprinkler	120 gph
1/2-inch hose and nozzle	240-300 gph
5/8-inch hose and nozzle	270-330 gph
3/4-inch hose and nozzle	300-360 gph
Private Homes	
For each member of family including kitchen, laundry and bath	40 gpd
Public Buildings	gph per Fixture
Hotel	50
Apartment houses	20
Hospitals	25
Office buildings	40
Mercantile buildings	35
1-1/2-inch fire hose and nozzle	2400
Day school	50
Schools and Camps	
Schools	15-17
Camp	40
With hot and cold running water, kitchen, laundry, shower, bath and flush toilets	

Table 7-24. Consumption of Water in Condenser Cooling of 1000-MW Electric Power Plants

	Cooling Water Budget in Acre-Feet Per Year[a] For 1000-Megawatt Electric Reference Plants		
	Fossil-Fueled	Nuclear (HTGR)	Nuclear (LWR)
Once-Through Cooling			
Total Water Intake	540,000	670,000	890,000
Total Water Consumption	5,900	7,300	9.300
Cooling Pond			
Evaporation Loss	8,500	10,000	14,000
Drift Loss	Negligible	Negligible	Negligible
Purge	Variable	Variable	Variable
Total Water Intake			
Excluding Purge	8,500	10,000	14,000
Total Water Consumption	8,500	10,000	14,000
Spray Pond			
Evaporation Loss	8,500	10,000	14,000
Drift Loss	1,100	1,300	1,800
Purge	Variable	Variable	Variable
Total Water Intake			
Excluding Purge	9,600	11,300	15,800
Total Water Consumption	9,600	11,300	15,800
Evaporative Towers			
Evaporation Loss	8,700	11,000	14,000
Drift Loss	110	130	180
Blowdown	4,300	5,400	7,100
Total Water Intake	13,000	17,000	21,000
Total Water Consumption	8,800	11,000	14,000

[a] Average values generally applicable throughout the United States; a temperature rise across the condenser of $20°F$ is assumed throughout and annual consumption values are computed at a plant load factor of 0.80.

Table 7-25. Estimated Cooling Pond Area and Water Consumption for 1000-MWe Power Plants (Patterson et al., 1971)

Location	Seattle, Washington	Yuma, Arizona	Houston, Texas	Miami, Florida	Kansas City Missouri	New York, New York	Average of the 6 Locations
Natural Equilibrium Temperature, July, °F[a]	69.2	83.6	85.9	84.6	82.1	76.0	-
Maximum Pond[b] Loading (Millions of Btu/hr/ac)	8.8	4.1	2.5	3.5	4.6	6.9	-
Pond Area Required[c] in Acres							
Fossil-Fueled Plant	480	1,000	1,700	1,200	910	610	1,000
Nuclear (HTGR)	590	1,300	2,100	1,500	1,100	750	1,200
Nuclear (LWR)	790	1,700	2,800	2,000	1,500	1,000	1,600
Yearly Evaporation[d] in ac-ft							
Fossil-Fueled Plant	5,800	10,000	11,000	9,600	8,100	6,100	8,500
Nuclear (HTGR)	7,100	13,000	13,000	12,000	9,700	7,500	10,000
Nuclear (LWR)	9,500	18,000	18,000	16,000	13,000	10,000	14,000

[a]Taken as representative of a summer month.
[b]Based on a limitation of 87°F at the plant intake in July.
[c]Based on heat rejection rates.
[d]Based on estimated evaporation during average month and a load factor of 0.80.

Table 7-26. Unit Water Requirements for Producing Energy (Water Resources Council, 1974)

Energy Source	Standard Unit	Consumption of Water	Water Needed (gal/million Btu)	Water Uses of Consideration
Western Coal Mining	ton	6-14.7 gal/ton	0.25-0.61	Dust control
Eastern Surface Mining	ton	15.8-18.0 gal/ton	0.66-0.75	Dust control
				Coal washing
Oil Shale	barrel	145.4 gal/bbl	30.1	Processed shale disposal
				Shale oil upgrading
				Power requirements
				Retorting
				Mining and crushing
				Revegetation
				Sanitary use
				Associated urban
Coal Gasification	MSCF[a]	72-158 gal/MSCF	72-158	Process use
				Cooling use
Coal Liquefaction	barrel	175-1,134 gal/bbl	31-200	Process use
				Cooling use
Nuclear	kWh	0.80 gal/kWh	234.46	Cooling
				Uranium mining
Oil and Gas Production	barrel	17.3 gal/bbl	3.05	Well drilling
				Secondary and tertiary recovery
Refineries	barrel	43 gal/bbl	7.58	Process water
				Cooling water
Fossil-Fueled Power Plants	kWh	0.41 gal/kWh	120.16	Cooling water
Gas Processing Plants	MSCF[a]	1.67 gal/MSCF[a]	1.67	Cooling water

[a]Million standard cubic feet.

Table 7-27. Measurement of Aesthetics of Rivers (Leopold, 1973)

Descriptive Categories	Rating Value				
	1	2	3	4	5
Physical Factors					
River Width (ft) (at low flow)	<3	3-10	10-30	30-100	>100
Depth (ft)	<0.5	0.5-1	1-2	2-5	>5
Velocity (ft/sec)	<0.5	0.5-1	1-2	3-5	>5
Stream Depth (ft)	<1	1-2	2-4	4-8	>8
Flow Variability	Little variation		Normal	Ephemeral or large variation	
River Pattern	Torrent	Pool and riffle	Without riffles	Meander	Braided
Valley Height/Width	≤1	2-5	5-10	11-14	≥15
Streambed Material	Clay or silt	Sand	Sand and gravel	Gravel	Cobbles or larger
Bed Slope (ft/ft)	<0.0005	0.0005-0.001	0.001-0.005	0.005-0.01	>0.01
Drainage Area (mi²)	<1	1-10	10-100	100-1000	>1000
Stream Order	≤2	3	4	5	≥6
Erosion of Banks	Stable		Slumping		Eroding large-scale deposition
Sediment Deposition in Bed					
Width of Valley Flat (ft)	Stable <100	100-300	300-500	500-1000	>1000
Biological and Water Quality Factors					
Water Color	Clear colorless		Green tints		Brown
Turbidity (ppm)	<25	25-150	150-1000	1000-5000	>5000
Floating Material	None	Vegetation	Foamy	Oily	Variety
Water Condition (general)	Poor		Good		Excellent
Algae					
Amount	Absent				Infested
Type	Green	Blue-green	Diatom	Floating green	None
Larger Plants					
Amount	Absent				Infested
Kind	None	Unknown rooted	Elodea, duck weed	Water lily	Cattail

Table 7-27, continued

Descriptive Categories	Rating Value				
	1	2	3	4	5
River Fauna	None				Large variety
Pollution Evidence	None				Evident
Land Flora					
Valley	Open	Open w. grass, trees	Brushy	Wooded	Trees and brush
Hillside	Open	Open w. grass, trees	Brushy		
Diversity	Small				Great
Condition	Good				Overused
Human Use and Interest Factors					
Trash and **Litter**					
Metal (no/100 ft of river)	< 2	2-5	5-10	10-50	> 50
Paper	< 2	2-5	5-10	10-50	> 50
Other	< 2	2-5	5-10	10-50	> 50
Material Removable	Easily removed				Difficult removal
Artificial Controls (dams, etc.)	Free and natural				Controlled
Accessibility					
Individual	Wilderness				Urban or paved access
Mass Use	Wilderness				Urban or paved access
Local Scene	Diverse views and scenes				Closed or without diversity
Vistas	Vistas of far places				Closed or no **vistas**
View Confinement	Open or no obstructions				Closed by hills, cliffs or trees

Land Use	Wilderness	Grazed	Lumbering	Forest, mixed recreation	Urbanized
Utilities	Scene unobstructed by power lines				Scene obstructed by utilities
Degree of Change	Original				Materially altered
Recovery Potential	Natural recovery				Natural recovery **unlikely**
Urbanization	No buildings				Many buildings
Special Views	None				Unusual interest
Historic Features	None				Many
Misfits	None				Many

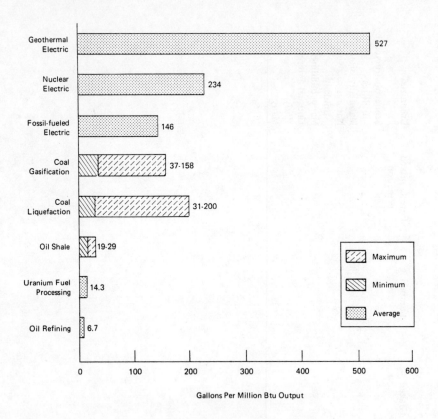

Figure 7-6. Water consumption in energy conversion and refining (DOI, 1974).

as "wild and scenic." These rivers receive special federal protection under the Scenic Rivers Act of 1968 (PL 90-542).

REFERENCES

Alpin, J. A. "The Effect of Explosives on Marine Life," *Calif. Fish Game* 33(1)23-27 (1947).

Chesapeake Biological Laboratory. "Effects of Underwater Explosions on Oysters, Crabs and Fish," Chesapeake Biological Laboratory Publ. 70:1-43 (1948).

Clark, J. *Coastal Ecosystem Ecological Considerations for Management of the Coastal Zone*, The Conservative Foundation, Washington, DC (1974).

Colston, N. V. "Characterization of Urban Land Runoff in Non-Point Sources of Water Pollution," Virginia Water Resources Center (1975).

Environmental Protection Agency, U.S. "Quality Criteria for Water," EPA 44019-76023 (1976).

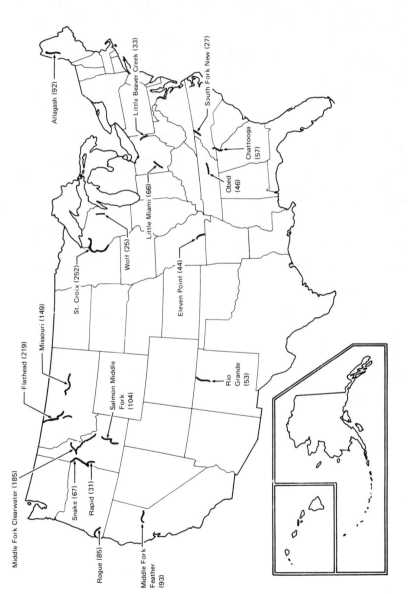

Figure 7-7. Wild and scenic rivers of the U.S. (river, miles designated) (National Geographic, 1977).

Environmental Protection Agency, U.S. "STORET Computer Print Out for Lake Champlain," 202B, Basin 4 (1976b).

Folk, M. R., and M. J. Lawrence. "Seismic Exploration: Its Nature and Effect on Fish," Fish and Marine Service Central Region Tech. Report Series No. CEN/T 73-9 (1973).

Hann, R. W., Jr. *Fundamental Aspects of Water Quality Management* (Westport, CT: Technomic Publishing Co., Inc., 1972).

Interior, U. S. Department of, Geological Survey. "Water Demands for Expanding Energy Development," Circular 703 (1974).

Leopold, L. B. "Quantitative Comparison of Some Aesthetic Factors Among Rivers, Geological Survey Circular 620, Washington, DC (1969, 1973).

National Geographic Magazine. Wild and Scenic Rivers of the United States (Map). 152 (1) (1977).

Navy, U.S. *U.S. Navy Diving Manual*, NAVSHIPS 0994-001-9010 (1970).

Omernik, J. M. "Nonpoint Source–Stream Nutrient Level Relationships: a Nationwide Study," EPA-600/3-77-105 (1977).

Patterson, J. W. *Directory of Federal and State Water Pollution Standards* (1976).

Stalnaker, C. B., and J. L. Arnette. "Methodologies for the Determination of Stream Resource Flow Requirements: an Assessment," U.S. Fish and Wildlife Service, Department of Interior (1976).

Thompson, J. A. "Biological Effects of the Ripple Rock Explosion," *Progress Report of Pacific Coast Station, Fish Res. Bd. Con.* 111: 3-8 (1958).

Todd, D. K. *The Water Encyclopedia* (Port Washington, NY: Water Information Center, 1970).

Water Resources Council. "Water Requirements, Availabilities, Constraints and Recommended Federal Actions, Project Independence (November 1974).

Young, G. A. "Guidelines for Evaluating the Environmental Effects of Underwater Explosion Tests," AD-758, Naval Ordinance Laboratory, White Oak, MD (1973).

CHAPTER 8

NOISE

Noise intrusion into a quiet environment would in most cases have greater impact than additional noise into a noisy environment. Table 8-1 gives typical ambient noise levels from quiet wilderness to the highest noise situations. The type of environment is listed on the left, while comparative noise sources are given on the right side of the table. Noise levels on the center scale are given in decibels (dBA). Table 8-2 presents typical noise levels for various phases of construction (in this table it is assumed that the noisiest location is 50 ft from the boundary). The column labeled I refers to all pertinent equipment at the site; whereas column II refers to minimum equipment at the site.

Table 8-3 lists typical noise sources, peak levels reported and decreasing noise levels at distances from source. The table assumes a 6-dBA decrease for every doubling of distance, and an atmospheric adsorption of one dBA per 100 ft, when measured noise levels were not available. Sources are grouped by similar working situations. Aircraft are reported for takeoff and landing. Weapons are reported for distances that noise levels of 75 and 140 dBA are carried over flat terrain.

Table 8-4 reports human behavior and physiological effects from noise levels listed in the first column. Figure 8-1 is a graphic display of noise as it interferes with communication. The dBA level is related directly to the distance between speakers.

Table 8-5 is used in prediction of human effects from day-night average sound levels of 55, 65 and 75 dBA. Reactions of communities are given for speech intelligibility, complaint level, annoyance and attitudes.

Table 8-1.   Typical Noise Level, dBA (DOD, 1975)

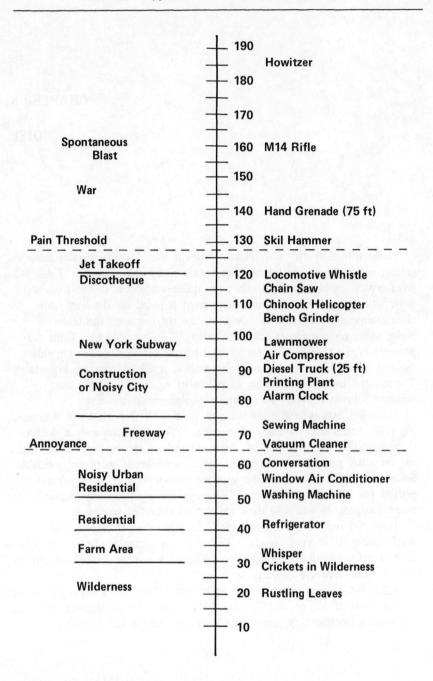

Table 8-2. Typical Noise Levels During Construction (Goff, Novak, 1977)

Type	Housing		Office Building, Hotel		Road, Highways		Commercial, Industrial	
Phase	I	II	I	II	I	II	I	II
Grand Clearing	83	83	84	84	84	84	84	83
Excavation	88	75	89	79	88	78	89	71
Foundation	81	81	78	78	88	88	77	77
Erection	81	65	87	75	79	78	84	72
Finishing	88	72	89	75	84	84	89	74

Table 8-3. Noise Sources, dBA
(DOD, 1975; Congress, 1972; FAA, 1975)

Source	Noise Level (Peak)	Distance from Source[a]			
		50 ft	100 ft	200 ft	400 ft
Office Machines					
Card Processor	93		77		
Card Sorter	82		67		
Keypunch	86		65		
Printer	80		64		
Binder	92		77		
Collator	90		68		
Folder	93		75		
Offset Press	87		72		
Paper Shredder	110		85		
Xerox	77		67		
Machinery					
Drying Tumbler	94	79	73	67	61
Laundry	88	73	67	61	55
Chainsaw	125	110	104	98	92
Rip Saw	102	87	81	75	69

Table 8-3 , continued

Source	Noise Level (Peak)	Distance from Source			
		50 ft	100 ft	200 ft	400 ft
Power Saw	100	85	79	73	67
Skil Drill	103	88	82	76	70
Planer	112	90	84	78	72
Sander	93	90	84	78	72
Air Chisel	125	110	104	98	92
Rock Drill	118	98	92	86	80
Skil Hammer	132	117	111	105	99
Riveter	92	77	71	65	59
Air Wrench	107	92	86	80	76
Elevator	105	90	84	78	72
Conveyor	104	89	83	77	71
Water Pump	98	76	70	64	58
Construction					
Heavy Trucks	95	84-89	78-83	72-77	66-71
Pickup Trucks	92	72	66	60	54
Dump Trucks	108	88	82	76	70
Concrete Mixer	105	85	79	73	67
Jackhammer	108	88	82	76	70
Scraper	93	80-89	74-82	68-77	60-71
Dozer	107	87-102	81-96	75-90	69-84
Paver	109	80-89	74-83	68-77	60-71
Generator	96	76	70	64	58
Shovel	111	91	85	79	73
Crane	104	75-88	69-82	63-76	55-70
Loader	104	73-86	67-80	61-74	55-68
Grader	108	88-91	82-85	76-79	70-73
Caterpillar	103	88	82	76	70
Dragline	105	85	79	73	67
Shovel	110	91-107	85-101	79-95	73-89
Dredging	89	79	73	66	60
Pile Driver	105	95	89	83	77
Ditcher	104	99	93	87	81
Fork Lift	100	95	89	83	77
Vehicles					
Snowmobile	94	78	72	66	60
Diesel Train	98	80-88	74-82	68-76	62-70
Mack Truck	91	84	78	72	66
Travelall	71	56	50	44	38
Jeep Wagoner	78	63	57	51	45
Bus	97	82	76	70	54
Compact Auto	90	75-80	69-74	63-68	57-62
Passenger Auto	85	69-76	63-70	57-64	51-58
Motorcycle	110	82	76	70	64

Table 8-3 , continued

Type Aircraft	Takeoff		Landing	
	dA	(EPNdB)[b]	dBA	(EPNdBA)
727,737,DC9,BAC111	94-100	92-96	85-90	97-104
707,720,DC8	100-105	–	94-100	–
747 Widebody	103	107-115	92	104-114
DC10, L1011	90	95-106	84	99-108
DC3, Propeller	85-90	–	75-82	–
Single-Engine Propeller	76-90	77-78	67-77	87-88
Multipropeller	79-93	–	70-80	–
Executive Jet	93-97	83-94	81-87	92-101
OH58 (Ranger Helicopter)	84	–	72	–
UH1 (Huey Helicopter)	77	–	77	–
C141 (Cargo Plane)	134	–	117	–

Type Weapon	mm	Distance for Decibel Level of:		
		140 dBA (ft)[c]	75 dBA	
			(ft)	(mi)
45 Pistol	–	75	18,000	3.4
M3 Machine Gun	–	75	18,000	3.4
M60 Machine Gun	7.6	50	9,950	1.8
MI Mortar	81	100	19,850	3.8
M72 Antitank	66	350	27,450	5.2
Pedestal-Mounted	152	240	23,760	4.5
M114 Howitzer (tow)	105	400	28,100	5.3
M107 Self-Propelled	175	700	30,780	5.8

[a]Assume 6 dBA decrease for every doubling of distance.
[b]EPNdB: Effective Perceived Noise Level
[c]Assume atmospheric absorption of 1dB/100 ft.

Table 8-4. Effects of Noise on Man

dBA Level	Potential Effect
20	No sound perceived
25	Hearing threshold
30	– –
35	Slight sleep interference
40	– –
45	– –
50	Moderate sleep interference
55	Annoyance (mild)
60	Normal speech level
65	Communication interference
70	Smooth muscles/glands react
75	Changed motor coordination
80	Moderate hearing damage
85	Very annoying
90	Affect mental and motor behavior
95	Severe hearing damage
100	Awaken everyone
105	– –
110	– –
115	Maximum vocal effort
120	– –
125	Pain threshold
130	Limit amplified speech
135	Very painful
140	Potential hearing loss high

Table 8-6 provides criteria for various sound levels as acceptable for a variety of land uses. Normally, a day-night level (L_{dn}) of 55 to 60 is acceptable in residential, hospital and motel zones. Figure 8-2 graphically displays the "acceptability" of dBA levels at a maximum. Generally, levels above 83 are considered noisy by most people. Levels above 80 dBA would probably bring community action.

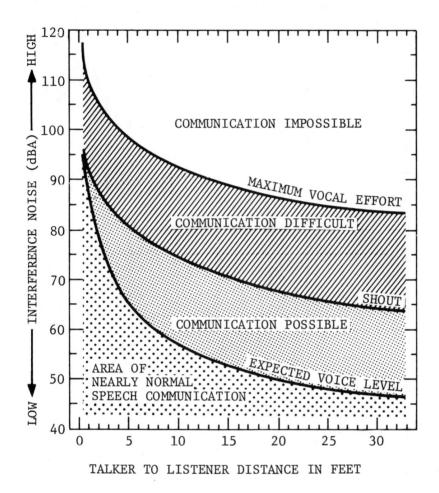

Figure 8-1. Speech interference levels (Congress, 1972).

Table 8-7 is a summary of methods used to predict noise impact and environmental analysis. While decibels is the most commonly understood noise measurement, other methodoligies are appropriate for certain environmental assessments. For example, human health and welfare effects are measured in L_{dn} (day-night levels) or Sound Level-Weighted Population (LWP). Structural damage prediction is based on peak pressure and weighted accelerations.

Table 8-5. Human Effects for Outdoor Day-Night Average Sound Level (CHABA, 1977)

Type of Effects / Noise Level	55 dBA	65 dBA	75 dBA
Speech – Indoors	No disturbance of speech with 100% sentence intelligibility (average) and a 5-dB margin of safety.	Slight disturbance of speech with 99% sentence intelligibility (average) and a 4-dB margin of safety.	Some disturbance of speech with sentence intelligibility (average) less than 99%.
– Outdoors	Slight disturbance of speech with 100% sentence intelligibility (average) at 0.35 meter,	Significant disturbance of speech 100% sentence intelligibility (average) at 0.1 meter,	Very significant disturbance of speech with 100% sentence intelligibility not possible at any distance,
	or	or	or
	99% sentence intelligibility (average) at 1.0 meter,	99% sentence intelligibility (average at 0.35 meter,	99% sentence intelligibility (average) at 0.1 meter,
	or	or	or
	95% sentence intelligibility (average) at 3.5 meters.	95% sentence intelligibility (average) at 1.2 meters.	95% sentence intelligibility (average) at 0.35 meter.
Average Community Reaction	None; 7 dB below level of significant "complaints and threats of legal action" and at least 16 dB below "vigorous action" (attitudes and other nonacoustical factors may modify this effect).	Significant; 3 dB above level of significant "complaints and threats of legal action" but at least 7 dB below "vigorous action" (attitudes and other nonacoustical factors may modify this effect).	Very severe; 13 dB above level of significant "complaints and threats of legal action" and at least 3 dB above "vigorous action" (attitudes and other nonacoustical factors may modify this effect).
High Annoyance	Depending on attitude and other nonacoustical factors, approximately 5% of the population will be highly annoyed.	Depending on attitude and other nonacoustical factors, approximately 15% of the population will be highly annoyed.	Depending on attitude and other onacoustical factors, approximately 37% of the population will be highly annoyed.
Attitudes Towards Area	Noise essentially the least important of various factors.	Noise is one of the most important adverse aspects of the community.	Noise is likely to be the most important of all adverse aspects of the community.

Table 8-6. Criteria for Outdoor Sound Levels for Analysis of
Environmental Noise Impact for Various Land Uses (CHABA, 1977)

Land Use	L_{dn} (dB)	L_{eq} (dB)
Residential[a]	55	
Hospital[a]	55	
Motel, Hotel[a]	60	
School Buildings and Outdoor Teaching Areas[a]		60
Church[b]		60
Office Buildings[b]		70
Theater		70
Playgrounds, Active Sports		70
Parks		60
Special Purpose Outdoors Areas		c

[a]15 dB - windows open
[b]25 dB - windows closed
[c]For outdoor amphitheaters or other critical land uses requiring special consideration, the hourly average sound level (L_h) due to the new intruding noise should not be allowed to be higher than 5 dB below the existing hourly average sound level in the absence of speaking in the amphitheater.

Effects on wildlife are more difficult to predict. Impacts depend on species, previous noise exposure, adaptability of the animals and type of noise (regular, irregular, sporadic, etc.). Generally, animals adapt to a regular, predictable noise, or one of a continuous nature, more readily than to sporadic noise bursts. Table 8-8 gives reactions, in behavior and physiology of animals to known noise levels ranging between 75 and 105 dBA. If population densities are known for the study area, and if noise level contours are plotted, an estimate can be made for numbers of animals potentially affected by noise.

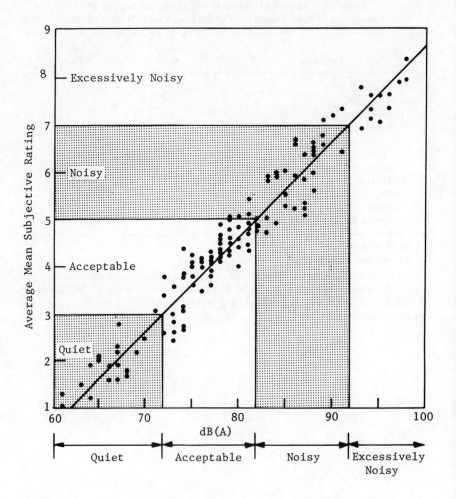

Figure 8-2. Average mean subjective rating as a function of maximum noise level in dBA (Congress, 1972).

Table 8-9 illustrates game behavior changes, due to noise from low flying aircraft. The legal definition of harassment would apply to all these predicted behavior changes. In general, the lower the aircraft, the more severe the reaction. Herd animals react more strongly to noise, than individuals alone. Wilderness species are most sentitive to noise exposure.

Table 8-7. Summary of Preparation of a Noise Impact Analysis (CHABA, 1977)

Type of Environment	Type of Criteria	Recommended Noise Measure	Assessment Methodology Used
General Audible Noises (including low-level impulse noise)	Potential for loss of hearing	Day-night average sound level	Population-weighted loss of hearing (PLH)
	Health and welfare effects on people, $L_{dn} > 55$	(a) Day-night average sound	(a) Sound level-weighted population (LWP) and noise impact index (NII)
	Environmental degradation/improvement on people/animals, $L_{dn} > 35$	(b) Word description	(b) Descriptions of the effects
Special Noises	Structural damage	(a) Peak pressure	(a) 200 Pa limit outside
Large, Impulse, Sonic Boom, Blast, Artillery	Annoyance due to auditory stimulation and building vibration	(b) Empirical formulas	(b) Listing of predicted damage as to amount and type
		(c) Peak acceleration (weighted)	(c) 1 meter/sec^2 inside
		Composite day-night average sound level using C-weighted sound exposure level for impulses	Sound level-weighted population (LWP) and noise impact index (NII)
Other	Other (infrasound, ultrasound, etc.)	Maximum sound pressure level	Discussion of possible effects No quantification made
Vibration	Structural damage	Peak acceleration (weighted)	1 meter/sec^2 for most structures 0.5 meter/sec^2 for sensitive structures 0.05 meter/sec^2 for certain ancient monuments
	Annoyance and complaints	RMS acceleration (weighted) vs time of exposure	Uses no complaint level for threshold of any adverse effects. Some quantification possible using vibration impact index

Table 8-8. Effects of Noise on Fish and Wildlife
(Banner and Hyatt, 1973; Bender, 1977; Helmer, 1976,
Klein, 1976; Committee on the Problem of Noise, 1963)

Species	Noise Level	Duration	Reaction
Cyprinodon varigatus[a]	20 dB/μb	11-12 days	Reduce viability Reduce survival Reduce growth
Fundulus similis[a]	20 dB/μb	11-12 days	Lethal to fry Reduce growth
Field mice	– –	– –	Stress Adrenal Hypertrophy
Dall sheep	75 dBA	min	Panic, run
Caribou	82-92 dBA	min	Nervous
Caribou	85-95 dBA	min	Run
Caribou	95-105 dBA	min	Panic
Waterfowl	80-85 dBA	min	Flock
Moose	82-92 dBA	min	Increase pace
Bison	85-95 dBA	min	Get up
Red Fox	80-85 dBA	min	Run
Birds	85 dBA	2 min	Scare

[a]Estuarine fish.

Figures 8-3 and 8-4 show FAA allowable approach and takeoff noise levels for large commercial-type aircraft. Aircraft are grouped by gross weight on the horizontal. Noise levels are given in Effective Perceived Noise Levels (EPNdB) in decibels. Generally, approach noise levels are all higher, ranging between 100 and 110 decibels.

Table 8-9. Aircraft Disturbance to Wildlife
(Calef and Lortie, 1973; Craighead and Craighead, 1972;
Davis, 1976; Geist, 1971; Hansen *et al.*, 1971; Heimer, 1976;
Klein, 1976; Milton, 1972; Renewable Resources Consultants, 1973;
Stephenson, 1975, U.S. DOD, 1975, U.S. DOI, 1975)

Elevation – Decibels – Species	100' 95-105	200' 82-92	300' 85-95	500' 81	1000' 75
	Typical Reaction				
Dall Sheep	ND[a]	ND	ND	ND	Panic
Grizzly Bear	Panic, stumble	Run	Run	Run	ND
Red Fox	ND	ND	ND	Run	ND
Caribou	Panic	Run	Nervous	None	None
Waterfowl	Startle	Move	Nervous	Flock	None
Moose	ND	Increase pace	None to startle	None	None
Bison	Run	Nervous	Get up	None	None

[a]ND: No data available.

Chapter 5 gives federal regulations for noise control, for ten different agencies of the U.S. Government. Table 8-10 provides specific noise levels allowed by selected states for off-road and recreational vehicles. Table 8-11 summarizes noise ordinances and laws by state. Most states have laws regulating motor vehicles and reacreational vehicles.

Table 8-12 is a summary of municipal noise ordinances, as of 1976. Major cities of all states are in the first column, population second, and types of noise control in following columns. Major federal actions would probably not have to comply with local noise ordinances.

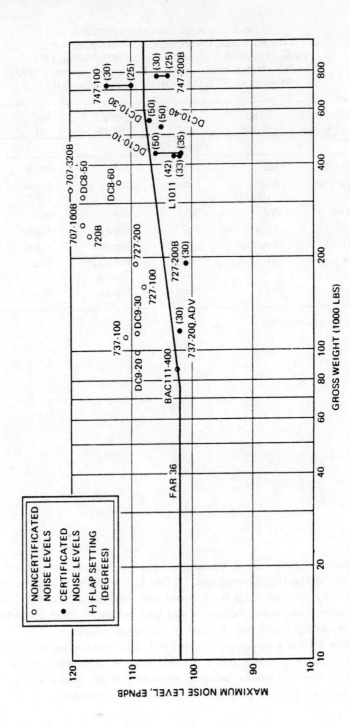

Figure 8-3. Noise limits (approach) and aircraft noise levels (FAA, 1976).

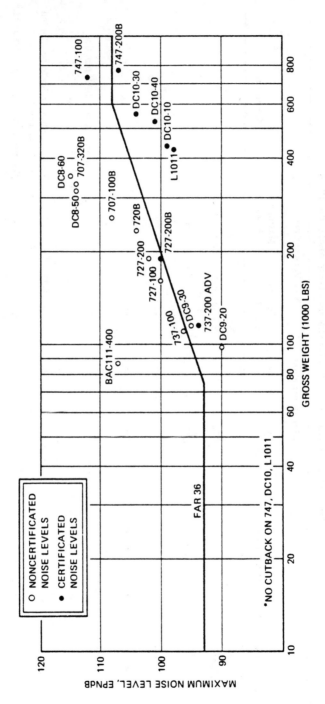

Figure 8-4. Noise limits (takeoff) and aircraft noise levels (with cutback) (FAA, 1976).

Table 8-10. State Recreational and Off-Road Vehicle Noise Regulations
(all levels in decibels measured at 50 ft unless noted otherwise) (EPA, 1975)

State	Vehicle Type	Vehicles in Operation		New Vehicle Sales		Comments
		Effective Date	Maximum Level	Date of Manufacture	Maximum Level	
Federal	Off-road	None	None	None	None	
California	Snowmobile	After 1972	82	Not specified	Not specified	
	Off-road, self-propelled	Not specified	Not specified	After 1-1-72	92	
				After 1-1-73	88	
				After 1-1-75	86	
Colorado			86 (over 35 mph)	After 1-1-71	86	
				After 1-1-73	84	
	Off-road, self-propelled	Not specified	82 (under 35 mph)	After 1-1-74	79	
				After 1-1-75	74	
Connecticut	Snowmobile	Before 1-1-75	82	—	—	Test procedures; SAE practice J192.[a]
		After 1-1-75	73	—	—	
	Off-road, self-propelled	Before 1-1-75	80	—	—	
		After 1-1-75	73	—	—	
Iowa	Snowmobile	Not specified	86	After 7-1-73	82	Test procedure—rules to be adopted by Commission.
Maine	Snowmobile	—	—	After 10-1-73	82	Test procedure: SAE practice J192.[a]
				After 2-1-75	78	
Massachusetts	Snowmobile	Not specified	73	Not specified	73	Test procedure: ISIA 1969[b] or other standard for measurement as registrar of motor vehicles adopts.
	Off-road, self-propelled	Not specified	73	Not specified	73	

*Executive Order 11989 (1977)

State	Vehicle					Test procedure
Michigan	Snowmobile	Not specified	82	After 2-1-72	82	Test procedure—SAE practice J192.[b]
New Hampshire	Off-road, self-propelled	After 7-1-73 After 7-1-78 After 7-1-83	82 73 70	—	—	Test procedure—ISIA 1969[b] or other standard of measurement as adopted by commissioner.
Oregon	Snowmobile	—	—	1975 1976-1978 After 1978	82 78	
	Off-road, self-propelled	Before 1975 1976 1976-1978 After 1978	94[c]/88[d] 91[c]/85[d] 88[c]/82[d] 83[c]/77[d]	—	-	
Vermont	Snowmobile	9-1-72 9-1-73	82 To be established	—	—	No test procedure given.
Wisconsin	Snowmobile	—	—	After 7-1-72 After 7-1-75	82 78	Test procedures SAE.[e] Practice J192.

[a] Society of Automotive Engineers, Recommended Practice J192 "Exterior Sound Level for Snowmobiles."
[b] International Snowmobile Industry Association (January 1969) "Procedure for Sound Level Measurements of Snowmobiles."
[c] Stationary at 25 ft.
[d] Moving at 50 ft.
[e] The logarithmic ratio of a particular quantity, such as sound pressure, intensity, or power, to a reference level, commonly the threshold of human hearing.

Table 8-11. State Noise Restrictions—1976 (Bragdon, 1976)

State	Motor Vehicle Mufflers	Motor Vehicle Sound Level Limits	Motorcycle Sound Level Limits	Off-Road Recreational Vehicle Sound Level Limits	Snowmobile Sound Level Limits	Motor-boat Mufflers	Status and Relationship to Local Noise Ordinances
Alabama	Yes	—	—	—	—	—	—
Arizona	Yes	—	—	—	—	Yes	—
Arkansas	Yes	—	—	—	—	—	—
California	Yes	Yes	Yes	Yes	Yes	Yes	Must develop model local noise ordinances. Local government must furnish copy of ordinance to state
Colorado	—	Yes, for over 6,000 lbs	Yes	Yes	—	—	Statutory standards enforced by citizen suit. Does not preempt "no less restrictive" standards
Connecticut	—	Yes	Yes	Yes	Yes	—	May adopt regulations. State must approve local noise ordinances.
Florida	—	Yes	Yes	—	—	—	May adopt regulations.
Hawaii	Yes	Yes	Yes	—	—	—	May adopt regulations.
Idaho	Yes	Yes	Yes	—	—	—	—
Illinois	—	—	—	—	—	—	Have adopted regulations. Relationship unknown.
Indiana	—	Yes	Yes	—	—	—	—
Iowa	Yes	—	—	—	Yes	—	—
Kansas	Yes	—	—	—	—	Yes	—
Kentucky	Yes	—	—	—	—	—	May adopt regulations. Local government cannot be stricter.
Louisiana	—	—	—	—	—	—	—
Maine	Yes	—	—	—	Yes	Yes	Must adopt standards.

		Must adopt limits	Must adopt limits				
Maryland	Yes	—	—	—	—	—	Have adopted regulations. Local government may be stricter.
Massachusetts	—	—	—	Yes	Yes	—	Have adopted regulations prohibiting "unnecessary emission" of noise
Michigan	—	—	—	—	—	—	—
Minnesota	—	Yes	Yes	—	Yes	—	Have adopted regulations. Local government cannot be stricter.
Missouri	Yes	—	—	—	—	—	—
Montana	—	—	Yes	—	Yes	—	—
Nebraska	Yes	Yes, for over 10,000 lb	—	—	—	—	—
Nevada	Yes	Yes	Yes	—	—	—	—
New Hampshire	—	—	—	Yes	Yes	—	Have adopted regulations.
New Jersey	Yes	N.J. Turnpike only	—	—	—	—	Local government may be stricter but requires state approval
New Mexico	—	—	—	—	Yes	—	Must adopt regulations.
New York	Yes	Yes, for over 10,000 lb	No	—	Yes	Yes	May adopt regulations. Local government may be stricter.
North Dakota	—	—	—	—	—	—	—
Ohio	—	—	—	Yes	Yes	—	May adopt regulations.
Oregon	Yes	Yes	Yes	—	Yes	—	Have adopted regulations.
Pennsylvania	Yes	Yes	Yes	—	Yes	—	May adopt regulations.
Vermont	—	—	—	Yes	Yes	—	—
Washington	Yes	Yes	Yes	—	Yes	—	Have adopted regulations. Local government may be stricter but requires state approval.
West Virginia	Yes	—	—	—	—	—	—
Wisconsin	Yes	—	—	—	Yes	—	—

Table 8-12. Municipal Noise Ordinances—1976 (Bragdon, 1976)

Jurisdiction	1970 Population	Nuisance	Zoning	Vehicle	Rec/Vehicle	Railroad	Aircraft	Construction	Building
ALABAMA									
Anniston	31,533	O	-	O	-	-	-	O	-
Birmingham	300,910	O	-	-	-	-	-	-	-
Irondale	3,166	X	O	-	-	-	-	-	X
Madison	3,086	-	X	-	-	-	X	-	-
Mobile	190,026	O	-	-	-	-	-	-	-
Montgomery	133,386	O	-	-	-	-	-	-	-
ALASKA									
Anchorage	48,081	O	-	X	X	-	-	-	-
Juneau	6,050	O	-	-	-	-	-	-	-
Ketchikan	6,994	O	-	-	-	-	-	-	-
ARIZONA									
Flagstaff	26,177	O	-	O	O	-	-	-	-
Phoenix	581,562	O	-	O	O	-	-	-	-
Scottsdale	67,823	X	X	X	-	-	X	-	-
Tempe	62,907	X	X	X	-	-	-	-	-
Tucson	262,933	X	X	-	-	-	-	-	-
ARKANSAS									
Little Rock	132,125	O	-	-	-	-	-	-	-
Pine Bluff	57,389	O	-	-	-	-	-	-	-
CALIFORNIA									
Alhambra	62,125	X	-	-	-	-	-	-	-
Amador	156	X	-	X	-	-	-	O	-
Anaheim	166,704	X	X	X	-	-	-	X	X
Arcadia	43,867	X	-	-	-	-	-	X	-
Belmont	23,667	X	-	-	-	-	-	-	-
Berkeley	116,716	X	-	-	-	-	-	-	X

City	Population							
Beverly Hills	33,416	X	X	–	–	X	–	X
Buena Park	63,646	–	O	–	–	–	X	X
Burbank	88,871	–	–	–	–	O	X	X
Burlingame	27,320	–	O	–	O	–	–	O
Capitola	7,175	–	O	–	–	O	–	O
Ceres	8,675	–	X	–	–	–	–	X
Chico	19,580	–	–	–	–	X	–	–
Commerce	10,662	–	X	X	–	–	X	X
Costa Mesa	72,660	–	–	–	–	X	X	X
Cotati	2,081	–	–	–	–	O	O	–
Cudahy	17,040	–	O	–	–	–	–	X
Culver City	37,600	–	O	–	–	X	–	X
Cupertino	18,216	–	O	–	–	–	–	O
Del Mar	4,475	–	O	–	–	O	–	O
Del Rey Oaks	1,830	–	–	–	–	O	–	O
Downey	88,442	–	O	X	X	X	–	X
Duarte	15,100	–	–	–	–	X	X	X
El Cajon	52,273	–	X	–	–	–	–	–
El Segundo	15,620	–	–	–	–	O	X	X
Escalon	1,834	–	X	–	–	X	X	X
Foster City	18,650	–	–	–	–	–	–	X
Fountain Valley	31,826	–	X	–	–	X	X	X
Fresno	165,972	–	–	–	–	O	X	X
Fremont	100,869	–	X	–	–	X	–	–
Cardena	41,021	X	–	–	X	O	X	X
Garden Grove	121,371	O	X	–	–	X	–	–
Glendale	132,752	–	–	–	–	–	X	X
Glendora	31,349	–	O	–	–	O	X	X
Gustine	3,546	X	O	–	–	X	X	X
Hayward	93,058	–	–	X	X	–	–	O
Hemet	12,252	X	–	–	–	O	X	O
Hermosa Beach	17,412	–	–	–	–	O	X	O
Huntington Beach	17,412	–	–	O	O	–	–	O
Huntington Park	33,744	–	–	–	–	–	–	O
Inglewood	89,985	–	O	X	X	–	X	X
Laguna Beach	15,100	–	–	X	X	–	X	–
Lakewood	82,973	–	X	X	X	–	X	O

Table 8-12, continued.

Jurisdiction	1970 Population	Nuisance	Zoning	Vehicle	Rec/Vehicle	Railroad	Aircraft	Construction	Building
CALIFORNIA (Continued)									
La Mesa	44,509	-	X	-	-	-	-	-	-
La Puente	31,450	X	-	-	-	-	-	O	-
Larkspur	10,487	X	-	X	X	X	-	-	-
Lodi	28,691	-	X	-	-	-	-	-	-
Lomita	19,784	X	X	-	-	-	-	-	-
Long Beach	358,633	-	-	X	-	-	X	X	X
Los Altos Hills	6,853	O	X	O	-	-	-	O	X
Los Angeles	2,816,061	X	X	X	X	-	-	O	-
Los Banos	9,188	-	-	X	-	-	-	-	-
Lynwood	43,353	X	X	O	X	-	-	-	-
Manteca	13,845	-	X	-	-	-	-	-	-
Menlo Park	26,826	O	O	-	-	-	-	-	-
Milpitas	32,400	-	-	-	-	-	-	O	-
Modesto	75,800	X	-	-	-	-	-	-	X
Monrovia	30,015	-	-	-	-	-	-	-	-
Monterey	26,302	X	X	-	-	-	-	-	-
Newark	27,153	X	X	-	-	-	-	X	X
Newport Beach	49,422	X	-	X	X	-	-	-	-
Norwalk	91,827	-	O	-	-	-	-	-	-
Novato	31,006	X	-	X	X	-	X	X	-
Oakland	361,561	O	X	-	-	-	-	-	-
Orange	77,365	X	X	-	-	-	-	X	-
Pacifica	36,020	O	-	-	-	-	-	-	-
Palmdale	10,600	-	-	O	O	-	-	O	-
Palo Alto	55,966	X	X	-	-	-	-	X	-
Pasadena	112,951	X	X	O	-	-	-	-	-
Perris	5,100	X	-	-	-	-	-	-	-
Petaluma	31,150	-	X	-	-	-	-	-	-
Placentia	30,200	X	-	-	-	-	-	-	-
Pleasant Hill	27,150	X	-	X	-	-	-	O	-

City	Population	1	2	3	4	5	6	7
Red Bluff	7,676	—	—	—	—	—	—	O
Redding	16,659	—	—	—	X	X	—	X
Redondo Beach	64,000	—	O	X	—	O	—	X
Richmond	79,043	—	—	X	—	X	X	—
Rocklin	3,039	—	X	—	X	—	X	—
Roseville	19,950	—	—	—	X	—	—	X
Ross	2,742	—	—	—	X	X	—	X
Sacramento	254,413	—	—	—	—	—	—	O
Salinas	58,893	—	—	—	O	O	X	O
San Anselmo	13,031	—	—	—	—	X	—	X
San Bernardino	104,251	—	X	—	X	—	—	O
San Bruno	38,750	—	—	—	—	—	—	X
San Carlos	26,053	—	—	—	—	—	X	—
San Clemente	17,063	—	—	—	—	—	—	O
San Diego	696,769	—	—	—	—	X	X	X
San Dimas	17,125	X	X	—	—	—	—	O
San Francisco	715,674	—	—	—	X	X	X	X
San Jose	445,779	—	X	—	—	—	—	—
San Juan Capistrano	11,000	—	—	O	X	—	—	X
San Leandro	68,698	—	—	—	—	X	—	O
San Marcos	3,896	—	—	—	—	—	X	X
San Mateo	78,991	—	—	—	X	—	—	O
San Rafael	38,977	X	X	—	—	X	X	O
Santa Barbara	70,215	—	—	X	—	X	—	O
Santa Clara	87,717	X	—	X	—	—	X	O
Santa Fe Springs	14,750	—	—	—	—	—	X	—
Santa Maria	32,749	—	—	—	—	—	—	X
Santa Monica	88,289	—	—	O	—	—	X	X
Santa Rosa	50,006	—	—	—	—	—	—	X
Saratoga	29,932	—	—	—	—	—	X	X
Sausalito	6,158	—	—	—	—	—	—	X
Simi Valley	59,832	—	—	—	—	—	X	X
South El Monte	13,442	—	—	—	—	X	—	X
South Gate	56,909	—	—	—	—	—	—	X
South Pasadena	22,629	—	—	—	—	—	—	O
Sunnyvale	95,408	—	O	—	—	O	X	O
Tracy	14,724	X	—	—	—	—	X	—

Table 8-12, continued.

Jurisdiction	1970 Population	Nuisance	Zoning	Vehicle	Rec/Vehicle	Railroad	Aircraft	Construction	Building
Torrance	134,584	X	X	X	–	–	–	O	–
Vallejo	74,800	X	–	–	–	–	–	–	–
Victorville	10,845	O	–	–	–	–	–	O	–
Walnut Creek	48,850	O	–	–	–	–	–	–	–
West Covina	74,000	X	–	X	–	–	–	–	–
Whittier	73,400	O	–	–	–	–	–	–	–
COLORDAO									
Arvada	49,083	O	X	X	–	–	–	–	–
Aspen	2,404	O	X	X	–	–	–	–	–
Aurora	74,974	–	X	–	–	–	–	–	–
Boulder	66,870	O	–	X	X	–	–	–	–
Colordao Springs	135,060	O	X	X	–	X	X	X	–
Denver	514,678	O	X	X	–	–	–	–	–
Dillon	182	–	–	O	–	–	–	–	–
Englewood	33,695	O	X	X	–	–	–	–	–
Fort Collins	43,337	O	X	X	X	–	–	X	–
Lakewood	92,787	X	X	X	X	–	–	X	–
Littleton	26,466	O	X	X	X	–	–	X	–
Wheat Ridge	29,795	O	–	–	–	–	–	–	–
CONNECTICUT									
Berlin	14,149	O	X	–	–	–	–	–	–
Bridgeport	156,542	X	X	X	–	–	–	X	X
Farmington	14,390	X	X	X	–	–	–	X	–
Hartford	158,017	O	–	–	–	–	–	–	O
New Haven	137,707	O	X	X	–	–	–	–	–
Stonington	15,590	O	X	X	–	–	–	–	–
Westport	27,414	–	X	–	–	–	–	–	–
DELAWARE									
Wilmington	80,386	O	X	X	–	–	–	–	–

		1	2	3	4	5	6	7
DISTRICT OF COLUMBIA								
District of Columbia	756,510	—	—	—	—	X	X	O
FLORIDA								
Anna Maria	1,400	—	—	—	—	—	—	O
Atlantis	844	—	—	—	—	—	X	X
Bal Harbor Village	2,104	—	—	—	—	—	—	O
Bay Harbor	4,723	—	—	—	—	—	—	X
Bay Lake	18	—	—	—	—	—	—	X
Boca Raton	28,506	—	O	—	—	—	X	X
Cape Canaveral	5,131	—	O	—	—	—	X	X
Clearwater	52,074	—	—	—	—	—	O	O
Cocoa Beach	11,555	—	O	—	—	—	—	—
Coral Gables	42,494	X	O	—	—	X	X	X
Dania	9,819	—	—	—	—	—	—	O
Daytona Beach	47,682	—	O	—	—	—	X	X
Deerfield Beach	19,577	—	O	—	—	X	X	X
Deland	11,641	—	—	—	—	—	—	—
Delray Beach	19,915	—	—	—	O	—	—	O
Edgewater	3,348	—	O	—	—	X	X	X
Fort Lauderdale	139,590	—	X	—	—	X	—	X
Fort Myers	32,563	—	—	—	—	—	—	O
Fort Pierce	31,752	—	—	—	—	—	X	O
Gainesville	64,510	—	—	—	—	X	X	X
Hallandale	32,292	—	—	—	—	—	X	X
Hialeah	102,452	—	—	—	—	O	O	O
Hialeah Gardens	1,076	—	O	—	—	—	—	X
Hollywood	106,873	—	O	—	O	O	—	O
Homestead	19,022	—	—	—	—	—	—	O
Indian Shores	891	—	—	—	—	—	—	O
Jacksonville	528,865	—	O	—	—	X	X	X
Lake Buena Vista	22	—	—	—	—	—	—	O
Lakeland	45,091	—	—	—	O	—	—	O
Lake Park	7,927	X	X	—	—	X	X	X
Lake Worth	25,934	—	—	—	—	—	—	O
Lauderdale by the Sea	2,941	—	—	—	—	—	—	O
Lighthouse Point	11,760	—	—	—	—	—	—	O
Madiera	4,769	—	—	—	—	X	X	X

Table 8-12, continued.

Jurisdiction	1970 Population	Nuisance	Zoning	Vehicle	Rec/Vehicle	Railroad	Aircraft	Construction	Building
FLORIDA (Continued)									
Margate	17,153	O	-	-	-	-	-	-	-
Melbourne	40,236	-	X	X	-	-	-	-	-
Miami	334,859	X	X	-	-	-	-	-	-
Miami Beach	89,741	O	X	-	-	-	-	-	-
Miami Shores	9,541	O	-	-	-	-	-	-	-
Miami Springs	13,384	O	-	-	-	-	-	-	-
Miramar	27,132	O	-	-	-	-	-	-	-
North Lauderdale	5,648	X	-	-	-	-	-	-	-
North Miami	42,970	X	-	-	-	-	-	-	-
North Palm Beach	12,056	O	-	-	-	-	-	-	-
Oakland Park	19,700	O	-	-	-	-	-	-	-
Oldsmar	2,090	O	X	-	-	-	-	-	-
Opa Locka	12,924	O	-	-	-	-	-	-	-
Orlando	97,565	O	X	-	-	-	X	-	-
Plantation	29,512	O	-	-	-	-	-	-	-
Plant City	15,781	O	-	-	-	-	-	-	-
Pinellas Park	28,526	O	-	-	-	-	-	-	-
Palm Beach Gardens	8,315	X	X	-	-	-	X	-	-
Pompano Beach	38,544	X	X	X	X	-	-	-	-
Lauderdale Beach	2,941	O	-	O	-	-	-	-	-
Riviera Beach	21,401	O	X	O	-	-	-	-	-
Redington Shores	2,111	O	-	-	-	-	-	-	-
St. Petersburg	216,232	X	X	X	-	-	-	-	-
Sarasota	44,638	O	-	-	-	-	-	-	-
South Daytona	7,825	-	X	-	-	-	-	-	-
Surfside	3,649	O	-	-	-	-	-	-	-
Tallahassee	72,586	-	-	X	-	-	-	-	-
Tampa	298,740	O	-	-	-	-	-	-	-
Tavares	3,673	O	-	-	-	-	-	-	-
Treasure Island	6,878	O	-	-	-	-	-	-	-

City	Population	1	2	3	4	5	6	7
Vero Beach	14,211	—	—	—	X	X	X	X
Virginia Gardens	2,592	—	—	—	—	—	—	O
West Miami	5,989	—	X	—	—	—	—	X
West Palm Beach	27,132	—	—	—	X	X	X	X
Winter Haven	16,136	—	X	—	X	X	X	X
GEORGIA								
Alma	3,756	—	—	—	—	O	—	O
Atlanta	497,421	—	—	—	—	—	—	O
Camilla	4,987	—	X	—	—	O	X	O
Carrolton	13,520	—	—	—	—	—	—	—
Claxton	2,669	—	—	X	—	O	X	X
College Park	18,203	—	X	—	—	O	X	O
Columbus	154,168	—	—	—	—	—	—	—
Cordele	10,733	—	—	—	—	—	O	O
Dacala	782	—	—	—	—	—	—	O
Danielsville	370	—	—	—	O	—	—	O
Decatur	21,943	—	—	—	—	—	—	O
Dover	220	—	—	—	—	—	—	O
Flowery Branch	761	—	O	—	O	O	—	O
Forest Park	19,994	—	—	—	—	—	—	O
Griffin	22,734	—	O	—	O	O	—	O
Hapeville	9,567	—	—	—	—	—	—	O
Kingsland	1,831	—	—	—	—	—	—	O
Lake City	2,306	—	—	—	O	O	—	O
Louisville	2,691	—	—	—	—	—	—	O
Macon	122,423	—	—	—	O	O	—	O
Moultrie	14,400	—	—	—	X	X	X	X
Newnan	11,205	—	—	—	O	X	O	O
Peachtree City	793	—	—	—	—	—	—	—
Rincon	1,854	—	—	—	—	—	—	O
Riverdale	2,521	—	X	—	X	X	O	O
Savannah	118,349	—	—	—	X	X	X	X
Tyrone	136	—	—	—	—	—	—	—
Warner Robins	33,491	—	X	—	X	X	X	O
Waynesboro	5,530	—	—	—	—	—	—	O
HAWAII								
Honolulu	324,871	—	—	—	X	X	X	O

Table 8-12, continued.

Jurisdiction	1970 Population	Nuisance	Zoning	Vehicle	Rec/Vehicle	Railroad	Aircraft	Construction	Building
IDAHO									
Boise	74,990	O	O	O	—	—	—	—	—
Idaho Falls	35,776	—	—	X	—	—	—	O	—
Pocatello	40,036	O	—	X	—	—	—	—	—
ILLINOIS									
Arlington Heights	64,884	—	X	—	—	—	—	—	—
Carbondale	22,816	X	X	X	X	—	—	X	—
Chicago	3,369,359	X	X	X	O	—	—	—	—
Decatur	90,397	O	—	—	—	—	—	—	—
Des Plaines	57,239	O	X	X	X	—	X	X	—
Downers Grove	32,751	X	—	X	—	—	—	—	—
Joliet	80,378	X	—	O	—	—	—	—	—
Marengo	4,235	X	—	X	—	—	—	—	—
Moline	46,237	—	—	X	—	—	—	—	—
Northbrook	27,297	—	—	—	—	—	X	—	X
Park Ridge	42,466	X	—	X	X	—	—	—	—
Peoria	126,963	X	—	X	X	—	—	O	—
Rockford	147,370	O	—	X	X	—	—	O	—
Savanna	4,942	O	—	O	—	—	—	—	—
South Holland	12,619	O	—	—	—	X	—	—	—
Urbana	32,800	O	X	X	X	—	—	X	—
INDIANA									
Evansville	138,764	O	X	X	X	—	X	O	—
Gary	175,415	O	X	O	—	—	—	—	—
Hammond	107,888	O	X	X	X	—	X	—	—
Indianapolis	745,739	X	—	—	—	—	X	—	O
Logansport	19,255	X	—	X	—	—	—	—	—
Lowell	5,822	O	—	—	—	—	—	—	—
Ogden Dunes	982	—	X	O	—	—	—	—	—
South Bend	125,580	O	—	O	—	—	—	O	—

	Population							
IOWA								
Bedford	2,361	—	—	—	—	0	—	0
Cedar Falls	29,597	—	0	—	—	X	X	0
Council Bluffs	60,348	—	0	—	0	0	—	0
Davenport	98,469	—	0	—	—	0	—	0
Des Moines	200,587	—	0	—	—	0	—	0
Dubuque	62,309	—	—	—	—	X	X	—
Pella	6,668	—	—	—	—	X	—	0
Sioux City	82,925	—	—	—	—	0	0	0
Storm Lake	8,591	—	—	—	—	X	X	0
Waterloo	75,533	—	—	—	—	—	—	0
KANSAS								
Lawrence	45,698	—	—	—	—	0	—	0
Prairie Village	28,138	—	X	—	X	X	X	0
Wichita	276,534	0	—	—	—	0	—	0
KENTUCKY								
Covington	52,535	—	0	—	0	0	—	X
Lexington	108,137	—	—	—	—	—	—	0
Louisville	361,472	—	X	X	X	X	—	—
Newport	25,998	—	—	—	—	0	—	0
LOUISIANA								
Baton Rouge	165,963	—	0	—	0	0	—	0
New Orleans	593,471	—	—	—	—	—	0	0
MARYLAND								
Baltimore	905,759	—	—	—	0	—	X	0
Cumberland	29,724	—	—	—	—	—	—	0
Rockville	41,564	—	—	—	—	—	—	0
MASSACHUSETTS								
Acton	14,770	—	—	—	—	—	0	—
Boston	641,070	—	—	—	—	X	X	X
Concord	16,148	—	0	—	0	0	—	0
Fall River	96,898	—	—	—	—	—	0	0
Milford	19,352	—	—	—	—	—	X	—

Table 8-12, continued.

Jurisdiction	1970 Population	Nuisance	Zoning	Vehicle	Rec/Vehicle	Railroad	Aircraft	Construction	Building
Newton	91,263	O	–	O	–	–	–	–	–
Pittsfield	57,020	X	–	X	–	–	–	–	–
Springfield	163,905	O	X	–	–	–	–	–	–
Worcester	176,572	O	–	–	–	–	–	–	–
MICHIGAN									
Ann Arbor	99,797	O	X	X	–	–	–	–	O
Augusta Township	1,016	O	–	–	–	–	–	–	–
Beverly Hills	13,598	O	–	–	–	–	–	–	–
Birmingham	26,170	O	–	X	–	–	–	–	–
Comstock	5,003	X	–	X	X	–	–	–	–
Dearborn	104,199	O	–	X	–	–	O	–	–
Detroit	1,512,893	O	–	–	–	–	–	–	–
Farmington	10,329	O	–	–	–	–	–	–	–
Cladwin	3,624	X	–	X	–	–	–	–	–
Grand Rapids	197,649	X	X	X	X	–	–	X	X
Harbor Springs	5,261	X	X	X	X	X	–	X	–
Kalamazoo	85,555	O	X	X	X	–	–	X	–
Meridian Township	23,817	X	X	X	X	–	–	–	X
Milford	4,699	–	X	–	–	–	–	–	–
Pontiac	85,279	O	X	–	–	–	–	–	–
Ravenna	851	O	–	–	–	O	–	–	–
Saginaw	91,849	O	O	O	–	O	–	O	–
Troy	39,419	O	–	O	–	–	–	–	–
Warren	179,260	O	X	O	–	–	–	–	–
Westland	86,749	X	X	–	–	–	–	–	–
Wyoming	56,560	O	–	–	–	–	–	–	–
MINNESOTA									
Bloomington	81,970	O	X	O	X	–	–	O	–
Brooklyn Park	13,692	X	X	X	X	–	–	–	–

City	Population	1	2	3	4	5	6	7	8
Cannon Falls	2,155	—	—	—	—	—	X	—	—
Columbia Heights	23,837	—	—	—	—	—	—	X	—
Gilman	798	—	—	—	—	—	—	—	O
Minneapolis	434,400	O	X	—	—	—	X	X	O
Rochester	53,766	—	—	—	—	—	—	X	O
St. Paul	309,828	—	—	—	—	—	—	—	O
MISSISSIPPI									
Jackson	153,968	—	—	—	—	—	—	—	O
MISSOURI									
Bridgeton	19,992	—	—	—	—	—	—	—	O
Gladstone	23,422	—	X	—	—	—	X	—	O
Grandview	17,456	—	O	—	—	—	O	X	O
Independence	111,662	—	—	—	—	—	O	X	O
Kansas City	507,330	—	X	—	—	O	X	—	O
St. Louis	622,236	—	—	—	—	—	X	—	O
Springfield	120,096	—	—	—	—	—	O	—	O
Waynesville	3,376	—	—	—	—	—	O	—	O
MONTANA									
Billings	61,581	—	—	—	—	—	—	—	O
Great Falls	60,091	—	X	X	X	X	X	X	O
Helena	22,730	—	X	—	X	X	X	—	O
Livingston	6,883	—	—	—	—	—	O	—	O
Missoula	29,497	—	—	—	—	X	X	X	X
NEBRASKA									
Beatrice	12,787	—	—	—	—	—	—	—	O
Lincoln	149,518	—	—	—	X	—	X	X	—
McCook	8,285	—	—	—	—	—	X	X	O
Omaha	346,929	—	O	—	—	—	O	—	O
Scottsbluff	14,507	O	O	—	—	—	O	—	O
Sidney	6,258	—	—	—	—	—	O	—	O
NEVADA									
Las Vegas	125,787	—	—	—	—	—	O	X	O

Table 8-12, continued.

Jurisdiction	1970 Population	Nuisance	Zoning	Vehicle	Rec/Vehicle	Railroad	Aircraft	Construction	Building
NEW HAMPSHIRE									
Berlin	15,256	0	-	-	-	-	-	-	-
Concord	30,022	0	-	-	-	-	-	-	-
Manchester	87,754	0	-	-	-	-	-	-	-
NEW JERSEY									
Absecon	6,094	0	-	-	-	-	-	-	-
Asbury Park	16,533	0	-	-	-	-	-	-	-
Bayonne	72,743	X	X	-	-	-	-	-	-
Belleville	34,643	X	X	-	-	-	-	-	-
Berkeley Heights	13,078	X	X	-	-	-	-	X	X
Bloomfield	52,059	0	-	-	-	X	-	-	-
Boonton	9,261	X	X	-	-	-	-	-	-
Bordentown	4,490	0	-	-	-	-	-	-	-
Brigantine	6,741	0	-	-	-	-	-	-	-
Burlington	11,991	0	-	-	-	-	-	-	-
Camden	102,551	0	-	-	-	-	-	-	-
Cape May	4,392	0	-	-	-	-	-	-	-
Cedar Grove	15,582	X	X	-	-	-	-	-	-
Clifton	82,437	X	X	-	-	-	-	-	-
Clinton	1,742	0	-	-	-	-	-	-	-
Corbin	258	0	-	-	-	-	-	-	-
Dover	15,039	0	-	-	-	-	-	-	-
East Orange	75,471	0	-	-	-	-	-	-	-
Elizabeth	112,654	0	X	-	-	-	-	-	-
Ewing	32,831	0	-	-	-	-	-	-	-
Fairlawn	37,975	0	X	-	-	-	-	-	-
Gloucester	14,707	0	X	-	-	-	-	-	-
Hackensack	36,008	0	-	-	-	-	-	-	-
Hammonton	11,464	0	X	-	-	-	-	-	-
Hanover	10,700	-	X	-	-	-	-	-	-

City	Population								
Harrison	11,811	O	-	-	-	-	-	-	-
Hasbrouck Heights	13,651	O	-	-	-	-	-	-	-
Hawthorne	9,173	-	X	-	-	-	-	-	-
Hightstown	5,431	O	-	-	-	-	-	-	-
Hoboken	45,380	-	X	-	-	-	-	-	-
Irvington	59,743	O	X	-	-	-	-	-	-
Jersey City	260,545	O	-	-	-	-	-	-	-
Lakewood	17,874	O	X	O	-	-	X	O	-
Linden	41,409	O	-	-	-	-	-	O	-
Long Branch	31,774	O	-	O	-	-	-	-	-
Margate	10,576	O	-	-	-	-	-	-	-
Maywood	11,087	X	-	-	-	-	-	-	-
Morristown	17,662	O	-	-	-	-	-	-	-
Newark	382,417	O	-	-	-	-	-	-	-
Newton	7,297	O	-	-	-	-	-	-	-
North Haledon	7,614	O	-	-	-	-	-	-	-
North Wildwood	3,914	O	-	-	-	-	-	-	-
Nutley	31,913	O	-	-	-	-	-	-	-
Ocean City	10,575	O	-	-	-	-	-	-	-
Orange City	32,566	O	-	-	-	-	-	-	-
Passaic	55,124	O	-	-	-	-	-	-	-
Paterson	144,824	O	-	-	-	-	-	-	-
Pemberton Borough	1,576	O	-	-	-	-	-	-	-
Perth Amboy	38,798	O	-	-	-	-	-	-	-
Plainfield	46,862	O	-	-	-	-	-	-	-
Pleasantville	13,778	O	X	-	-	-	-	-	-
Princeton	12,311	X	X	-	-	-	-	-	-
Rahway	29,114	O	X	-	-	-	-	-	-
Ridgefield Park	14,453	O	-	-	-	-	-	-	-
Salem	7,648	O	-	-	-	-	-	-	-
Secaucus	13,228	O	-	-	-	-	-	-	-
South Amboy	9,338	O	X	X	-	-	-	O	-
Sparta	10,819	X	-	-	-	-	-	O	O
Summit	23,620	O	-	-	-	-	-	-	-
Trenton	104,638	O	-	-	-	-	-	-	-
Vineland	47,399	O	-	-	-	-	-	-	-
Wayne	49,141	O	-	-	-	-	-	-	-
Westfield	33,720	O	-	-	-	-	-	-	-

Table 8-12, continued.

Jurisdiction	1970 Population	Nuisance	Zoning	Vehicle	Rec/Vehicle	Railroad	Aircraft	Construction	Building
NEW JERSEY (Continued)									
West Orange	43,915	X	X	X	X	–	–	–	–
Wharton	11,105	–	X	–	–	–	–	–	–
Wildwood	4,110	O	–	–	–	–	–	–	–
Woodbridge	78,846	X	–	–	–	–	–	–	–
NEW MEXICO									
Albuquerque	243,751	O	O	O	O	–	O	O	–
Gallup	13,779	O	–	O	–	–	–	–	–
Los Alamos	11,310	O	X	X	–	–	–	–	–
NEW YORK									
Albany	115,781	–	O	–	–	–	–	–	–
Auburn	34,599	–	X	–	–	–	–	–	–
Binghamton	64,123	–	X	–	–	–	–	–	–
Buchanan	2,110	–	X	–	–	–	–	–	–
Buffalo	462,768	O	–	O	–	–	–	–	–
Canandaigua	10,488	–	–	–	–	–	–	–	–
Clifton Springs	2,058	–	O	O	–	–	–	–	–
Corning	15,972	O	–	–	–	–	–	–	–
Cortland	19,621	–	X	–	–	–	–	–	–
Freeport	40,374	O	–	–	–	–	–	–	–
Geneva	16,763	O	–	–	–	–	–	–	–
Hammondsport	1,066	O	–	–	–	–	–	–	–
Hempstead	39,411	O	–	–	–	–	X	–	–
Hornell	12,144	O	–	–	–	–	–	O	–
Huntington	12,601	O	–	–	–	–	–	O	–
Islip	7,692	O	–	–	X	–	–	–	–
Ithaca	26,226	O	–	–	–	–	–	–	–
Lake George	1,506	O	O	–	–	–	–	–	–
Lynbrook	23,776	O	–	–	–	–	–	–	–

City	Population	1	2	3	4	5	6	7	8
Lyons	4,496	O	–	O	–	–	–	–	–
Macedon	1,168	O	–	–	O	–	–	–	–
Mamaroneck	18,909	O	–	X	–	–	–	–	–
Marion	850	O	–	O	–	–	–	–	–
Montour Falls	1,534	O	–	–	–	–	–	–	–
New Rochelle	75,385	O	X	X	–	–	–	–	X
New York City	7,895,563	O	–	–	–	–	–	–	–
Niagara Falls	85,615	O	X	–	–	–	–	–	–
Niskayuna	6,186	–	–	–	–	–	–	–	–
Ossining	21,659	O	–	–	–	–	–	–	–
Penn Yan	5,168	O	–	–	–	–	–	–	–
Phelps	1,989	O	–	–	–	–	–	–	–
Rochester	296,233	X	–	O	–	–	–	–	–
Smithtown	12,000	X	–	O	–	–	–	O	–
Sodus	1,831	O	–	–	–	–	–	–	–
Southampton	4,904	O	–	–	–	–	–	–	–
Utica	91,611	O	–	O	–	–	–	–	–
Watkins Glen	2,716	X	–	O	–	–	–	–	–
White Plains	50,125	O	–	–	–	–	–	–	–
Williamstown	1,919	X	X	O	–	–	–	–	–
Wolcott	1,617	X	X	–	–	–	–	–	–
Wallkill	1,849	X	X	X	–	–	–	–	–
Yonkers	204,297	O	–	–	–	–	–	–	–
NORTH CAROLINA									
Aberdeen	1,592	O	–	–	–	–	–	–	–
Asheville	57,681	O	–	–	–	–	–	–	–
Aurora	620	O	–	–	–	–	–	–	–
Belmont	4,814	O	–	–	–	–	–	–	–
Benson	2,267	O	–	–	–	–	–	–	–
Boone	8,754	O	–	–	–	–	–	–	–
Burlington	35,930	O	–	–	–	–	–	–	–
Carolina Beach	1,663	O	–	–	–	–	–	–	–
Carrboro	3,472	X	–	–	–	–	–	–	–
Chapel Hill	25,537	X	–	X	–	–	–	–	–
Concord	18,464	O	–	–	–	–	–	O	–
Conetoe	160	O	–	–	–	–	–	–	–
Durham	95,438	O	–	O	–	–	–	O	–

Table 8-12, continued.

Jurisdiction	1970 Population	Nuisance	Zoning	Vehicle	Rec/Vehicle	Railroad	Aircraft	Construction	Building
Fayetteville	53,510	0	–	0	–	–	–	0	–
Forest City	7,179	0	–	–	–	–	–	–	–
Franklin	2,336	0	–	–	–	–	–	–	–
Fuquay-Varina	3,576	0	–	–	–	–	–	–	–
Gastonia	47,143	0	–	–	–	–	–	–	–
Gibsonville	2,019	0	–	–	–	–	–	–	–
Goldsboro	26,810	0	–	–	–	–	–	–	–
Greensboro	144,076	0	–	0	–	–	–	–	–
Hickory	20,569	0	–	–	–	–	–	–	–
High Point	63,204	0	–	–	–	–	–	–	–
Kings Mountain	8,405	0	–	–	–	–	–	–	–
Kinston	22,309	0	–	–	–	–	–	–	–
Kure Beach	394	0	–	–	–	–	–	–	–
Laurinburg	8,859	0	–	–	–	–	–	–	–
Lumberton	16,961	0	–	–	–	–	–	–	–
Madison	2,081	0	–	–	–	–	–	–	–
Manteo	547	0	–	–	–	–	–	–	–
Marion	3,335	0	–	–	–	–	–	–	–
Monroe	11,282	0	–	–	–	–	–	–	–
Mt. Pleasant	1,174	0	–	0	–	–	–	–	–
New Bern	14,660	0	–	–	–	–	–	–	–
Newton	7,857	0	–	0	–	–	–	–	–
Raleigh	123,793	0	–	–	–	–	–	–	–
Red Springs	3,383	0	–	–	–	–	–	–	–
Roanoke Rapids	13,508	0	–	–	–	–	–	–	–
Rocky Mount	34,284	0	–	–	–	–	–	–	–
Roper	649	0	–	–	–	–	–	–	–
Salisbury	22,515	0	–	–	–	–	–	–	–
Seaboard	611	0	–	–	–	–	–	–	–
Silver City	4,689	0	–	–	–	–	–	–	–
Southern Pines	5,937	0	–	–	–	–	–	–	–

City	Population								
Statesville	19,996	–	–	–	–	–	–	–	O
Tarboro	9,425	–	–	–	–	–	–	X	O
Thomasville	15,230	–	–	–	–	–	–	–	O
Valdese	3,182	–	–	–	–	–	–	–	O
Wake Forest	3,148	–	–	–	–	–	–	–	O
Walnut Cove	1,213	–	–	–	–	–	–	–	O
Warsaw	2,701	–	–	–	–	–	–	–	O
Washington	8,961	–	–	–	–	–	–	–	O
Wilmington	46,169	–	–	–	–	–	X	X	O
Winston-Salem	132,913	X	–	–	–	–	–	X	O
Winton	917	–	–	–	–	–	–	–	O
NORTH DAKOTA									
Bismark	34,703	–	–	–	–	–	–	–	O
Minot	32,290	X	–	–	X	–	X	–	X
OHIO									
Akron	275,425	–	–	–	–	O	–	–	O
Amherst	9,902	–	–	–	–	–	–	–	O
Cincinnati	452,524	–	–	–	–	–	X	X	O
Cleveland	750,903	–	O	–	–	–	X	X	O
Columbis	540,025	–	–	–	–	–	–	X	O
Dayton	243,601	–	–	–	–	–	–	X	O
Mansfield	50,743	–	–	–	–	–	X	–	X
Middleburg Heights	12,367	X	–	–	X	X	X	X	–
Shaker Heights	36,306	–	–	–	–	–	X	–	O
Springfield	81,941	–	–	–	–	–	–	–	O
Toledo	383,818	–	X	–	–	X	X	X	O
University Heights	17,055	–	–	–	–	–	–	–	O
OKLAHOMA									
Oklahoma City	368,856	–	–	–	–	–	–	X	O
Tulsa	330,350	–	–	–	–	–	–	–	O
OREGON									
Albany	18,181	–	–	–	–	–	X	X	X
Ashland	12,342	–	–	–	–	–	O	–	O
Astoria	10,244	–	–	–	–	–	–	–	O

Table 8-12, continued.

Jurisdiction	1970 Population	Nuisance	Zoning	Vehicle	Rec/Vehicle	Railroad	Aircraft	Construction	Building
Beaverton	18,577	X	X	X	–	–	–	–	–
Bend	13,710	O	–	O	–	–	–	–	–
Bandon	1,832	O	–	O	–	–	–	–	–
Central Point	4,004	O	–	O	–	–	–	O	–
Coos Bay	13,466	O	–	O	–	–	–	–	–
Corvallis	35,153	O	–	–	–	–	–	O	–
Dallas City	10,423	O	–	O	–	–	–	–	–
Eugene	76,346	O	X	X	–	–	–	–	–
Grants Pass	12,455	O	X	–	–	–	–	–	–
Hillsboro	14,675	X	X	X	–	–	–	–	–
Klamath Falls	15,775	O	–	–	–	–	–	–	–
Lake Oswego	14,573	X	X	X	–	–	–	–	–
Medford	28,454	X	–	–	–	–	–	–	–
Milwaukie	16,379	O	–	O	–	–	–	–	–
Pendleton	13,197	O	–	–	–	–	–	–	–
Portland	380,620	O	X	X	X	–	–	X	–
Silverton	4,301	–	X	–	–	–	–	–	–
Toledo	2,818	O	–	–	–	–	–	–	–
Tualatin	768	O	–	–	–	–	–	–	–
Yachats	414	O	–	–	–	–	–	–	–
PENNSYLVANIA									
Allentown	109,527	X	X	X	–	–	X	–	–
Bethlehem	72,686	O	X	–	–	–	–	–	–
Dubois	10,112	O	–	–	–	–	–	–	–
Erie	129,231	O	–	–	–	–	–	–	–
Girard	2,631	–	X	–	–	–	–	–	–
Harrisburg	68,061	X	X	X	X	–	–	–	–
Muhlenberg Township	5,212	O	–	–	–	–	–	–	–
Philadelphia	1,950,098	O	–	–	–	–	–	–	–
Pittsburgh	520,117	O	–	–	–	–	–	–	–

City	Population								
Scranton	103,564	—	—	—	—	—	—	—	O
State College	33,778	—	—	—	—	—	X	X	X
West Mifflin	28,070	—	—	—	—	—	—	X	O
RHODE ISLAND									
Cranston	74,287	—	—	—	—	—	—	X	—
East Providence	48,151	—	—	—	—	—	—	X	—
Pawtucket	76,984	X	X	—	—	—	—	X	X
Providence	179,116	—	—	—	—	—	—	—	O
Warwick	83,694	—	—	—	—	—	X	X	—
SOUTH CAROLINA									
Columbia	113,542	—	—	X	—	—	X	X	—
Florence	25,997	—	—	—	—	—	X	X	—
SOUTH DAKOTA									
Lemmon	2,456	—	—	—	—	—	X	—	—
Sioux Falls	72,488	—	—	—	—	—	O	O	—
TENNESSEE									
Chattanooga	119,923	—	O	—	—	—	O	—	O
Kingsport	31,939	—	O	—	O	—	O	—	O
Knoxville	276,293	—	—	—	—	X	X	—	—
Memphis	623,530	—	O	—	—	—	O	X	O
Nashville	448,003	—	—	—	—	—	O	X	—
TEXAS									
Amarillo	127,010	—	—	—	—	—	X	X	O
Austin	193,862	—	—	—	—	—	—	—	O
Beaumont	117,548	—	O	—	—	—	—	—	O
Corpus Christi	204,525	—	—	—	O	—	O	—	O
Dallas	844,401	—	—	—	—	—	—	X	O
El Paso	322,261	—	O	—	O	—	—	—	O
Fort Worth	393,476	—	—	—	—	—	O	—	O
Garland	81,437	—	—	—	O	—	O	—	O
Houston	1,232,802	—	—	—	—	—	—	—	O

Table 8-12, continued.

Jurisdiction	1970 Population	Nuisance	Zoning	Vehicle	Rec/Vehicle	Railroad	Aircraft	Construction	Building
TEXAS (Continued)									
Irving	97,457	O	-	O	-	-	-	O	-
Killen	35,507	O	-	O	-	-	-	-	-
Mineral Wells	18,411	O	-	O	-	-	-	O	-
Odessa	78,380	O	X	O	-	O	O	O	-
Saginaw	2,382	O	-	O	-	-	-	O	-
San Antonia	654,153	O	-	-	-	-	-	-	-
Texarkana	30,497	O	-	O	-	-	-	O	-
Wichita Falls	96,265	O	-	O	-	-	-	O	-
UTAH									
Murray	21,206	X	-	X	-	-	-	X	-
Ogden	69,478	X	X	X	-	-	-	X	-
Provo	53,131	X	-	X	-	-	-	X	X
Roosevelt	2,005	O	-	-	-	-	-	-	-
Salt Lake City	175,885	X	X	X	X	X	-	X	-
VIRGINIA									
Alexandria	110,927	X	X	X	-	-	-	-	-
Arlington	174,284	O	X	X	-	-	-	-	-
Chesapeake	89,580	O	O	-	-	-	-	-	-
Fairfax	21,970	-	X	-	-	-	-	-	-
Hampton	120,779	O	O	O	O	-	-	O	-
Newport News	138,177	X	X	O	-	-	-	O	-
Norfolk	307,951	O	-	O	-	-	-	O	-
Richmond	249,621	O	O	-	-	-	-	-	-
Roanoke	92,115	X	X	-	-	-	-	-	-
Virginia Beach	172,106	-	X	-	-	-	-	-	-

WASHINGTON								
Bellevue	61,102	–	X	–	–	–	–	–
Cheney	6,718	X	X	–	–	–	–	–
Colfax	2,664	X	X	X	X	X	X	O
College Place	4,510	O	–	X	–	–	–	–
Kennewick	15,212	X	X	X	X	X	X	O
Medina	3,455	X	–	–	X	–	X	X
Pullman	20,509	–	X	X	X	X	X	O
Renton	25,878	X	X	O	O	O	X	–
Richland	26,290	–	–	O	–	–	O	–
Seattle	530,831	O	X	X	O	O	X	X
Snohomish	5,174	X	–	X	–	–	X	–
Spokane	170,516	O	X	O	O	O	X	–
Tacoma	154,581	–	O	–	–	–	–	X
Walla Walla	23,619	O	X	O	O	O	O	–
Yakima	45,588	O	–	O	O	O	O	–
WISCONSIN								
Janesville	46,426	O	–	–	–	–	–	–
Madison	173,258	X	X	X	O	O	O	–
Milwaukee	717,372	X	X	X	X	X	O	O
Racine	95,162	X	X	X	–	X	O	–
Sparta	6,258	O	–	O	O	–	O	–
WYOMING								
Casper	39,361	–	O	O	–	–	–	–
Cheyenne	40,914	X	–	X	X	X	X	–
Lander	7,112	O	–	O	X	X	X	–
Powell	4,807	O	–	–	X	X	X	–
Riverton	7,995	–	–	–	–	X	–	–
Worland	5,055	O	–	–	–	–	–	–

Key: X = Regulation includes acoustical criteria
     O = Regulation does not include acoustical criteria
     – = No regulation

REFERENCES

Banner, A. and M. Hyatt. "Effects of Noise on Eggs and Larvae of Two Estuarine Fishes," *Trans. Am. Fish Soc.* 102(1):134-136 (1973).

Bender, A. "Noise Impact on Wildlife: An Environmental Impact Assessment," Automation Industries, Inc. Silver Springs, MD (1977).

Bragdon, C. R. "Municipal Noise Ordinances—1976," *Sound and Vibration* (December 1976).

Calef, G. W., and G. M. Lortie. "Observations on the Porcupine Caribou Herd," Environmental Impact Assessment of the Portion of the Mackenzie Gas Pipeline from Alaska to Alberta (1973).

CHABA Working Group 69. "Guidelines for Preparing Environmental Impact Statements on Noise," U.S. Department of Defense (1977).

Committee on the Problem of Noise. Noise Final Report. (London: Her Majesty's Stationery Office, 1968).

Congress, U.S. "Report to the President and Congress on Noise," Senate Document 92-63. 92nd Congress (1972).

Craighead, F.C., and J. J. Craighead. "Grizzly Bear Prehibernation and Denning Activities as Determined by Radio-Tracking," *Wildlife Monographs* No. 32 (1972).

Davis, J. "Memorandum to Robert Fedeler," *Alaska Fish and Game* (1976).

Department of Defense, U.S., U.S. Army Environmental Hygiene Agency. "Noise Hazard Evaluation," (1975).

Department of Interior, U.S. "Alaska Natural Gas Transportation System," Draft Environmental Impact Statement, Parts I and II (1975).

Environmental Protection Agency, U.S., Office of Noise Abatement and Control. "Noise Source Regulation in State and Local Noise Ordinances" (1975).

Executive Order 11989. "Off-road Vehicles on Public Lands," (1977).

Federal Aviation Administration, U.S. Department of Transportation. "Final Amendments to FAR 36," Noise Standards 14 CFR, 21, 36, 91 (1976).

Federal Aviation Administration, U.S. Department of Transportation. "FAA Advisory Circular 36-1A" (1975).

Geist, V. "Is Big Game Harrassment Harmful?" *Oil Week* 14:12-13 (1971).

Goodfriend, L. S., and F. M. Kessler. "Industrial Noise Pollution," in *Pollution Engineering and Scientific Solutions*, E.S. Barrekette, Ed. (New York: Plenum Press, 1973).

Goff, R. J. and E. W. Novak. Environmental Noise Impact Analysis for Military Activities: Users Manual. Technical Report N-30. Construction Engineering Research Laboratory (1977).

Hansen, H. A., P. E. Shepherd, J. G. King and W. A. Troyer. "The Trumpeter Swan in Alaska," *Wildlife Monographs* No. 26 (1971).

Heimer, W. E. "Dall Sheep Reaction to Noise," Letter, Alaska Department of Fish and Game, Fairbanks (1976).

Klein, D. R. "The Reaction of Some Northern Mammals to Aircraft Disturbances," Alaska Cooperative Wildlife Research Unit (unpublished data) (1976).

Milton, J. P. "The Web of Wilderness," *The Living Wilderness, Special Alaska Issue,* 35(116):14-19 (1972).

Renewable Resources Consulting Services. "A Study of the Reactions of Caribou, Moose and Grizzly Bear to Aircraft Disturbance," Edmonton, Alberta (1973).

Stephenson, R. O. "Biologist Tells of Methods Used to Count Wolves," *Alaska Wildlife Digest* (Spring 1975).

CHAPTER 9

PHYSICAL RESOURCES

INTRODUCTION

In an environmental impact statement, the action rarely has an impact on physical resources. Usually, it is the physical foundation that would affect the action or cause it to be modified. Physical features and data are more often included in descriptive chapters, and are used by engineers in design of structures. The physical resources discussed in the chapter include: topography, geology, soils, fire, earthquakes, volcanic areas and minerals.

Table 9-1 describes the range and availability of topographical maps of the U.S. Geological Survey (Department of the Interior). For site-specific environmental statements, usually 7.5-minute maps of the area would be one of the first data collection steps. The "scale" column allows for comparison with other map and aerial photo data available. Column "quadrangle size" provides for study area coverage, or for estimating how many maps will be needed to cover the particular study area. Topographical maps provide needed data on slope, elevation, watersheds, rough vegetative and urbanization patterns. The black and white topographical maps often make the best base maps of the study area, over which data are plotted.

Physical subdivisions on the largest scale are shown on Figure 9-1. The heavy lines separate geological divisions of the U.S, while lighter lines illustrate the subdivisions within each region. U.S. vegetative and soil regions generally follow these physical baselines.

Figure 9-2 illustrates major soil orders of the U.S., on the broadest classification system. The two pages of key to Figure 9-2 are based on the soil orders and suborders of the Soil Conservation Service (Department of the Interior). The pattern, *i.e.,* white = albisols, illustrates the orders of soils, while letter, number notation indicates suborders of soils.

549

Table 9-1. U.S. Geological Maps: Topographical (DO I, 1972a)

Series	Scale	1-Inch Equals	Quadrangle Size (lat-long)	Quadrangle Size (mi²)	Paper Size
United States:					
7.5-minute	1:24,000	2,000 ft	7 1/2' x 7 1/2'	49-70	22 x 27 / 23 x 27
15-minute	1:62,500	0.98 mi	15' x 15'	197-282	17 x 21 / 19 x 21
1:63,360 (Alaska)	1:63,360	1.00 mi	15' x 20'-30'	207-281	17 x 21 / 18 x 21
30-minute	1:125,000	1.97 mi	30' x 30'	789-1,082	17 x 21
1-degree	1:250,000	3.94 mi	1° x 1°	3,173-4,335	17 x 21
1:250,000	1:250,000	3.94 mi	1° x 2°	6,346-8,669	22 x 29 / 22 x 32
Reconnaissance (Alaska)	1:250,000	3.94 mi	1° x 2°-3°	4,580-7,310	22 x 34
1:250,000 (Alaska)	1:250,000	3.94 mi	1° x 2°-3°	4,580-7,310	23 x 30
1:250,000 (Hawaii)	1:250,000	3.94 mi	1° x 1°30'-1°35'	6,730-7,104	23 x 30
1:1,000,000	1:1,000,000	15.78 mi	4° x 6°	73,734-102,759	24 x 29
1:1,000,000	1:1,000,000	15.78 mi	4° x 12°	78,960-122,066	27 x 27 / 26 x 30
Puerto Rico:					
7.5-minute	1:20,000	0.31 mi	7 1/2' x 7 1/2'	71	31 x 36
Special	1:30,000	0.47 mi			
Virgin Islands of the United States:					
1:24,000	1:24,000	2,000 ft	7 1/2' x 6'	56	20 x 27
7.5-minute	1:24,000	2,000 ft	7 1/2' x 7 1/2'	71	23 x 27

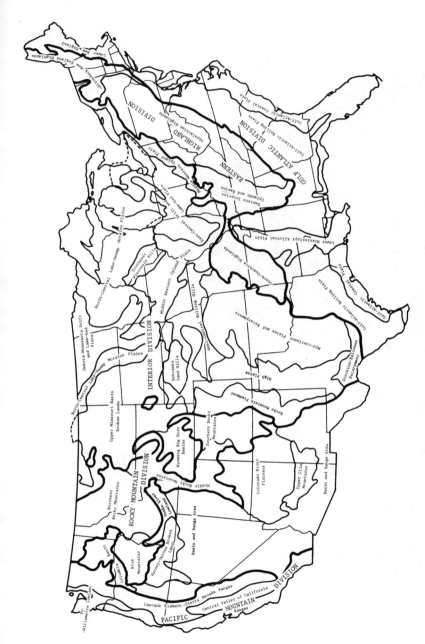

Figure 9-1. Physical divisions of the U.S. (Hammond, 1965).

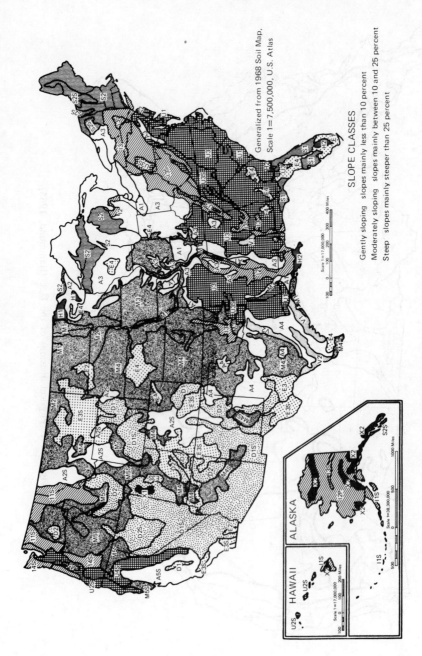

Generalized from 1968 Soil Map,
Scale 1=7,500,000, U.S. Atlas

SLOPE CLASSES

Gently sloping slopes mainly less than 10 percent
Moderately sloping slopes mainly between 10 and 25 percent
Steep slopes mainly steeper than 25 percent

Figure 9-2. Soil orders of the U.S.

Key to Figure 9-2

SOIL ORDERS AND SUBORDERS OF
THE UNITED STATES AND THEIR UTILIZATION

(USDA–SOIL CONSERVATION SERVICE.)

ALFISOLS . . . Soils with gray to
brown surface horizons, medium to
high base supply, and subsurface
horizons of clay accumulation;
usually moist but may be dry
during warm season

A1 AQUALFS (seasonally saturated with
water) gently sloping; general crops
if drained, pasture and woodland if
undrained (Some Low-Humic Gley
soils and Planosols)

A2 BORALFS (cool or cold) gently sloping; mostly woodland, pasture, and
some small grain (Gray Wooded
soils)

A2S BORALFS steep; mostly woodland

A3 UDALFS (temperate or warm, and
moist) gently or moderately sloping; mostly farmed, corn, soybeans,
small grain, and pasture (Gray-
Brown Podzolic soils)

A4 USTALFS (warm and intermittently
dry for long periods) gently or moderately sloping; range, small grain,
and irrigated crops (Some Reddish
Chestnut and Red-Yellow Podzolic
soils)

A5S XERALFS (warm and continuously dry
in summer for long periods, moist
in winter) gently sloping to steep;
mostly range, small grain, and irrigated crops (Noncalcic Brown soils)

ARIDISOLS . . .Soils with pedogenic
horizons, low in organic matter,
and dry more than 6 months of the
year in all horizons

D1 ARGIDS (with horizon of clay accumu-
lation) gently or moderately sloping;
mostly range, some irrigated crops
(Some Desert, Reddish Desert, Reddish
Brown, and Brown soils and associated
Solonetz soils)

D1S ARGIDS gently sloping to steep

D2 ORTHIDS (without horizon of clay
accumulation gently or moderately
sloping; mostly range and some irrigated crops (Some Desert, Reddish
Desert, Sierozem, and Brown soils,
and some Calcisols and Solonchak
soils)

D2S ORTHIDS gently sloping to steep

ENTISOLS . . .Soils without pedogenic horizons

E1 AQUENTS (seasonally saturated with
water) gently sloping; some grazing

E2 ORTHENTS (loamy or clayey textures)
deep to hard rock; gently to moderately
sloping; range or irrigated farming
(Regosols)

E3 ORTHENTS shallow to rock;
mostly range

E4 PSAMMENTS (sand or loamy sand
textures) gently to moderately sloping; mostly range in dry climates,
woodland or cropland in humid
climates (Regosols)

HISTOSOLS . . .Organic soils

H1 FIBRISTS (fibrous or woody peats,
largely undecomposed) mostly
wooded or idle (Peats)

H2 SAPRISTS (decomposed mucks) truck
crops if drained, idle if undrained
(Mucks)

INCEPTISOLS . . . Soils that are
usually moist, with pedogenic horizons of alteration of parent materials
but not of accumulation

11S ANDEPTS (with amorphous clay or
vitric volcanic ash and pumice)
gently sloping to steep; mostly woodland; in Hawaii mostly sugar cane,
pineapple, and range (Ando soils,
some Tundra soils)

12 AQUEPTS (seasonally saturated with
water) gently sloping; if drained,
mostly row crops, corn, soybeans,
and cotton, if undrained, mostly
woodland or pasture (Some Low-
Humic Gley soils and Alluvial soils)

12P AQUEPTS (with continuous or sporadic
permafrost) gently sloping to
steep; woodland or idle (Tundra
soils)

13 OCHREPTS (with thin or light-colored
surface horizons and little organic
matter) gently to moderately sloping;
mostly pasture, small grain, and hay
(Sols Bruns Acides and some Alluvial
soils)

13S OCHREPTS gently sloping to steep;
woodland, pasture, small grains

14S UMBREPTS (with thick dark-colored
surface horizons rich in organic matter)
moderately sloping to steep; mostly
woodland (Some Regosols)

MOLLISOLS . . .Soils with nearly
black, organic-rich surface horizons
and high base supply

Key to Figure 9-2

KEY (Continued)

M1   AQUOLLS (seasonally saturated with water) gently sloping; mostly drained and farmed (Humic Gley soils)

M2   BOROLLS (cool or cold) gently or moderately sloping, some steep slopes in Utah; mostly small grain in North Central States, range and woodland in Western States (Some Chernozems)

M3   UDOLLS (temperate or warm, and moist) gently or moderately sloping; mostly corn, soybeans, and small grains (Some Brunizems)

M4   USTOLLS (intermittently dry for long periods during summer) gently to moderately sloping; mostly wheat and range in western part, wheat and corn or sorghum in eastern part, some irrigated crops (Chestnut soils and some Chernozems and Brown soils)

M4S   USTOLLS moderately sloping to steep; mostly range or woodland

M5   XEROLLS (continuously dry in summer for long periods, moist in winter) gently to moderately sloping; mostly wheat, range, and irrigated crops (Some Brunizems, Chestnut, and Brown soils)

M5S   XEROLLS moderately sloping to steep; mostly range

SPODOSOLS . . .Soils with accumulations of amorphous materials in subsurface horizons

S1   AQUODS (seasonally saturated with water) gently sloping; mostly range or woodland; where drained in Florida, citrus and special crops (Ground-Water Podzols)

S2   ORTHODS (with subsurface accumulations of iron, aluminum, and organic matter) gently to moderately sloping; woodland, pasture, small grains, special crops (Podzols, Brown Podzolic soils)

S2S   ORTHODS steep; mostly woodland

ULTISOLS . . . Soils that are usually moist, with horizon of clay accumulation and a low base supply

U1   AQUULTS (seasonally saturated with water) gently sloping; woodland and pasture if undrained, feed and truck crops if drained (Some Low-Humic Gley soils)

U2S   HUMULTS (with high or very high organic-matter content) moderately sloping to steep; woodland and pasture if steep, sugar cane and pineapple in Hawaii, truck and seed crops in Western States (Some Reddish-Brown Lateritic soils)

U3   UDULTS (with low organic-matter content; temperate or warm, and moist) gently to moderately sloping; woodland, pasture feed crops, tobacco, and cotton (Red-Yellow Podzolic soils, some Reddish-Brown Lateritic soils)

U3S   UDULTS moderately sloping to steep; woodland, pasture

U4S   XERULTS (with low to moderate organic-matter content, continuously dry for long periods in summer) range and woodland (Some Reddish-Brown Lateritic soils)

VERTISOLS . . .Soils with high content of swelling clays and wide deep cracks at some season

V1   UDERTS (cracks open for only short periods, less than 3 months in a year) gently sloping; cotton, corn, pasture, and some rice (Some Grumusols)

V2   USTERTS (cracks open and close twice a year and remain open more than 3 months); general crops, range, and some irrigated crops (Some Grumusols)

AREAS with little soil . . .

X1 Salt flats

X2 Rock land (plus ice fields in Alaska)

SOURCE: Wolfanger, L. A. 1971, Soil Orders and Suborders of the United States (in) Smith, Guy-Harold, ed. 1971. Conservation of Natural Resources, 4th Edition. John Wiley & Sons, Inc. New York

Table 9-2 defines another broadly used soil classification system of the Soil Conservation Service (SCS), based on soil capability from I to VIII for supporting crops, forests or grazing. Table 9-3 shows soil types, the smallest unit of soil classification of the SCS. Data on Table 9-3 are typically found on a county basis in SCS publications entitled "Soil Surveys." Older soils surveys give data as to crop usage, slope, drainage, plasticity and productivity, as well as soil maps of the county. Newer soil surveys include soil information, such as suitability for engineering structures, dams, roads and houses. Not all counties have soil surveys. A list of counties with soil surveys completed is updated regularly by the SCS.

Table 9-2. USDA—Soil Conservation Service—Soil Capability Classes

The Soil Conservation Service has developed a grouping of soil types into capability classes. The classes range from I for excellent soils to VIII for poor soils. Generally, soils are mapped by a color code by SCS personnel. Soils which are excellent for farming are also excellent for construction, in most cases. For this reason many of our best soils are irreversibly lost to building and urbanization. Mapping soils of the study area can help predict how much good to excellent farmable acres will be converted by the proposed project. Definitions of soil classes follow:

Class I—Soils that have few limitations that restrict their use. Suitable for cultivation.

Unit I-4—Deep, well-drained, nearly level, upland soils.

Unit I-6—Nearly level, well-drained, silty soils on flood plains and low terraces.

Class II—Soils that have some limitations that reduce the choice of plants or require moderate conservation practices. Suitable for cultivation.

Subclass IIe—Nearly level to gently sloping soils, subject to erosion if tilled.

Subclass IIw—Moderately wet soils.

Class III—Soils that have severe limitations that reduce the choice of plants, require special conservation practices, or both. Suitable for cultivation.

Subclass IIIw—Wet soils that require artificial drainage if tilled.

Subclass IIIs—Soils that are severely limited by sandiness.

Class IV—Soils that have very severe limitations that restrict the choice of plants, require very careful management, or both. Marginal soils.

Subclass IVe[a]—Soils severely limited by risk of erosion if tilled.

Subclass IVw[b]—Soils severely limited for use as cropland because of excess water.

Table 9-2, continued.

Class V—Soils that have little or no erosion hazard but have other limitations that are impractical to remove and that limit their use largely to pasture, woodland or wildlife food and cover. Level but wet.

Subclass Vw—Soils limited in use to grazing or woodland because of poor internal drainage.

Class VI—Soils that have severe limitations that make them generally unsuitable for cultivation and limited by steepness, drought or moisture. Suitable for grazing and forestry uses.

Class VII—Soils with very severe limitations that restrict their use to pasture or trees.

Subclass VIIe—Hilly, steep, erosive.
Subclass VIIs —Stony, rolling, steep, shallow to bedrock.

Class VIII—Soils with no agricultural use, mountains.

^{a}e: erodible.
^{b}w: wet

Figure 9-3 illustrates the common soil or grain size limits of the Department of Agriculture (USDA), in comparison to other soil classification systems. Soils are usually described in terms of "sands," "silts" or "clay" content, which mean specific size classes. Sieve sizes and particle sizes for these commonly used terms in highway, agriculture and foundation work are found on Figure 9-3. Table 9-4 gives another comparison of soil classification systems. The first texture column is after the SCS(U.S. Department of Agriculture). The second column, Unified system, is more common in determining foundation suitability. The third column is that used by the American Association of State Highway Officials for highway design. The last column describes general soil properties, which these systems or nomenclature share.

Table 9-5 lists specific soil properties for the "Unified Soil Classification System," which is used in construction, rather than for agricultural use. Compaction, drainage, frost heave and expansion potential columns are all used for siting of facilities. These are physical features which would affect the action, if a site has been ill chosen.

Once soils have been described, the impact assessment follows. One impact from almost all constructions projects is erosion. Figures 9-4 to 9-6 and Tables 9-6 through 9-10 are used to predict soil loss per acre per year. This is followed by an example of its use, for a theoretical strip mine. Table 9-11 follows, with a state-by-state summary of required mitigation efforts to reclaim strip-mined lands.

Table 9-3. Typical Data Available from Soil Surveys (USDA, 1977)

Major Soil Type	Soil Drainage	Topography	Suitability of Area Soils for:				
			Septic Systems	Single-family Dwellings	Highways	Excavation	Agriculture
Glenelg	Good	Rolling upland	Good except on steep slopes	Good	Good	Good (bedrock hazard on steep slopes)	Good if slopes not severe
Manor	Good to excessive	Rolling upland	Good except on steep slopes	Good	Good to fair stability	Good (bedrock hazard on steep slopes)	Fair-good, shallow, sloping
Elioak	Good	Rolling upland	Fair (moderately slow permeability)	Good	Good to fair stability	Good (bedrock hazard on steep slopes)	Good if slopes not severe
Chester	Good	Rolling upland	Very good except on steep slopes	Good	Good	Good (bedrock hazard on steep slopes)	Very good
Brandywine	Excessive	Hilly-steep upland	Good except on steep slopes	Good	Good to fair stability, bedrock hazard	Poor (bedrock hazard)	Poor
Mt. Airy	Excessive	Rolling–steep upland	Poor (bedrock hazard)	Good	Fair stability	Poor (shallow depth to bedrock)	Fair (especially pasture-forage)
Lingapore	Good to excessive	Upland ridges	Good	Good	Fair stability	Poor (shallow depth to bedrock)	Fair to poor
Belvoir	Poor to fair	Upland flats and drainage-way heads	Very poor drainage	Poor (high water table)	Poor (high water table)	Poor (high water table)	Poor

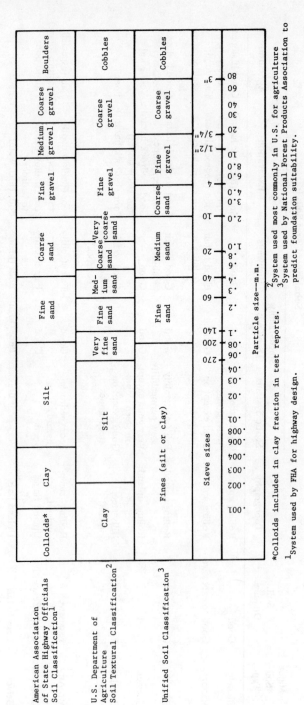

Figure 9-3. A comparison of grain-size limits in the three classification systems.

Table 9-4. Soil Properties Comparisons of Three Classification Systems[a]

USDA Texture Class and Symbol	Unified Symbol	AASHO Symbol	Soil Properties Related to Classifications
Clay; silty clay, c; sic	CH	A-7	High, shrink-swell clays
	MH	A-7	Mica, iron oxide, kaolinitic clays
	CL	A-7	Low LL, generally $<$45 pct clay
Silty clay loam, sicl	CL	A-7	Low LL, plastic (A-6 if clay $<$30 pct)
	ML-CL	A-7	Low LL, moderately plastic (A-6 if clay $<$30 pct)
	CH	A-7	High LL, high, shrink-swell clays
	MH	A-7	High LL, mica, iron oxide, kaolinitic
Clay loam, cl	CL	A-6 or A-7	Low LL, plastic
	ML-CL	A-6	Low LL, moderately plastic
	CH	A-7	High LL, high, shrink-swell clays
	MH	A-7	High LL, mica, iron oxide, kaolinitic
Loam, l	ML-CL	A-4	Moderately plastic (A-6 if clay $>$21 pct)
	CL	A-6	Plastic (A-4 if clay $<$22 pct)
	ML	A-4	Low plasticity (A-7 if clay $>$21 pct)
Silt loam, sil	ML-CL	A-4	Moderately plastic (A-6 if clay $>$21 pct)
	ML	A-4	Low plasticity (A-7 if clay $>$21 pct)
	CL	A-6	Plastic
Silt, si	ML	A-4	Low plasticity
Sandy clay, sc	CL	A-7	Fines $>$50 pct
	SC	A-7	Fines 50 pct or less
Sandy clay loam, scl	SC	A-6	Plastic, fines 36-50 pct
	SC	A-2-6	Plastic, fines 35 pct or less
	CL	A-6	Plastic, fines $>$50 pct
Sandy loam, sl	SM	A-2-4 or A-4	Low plasticity
	SC	A-2-4	Plastic
	SM-SC	A-2-4	Moderately plastic
Fine sandy loam, fsl	SM	A-4	Nonplastic, fines 50 pct or less
	ML	A-4	Nonplastic, fines $>$50 pct
	ML-CL	A-4	Moderately plastic, fines $>$50 pct
	SM-SC	A-4	Moderately plastic, fines 50 pct or less
Very fine sandy loam, vfsl	ML-CL	A-4	Moderately plastic
	ML	A-4	Low plasticity
Loamy sands, ls; lfs; lvfs	SM	A-2-4	Nonplastic, fines 35 pct or less
	SM-SC	A-2-4	Moderately plastic, fines 35 **pct** or less
	SM	A-4	Low plasticity, fines $>$35 pct
	ML	A-4	Little or no plasticity
Sand, fine sand, s; fs	SP-SM	A-3	Fines approx. 5-10 pct
	SM	A-2-4	Fines approx. $>$10 pct
	SP	A-3	Fines $<$5 pct
Very fine sand, vfs	SM	A-4	Low plasticity
	ML	A-4	Little or no plasticity
Coarse sand, cs	SP; GW	A-1	Fines $<$5 pct
	SP-SM	A-1	Fines 5-12 pct
	SM	A-1	Fines 13-25 pct
	SM	A-2-4	Fines $>$25 pct
Gravel, G	GP; GW	A-1	Fines $<$5 pct
50 pct passes No. 200	GM or GC	A-1	Fines 5-25 pct
50 pct of coarse	GM or GC	A-2	Fines 26-35 pct
passes No. 4 sieve	GM	A-4	Fines $>$35 pct
	GC	A-6	Fines $>$35 pct

[a]This table may be used as a guide in classifying soils for which no engineering test data are available. The symbol $>$means "greater than"; the symbol $<$means "less than." pct = %.

Table 9-5. Types of Soils and Their Design Properties for Foundations (NFPA, 1976).

Soil Group	Unified Soil Classification System Symbol	Soil Description	Allowable Bearing (lb/ft²) with Medium Compaction or Stiffness	Drainage Characteristics [a]	Frost Heave Potential	Volume Change Potential Expansion
Group I—Excellent	GW	Well-graded gravels, gravel sand mixtures, little or no fines	8,000	Good	Low	Low
	GP	Poorly graded gravels or gravel sand mixtures, little or no fines	8,000	Good	Low	Low
	SW	Well-graded sands, gravelly sands, little or no fines	6,000	Good	Low	Low
	SP	Poorly graded sands or gravelly sands, little or no fines	5,000	Good	Low	Low
	GM	Silty gravels, gravel-sand-silt mixtures	4,000	Good	Medium	Low
	SM	Silty sand, sand-silt mixtures	4,000	Good	Medium	Low
Group II—Fair to Good	GC	Clayey gravels, gravel-sand-clay mixtures	4,000	Medium	Medium	Low
	SC	Clayey sands, sand-clay mixture	4,000	Medium	Medium	Low
	ML	Inorganic silts and very fine sand, rock flour, silty or clayey fine sands or clayey silts with slight plasticity	2,000	Medium	High	Low
	CL	Inorganic clays or low to medium plasticity, gravelly clays, sands, clays, silty clays, lean clays	2,000	Medium	Medium	Medium [b]

Group III—Poor	CH	Inorganic clays of high plasticity, fat clays	2,000	Poor	Medium	High[b]
	MH	Inorganic silts, micaceous or diatomaceous fine sandy or silty soils, elastic silts	2,000	Poor	High	High
Group IV—Unsatisfactory	OL	Organic silts and organic silty clays of low plasticity	400	Poor	Medium	Medium
	OH	Organic clays of medium to high plasticity, organic silts	0	Unsatisfactory	Medium	High
	PT	Peat and other highly organic soils	0	Unsatisfactory	Medium	High

[a]The percolation rate for good drainage is over 4 inches per hour, medium drainage is 2 to 4 inches per hour, and poor is less than 2 inches per hour.

[b]Danger expansion might occur if these two soil types are dry but subject to future wetting.

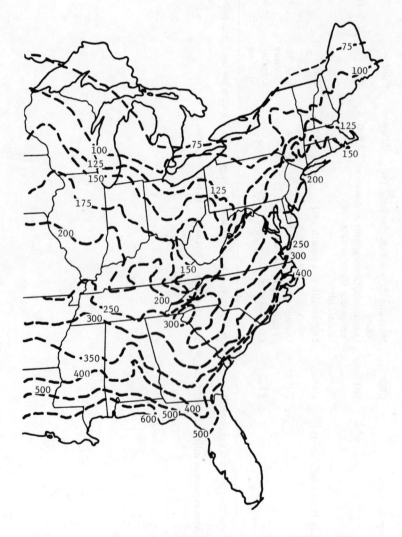

Figure 9-4. Rainfall-erosion losses from eastern U.S. (USDA, 1965).

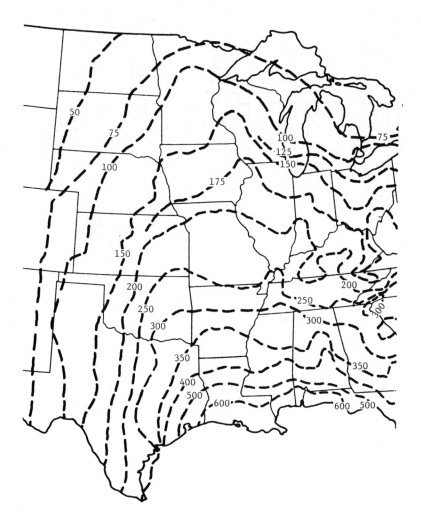

Figure 9-5. Rainfall-erosion losses from the midwest.

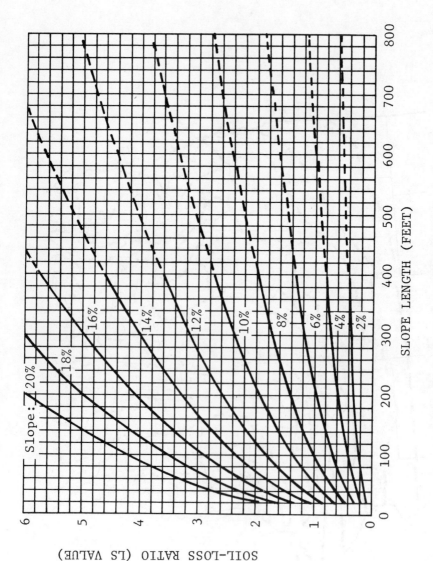

Figure 9-6. Slope-effect chart (topographic factor, LS).

Table 9-6. Typical Soils Data and K Values for Site-Specific Analysis

Soil Series[a]	Horizon[b]	USDA Texture Range [c]	K-Value[d]
Abbottstown	A	1, sil	0.43
	B	1, sil, sicl	0.43
	C	1	0.43
Adelphia	A	sl, fsl	0.32
	B	1, scl, fsl	0.43
	C	sl, ls	0.43
Albrights	A	sil, gsil, gl	0.43
	B	sicl, cl, scl	0.43
	C	1	0.43
Aldino	A	sil	0.43
	B	sicl, sil	0.43
	C	1, sil	0.43
Allegheny	A	1, fls, sil	0.32
	B	cl, sil, sicl	0.28
	C	cl, 1, scl	0.28
Alluvial Land	A	variable	0.28
	B	variable	0.28
	C	variable	0.28
Altavista	A	fsl, sl, 1	0.32
	B	sil, cl	0.43
	C	gsl	0.43
Andover	A	1, gl, sl	0.43
	B	cl, 1, gcl	0.43
	C	gl, gscl	0.43
Armaugh	A	sil, sicl	0.43
	B	sicl, sic, c	0.28
	C	sic, sicl, cl	0.17
Ashby	A	shl, sil	0.28
	B	sil	0.24
	C	shale	– –
Ashton	A	1, sil, fsl	0.28
	B	sil, sicl	0.28
	C	fsl, 1, sil	0.28
Athol	A	1, sil	0.37
	B	sil, cl, scl	0.28
	C	gl, (variable)	0.28

[a]Over 6,000 in U.S.
[b]A: surface material; B: intermediate; C: parent material.
[c]Silt, loam, clay, etc.   (Table 9-4).
[d]Erodibility: 0.43: highly erodible; 0.28: moderate; 0.17: low.

Table 9-7.   Indications of the General Magnitude
of the Soil-Erodibility Factor, K^a

| Texture Class | Organic Matter Content | | |
| | <0.5% | 2% | 4% |
	K	K	K
Sand	0.05	0.03	0.02
Fine Sand	0.16	0.14	0.10
Very Fine Sand	0.42	0.36	0.28
Loamy Sand	0.12	0.10	0.08
Loamy Fine Sand	0.24	0.20	0.16
Loamy Very Fine Sand	0.44	0.38	0.30
Sandy Loam	0.27	0.24	0.19
Fine Sandy Loam	0.35	0.30	0.24
Very Fine Sandy Loam	0.47	0.41	0.33
Loam	0.38	0.34	0.29
Silt Loam	0.48	0.42	0.33
Silt	0.60	0.52	0.42
Sandy Clay Loam	0.27	0.25	0.21
Clay Loam	0.28	0.25	0.21
Silty Clay Loam	0.37	0.32	0.26
Sandy Clay	0.14	0.13	0.12
Silty Clay	0.25	0.23	0.19
Clay	—	0.13-0.29	—

[a]The values shown are estimated averages of broad ranges of specific soil values.
When a texture is near the borderline of two texture classes, use the average of
the two K values. For specific soils, use Soil Conservation Service K-value tables.

Table 9-8.   Factor P Values for Components of
Erosion and Sediment Control Systems

Component	Factor P Value
Small Sediment Basin	
0.04 basin/ac	0.50
0.06 basin/ac	0.30
Downstream Sediment Basin	
With chemical flocculants	0.10
Without chemical flocculants	0.20
Erosion-Reducing Structures	
Normal rate usage	0.50
High rate usage	0.40
Strip Building	0.75

Table 9-9. Maximum Permissible C Values (T/RKLS) For Indicated
Gradient and Slope Length With Straight And
With Contoured Rows (USDA, 1965)

Gradient (%)	Values for Slope Length (ft) of							
	60	80	100	150	200	250	300	400
	Straight Row							
2	0.45	0.35	0.33	0.26	0.22	0.20	0.17	0.15
4	0.22	0.19	0.17	0.13	0.11	0.10	0.092	0.081
6	0.13	0.11	0.10	0.083	0.072	0.065	0.058	0.050
8	0.089	0.077	0.068	0.055	0.048	0.043	0.039	0.034
10	0.064	0.056	0.050	0.040	0.035	0.030	0.028	0.024
12	0.048	0.042	0.037	0.030	0.026	0.023	0.021	0.018
14	0.038	0.033	0.029	0.024	0.020	0.018	0.017	0.014
16	0.030	0.026	0.024	0.019	0.016	0.015	0.013	0.012
18	0.025	0.022	0.019	0.016	0.014	0.012	—	—
20	0.021	0.018	0.016	0.013	0.011	—	—	—
	Contoured							
2	0.75	0.58	0.57	0.43	0.37	0.33	0.28	0.25
4	0.44	0.38	0.34	0.26	0.22	0.20	0.18	0.16
6	0.26	0.22	0.20	0.17	0.14	0.13	0.12	0.10
8	0.15	0.13	0.11	0.092	0.080	0.072	0.065	0.057
10	0.11	0.093	0.083	0.067	0.058	0.050	-0.047	0.040
12	0.08	0.070	0.062	0.050	0.043	0.038	0.035	0.030
14	0.048	0.041	0.036	0.030	0.025	0.022	0.021	0.018
16	0.038	0.032	0.030	0.024	0.020	0.019	0.016	0.015
18	0.031	0.027	0.024	0.020	0.018	0.015	—	—
20	0.023	0.020	0.018	0.014	0.012	—	—	—

Table 9-10. Average Factor C Values for Various
Surface Stabilizing Treatments

Treatment	Factor C Values Time Elapsed Between Seeding and Building	
	None	6 Months
Seed, fertilizer and straw mulch Straw disked or treated with asphalt or chemical straw tack	0.35	0.23
Seed and fertilizer	0.64	0.54
Chemical treatment	0.89	—
Seed and fertilizer with chemicals	0.52	0.38

SOIL LOSS PREDICTION METHOD

The universal soil loss equation can be applied all over the U.S. to predict tons of soil lost per acre. Originally, the equation was used for agricultural erosion predictions, but now can also be used to predict silt loads in rivers and soil losses from construction sites. While the information which follows is "universal" and does provide a useful guide to most U.S. soils, more precise site data would give a more accurate soil loss estimate.

The equation is:

$$A = RKLSCP$$

where A = estimated average annual soil loss, ton/ac

> R = rainfall and runoff erosivity index. Its local value can generally be obtained by interpolating between the isovalue lines of Figures 9-4 and 9-5. (Exceptions are the Coastal Plains of the Southeast. R values presently used in the Coastal Plains do not exceed 350: In the Northwest, the map values must be increased to account for effect of runoff from thaw and snowmelt. Estimated adjustments for specific locations can be obtained from the Soil Conservation Service.)

> K = soil-erodibility factor. It is the average soil loss per unit of R under arbitrarily selected "basic" conditions, and depends on soil properties. The value of K for most of the U.S. mainland soils can be obtained from local offices of the Soil Conservation Service (example: Table 9-6). Gross approximations based primarily on soil texture can be obtained from Table 9-7.

> LS = slope-effect on erosion. The factor LS is the expected ratio of soil loss per unit area on a field slope to corresponding loss from the basic 9% slope, 72.6 ft long. This ratio, for specific combinations of slope length and gradient, may usually be taken directly from the slope-effect chart (Figure 9-6). For example, a 10% slope, 260 ft long, would have an LS ratio of 2.6.

When the equation is used as a guide for selection of practices on an area where several slopes are combined into a single field, the slope characteristics of the most erosive significant segment of the field should be used for Figure 2. Use of field averages on such slope complexes would underestimate soil movement on significant parts of the field.

> C = cover and management factor. C values range from 0.001 for well-managed woodland to 1.0 for tilled, continuous fallow. C for a given cropping and management system varies with rainfall distribution and planting dates. Generalized values for illustrative purposes are given in Table 9-8. Local values can be computed by a procedure published in Agriculture Handbook No. 282, or computed values may be obtained from the Soil Conservation Service. Values following construction can be estimated from Table 9-9.

Table 9-11. Matrix of Information on State Surface-Mined Area Reclamation Programs (December 1975) (Imhoff _et al.,_ 1975)

STATE	\<br\>STAGE OF PROGRAM DEVELOPMENT			STATE LAW			RECLAMATION--MAIN ACTIONS REQUIRED AND STANDARDS SET					
	ACT(s)	RULES AND REGULATIONS	TECHNICAL GUIDELINES	TITLE OF ACT(s)	ADMINISTERING AGENCY(ies)	MINERAL OR COMMODITY COVERED	CONTROL WATER FLOW AND QUALITY	CONSERVE AND REPLACE TOPSOIL	BACKFILL AND GRADE	REDUCE HIGHWALL OR PITWALL	BURY OR NEUTRALIZE TOXIC WASTES	REVEGETATE FOR BENEFICIAL USE
Alabama	X	X	--	Alabama Surface Mining Act of 1969 & Alabama Surface Mining Reclamation Act of 1975	Department of Industrial Relations and Surface Mining Reclamation Commission	All minerals except limestone, marble, & dolomite (coal covered by 1975 Act)	X	X	Strike-off top of spoil ridges to width ≥ 15 ft & cover coal seam with spoil to depth of ≥ 10 ft	Eliminate coal mine highwall, except at final cut	With 2 ft of earth or permanent water body	Standards for forests, grasses, & legumes; soil additives may be required
Alaska	NOTE: On State lands, reclamation requirements are established by the State of Alaska--on a case-by-case basis--as part of the terms of leases to mine operators. Most of the mineral deposits of Alaska lie on State or Federal lands (where reclamation requirements are a condition of leasing).											
Arizona	NOTE: The State of Arizona applies standard reclamation requirements to State Lands as a condition of mineral leases. Arizona also contains Federal lands where reclamation requirements are a condition of mineral leases. Some local units of government use land-use controls (e.g., zoning) and activity permits (e.g., minerals proceeding) to encourage reclamation.											
Arkansas	X	X	X	The Arkansas Open Cut Land Reclamation Act of 1971	Department of Pollution Control & Ecology	All minerals	X	Standards vary according to original natural conditions	All grades will be ≤ 33%; blade & grade to approximate original surface conditions	X	With 3 ft of earth or permanent water body	X
California	X	--	--	Surface Mining & Reclamation Act of 1971	Department of Pollution Control & Ecology	All minerals	X	--	--	--	--	--

Table 9-11, Continued

STATE	ACT(s)	RULES AND REGULATIONS	TECHNICAL GUIDELINES	TITLE OF ACT(s)	ADMINISTERING AGENCY(ies)	MINERAL OR COMMODITY COVERED	CONTROL WATER FLOW AND QUALITY	CONSERVE AND REPLACE TOPSOIL	BACKFILL AND GRADE	REDUCE HIGHWALL OR PITWALL	BURY OR NEUTRALIZE TOXIC WASTES	REVEGETATE FOR BENEFICIAL USE
	STAGE OF PROGRAM DEVELOPMENT			STATE LAW			RECLAMATION—MAIN ACTIONS REQUIRED AND STANDARDS SET					
Colorado	X	--	--	Colorado Open Mining Land Reclamation Act of 1973	Department of Natural Resources	Coal, sand, gravel, quarry aggregate, & construction limestone	X	--	Strike-off top of spoil ridges to width of >15 ft; achieve level or undulating skyline	--	--	X (Exceptions for unsuitable areas)
Connecticut	NOTE: Local governmental land-use controls and permit activities may be applicable to mining and reclamation.											
Delaware	NOTE: Local governmental land-use controls and permit activities may be applicable to mining and reclamation.											
Florida	X	--	--	Chapter 211, II Florida Statutes	Department of Natural Resources	All minerals	X (Lakes shall support fish or recreation)	X	All grades will be < 25%; blend peaks, ridges, & valleys; develop uninterrupted drainage	--	--	Plant coverage >80%; bare areas <1/4 acre
Georgia	X	X	X	Georgia Surface Mining Act of 1968, as amended	Department of Natural Resources	All minerals	X	X	Blend peaks, ridges, & valleys into a rolling topography suitable for plant growth	X (Except in solid rock)	With 2 ft of soil supporting vegetation	Attain high quality permanent cover

State					Law	Agency	Minerals covered		Topsoil	Grading	Final grade	Cover material	Revegetation
Hawaii	X	--	--	X	Chapter 181, Subtitle 3, Hawaii Statutes	Department of Land & Natural Resources	All minerals except sand, rock, gravel & construction materials	X	If necessary for end-use objective	Strike-off peaks & ridges of spoil & fill depressions	--	--	Quick cover grass crop, followed by reforestation, or conversion to farming
Illinois	X	X		X	Surface-Mined Land Conservation & Reclamation Act	Department of Mines & Minerals	All minerals	X	Row crops, 18"; Other uses, replace as practicable	Varies by planned use i.e. original grade for row crops; $\leq 30\%$ forest & wildlife; $\leq 50\%$ hay & pasture	To grade of $\leq 50\%$	With ½ ft of water or suitable material	Replant row crops if soils suitable. Detailed standards for other uses
Indiana	X	X		X	Chapter 344, Acts of 1967, Indiana Statutes	Department of Natural Resources	Coal, clay, & shale	X	--	Grades; row crops $<8\%$, pasture & hay $\leq 25\%$, forest & range $<33\%$ (slope lengths limited)	To grade of $<33\%$ or create lake in pit	With 2 ft of soil, overburden, or water	X
Iowa	X	X		X	An Act Relating to Surface Mining, as amended	Department of Soil Conservation	All minerals	X	In coal mine reclamation, strata more suitable than top soil may be used	Grade spoil to $\leq 25\%$, except where original land was steeper, then, blend with adjacent land	To grade of $\leq 33\%$	With 2 ft of spoil	X (Detailed guidelines available)
Kansas	X	X		X	Mined-Land Conservation & Reclamation Act	State Corporation Commission	Coal	X	As necessary to provide plant growth material	Rolling topography traversable for planned use; grade $<25\%$ (slope lengths limited)	To grade of $<25\%$ unless supported, as by a lake	With 2 ft of spoil or permanent water body	X

Table 9-11, continued

STATE(s)	RULES AND REGULATIONS	TECHNICAL GUIDELINES	TITLE OF ACT(s)	ADMINISTERING AGENCY(ies)	MINERAL OR COMMODITY COVERED	CONTROL WATER FLOW AND QUALITY	CONSERVE AND REPLACE TOPSOIL	BACKFILL AND GRADE	REDUCE HIGHWALL OR PITWALL	BURY OR NEUTRALIZE TOXIC WASTES	REVEGETATE FOR BENEFICIAL USE
						STATE LAW		RECLAMATION—MAIN ACTIONS REQUIRED AND STANDARDS SET			
Kentucky	X	X	Chapter 350, Kentucky Revised Statutes	Department for Natural Resources & Environmental Protection	All minerals	Detailed standards	--	Approximate original contour; grade bench tables to $\leq$10%	Auger mining face to $\leq$45°; other mining, backfill & cover coal to 4 ft	With 4 ft of overburden	X (Detailed guidelines available, e.g., time of planting)
Louisiana								NOTE: Local governmental land-use controls and permit activities may be applicable to mining and reclamation.			
Maine	X	--	1) Mining & Rehabilitation of Land Act, & 2) Site Location of Development Act	Department of Environmental Protection	All minerals (sand & gravel are covered only by Site Act)	X	X	X	--	--	X
Maryland	X	X	Maryland Strip Mining Law	Energy & Coastal zone Administration	Coal	X (pH range 6.8 to 8.5)	X	Area, approximate contour; terracing, grade the bench to <9% & outer slope grade to <70%	Eliminate highwall by backfill & cut	With 2 ft of overburden	Quick cover grass crop, followed by vegetation for end uses
Massachusetts								NOTE: Local governmental land-use controls and permit activities may be applicable to mining and reclamation.			

State				Enabling Act	Administering Agency	Minerals Covered		Specific Criteria	Grading	Slope of Face	Cover	Revegetation
Michigan	X	–	–	Mine Reclamation Act of 1970 as amended	Department of Natural Resources	All minerals except clay, gravel, marl, peat, or sand	–	–	–	–	–	–
Minnesota	X	–	–	Mineland Reclamation Act of 1971 as amended	Department of Natural Resources	Metallic minerals	–	–	–	–	–	–
Mississippi	NOTE: Local governmental land-use controls and permit activities may be applicable to mining and reclamation.											
Missouri	X	–	–	1) Reclamation of Mining Lands & 2) The Land Reclamation Act	Department of Natural Resources	Act 1) coal & barite; Act 2) clay, limestone, sand & gravel	–	–	Act 1) traversable for farming Act 2) traversable for intended uses & strike-off top of spoil ridges to width of >20 ft (forest & pasture)	Act 1) slope of face will be ≤25%	With 4 ft of earth supportive of vegetation	Appropriate to type of end use declared
Montana	X	X	X (Partial)	1) Montana Strip & Underground Mine Reclamation Act, & 2) Open Cut Mining Act, & 3) Montana Hard-Rock Mining Reclamation Act	Department of State Lands	Act 1) Coal & uranium; Act 2) bentonite, clay, phosphate rock, scoria, & sand & gravel; Act 3) other minerals	X	Act 1) specific criteria, e.g., pH range of 6.0 to 9.0	Act 1) grade to ≤20%	Act 1) slope of face will be ≤20%	Act 1) backfill with 8 ft of overburden	Suitable, permanent, diverse & primarily native species

Table 9-11, continued

STATE	STAGE OF PROGRAM DEVELOPMENT			STATE LAW			RECLAMATION—MAIN ACTIONS REQUIRED AND STANDARDS SET					
	RULES AND REGULATIONS	TECHNICAL GUIDELINES		TITLE OF ACT(s)	ADMINISTERING AGENCY(ies)	MINERAL OR COMMODITY COVERED	CONTROL WATER FLOW AND QUALITY	CONSERVE AND REPLACE TOPSOIL	BACKFILL AND GRADE	REDUCE HIGHWALL OR PITWALL	BURY OR NEUTRALIZE TOXIC WASTES	REVEGETATE FOR BENEFICIAL USE
Nebraska	NOTE: Local governmental land-use controls and permit activities may be applicable to mining and reclamation.											
Nevada	NOTE: Local governmental land-use controls and permit activities may be applicable to mining and reclamation.											
New Hampshire	NOTE: Local governmental land-use controls and permit activities may be applicable to mining and reclamation.											
New Jersey	NOTE: Local governmental land-use controls and permit activities may be applicable to mining and reclamation.											
New Mexico	X	X	--	New Mexico Coal Surfacemining Act	Bureau of Mines & Mineral Resources	Coal	X	X	Topography will be "gently undulating" or consistent with proposed end use	--	X	To serve selected end use
New York	X	--	--	N.Y. State Mined Land Reclamation Law	Department of Environmental Conservation	All minerals & mined topsoil	X	X	X	To be safe, stable & compatible with surrounding terrain	X	X
North Carolina	X	--	--	The Mining Act of 1971	Department of Natural & Economic Resources	All minerals	X	--	Minimizing earth slides & consistent with future land use	--	X	X (With appropriate local or State agency approval)

State			Law	Agency	Minerals		Plant growth material	Topography/Contour			
North Dakota	X	--	--	N. Dakota Century Code; Reclamation of Strip-Mined Land	Public Service Commission	Coal	X	Replace all available plant growth material, up to 5 ft thickness	Approximate original contour, or serve approved end use	Slope of face will be ≤35%	--	X
Ohio	X	X	--	1) Strip Mine Law, & 2) Surface Mine Law	Department of Natural Resources	Act 1) Coal, Act 2) All other minerals	X	X (or other plant-growth materials)	Approximate original contour, or serve approved end use	X	X	X
Oklahoma	X	--	--	Mining Lands Reclamation Act	Department of Mines	All minerals	--	--	Topography will be traversable for approved end use; slope of box cut overburden will be ≤25°	Suitable to serve end-use objective	With 3 ft of overburden	X (Exemptions; soils with poor texture, toxicity, & nutrient deficiency)
Oregon	X	X	--	Oregon Mined Land Reclamation Act, as amended	Department of Geology & Mineral Industries	All minerals	X	--	As appropriate for planned subsequent beneficial use	As appropriate for planned subsequent beneficial use	--	X
Pennsylvania	X	X	--	Surface Mining Conservation & Reclamation Act, as amended	Department of Environmental Resources	All minerals	X	X (12" of soil, conditions permitting, or all available topsoil)	Approximate original contour; terrace; or serve approved end use	Eliminate highwall	Varies with existing conditions	X
Rhode Island												
South Carolina	X	X	--	S. Carolina Mining Act	Land Resources Conservation Commission	All minerals	X	--	Minimizing slides & consistent with future land use	--	X	X (With appropriate local or state agency approval)

NOTE: Local governmental land-use controls and permit activities may be applicable to mining and reclamation.

Table 9-11, continued

STAGE OF PROGRAM DEVELOPMENT			STATE LAW			RECLAMATION--MAIN ACTIONS REQUIRED AND STANDARDS SET					
STATE	ACT(s) RULES AND REGULATIONS	ACT(s) TECHNICAL GUIDELINES	TITLE OF ACT(s)	ADMINISTERING AGENCY(ies)	MINERAL OR COMMODITY COVERED	CONTROL WATER FLOW AND QUALITY	CONSERVE AND REPLACE TOPSOIL	BACKFILL AND GRADE	REDUCE HIGHWALL OR PITWALL	BURY OR NEUTRALIZE TOXIC WASTES	REVEGETATE FOR BENEFICIAL USE
South Dakota	X	- -	Surface Mining Land Reclamation Act, as amended	Department of Agriculture	All minerals	X	X	"Achieve contour most beneficial to the proposed land use"	Slope will be $\leq 14°$	With 8 ft of compacted material or permanent water body	To create self-regenerative growth without irrigation
Tennessee	X	X	The Tenn. Surface Mining Act	Department of Conservation	All minerals except dimension stone, limestone, & marble	Detailed standards are in effect	X	Contour, fill benches prohibited on slopes >28°; Area, approximate original land surface	Eliminate highwall with complete backfill, sloped to bench $\leq 35°$	With 4 ft of compacted material or permanent water body	Where approved, permanent growth serving purpose at least as useful as pre-mining
Texas	X	- -	Texas Surface Mining & Reclamation Act	Railroad Commission of Texas	Coal, lignite, & uranium	X	Use stratum best for plant growth	Approximate original contour	X	X	Establish diverse self-regenerative cover suitable for approved end use
Utah	X	- -	Mined Land Reclamation Act of 1975	Department of Natural Resources	All minerals (including oil-shale &	X	X	X (where "practical")	- -	X	X (Priority to

State				Law	Agency	Minerals						
Vermont	X	--	--	Vermont's Land Use & Development Law	District Environmental Commissions & the Environmental Board	All minerals	--	--	--	--	--	--
Virginia	X	X	X	1) 45.1-198, & 2) Title 45.1-180, chap. 16	Department of Conservation & Economic Development	Act 1) coal, Act 2) all other minerals	X	--	"...retain spoil on bench insofar as feasible..."	"...reduce ...to the maximum extent practicable..."	With 4 ft of material suitable for plant growth	X
Washington	X	X	--	Surface-Mined Land Reclamation Act	Department of Natural Resources	All minerals	X	--	Conform to surrounding land area	Grade of wall in unconsolidated, <66%; wall slope in rock, <45°	With 2 ft of clean fill	X
West Virginia	X	X	X	Article 6, Chap. 20, Code of W.V., as amended	Department of Natural Resources	All minerals	Standards set forth in Drainage Handbook for Surface Mining	X	Fill benches denied on grades >65%; contour mined areas will be suitable for farm machinery	X	With 4 ft of material suitable for plant growth	Detailed standards
Wisconsin	X	--	--	Metallic Mining Reclamation Act	Department of Natural Resources	Metallic minerals	X	X	X	-- --	X	X
Wyoming	X	X	--	Wyoming Environmental Quality Act of 1973	Department of Environmental Quality	All minerals	X	Use most suitable plant growth materials	Approximate original contour; terrace; or serve approved end use	Stabilize; slope; minimize effect on landscape	X	X

Source: Imhoff, E.A., T.O. Friz, and J.R. LaFevers, A Guide to State Programs for the Reclamation of Surface Mined Areas, Geological Survey Circular 731.

P = factor for supporting practices. Its value can be obtained from Table 9-10. With no support practices, P=1.0. Support practices are erosion control factors during construction.

Example Soil Loss Problem

Using the soil loss equation, a theoretical strip mine of 10,000 acres in steep Kentucky mountain soils is computed. The R factor for rainfall is 200 from Figure 9-4. The K factor for a clay loam with very low organic content is 0.28 (Table 9-7). Since the steepest land has 20% slopes, from Figure 9-6 at 200 ft, the LS value is 6. The C value for at least six months will be 1.0 when the land is bare. After the strip mining is complete, slopes will be seeded and fertilized. The C factor is then reduced to 0.54 (Table 9-9). A downstream sediment basin is used during mining with chemical flocculants to settle silt. After the area is mined, the watershed is seeded and the sediment basin structure removed. During the mining period, the P factor is 0.2 (Table 9-10). With no supporting practices the P factor becomes 1, six months later.

Thus two equations for the year are appropriate:

$$A_1 = 200 \times .28 \times 6 \times 1 \times .2 = 67.2$$

$$A_2 = 200 \times .28 \times 6 \times .54 \times 1 = 181.4$$

$$67.2 \ A_1 = \text{ton/ac/} \frac{\text{yr}}{2} \text{ during mining for six months}$$

$$181.4 \ A_2 = \text{ton/ac/} \frac{\text{yr}}{2} \text{ during six months following mining operation}$$

$$A_1 + A_2 = \text{amount of soil lost per acre} \times 10,000 \text{ acres for the year}$$
$$= 2.5 \text{ million tons.}$$

The soil loss equation and supporting data tables were designed to predict long-time average losses for specific conditions. Specific-year losses may be substantially greater or smaller than the annual averages because of differences in the number, size and timing of erosive rainstorms and in other weather parameters.

FIRE DATA

The U.S. Department of the Interior (DOI), Bureau of Land Management (BLM), state offices and the Denver Service Center have fire reports on all fires on public lands. In addition, statistics are computerized for regions and can be requested by description of latitude and longitude. Western BLM state offices, locations and fire numbers are shown on Table 9-12.

Table 9-12. BLM State Fire Code and Fire Numbers (DOI, 1975[a])

Office	Code	Fire Numbers	Office	Code	Fire Numbers
ARIZONA			**NEW MEXICO**		
St. George	01	0001-0045	Socorro	02	4651-4700
Phoenix	02	0046-0090	Las Cruces	03	4701-4750
Safford	04	0091-0135	Roswell	06	4751-4800
Yuma	05	0136-0150	**OREGON OR WASHINGTON**		
CALIFORNIA			Lakeview	01	4801-5050
Bakersfield	01	0151-0300	Burns	02	5051-5350
Susanville	02	0301-0600	Vale	03	5351-5900
Redding	03	0601-0650	Princeville	05	5901-6200
Folsom	04	0651-0700	Baker	06	6201-6400
Ukiah	05	0701-0750	Salem	08	6401-6450
Riverside	06	0751-0800	Eugene	09	6451-6500
COLORADO			Roseburg	10	6501-6550
Craig	01	0801-0925	Medford	11	6551-6800
Montrose	03	0926-1025	Coos Bay	12	6801-6850
Canon City	05	1026-1075	Spokane	13	6851-6900
Grand Junction	07	1076-1200	**UTAH**		
IDAHO			Salt Lake City	02	6901-6950
Boise	01	1201-1550	Fillmore	03	6951-7000
Burley	02	1551-1900	Cedar City	04	7001-7050
Idaho Falls	03	1901-2100	Richfield	05	7051-7100
Salmon	04	2101-2200	Monticello	06	7101-7150
Shoshone	05	2201-2550	Price	07	7151-7200
Coeur d'Alene	06	2551-2600	Vernal	08	7201-7250
MONTANA			Kanab	11	7251-7300
Malta	01	2601-2700	**WYOMING**		
Miles City[a]	02	2701-2800	Worland	01	7301-7360
Billings	04	2801-2850	Rawlins	03	7361-7450
Dillon	05	2851-2950	Rock Springs	04	7451-7550
Lewistown	06	2951-3100	Casper	06	7551-7600
Missoula	07	3101-3150	**ALASKA**		
NEVADA			Anchorage	01	7601-8475
Elko	01	3151-3500	Fairbanks	02	8476-9350
Winnemucca	02	3501-3650	**BOISE INTERAGENCY FIRE CENTER**		
Carson City	03	3651-4000	Forest Service		9351-9650
Ely	04	4001-4200	National Park Service		9651-9700
Las Vegas	05	4201-4500	Bureau of Indian Affairs		9701-9750
Battle Mountain	06	4501-4600	All Other Agencies		9751-9800
NEW MEXICO					
Albuquerque	01	4601-4650			

[a]Lake States Office and Makotopi Project.

Fires are reported for both wildfires and control burns in most western states. Fire "classes" are by size of fire:

- Class A – 0 - .25 acres
- Class B – .26 - 9 acres
- Class C – 10 - 99 acres
- Class D – 100 - 299 acres
- Class E – 300 - 999 acres
- Class F – 1,000 - 4,999 acres
- Class G – 5,000 acres or more

Fire reports contain location and ownership of land burned, and costs of suppress fires and causes are coded statistically. There are 30 typical causes listed for fires. Land is classified into a value class to code a value-at-risk scale. Suppression efforts in terms of men, equipment, time, retardants and total force are recorded.

The amount of damage is recorded by severity of burn, acres burned and value. Table 9-13 gives estimated dollar value per acre for soil loss, watershed, location, timber, recreation, wildlife and grazing damage. Real estate value would be available from the county tax assessor.

Although a large majority of western fires (Figure 9-7) are caused naturally by lightning, there are potential risks from man's actions. Some EIS actions which may increase fire potential are: water withdrawal, aircraft use, exhaust from equipment, land clearing, slash burning, blasting, military maneuvers, power lines and accidents ranging from construction crew's smoking, explosions and oil spills.

Another physical factor, which may affect the proposed action is earthquake risk. Figure 9-8 illustrates national risk areas, based on velocity. The low risk areas are shown as 0.10 isopaths, representing effective peak velocity of 3 in./sec, ranging to high risk areas of 0.40, on the West Coast. Figure 9-9 illustrates potential earthquake risk of fractions of g, or accelerations due to gravity. High risk areas are 0.40. Figure 9-10 combines these factors to a "shaking hazard," with contours showing maximum shaking expected in a 50-year period. For example, a contour at 60% of gravity means a 90% certainty that the region will not experience ground shaking more than 60% of the force of gravity. Figure 9-11 combines all earthquake data to a seismic risk map, of minor, moderate or major risk areas. Actions located in "major" areas should include consideration of local seismicity data. Historical seismicity data are available for specific locations, by latitude and longitude, from the Environmental Data Service, NOAA, Department of Commerce, Boulder, Colorado. Table 9-14 shows some of the larger earthquakes in the U.S., lower 48 states only. Richter

Table 9-13. BLM Guide for Resource Damage
Estimates from Fires (DOI, 1975[b])

Description of Resource in Place	Dollar Damage per Acre by Severity of Burn		
	Severe (1)	Medium (2)	Light (3)
Soil Resource			
– has a high degree of instability and is subject to potentially critical wind or water erosion loss. Erosion condition class severe as determined for unit resource analysis maps.	20-25	10-20	5-10
– is unstable and erosion potential is high. Erosion condition class *Critical* as determined for URA maps.	10-15	5-10	5
– is somewhat unstable and erosion is moderate. Erosion condition class *Moderate*.	5-10	5	3-5
– poses little nongeologic erosion potential. Erosion condition class *Slight*.	5	3-5	<3
– is stable and area has no erosion potential. Erosion condition class *Stable*.	3-5	<3	<3
Watershed Resource			
– is a domestic watershed directly serving a standard metropolitan statistical area.	30-40	20-30	10-15
– is a domestic watershed directly serving a nonmetropolitan statistical area.	20-30	10-15	5-10
– is part of an established hydroelectric and/or irrigation river basin.	5-10	3-5	<3
Location Resource			
– is part of or immediately adjacent to a standard metropolitan statistical area and/or may be an integral portion of area's complex and base.	20-30	10-20	5
– is part of a populated area and community complex.	10-20	5-10	3-5
– has a high and real potential of becoming an integral part of a community.	5-10	3-5	<3
– has no potential for populated community importance in foreseeable future.	3-5	<3	<3
Timber Resource[a]			
– is an integral part of a formal management plan and cutting cycle.	80-100	40-80	20-40
– has present or foreseeable commercial demand.	40-60	20-40	10-20
– is of sparse commercial or any age commercial demand.	20-40	10-20	3-5
– is of sparse commercial or any age noncommercial timber.	20-40	10-20	3-5
– has no growth on site and is not generally suited for timber.	<3	<3	<3

Table 9-13. Continued

Description of Resource in Place	Dollar Damage per Acre by Severity of Burn		
	Severe (1)	Medium (2)	Light (3)
Recreation Resource			
— has unique or specific recreation value and is being used heavily.	20-30	10-20	5-10
— is presently receiving heavy use.	10-20	5-10	3-5
— is presently receiving moderate use.	5-10	3-5	<3
— is presently receiving light use.	3-5	<3	<3
Wildlife Resource			
— is a critical limiting habitat for fish and/or wildlife.	30-60	10-30	5-10
— receives seasonal use by fish and/or wildlife.	15-25	10-15	3-5
— has potential for increased fish and wildlife population.	5-15	3-5	<3
— has no potential for future wildlife.	<3	<3	<3
Grazing Resource[a]			
— is an integral part of a scientific range study.	20-30	10-20	5-10
— is an integral part of a grazing allotment.	5-10	5	3-5
— is producing forage vegetation but is not presently an integral part of a grazing allotment.	5	3-5	<3
— is producing no forage vegetation.	0	0	0

[a]Calculate actual volume and value of commercial timber lost and add value to the total dollar damage determined for the area.

magnitudes can be compared with length and width of measured displacement across the zone of quake. Figure 9-12 shows the direct relationship between energy released and magnitude on the Richter scale from 4 to 10.

In earthquake-prone areas, projects should be sited correctly and designed to resist horizontal and vertical gravity forces. Figure 9-13 provides some design and location factors for siting structures on faults. Comparison of historical data of quakes, such as time since last displacement (Figure 9-12) and displacement (Table 9-14) distances, can result in prediction of necessary design for structures. While the EIS writer need not design the action, he must assess the potential safety of structures located in danger areas.

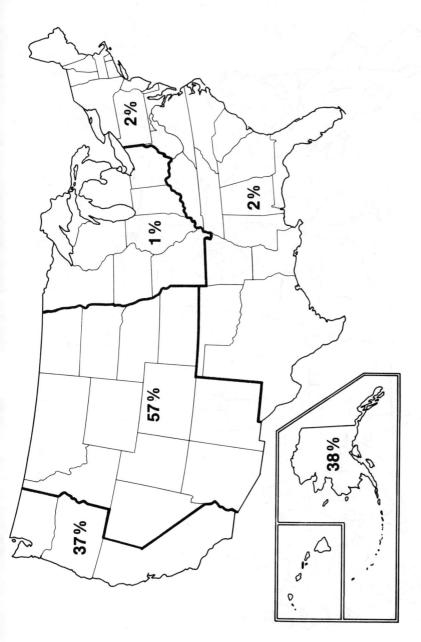

Figure 9-7. Percentages of fires caused by lightning (Taylor, 1973; Barney, 1971).

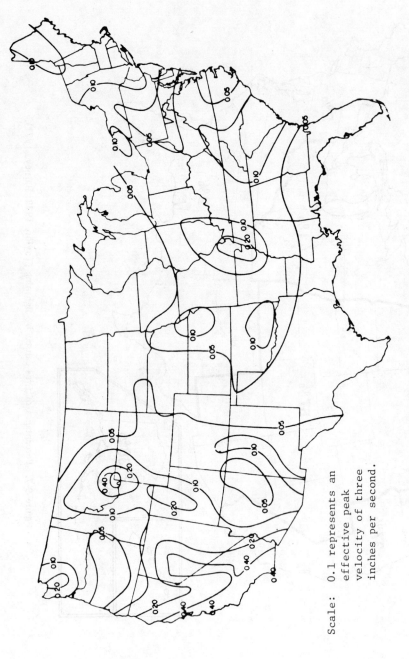

Scale: 0.1 represents an effective peak velocity of three inches per second.

Figure 9-8. Potential earthquake risk (velocities) (Donovan, 1977).

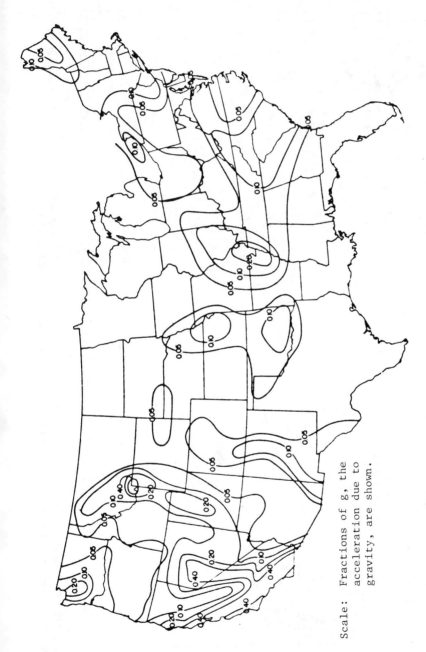

Scale: Fractions of g, the
acceleration due to
gravity, are shown.

Figure 9-9. Potential earthquake risk (accelerations) (Donovan, 1977).

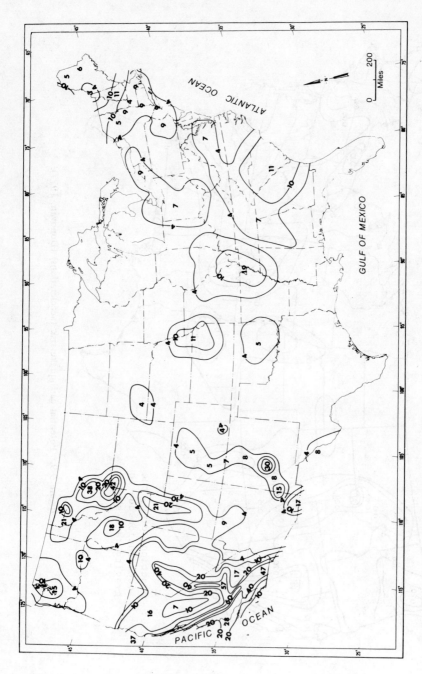

Figure 9-10. Probable levels of earthquake shaking hazards. Maximum amount of shaking is likely to occur at least once in a 50-year period. Source: U.S. Geological Survey, Department of the Interior, 1976 (DOI, 1977a).

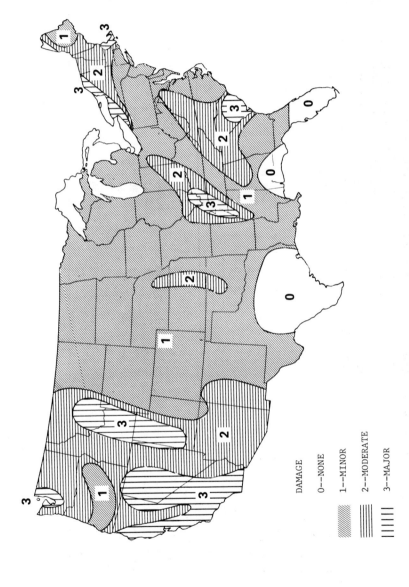

Figure 9-11. Prediction: seismic risk map (DOC, 1969).

Table 9-14. Length and Amount of Displacement Related to Earthquakes (Flawn, 1970)

Date	Location	Richter Magnitude	Length (mi)	Observed Displacement		
				Maximum Vertical Component	Maximum Horizontal Component	Maximum Total Across Zone
1857	Fort Tejon, California	7.75	40-250	–	Large	–
1868	Hayward, California	7	–	–	Some	–
1872	Owens Valley, California	7.25	50	13 ft	18 ft	–
1899	San Jacinto, California	6.75	2	–	–	–
1906	San Francisco, California	8.3	190 or 270	3 ft	21 ft	16 ft
1915	Pleasant Valley, Nevada	7.6	24	15 ft	–	15 ft
1932	Cedar Mountains, Nevada	7.3	38	24 in.	34 in.	35 in.
1934	Excelsior Mountains	6.5	0.85	5 in.	–	5 in.
1934	Colorado River Delta, Baja, California	7.1	–	–	–	–
1940	Imperial Valley, California	7.1	40	–	19 ft	19 ft
1947	Manix, California	6.2	1	–	3 in.	3 in.
1950	Fort Sage Mountains, California	5.6	5.5	5-8 in.	–	8 in.
1951	Superstition Hills, California	5.6	1.9	–	Slight	Slight
1952	Kern County, California	7.2	40	4 ft	2-3 ft	3.6 ft
1954	Rainbow Mountains, Nevada	6.6	11	12 in.	–	12 in.
1954	Fallon, Nevada	6.8	14	30 in.	–	30 in.
1954	Fairview Peak, Nevada	7.2	35	14 ft	12 ft	18.5
1954	Dixie Valley, Nevada	6.9	31	7 ft	7 ft	7 ft
1956	San Miguel, Baja, California	6.8	12	36 in.	31 in.	36 in.
1966	Parkfield, California	5.6	25	–	4 in.	4 in.

COMPARATIVE SIZE AND DAMAGE OF EARTHQUAKES ON RICHTER SCALE

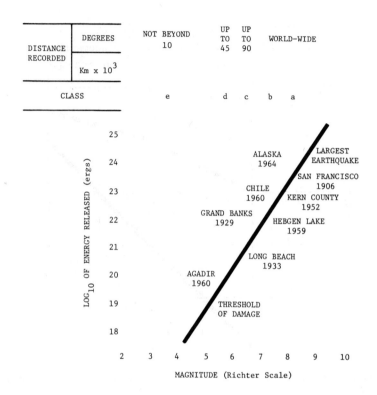

Figure 9-12. Energy release on the Richter Scale for earthquakes.

Figure 9-14 shows another danger area, the zone of volcanic activity. A line of active volcanoes is found along Alaska's southern coast, and another line from Oregon to Northern California. While volcanic areas of eastern Oregon, Idaho and Nevada are no longer active, the EIS would normally note location of actions within these zones.

Many environmental impact statements involve large tracts of public lands, and converting these lands to other uses, such as grazing, timber production, military bases, etc. Alternatives should include using that land for some other productive use. In many cases, "short-term uses" vs "long-term losses" is a very difficult section to write. Mineral production can be used for both of those comparative sections of an EIS. The land may serve as a potential for future mining of a valuable nonrenewable resource.

LOCATION OF STRUCTURES ON FAULTS

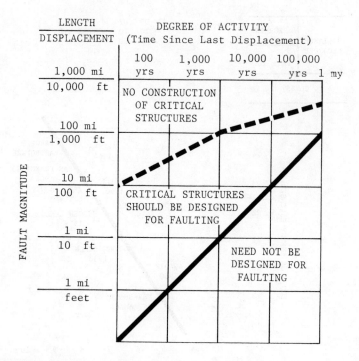

Figure 9-13. Physical criteria for site selection and evaluation (Albee and Smith, 1967).

Committment of the land, for example, to a military use such as bombing, could restrict future exploration for minerals. Therefore, a short-term use could foreclose long-term options.

Table 9-15 shows mineral production and value by state. The EIS writer notes the potential loss of the resource in dollars or acres. If the site has an important metal or mineral, the next step is to order location maps of those minerals. Table 9-16 gives references for available U.S. mineral maps of the U.S. Geological Survey.

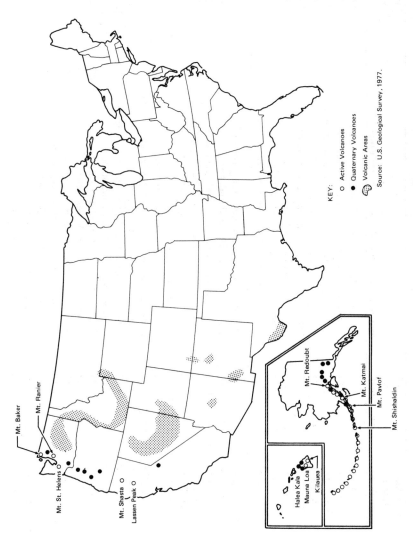

Figure 9-14. Volcanoes of the U.S. (DOI, 1977b).

Table 9-15. State Mineral Production (DOI, 1976)

State	Value (thousands $)	Rank	% of U.S. total	Principal Minerals, in Order of Value	Value of Mineral Production/sq mi $	Rank
Alabama	764,746	19	1.39	Coal, petroleum, cement, stone	14,818	16
Alaska	448,437	23	0.81	Petroleum, sand and gravel, natural gas, stone	765	50
Arizona	1,562,234	9	2.83	Copper, molybdenum, sand and gravel, cement	13,715	18
Arkansas	406,821	26	0.74	Petroleum, bromine, stone, natural gas	7,660	27
California	2,797,080	3	5.07	Petroleum, cement, sand and gravel, natural gas	17,626	13
Colorado	750,299	20	1.36	Petroleum, perlite, coal, sand and gravel	7,197	29
Connecticut	35,362	47	0.06	Stone, sand and gravel, feldspar, lime	7,060	30
Delaware	3,793[a]	50	(b)	Sand and gravel, magnesium compounds, clays, gem stones	1,844	44
Florida	1,043,895	14	1.89	Phosphate rock, petroleum, stone, cement	17,826	12
Georgia	363,100	29	0.66	Clays, stone, cement, sand and gravel	6,167	32
Hawaii	42,042	44	0.08	Stone, cement, sand and gravel, pumice	6,518	31
Idaho	208,558	31	0.38	Silver, phosphate rock, zinc, sand and gravel	2,496	39
Illinois	1,149,210	11	2.08	Coal, petroleum, stone, sand and gravel	20,376	9
Indiana	440,690	24	0.08	Coal, cement, stone, petroleum	12,143	20
Iowa	176,720	32	0.32	Cement, stone, sand and gravel, gypsum	3,139	37
Kansas	889,398	18	1.61	Petroleum, natural gas, natural gas liquids, cement	10,812	22
Kentucky	2,563,210	4	4.65	Coal, stone, petroleum, natural gas	63,454	8
Louisiana	8,146,578	2	14.77	Petroleum, natural gas, natural gas liquids, sulfur	167,891	1
Maine	36,348	45	0.07	Cement, sand and gravel, zinc, stone	1,094	48
Maryland	172,880	33	0.31	Coal, stone, cement, sand and gravel	16,345	14
Massachusetts	62,109	43	0.11	Stone, sand and gravel, lime, clays	7,522	28
Michigan	1,040,067	15	1.89	Iron ore, petroleum, cement, copper	17,866	11
Minnesota	1,026,366	16	1.86	Iron ore, sand and gravel, stone, cement	12,209	19
Mississippi	391,155	28	0.71	Petroleum, natural gas, sand and gravel, cement	8,198	26
Missouri	691,049	21	1.25	Lead, cement, stone, zonc	9,916	23
Montana	574,801	22	1.04	Petroleum, copper, coal, cement	3,907	34

State	Value	Rank	%	Principal minerals	Value	Rank
Nebraska	98,634	42	0.18	Petroleum, cement, sand and gravel, stone	1,217	47
Nevada	257,876	30	0.47	Copper, gold, sand and gravel, diatomite	2,333	40
New Hampshire	13,691	48	0.02	Sand & gravel, stone, clays, gem stones	1,472	45
New Jersey	140,748	37	0.26	Stone, sand and gravel, zinc, magnesium compounds	17,962	10
New Mexico	1,941,544	8	3.52	Petroleum, natural gas, copper, natural gas liquids	15,958	15
New York	440,573	25	0.80	Cement, stone, zinc, salt	8,887	25
North Carolina	155,869	35	0.28	Stone, sand and gravel, cement, feldspar	2,964	38
North Dakota	159,427	34	0.29	Petroleum, coal, natural gas liquids, sand and gravel	2,256	41
Ohio	1,107,670	12	2.01	Coal, stone, lime, cement	26,871	7
Oklahoma	2,123,690	7	3.85	Petroleum, natural gas, natural gas liquids, cement	30,374	6
Oregon	103,920	40	0.19	Stone, sand and gravel, cement, nickel	1,072	49
Pennsylvania	2,374,512	6	4.30	Coal, cement, stone, lime	52,379	4
Rhode Island	5,982	49	0.01	Stone, sand and gravel, gem stones	4,928	33
South Carolina	105,171	39	0.19	Cement, stone, clays, sand and gravel	3,387	36
South Dakota	102,627	41	0.19	Gold, cement, stone, sand and gravel	1,332	46
Tennessee	395,608	27	0.71	Coal, stone, zinc, cement	9,365	24
Texas	13,711,144	1	24.85	Petroleum, natural gas, natural gas liquids, cement	51,288	5
Utah	952,045	17	1.72	Copper, petroleum, coal, gold	11,212	21
Vermont	35,453	46	0.06	Stone, asbestos, sand and gravel, talc	3,690	35
Virginia	1,058,207	13	1.92	Coal, stone, cement, sand and gravel	25,926	8
Washington	143,916	36	0.26	Cement, sand and gravel, stone, coal	2,110	42
West Virginia	2,403,177	5	4.36	Coal, natural gas, stone, cement	99,383	2
Wisconsin	114,763	38	0.21	Stone, sand and gravel, iron ore, cement	2,044	43
Wyoming	1,437,200	10	2.60	Petroleum, sodium compounds, coal, uranium	14,678	17
Total	55,172,000		100.00		15,262	

aIncomplete total.
bLess than 0.5%.

Table 9-16. Mineral Resource Maps of
the United States (DOI, 1971-1976)

Publication No.	Mineral	Year	Scale
MR13	Copper	1962	1:3,168,000
MR14	Borates	1962	1:3,168,000
MR15	Lead	1962	1:3,168,000
MR16	Vanadium	1962	1:3,168,000
MR17	Asbestos	1962	1:3,168,000
MR18	Pyrophyllite, kyanite	1962	1:3,168,000
MR19	Zinc	1962	1:3,168,000
MR20	Antimony	1962	1:3,168,000
MR21	Uranium	1962	1:3,168,000
MR22	Bismuth	1962	1:3,168,000
MR23	Manganese	1962	1:3,168,000
MR24	Gold	1962	1:3,168,000
MR25	Tungsten	1962	1:3,168,000
MR26	Chromite	1962	1:3,168,000
MR27	Magnesite, brucite	1962	1:3,168,000
MR28	Thorium	1962	1:3,168,000
MR29	Titanium	1962	1:3,168,000
MR30	Mercury	1962	1:3,168,000
MR31	Talc, soapstone	1962	1:3,168,000
MR32	Gold, silver[a]	1962	1:2,500,000
MR33	Gypsum, anhydrite	1962	1:3,168,000
MR34	Silver	1962	1:3,168,000
MR35	Beryllium	1962	1:3,168,000
MR36	Niobium, tantalum	1963	1:3,168,000
MR37	Kaolinitic clay	1963	1:3,168,000
MR38	Placer gold[a]	1964	1:2,500,000
MR40	Iron[a]	—	1:2,500,000
MR41	Industrial minerals[a]	1964	1:2,500,000
MR43	Barite	1965	1:3,168,000
MR44	Tin	1965	1:3,168,000
MR51	Iron	1967	1:3,168,000
MR52	Antimony[a]	1970	1:2,500,000
MR53	Bismuth[a]	1970	1:2,500,000
MR54	Mercury[a]	1970	1:2,500,000
MR55	Molybdenum	1970	1:3,168,000
MR56	Uranium, thorium[a]	1970	1:2,500,000
PB233 217/AS	Metallic minerals[a]	1972	——
MR60	Fluorite	1974	1:3,168,000
MR61	Cobalt[a]	1974	1:2,500,000
MR62	Copper[a]	1974	1:2,500,000
MR64	Platinum[a]	1975	1:2,500,000
MR65	Tin[a]	1974	1:2,500,000
MR66	Tungsten[a]	1975	1:2,500,000
MR67	Zinc[a]	1975	1:2,500,000
MR68	Chromite[a]	1975	1:2,500,000
MR69	Lead	1975	1:2,500,000

[a]Alaska

Table 9-17 gives the user comparative data for the importance and value of the minerals present in the study area. Both world and U.S. production are given. Supply and demand figures are given for each mineral or metal. The second half of Table 9-17 is devoted to data to help the user interpret impacts of mining minerals. The crude ore, waste and ratio of material handled to marketable products, gives the user a quantifiable waste of resources. It helps to identify restoration or by-products left, after the mining, as an environmental "cost". The dollar value column gives "benefits" of that action. The last two columns compare mining techniques used to extract the minerals. Those that show 100% strip mined (*i.e.,* gypsum) do the greatest environmental damage. Those that are removed by drilling and blasting, however, would have noise as an impact. Table 9-18 gives alternate locations of mineral productions.

Table 9-17. U.S. Minerals Supply–Demand and World Production (DOI, 1976)

MINERAL/METAL	UNIT MEASURE	WORLD PRODUCTION*	U.S. PRODUCTION*	U.S. % OF WORLD PROD.	TOTAL NET* SUPPLY**	DEMAND* U.S. 1974	DEMAND YEAR 2000	MATERIAL HANDLED BY MINES (1000 ton) CRUDE ORE	WASTE	RATIO***	$ VALUE[k] PER TON*	MINING (%) STRIP	DRILL & BLAST
Carbon: black	million lb.	7,916	3,390	43	—	—	—	—	—	—	—	—	—
Bituminous coal	1000 ton	2,327,860	587,928	25	551,263[g]	547,161	1,000,000[g]	—	—	—	—	—	—
Lignite coal	1000 ton	918,099	15,478	2	—	—	—	—	—	—	—	—	—
Anthracite	1000 ton	206,258	6,617	3	—	—	—	—	—	—	—	—	—
Gashouse coke	1000 ton	8,964	—	—	5,448[g]	5,448	2,000	—	—	—	—	—	—
Oven coke	1000 ton	408,741	61,581	15	—	—	—	—	—	—	—	—	—
Natural gas[a]	million cu.ft.	47,137,672[a]	21,600,522[a]	46	—	21,512[h]	49,000[h]	—	—	—	—	—	—
Peat	1000 ton	220,344	731	—	—	—	—	—	—	—	—	—	—
Petroleum (crude)	1000 barrels	20,537,727	3,202,585	16	—	—	—	—	—	—	—	—	—
Asbestos	1000 ton	4,536	113	3	824	846	2,430	1,470	371	17:1	8.08	—	66
Barite	1000 ton	4,789	1,106	23	1,871	—	—	1,960	2,370	4:1	9.05	58	25
Cement	1000 ton	776,210	82,888	11	—	83	—	—	—	—	7.49	—	0
Clay, China	1000 ton	17,715	6,393	36	58,680[e]	61,087[e]	174,000[e]	54,200[e]	46,300[e]	2:1	—	—	—
Diamond	1000 carats	44,085	—	—	—	—	—	—	—	—	—	—	—
Feldspar	1000 ton	3,174	854	27	—	—	—	1,190	163	2:1	10.54	—	93
Fluorspar	1000 ton	5,082	201	4	1,531	—	—	612	129	3:1	28.71	0	100
Graphite	1000 ton	432	—	—	—	—	—	—	—	—	—	—	100
Gypsum	1000 ton	66,109	11,999	18	25,985	—	—	12,400	12,400	1:1	4.32	100	81
Lime	1000 ton	121,640	21,645	18	—	21,606	—	—	—	—	—	—	—
Magnesite	1000 ton	10,195	—	—	—	—	—	—	—	—	—	100	100
Mica[b]	1000 lb.	520,946	273,932	53	230,000[f]	—	—	—	—	—	9.04[j]	—	10
Nitrogen (Agric.)	1000 ton	45,037	10,088	22	10,660	14,946	—	155,000	242,000	9:1	3.29	97	5
Phosphate rock	1000 ton	121,601	45,686	38	6,084	6,084	14,455	—	—	—	—	—	—
Potash	1000 ton	26,068	2,552	10	—	—	—	3,930	141	1:1	2.41	—	14
Pumice	1000 ton	14,422	3,964	28	—	—	—	—	—	—	—	—	—
Pyrites	1000 long ton	23,368	424	2	—	—	—	—	—	—	—	—	—
Salt	1000 ton	172,228	46,423	27	49,373	49,373	158,900	13,400	737	1:1	7.38	—	100
Strontium	1000 long ton	108	—	—	—	—	—	—	—	—	—	—	—
Sulfur	1000 long ton	50,861	11,419	22	10,968	10,014	30,000	—	—	—	—	—	—
Talc, soapstone	1000 ton	6,023	1,268	21	1,102	—	—	—	—	—	—	99	75
Vermiculite	1000 ton	554	341	62	—	—	—	—	—	—	—	—	58

Mineral	Unit												
Antimony^c	ton	77,751	661	1	45,000	18,041	48,000	--	--	--	--	--	100
Arsenic	ton	54,764	--	--	--	--	--	--	--	--	--	--	--
Bauxite	1000 long ton	76,989	1,949	3	--	--	--	3,140	9,720	5:1	10.48	--	87
Bismuth	1000 lb.	8,556	--	--	15,000	--	--	--	--	--	--	--	--
Cobalt	ton	33,504	--	--	--	--	--	--	--	--	--	--	94
Copper^c	1000 ton	8,105	1,594	20	--	--	--	293,000	765,000	569:1	9.01	99	100
Gold	1000 troy oz.	39,780	1,127	3	--	--	--	4,290^i	9,250^i	19:1^i	23.00^i	87-98	82
Iron ore	1000 long ton	879,414	84,355	10	130,691	138,160	--	240,000	252,000	6:1	5.80	92	29
Lead^c	1000 ton	3,845	664	17	--	--	--	10,500	2,640	18:1	41.88	<1	9
Mercury	1000 76-lb. flask	262	2	1	62	59	102	31	564	131:1	16.94	99	100
Molybdenum^c	1000 lb.	188,274	112,011	60	39,658	63,476	188,000	--	--	--	--	--	12
Nickel^c	1000 ton	826	17	2	241	--	--	--	--	--	--	--	0
Platinum	1000 troy oz.	5,759,822	12,657	--	4,711	1,981	3,157	629	268	0.1:1	--	--	70
Silver	1000 troy oz.	295,562	33,762	11	--	177,015	420,000	762	149	--	81.92	14	93
Tungsten	1000 lb.	82,357	7,381	9	17,745	16,298	76,400	6,320	144,000	8969:1	36.49	13	21
Uranium oxide	ton	24,176	11,528	48	14,000	11,900	73,113	--	--	--	--	99	50
Vanadium^c	ton	22,149	4,870	22	--	--	--	--	--	--	--	--	--
Zinc^c	1000 ton	6,384	500	8	--	--	--	--	--	--	--	--	--
Aluminum	1000 ton	14,517	4,903	34	5,247	6,294	28,400	--	--	--	--	--	--
Cadmium	ton	18,780	3,333	18	5,204	2,194	7,100	--	--	--	--	--	--
Copper	1000 ton	8,148	1,570	19	2,764	--	--	--	--	--	--	--	--
Pig iron	1000 ton	566,534	95,477	17	96,182	--	--	--	--	--	--	--	--
Lead	1000 ton	3,821	684	18	1,426	1,599	2,730	--	--	--	--	--	--
Selenium	1000 lb.	2,621	644	25	--	--	--	--	--	--	--	--	--
Steel^d	1000 ton	779,349	145,720	19	155,478	--	--	8,270	--	--	--	--	--
Tin	long ton	225,501	6,000	3	51,000	1,673	--	--	--	--	--	--	0
Zinc	1000 ton	5,968	555	9	1,340	--	3,090	--	2,410	26:1	36.70	2	99

*1974

**includes primary shipments, stockpile, imports minus exports

***units of material handled to units of marketable product

a - marketable
b - includes scrap
c - ore and concentrate
d - ingots and castings
e - all clays

f - minus scrap
g - included above
h - dry residual, excludes extraction loss
i - lode ore
j - scrap
k - principal mineral product + byproduct

Source: USGS, 1976; Minerals Yearbook, 1974.

Table 9-18. Minerals Produced in the United States (DOI, 1976)

Mineral	Principal Producing States, in Order of Quantity
Antimony ore and concentrate	Idaho, Montana, Nevada
Aplite	Virginia
Asbestos	California; Vermont, Arizona, North Carolina
Asphalt (native)	Texas, Utah, Alabama, Missouri
Barite	Nevada, Missouri, Georgia, Arkansas
Bauxite	Arkansas, Alabama, Georgia
Beryllium concentrate	Utah
Boron minerals	California
Bromine	Arkansas, Michigan, California
Calcium-magnesium chloride	Michigan and California
Carbon dioxide (natural)	New Mexico, California, Colorado, Utah
Cement	California, Texas, Pennsylvania, Michigan
Clays	Georgia, Texas, Ohio, North Carolina
Coal	Kentucky, West Virginia, Pennsylvania, Illinois
Copper (mine)	Arizona, Utah, New Mexico, Montana
Diatomite	California, Nevada, Washington
Emery	New York
Feldspar	North Carolina, Connecticut, Georgia, California
Fluorspar	Illinois, Montana, Texas, Nevada
Garnet, abrasive	Idaho and New York
Gold (mine)	South Dakota, Nevada, Utah, Arizona
Graphite	Texas
Gypsum	California, Michigan, Texas, Iowa
Helium	Kansas, Texas, Oklahoma, Arizona
Iodine	Michigan
Iron ore	Minnesota, Michigan, California, Wyoming
Kyanite	Virginia, Georgia, Florida
Lead (mine)	Missouri, Idaho, Colorado, Utah
Lime	Ohio, Pennsylvania, Missouri, Texas
Lithium minerals	North Carolina, Nevada, California
Magnesite	Nevada
Magnesium chloride	Texas
Magnesium compounds	Michigan, California, New Jersey, Florida
Manganiferous ore	Minnesota and New Mexico
Manganiferous residuum	New Jersey
Marl, greensand	New Jersey
Mercury	California, New York, Nevada, Alaska
Mica, scrap	North Carolina, Alabama, Georgia, South Carolina
Molybdenum	Colorado, Arizona, New Mexico, Utah
Natural gas	Texas, Louisiana, Oklahoma, New Mexico
Natural gas liquids	Texas, Louisiana, Oklahoma, New Mexico
Nickel	Oregon
Olivine	Washington and North Carolina

Table 9-18. Continued.

Mineral	Principal Producing States, in Order of Quantity
Peat	Michigan, Illinois, Indiana, Florida
Perlite	New Mexico, Arizona, California, Nevada
Petroleum, crude	Texas, Louisiana, California, Oklahoma
Phosphate rock	Florida, Idaho, Tennessee, North Carolina
Platinum-group metals	Alaska
Potassium salts	New Mexico, Utah, California
Pumice	Oregon, California, Arizona, New Mexico
Pyrites ore and concentrate	Tennessee, Colorado, Arizona
Rare-earth metal concentrate	California, Georgia, Florida
Salt	Louisiana, Texas, New York, Ohio
Sand and gravel	Alaska, California, Michigan, Illinois, Texas
Silver (mine)	Idaho, Arizona, Montana, Utah
Sodium carbonate (natural)	Wyoming and California
Sodium sulfate (natural)	California, Colorado, Nevada
Staurolite	Florida
Stone	Pennsylvania, Illinois, Texas, Florida
Sulfur (Frasch)	Texas and Louisiana
Talc, soapstone, pyrophyllite	New York, Montana, Vermont, Texas
Tin	Colorado, New Mexico, Alaska
Titanium concentrate	New York, Florida, New Jersey, Georgia
Tripoli	Illinois, Oklahoma, Arkansas, Pennsylvania
Tungsten concentrate	California, Colorado, Nevada
Uranium	New Mexico, Wyoming, Colorado, Utah
Vanadium	Arkansas, Colorado, Idaho, Utah
Vermiculite	Montana and South Carolina
Wollastonite	New York
Zinc (mine)	New York, Missouri, Tennessee, Colorado
Zircon concentrate	Florida and Georgia

REFERENCES

Agriculture, U.S. Department of, Agriculture Research Service. *Agriculture Handbook* No. 282 (1965).

Agriculture, U.S. Department of, Soil Conservation Service. "List of Published Soil Surveys" (1977).

Albee, A. L., and J. L. Smith. "Geologic Site Criteria for Nuclear Power Plant Location," *Soc. Min. Eng. Trans.* (December 1967).

Barney, R. "Selected Interior Alaska Wildfire Statistics with Long-Term Comparisons," USDA Forest Service, Research Note, PNW 154 (1971).

Commerce, U.S. Department of, National Oceanographic Atmospheric Administration. "National Ocean Survey," Washington, D.C. (1969).

Donovan, N. C. Paper to American Society of Civil Engineers, *Technol. Rev.* (May 1977).

Flawn, P. T. *Environmental Geology* (New York: Harper and Row, 1970).

Hammond, E. H. Physical, Subdivisions Map, *The National Atlas of the United States* (1965).

Imhoff, E. A., T. O. Friz and J. R. LaFevers. "A Guide to State Programs for the Reclamation of Surface Mined Areas," *U.S. Geol. Surv. Circ.* 731 (1975).

Interior, U.S. Department of, Bureau of Land Management. "Fire Code Numbers" (1975a).

Interior, U.S. Department of, Bureau of Land Management. "Fire Value of Resources Lost," U.S. Government Printing Office 1975-680-603/528 Reg. 8 (1975b).

Interior, U.S. Department of, Bureau of Mines. *Minerals Yearbook:* Vol. I, *Metals, Minerals, and Fuels* (Washington, D.C.: U.S. Government Printing Office, 1976).

Interior, U.S. Department of, Geological Survey. "Map Scales," Reston, Va (1972a).

Interior, U.S. Department of, Geological Survey. "Publications of the Geological Survey 1962-1970," Reston, Va (1972b).

Interior, U.S. Department of, Geological Survey. "Publications of the Geological Survey, Annual Supplements" (1971-1976).

Interior, U.S. Department of, Geological Survey. "Earthquake Shaking Hazards (Map)," Reston, Va (1977a).

Interior, U.S. Department of, Geological Survey. "Volcanoes of the U.S. (Map)," Reston, Va (1977b).

National Forest Products Association. "The All Weather Wood Foundation System Basic Requirements," *Tech. Rep.* No. 7, Washington, D.C. (1976).

Taylor, A. R. "Ecological Aspects of Lightning in Forests," *Proc. Tall Timbers Fire Ecol. Conf.* 13:455-482 (1974).

Wolfanger, L. A. "Soil Orders and Suborders of the United States," in *Conservation of Natural Resources,* 4th ed., G. H. Smith, Ed. (New York: John Wiley and Sons, Inc., 1971).

CHAPTER 10

ECOSYSTEMS

INTRODUCTION

Potential projects that will alter ecosystems can vary from small on-site disturbances to long-range plans that will cut across several major biomes. Examples of the latter type include interstate highway systems, pipelines, transmission lines or nationwide coal removal programs. If an impact is localized, an on-site visit be biologists may be necessary. However, a large multistate impact project cannot be effectively covered by a site visit or even a series of field trips.

The biologist on the interdisciplinary team can use the biome approach for large-scale projects. While literature on ecosystems in textbooks is biome-oriented, journal articles and other scientific data sources are usually more specific to a particular location and ecosystem. The ecological principles are generally applicable throughout the similar biome types. For example, data gathered from a deciduous forest in Tennessee can be used for deciduous forest impacts in Kentucky or Virginia. Major biomes of the United States are shown in Figure 10-1.

UNITS OF ECOLOGICAL ASSESSMENT

The biome is the largest, most general ecological unit used for biological impact assessment. Some biomes are more restricted than others, some more fragile. The fragile or sensitive to disturbance-type of biomes include deserts and tundra. Because of agricultural conversions, large biomes, such as the grasslands or true prairie, no longer exist as vast undisturbed ecosystems in the United States.

The next smaller unit of ecological assessment is the community. For example, within the deciduous biome, the proposed project may be located within an oak/hickory or birch/beech/maple community. These trees describe the dominant association or major tree species of the area.

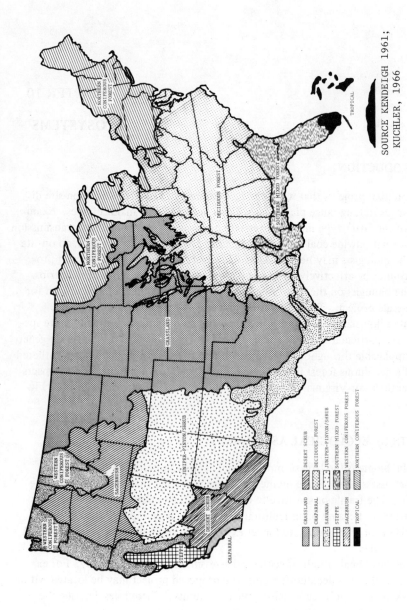

Figure 10-1. Biomes of the United States.

To complete the community, dominant animal types are usually described within their habitat. To understand the community structure and function is to understand the ecosystem relationships. If the impact of the project affects one component of the community, related or dependent biota will be altered secondarily.

Food relationships are among the easiest to determine. Upland and wetland food chains are shown in Tables 10-1 and 10-2. If a project will remove the vegetative species shown on the horizontal axis, the dependent animal species (vertical axis) will be secondarily impacted by reduced food sources. If the animal feeds on many different available food sources, the impact is less severe. If the animal depends on only a very few species, removal of those plants would eventually cause reductions in wildlife populations. Habitat requirements, such as cover, water, den sites and territorial space, are more difficult to determine.

At the base of every food chain, the total community depends on primary productivity or food conversion from the sun's energy. Not all of this productivity is used directly as food for animals. Some energy is used for plant community respiration and maintenance. Some plant material is not used directly, but only used secondarily as detritus, or as dead organic matter for nutrient recycling and soil enrichment.

ECOSYSTEM PRODUCTIVITY RATES

Table 10-3 shows general quantitative factors for various ecosystem primary productivity rates. While these rates vary from site to site, the table allows for quantitative analysis of impacts of sites, where no site-specific data are known. Productivity is the amount of green plant material produced over a year's growing season by all plants in the community. Standing crop is the amount of vegetation in place at one time. In general, annual productivity rates depend on: (1) length of growing season, (2) moisture available, and (3) soil fertility.

As can be seen in Table 10-3, the colder, short summer season ecosystems, such as tundra, are very low in primary productivity, usually less than one ton per acre. As one moves south, days are longer as is productivity rate. Prairie or grassland temperate ecosystems average 6 to 7 tons per acre, while tropical ecosystems average 13 tons per acre. Moisture also influences the productivity rate. For example, northern conifers' productivity rate is about 5 tons per acre and western conifers, which receive heavy rains, produce 11 tons per acre. Table 10-3 also shows similar plant communities on different soil types; some are more productive than others.

Net primary productivity rates are one way of quantifying impacts of proposed projects. One method is to predict total immediate impact of vegetative removal by multiplying acres disturbed by the annual productivity rate.

Table 10-1. Plant and Animal Food Chains on Uplands

ANIMALS / PLANTS*	OAK	PINE	BLACKBERRY	WILD CHERRY	DOGWOOD	GRAPE	POISON IVY	CEDAR	PRICKLYPEAR	MAPLE	BLUEBERRY	HACKBERRY	BIRCH	MESQUITE	ELDERBERRY	SERVICEBERRY	SUMAC	ASPEN	FIR	SAGEBRUSH	BEECH	WILLOW	SPRUCE	MANZANITA	ALDER	BRISTLEGRASS	RAGWEED	PANICGRASS	KNOTWEET	FILAREE	SUNFLOWER	CRABGRASS	CLOVER	BROMEGRASS	DOVEWEED	CORN	WHEAT	OATS	BARLEY	SORGHUM	APPLE
Blue grouse		X									X								X																						
Spruce grouse													X						X																						
Franklin grouse		X									X											X	X																		
Ruffed grouse	X		X	X	X	X					X		X					X		X	X																				
Prairie chicken		X																X									X		X				X			X	X	X			
Sharp-tailed grouse				X						X			X									X			X						X		X				X				
Hungarian partridge																										X	X		X					X		X	X	X	X		
Bobwhite quail	X																									X	X	X			X				X	X	X			X	
California quail																														X			X						X		
Gambel quail														X																											
Ring-necked pheasant			X			X																					X									X	X	X	X		X
Wild turkey	X	X			X	X											X										X	X				X				X		X		X	
Mourning dove																										X	X		X		X	X			X	X	X				
Red-shafted flicker	X																																								
Yellow-shafted flicker							X																																		
Pileated woodpecker				X		X									X																										
Red-bellied woodpecker	X					X																														X					
Red-headed woodpecker	X																																			X					
Horned lark																										X	X		X	X							X	X			
Blue jay	X	X																																		X					
Steller jay	X														X																										
Scrub jay	X	X		X																																X	X				
Crow																X																				X	X	X	X	X	
Chickadee		X																																							
Titmouse	X																				X																				
Nuthatch	X	X																																							
Mockingbird						X						X																													
Catbird			X	X			X																																		
Brown thrasher	X		X	X											X																										
Robin			X	X	X	X		X				X					X																								
Cedar waxwing				X	X	X		X																																	
Meadowlark																										X										X	X	X			
Cowbird																										X	X	X							X	X	X	X			
Cardinal			X		X	X																				X										X					
Song sparrow																										X	X	X	X												
Black bear	X			X		X					X										X																				X
Raccoon	X					X																														X					
Woodchuck																										X		X			X	X		X							
Red squirrel	X	X								X						X			X		X		X																		
Gray squirrel	X	X								X											X																				
Fox squirrel	X									X											X															X	X				
Flying squirrel	X																				X																				
Porcupine		X								X			X						X		X		X																		
Jackrabbit														X						X						X		X		X		X	X								
Cottontail		X			X				X					X			X																				X				
13-lined ground squirrel																										X	X		X	X		X	X								
White-tailed deer	X	X	X							X	X								X			X	X													X					
Mule deer	X	X		X				X				X				X			X	X				X							X			X							
Antelope								X	X											X																					

*Plant provides at least 5–10% of diet.

Source: Martin, A.C., H. S. Zim, and A. L. Nelson, American Wildlife and Plants: A Guide to Wildlife Food Habits, Dover, New York, 500 pp., 1961.

Table 10-2. Plant and Animal Food Chains in Wetlands

ANIMALS \ PLANTS*	ALGAE	HORSETAIL	CATTAIL	BURREED	EELGRASS	PONDWEED	WIDGEONGRASS	NAIAD	ARROWHEAD	WATERWEED	WILD CELERY	SALTGRASS	CORDGRASS	RICE CUTGRASS	WILD RICE	WILD MILLET	CHUFA	BULLRUSH	SPIKERUSH	SAWGRASS	ARROW-ARUM	DUCKWEED	PICKEREL WEED	SMARTWEED	GLASSWORT	WATERSHIELD	WATERLILY	COWLILY	COONTAIL	GRASSES	WHEAT	BARLEY	OATS	RICE	SORGHUM	CORN	ALFALFA	SEDGE	MUSKGRASS	PANICGRASS	POPLAR	WILLOW	BIRCH	HAZELNUT	SERVICEBERRY	SWEETGUM	ASPEN
Swans	X	X		X		X	X		X		X							X	X					X	X					X	X	X															
Canada goose						X	X					X	X					X	X						X					X						X											
Brant					X							X																																			
Snow goose			X			X	X						X																		X	X															
Mallard						X	X	X	X						X	X		X	X			X		X																							
Black duck						X	X	X			X		X		X			X	X					X										X	X												
Gadwall	X					X	X	X										X	X																												
Baldpate					X	X	X							X				X	X										X																		
Pintail						X	X								X	X	X	X							X													X	X								
Green-winged teal						X	X								X	X		X				X		X																							
Blue-winged teal						X	X									X		X				X		X														X	X	X							
Shoveller						X	X									X		X				X		X																X							
Wood duck				X							X	X			X			X	X		X	X		X																							
Redhead						X	X	X							X		X				X						X		X										X								
Ring-necked duck						X	X																				X												X								
Canvasback						X	X	X	X		X								X								X																				
Scaup						X	X	X										X																					X								
Goldeneye						X												X																													
Bufflehead						X												X																													
Ruddy duck						X	X	X																																							
Coot	X										X				X		X	X				X					X									X			X								
Sandhill crane																														X	X	X	X	X													
Virginia rail						X												X												X								X									
Sora															X	X																		X	X												
Purple gallinule															X																																
Avocet																																															
Redwing																		X				X		X							X	X	X	X	X		X			X								
Beaver				X					X					X													X	X												X	X	X	X	X	X		
Muskrat		X	X																								X			X								X			X	X	X	X	X	X	X
Moose	X																										X														X	X	X	X			X

*Plants which provide at least 5-10% of animals diet.

Source: Martin, A.C., H.S. Zim, and A.L. Nelson, American Wildlife and Plants: A Guide to Wildlife Food Habits, Dover, New York, 500 pp., 1961.

Table 10-3. World Productivity for Land Areas (Rodin *et al.*, 1975; Olson, 1975)

Terrestrial Ecosystems	Net Primary Productivity (ton/ac)
Polar deserts	0.02-0.4
Tundras	0.7-1.1
Polar bogs	1.0
Polar floodplain	0.8
Mountainous polar	0.7
Mountainous tundra	0.3-4.5
Maritime herbaceous; herb-wood	4.5
Open forest-tundra; northern taiga	2.2
Same, on gley-permafrost	1.8
Middle taiga forest	3.1
Same, on permafrost	2.7
Southern taiga	3.3
Same, on yellowish-podzolic soils	4.5
Same, on turf-calcareous and turf-gley soils	4.5
Same, on taiga bog soils	1.8
Broadleaf forest	3.6
Mixed-forest yellow soils	4.5
Bogs	1.6
Humid boreal floodplains	2.7
Mountain-taiga; montane conifer	2.7
Same, on mountain permafrost; subalpine	2.2
Mountain meadows or forest on gray mountain	3.3
Mountain meadows	5.4
Broadleaf forests on brown forest soils	5.8
Same, on redzinas	5.4
Herbaceous prairie	6.7
Cool conifers	5.4
Coastal conifers	11.2
Northern broadleaved forest	3.6
Central broadleaved forest	5.8
Central broadleaved forest (redzina soils)	5.4
Montane evergreen	8.0
Broadleaf forests, swampy (wetland)	5.8-6.1
Bogs	11.2
Humid subboreal floodplains	5.4
Mountain forest	5.4
Steppe, on typical and leached chernozems	5.8
Same, on ordinary and southern chernozems	3.6
Same, on solonets chernozems	3.6
Steppified formations	2.2
Halophytic formations	1.8
Psammophytic formations	3.6
Dry steppe	4.0
Desert steppe	2.2
Dry and desert steppe on chestnut and solonets complexes	2.2
Same, on solonets	2.2
Herbaceous bog on meadow-bog soils	3.1
Semiarid subboreal floodplains	5.4
Mountain dry steppe on mountain chestnut	3.1
Mountain steppe on mountain cherozems	4.5

Mountain meadow steppe	4.9
Steppified desert on brown semidesert	1.8
Same, on brown-soil and solonets complexes	1.6
Same, on solonets	1.4
Desert on gray-brown	0.7
Psammophytic formations on sand (in desert)	2.2
Halophytic formations (in desert)	0.2
Arid subboreal floodplains	5.8
Mountain desert on brown mountain semidesert	1.3
Same, on desert highland	0.7
Broadleaf forest on red and yellow soils; lowland evergreen	8.9
Same, on red renzinas and terra rossa	7.1
Herbaceous prairie on reddish black soils and rubrozems	5.8
Broadleaf forest, swampy evergreen	11.2
Meadow-bog and bog	58.0
Humid subtropical floodplains	17.8
Mountain broadleaf forest on mountain yellow and red soils	8.0
Xerophytic forest	7.1
Shrub-steppe formations on gray-brown soils	4.5
Same, on gray-brown solonets soils	2.7
Same, on subtropical chernozemlike and coalesced soils	3.6
Psammophytic formations on sandy soils and sand	2.2
Halophytic formations on solonchak soils	0.2
Semiarid subtropical floodplains	26.8
Mountain xerophytic forest	6.7
Mountain shrub-steppe	3.6
Steppified desert on serozems	4.5
Desert on subtropical desert soils	0.4
Psammaophytic formations on sand	2.7
Desert on takyr soils	0.4
Halophytic formations on solonchak	0.04
Arid subtropical floodplains	40.2
Mountain desert on mountain serozems	5.4
Same, on subtropical mountain desert soils	0.4
Humid evergreen forest	13.4
Same, on dark-red soils	12.0
Seasonally humid evergreen and secondary tall-grass savanna	7.1
Same, on black tropical soils	6.7
Bog formations	66.9
Humid tropical floodplain	31.2
Mangrove forest	4.5
Humid tropical mountain forest	15.6
Seasonally humid tropical mountain forest	9.8
Xerophytic forest on ferralitized brownish-red soils	7.6
Grass and shrub savanna	5.4
Same, on tropical black soils	4.9
Same, on tropical solonets soils	3.1
Meadow and swamp savanna	6.2
Mountain savanna	5.4
Desertlike savanna	1.8
Desert on tropical desert soils	0.4
Desert on tropical coalesced soils	0.1
Arid tropical floodplain	17.8
Mountain desert on tropical mountain desert soils	0.04
Earth's total land area (without glaciers, streams, lakes)	5.7
Glaciers	0
Lakes and streams	2.2

The second method is to predict a recovery rate for the ecosystem, providing the initial disturbance is only temporary, not a permanent facility. A general rule of thumb is the lower the productivity rate, the slower the recovery of the ecosystem.

Secondary productivity rates, or animal populations dependent on the vegetative production, are not as simply quantified. Animal populations are usually measured as density factors (animal units per area unit), rather than annual production rates. Table 10-4 shows typical wildlife densities in the United States. Small birds and mammals usually number 5 to 10 per acre. Gamebirds, squirrels, rabbits, etc., usually need one to 10 acres of habitat. Larger, big game animals require larger acreages and, therefore, have lower densities. Predators need the largest territories and, therefore, have the largest densities.

IMPACT ON WILDLIFE POPULATIONS

The greatest error often made in EISs is the general statement that "as habitat is destroyed, the wildlife will move over to adjacent areas of similar vegetative cover." This is simply not true. Nor is it true that the wildlife die instantly as heavy construction equipment moves onto the site. Neither of these oversimplified scenarios describes the impact of the project development.

First, assume all the surrounding habitat is full of wildlife, or at its carrying capacity. This assumption is almost always correct because natural overproduction of young is the rule of wildlife populations. Constant competition for food, space, nesting sites and cover reduces the number of survivors. Therefore, the resultant density of animals is just about what that habitat can naturally support. Now, the scenario more closely follows as the bulldozers move in, construction begins and food and vegetative cover are removed in a short time. Small or slow-moving animals may be killed by heavy equipment. Larger mobile species will move and seek cover in adjacent habitat. However, that habitat now has twice the animals it can support. The competition increases suddenly; food, shelter, nesting sites and other limiting factors, over a period of time, perhaps a year, take their toll on the surplus animals, until the carrying capacity is again reached. The overall result is a loss of population over time.

Field sampling at a project site would only give the standing crop estimate of animals present. True animal densities could only be measured over all seasons. Usually, the EIS process does not allow time for this type of sampling over time. Therefore, a table, such as Table 10-4, can be prepared from literature search, for the most important species, or for representatives of the area. Impacts on wildlife populations can then be quantified. The

Table 10-4. Typical Wildlife Densities (per acre)

Animal or Group	Range	Average	Region	Source
Gamebirds	0.0005-0.35	0.14	US[a]	---
Doves	---	0.04	US	Giles, 1969
Quail (bobwhite)	0.11-1.0	0.35	US	Allen, 1962
Quail (scaled)	---	0.0005	SW[b]	Allen, 1962
Ruffed Grouse	---	0.25	NE[c]	Allen, 1962
Pheasant	---	0.2	Midwest	Allen, 1962
Ptarmigan	0.03-0.003	0.016	AK[d]	Weeden, 1963
Songbirds	3-4	3.5	US	Kendeigh, 1961
Sparrow	0.16-0.7	0.4	SE[e]	Kendeigh, 1961
Meadowlark	0.12-0.16	0.14	SE	Kendeigh, 1961
Cardinal	0.12-0.5	0.3	SE	Kendeigh, 1961
Wren	---	0.2	SE	Kendeigh, 1961
Bluejay	0.08-0.1	0.09	SE	Kendeigh, 1961
Thrush	0.04-0.5	0.3	SE	Kendeigh, 1961
Woodpecker	0.02-0.1	0.06	SE	Kendeigh, 1961
Ovenbird	---	0.8	NE	Kendeigh, 1961
Vireo	---	0.8	NE	Kendeigh, 1961
Birds	---	0.09	Arctic	Kendeigh, 1961
Birds	0.37-1.08	0.7	SW	Kendeigh, 1961
Waterfowl	1.7-4.6	3	US	Beard, 1953
Wood Duck	1-7	3.5	SE	Arner, 1966
Small Mammals	1-25	5	US	---
Beaver	0.5-0.6	0.5	US	---
Squirrel	1-3	1	US	Kendeigh, 1961
Chipmunk	1-10	5	US	Kendeigh, 1961
Mice, Shrews	10-35	20-25	US	Kendeigh, 1961
Wood Rat	2-5	3	SW	Kendeigh, 1961
Ground Squirrel	---	16	SW	Kendeigh, 1961
Mice, Rats	---	3.4	SW	Kendeigh, 1961
Cottontail	0.25-10	1	US	Allen, 1962
Jackrabbit	---	0.2	SW	Kendeigh, 1961
Snowshoe Hare	0.43-2.4	1-2	AK	Ernest, 1974
Raccoon	0.05-0.1	0.07	US	---
Muskrat	1-10	5	Midwest	Errington, 1967
Big Game	0.001-1.0	0.1	US	---
Dall Sheep	0.0013-0.0037	0.002	AK	AKDFG,[f] 1976
Moose	0.001-0.008	0.005	AK	AKDFG, 1976
Antelope	0.02-0.002	0.01	West	Kendeigh, 1961

Table 10-4. continued

Animal or Group	Range	Average	Region	Source
Mule Deer	0.04-0.06	0.05	West	Allen, 1962
White-Tailed Deer	0.02-1	0.6	US	Taylor, 1965
Predators	0.00002-0.03	0.002	US	---
Wolf	0.00002-0.00005	0.000023	AK	Stephenson, 1975
Fox	0.0004-0.03	0.01	US	---
Mountain Lion	---	0.0002	West	Seton, 1909
Bear	---	0.0002	West	Seton, 1909
Bobcat	0.0003-0.00005	0.0004	US	Young, 1958
Grizzly Bear	---	0.0001	West	Cole, 1975
Coyote	0.0009-0.002	0.001	West	Gier, 1968
Lizards	---	2.6	West	Kendeigh, 1961
Snails/ Slugs	5000-6000	5500	Midwest	Kendeigh, 1961
Insects	---	113,000	Midwest	Kendeigh, 1961

[a]US: United States ranges in general.   [d]AK: Alaska
[b]SW: Southwestern states.   [e]SE: Southeastern states.
[c]NE: Northeastern states.   [f]Alaska Division Fish and Game.

total acreage disturbed by the project can be multiplied by average wildlife
population density. In addition, secondary acreage disturbance surrounding
the site will be altered temporarily during the construction period. Other
secondary impacts from the proposed project operation, such as air, noise,
water pollution, or related growth of industry or residential areas surrounding
the project may result in greater habitat loss than the project's initial construction. Often, the ecosystem which replaces the original one is different.
For example, native woodland species would be replaced by introduced and
urban-tolerant species.

Not all ecosystems disturbed are natural communities. More often, the
proposed project is located in agricultural landscapes. Here, the original
inhabitants of the biome have been replaced by cultivated crops and domestic livestock. The same principles of natural ecosystems apply, however.
The food chain is usually more simple, with man acting as the final consumer, or top predator. Agricultural impacts can also be quantified, in terms
of energy, productivity and potential yield. Table 10-5 lists typical U.S.
yields of crops per acre. These data can be made more specific to the location of the project by using county statistics from soil surveys or from U.S.
Department of Agriculture records of local crop production. Acres converted
to other uses are multiplied by average yield to estimate potential impacts
on the local market. These yield losses may be further quantified by multiplying by years of possible loss. For example, a right-of-way may be replanted

Table 10-5. U.S. Productivity for Agriculture (USDA, 1975)

Agricultural Systems	Yield (ton/ac)
Wheat	0.9
Winter wheat	1.0
Spring wheat	0.8
Rye	0.7
Rice (rough)	2.3
Corn-Grain	2.9
Corn-Silage	12.0
Oats	0.8
Barley	1.0
Sorghum (Silage)	10.7
Cotton	0.2
Sugarbeets	19.7
Sugar Cane	37.6
Tobacco	1.0
Peanuts	1.1
Soybeans	0.8
Snap Beans	1.8
Beets	6.0
Broccoli	3.7
Carrots	13.1
Peas	1.9
Potatoes	11.7
Tomatoes	6.9
Hay	2.1
Alfalfa	2.8

within a year, whereas a new facility may have a life expectancy of 50 years or more. Using Table 10-5, therefore, a 10-year loss of a barley crop would equal one year's production of sorghum silage for cattle feed.

Table 10-6 estimates the secondary productivity of pasture for domestic sheep and cattle. Highly productive pastures are found in the midwest, while poor grazing productivity is common in the desert southwest and dry sage-brush western states. Agricultural impacts are quantified by animal units per acre multiplied by acres converted to other uses by the project. In addition to potential grazers shown on Table 10-6, the EIS writer should note other herbivores which may be converted to animal unit equivalent (1000 lb live weight). These may include one horse, five antelope, four deer, one and four-tenths elk, or four caribou. In many areas of the west particularly, the local Bureau of Land Management offices have computed animal unit carry-ing capacity of range. This will aid the EIS in being more site-specific to the project study area.

Table 10-6. Agriculture Animal Units[a] by State

State	Acres of Pasture	No. of Cattle (1000s of head)	Sheep[b] (1000s ÷ 5)	Animal Unit/ Acre
Alabama	6,192	2,700	0.9	.44
Alaska	1,540	9	2.6	.008
Arizona	34,652	1,170	76	.04
Arkansas	6,372	2,680	1	.42
California	24,515	5,200	182	.22
Colorado	26,109	3,375	110	.13
Connecticut	176	110	1	.63
Delaware	57	33	0.4	.59
Florida	9,319	2,950	0.8	.32
Georgia	5,253	2,420	0.7	.46
Hawaii	1,042	250	–	.24
Idaho	8,495	2,150	112	.27
Illinois	4,642	3,200	39	.70
Indiana	3,262	2,125	36	.66
Iowa	7,316	7,350	74	1.01
Kansas	19,571	6,400	32	.33
Kentucky	8,185	3,750	8	.46
Louisiana	4,171	1,832	3	.44
Maine	342	138	2.6	.41
Maryland	623	444	3.4	.72
Massachusetts	202	107	1.3	.54
Michigan	2,210	1,640	28	.75
Minnesota	3,135	4,430	60	1.43
Mississippi	7,446	3,000	1.4	.40
Missouri	15,433	6,800	32	.44
Montana	46,782	3,340	136	.07
Nebraska	24,003	6,900	34	.29
Nevada	9,856	657	28	.07
New Hampshire	150	71	1	.48
New Jersey	185	117	2	.64
New Mexico	44,098	1,720	110	.04
New York	3,365	1,875	14.2	.56
North Carolina	3,117	1,120	2	.36
North Dakota	13,431	2,635	51	.20
Ohio	3,987	2,350	88	.61
Oklahoma	23,831	6,500	13	.27
Oregon	13,014	1,470	71	.12
Pennsylvania	2,239	1,960	25	.89
Rhode Island	20	12	0.5	.63
South Carolina	1,894	710	0.3	.38
South Dakota	27,218	4,950	145	.19
Tennessee	6,907	3,300	4	.48
Texas	111,526	16,600	497	.15

Table 10-6, continued

State	Acres of Pasture	No. of Cattle (1000s of head)	Sheep[b] (1000s ÷ 5)	Animal Unit/ Acre
Utah	9,477	900	132	.11
Vermont	736	336	1.3	.46
Virginia	4,534	1,750	35	.39
Washington	8,944	1,420	15	.16
West Virginia	2,431	540	26	.23
Wisconsin	5,464	4,640	18	.85
Wyoming	32,633	1,690	238	.06

[a]Animal unit = livestock converted to approximate standard equivalent to a mature 1000-lb cow

[b]Sheep s = 1 cow = animal unit

Aquatic ecosystem impact analysis is not the same as discussed previously for terrestrial ecosystems. However, primary and secondary productivity rates are useful determinants of impact of disturbance. While in terrestrial systems, removal of vegetation decreases productivity, manipulation of aquatic systems sometimes increases productivity. Two examples of this type of impact are increasing nutrients or increasing temperatures. These actions may cause eutrophication, or algal blooms, which are not necessarily beneficial.

Table 10-7 shows known primary and secondary productivity rates of various types of aquatic ecosystems around the world. In general, cold, deep, northern or high-altitude systems have low productivity rates. Tropical, warm, shallow and marshy aquatic systems have high productivity. Indian fish-rearing ponds have the highest production in the world—up to 35 tons per acre. Secondary productivity of all fish in the aquatic ecosystem ranges from a low of 4 pounds per acre to a high of 17 or 18 thousand per acre for fish culture systems, artificially maintained and fertilized by man. An action by man, such as damming a cold trout stream, could increase the overall productivity of the aquatic ecosystem, by replacing a limited trout fishery with a fast growing bass fishery. After a reservoir is filled, new fish growth is rapid for five to seven years. Then, fish production starts to decline, as well as resultant sport fishing. In altering a fish population, a quality factor must also be assessed, as well as the quantity change over time.

Table 10-8 and Figure 10-2 represent various standing crops of fish by species, since most fishermen are concerned with favored sport species, and not total biotic production rates. These standing crops are useful for projecting both immediate impacts of proposed projects and long range impacts resulting from replacing one population with another population. For example, changing a

Table 10-7. Aquatic Ecosystems Annual Productivity Rates

	Type of Ecosystem	Location	Primary Productivity (Plants)[a]		Secondary Productivity (Fish)	
			$(Kcal/m^2)$	(gO^2/m^2)	(ton/ac)	(lb/ac)
Lakes						
Naroch	Large, mesotrophic	USSR	1,600	—	1.5	38
Myastro	Intermediate	USSR	1,800	—	1.7	57
Batorin	Eutrophic	USSR	1,900	—	1.8	76
Ooty	Tropical	India	13,300	3,700	12.6	—
Kodai Kanal	Tropical	India	1,400	390	1.3	114
Yercaud	Tropical	India	10,200	2,800	9.6	4
Morske Oko	Oligotrophic	Czechoslovakia	—	—		29
Chad	Turbid	Africa	5,000	—	4.7	—
Krugloe	High latitude	USSR	50	—	0.05	—
Char	High latitude	Canada	75	—	0.07	—
Reservoirs						
Amaravathi	Man-made	India	11,300	3,100	10.7	143
Stanley	Man-made	India	8,100	2,300	7.7	56
Bhavanisagar	Man-made	India	8,200	2,300	7.7	25
Sathanur	Man-made	India	8,100	2,200	7.7	69
Krishnagiri	Man-made	India	5,600	1,600	5.3	19
Sandynulla	Man-made	India	8,100	2,300	7.7	40
Klicava	Man-made	Czechoslovakia	—	—		67
Rivers						
Danube	Free-flowing	Czechoslovakia	—	—		192-260
Bradska	Trout stream	Czechoslovakia	—	—		134-223[b]

Loucha	Trout stream	Czechoslovakia	—	—	—	107-125[c]
Thames	Polluted	England	2,000-4,000	—	1.9-4.2	1,879
Patuxent	Free-flowing	Maryland	800-1,200[d]		3.9-5.9	—
Other Fresh						
Ft. Moat	Fish ponds	India	22,000-37,000	6,000	20.9-35.1	803-1,820
Odathurai	Irrigation tank	India	8,500	2,300	8.0	77
Chetpat	Swamp	India	27,300	7,600	25.9	1,963
Ayyankulam	Pond	India	31,100	8,800	29.5	1,283
Danube	Oxbows, marsh	Czechoslovakia				232
Silver Springs	Large spring	Florida	20,800		19.7	—
Saline						
Long Island Sound	Coastal	New York	5,700		5.4	—
Estuary	Marsh	Georgia	10,300		9.8	—
Estuary	Marsh	Louisiana	9,800		6.0-11.0	1,100
Estuary	Aquaculture	Japan				17,500
Contental Shelf	Ocean	—	500-3,000		0.5-2.8	—
Ocean	Deep	—	<1,000		<0.9	—

[a] Assume 4.5 Kcal/g dry weight for plants
  1 g O_2 = 3.5 Kcal = 0.375 g C.
  1 g C = 9.4 Kcal = 2 g of organic matter.
[b] Trout and sculpin
[c] Trout only
[d] Assume 250 days at 3.2-4.8 g O_2/day
(Table modified from: Odum, 1971; Kojak and Hillbricht, 1972; Brylinsky and Mann. 1973.)

Table 10-8. Standing Crops of Fish (Carlander, 1955)

General Habitat	Pounds/Acre
River Backwaters and Oxbows	500
Midwestern Reservoirs	400
Other Reservoirs and Ponds	200-300
Warm-Water Lakes	125-150
Cold Trout Lakes	<50
Warm-Water Streams	9-43
Trout Streams	55
Southern Ponds	230-330

BY SPECIES	SCAVENGERS	Pounds/Acre
Gizzard Shad		100-350
Buffalo Fish		116-166
Smallmouth Buffalo		51
Bigmouth Buffalo		174
Black Buffalo		22
Carp		107-202
Chub Sucker		14-22
Spotted Sucker		8
Redhorse		8
Common Sucker		11
Golden Shiner		21-42
Minnows		22-40
Drum		7-28

INTERMEDIATE

Bluegill	116
Green Sunfish	29
Pumpkinseed	19
Redear Sunfish	31
Rock Bass	8
Warmouth	10
Longear Sunfish	3
White Crappie	21
Black Crappie	40
Yellow Perch	14
White Perch	12
Bullheads	30

PREDATORS

Largemouth Bass	20-25
Smallmouth Bass	4
Spotted Bass	1
Redeye Bass	9
White Bass	3
Yellow Bass	5
Bowfin	22
Gar	9
Eel	15
Channel Catfish	39
Flathead Catfish	22
Northern Pike	5-8
Mud Pickerel	1
Chain Pickerel	4
Walleye	6-12
Sauger	5
Trout	4-44
Whitefish	7

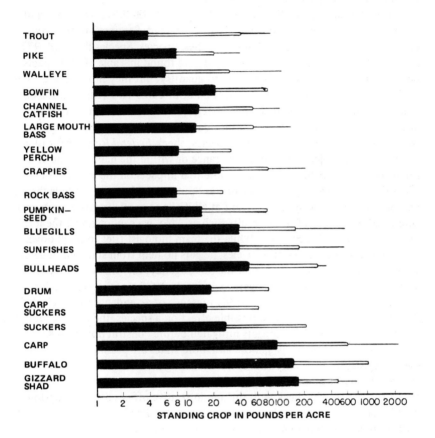

Figure 10-2. Standing Crops of Fish per Acre, by Species (Carlander, 1955)

trout stream to a reservoir may increase fish production five to six times. Adding nutrients or organic matter may cause a loss of clean water species and a replacement by highly productive scavenger species, such as buffalo or carp. Fishermen, however, often resent this change. Figure 10-2 shows the most favored sport fish on top, with naturally low-standing crops.

Game fish and wildlife are usually of great interest to both the local sportsmen and state and federal fish and wildlife agencies. Often these impacts are quantifiable, due to vast amounts of data and research on sport species. It is possible to mitigate many impacts on these species also, for the same reason. Research on management of these sport species usually points to methods to increase production and enhance the habitat. Fish and wildlife coordination efforts during the EIS process usually elicit responses from agencies to provide for popular game species in mitigation efforts.

Under the Endangered Species Act of 1973, (PL 93-205) certain rare and nongame species of plants and animals are protected. Section 7 of that law provides for protection of critical habitat of these species. Species listed in 1977 as officially "endangered" or "threatened" are found in Table 10-9. Impacts on these species are almost impossible to quantify, but they must be addressed in all EISs. Locate the proposed project on both Table 10-9 (Distribution column) and on Figure 10-3. Most endangered species are found in very limited habitats; many are concentrated in Florida, Texas, California, Hawaii and Nevada. (Table 10-9 omits Hawaiian species; check *Federal Register* for island species.) If the project falls within the range or within the habitat of an endangered species, the EIS should discuss potential impacts on the species. Most often the impact can only be discussed as "potential," because rarely is the endangered species known to be present at all. Calls to specialists, biologists and wildlife agencies often lead to results such as, "No, we cannot reveal the location of nest sites of species A." While the team biologist tries to track down the whereabouts of the elusive species, he gets no help from state and federal agencies. Then, as a comment from the same agency, the EIS is often called insufficient in the area of endangered species. In 1977 alone, several major federal projects were halted, due to the presence of an endangered species. If the EIS process does discover a possible effect on a species, the project should be altered or relocated, or impacts mitigated before construction begins.

In addition to federal laws, more and more states are passing endangered species legislation, to qualify for federal matching monies. Table 10-10 summarizes the status of state programs. These programs are evolving quickly, so the EIS writer should check with the administrative offices listed for up-to-date state legislation. Table 10-11 summarizes, by state, the plants and animals considered to be rare, threatened or endangered within that state's borders. All species listed are not yet legally protected by state law.

Table 10-9. Endangered, Threatened and Rare Species of the United States[a]
(September 1977)(DOI, 1973; DOI, 1974; DOI, 1975; DOI, 1976a; DOI, 1976b; DOI, 1976c; DOI 1977a; 1977b)

Common Name	Scientific Name	Distribution	Habitat
Endangered Fishes			
Shortnose sturgeon	*Acipenser brevirostrum*	Hudson River, one Florida specimen	Spawn river, Atlantic seaboard
Longjaw cisco	*Coregonus alpenae*	Lakes Michigan and Huron, eastern Lake Erie	20-60 fathoms, fresh lakes
Woundfin	*Plagopterus argentissimus*	Virgin River below Hurricane, Utah	Swift rivers
Greenback cutthroat trout	*Salmo clarki stomias*	Blackhollow Creek, Cache la Poudre River, few possible streams in Boulder & Larimer Counties, Colorado	Fresh cold streams and rivers
Lahontan cutthroat trout	*Salmo clarki henshawi*	California, Nevada	Streams
Paiute cutthroat trout	*Salmo clarki seleniris*	California	Streams
Humpback chub	*Gila cypha*	Green and Colorado Rivers, from Grand Canyon area northward to vicinity of Flaming Gorge Dam on Utah-Wyoming border	Flowing streams and rivers
Mohave chub	*Gila (Siphateles) mohavensis*	Lake Tuendae, Zzyzx Resort, 9 miles south of Baker, California; Owens River	Lakes, turbid, swift warm rivers
Colorado squawfish	*Ptychocheilus lucius*	Middle and lower Green River, main Colorado River above Lake Powell, and Salt River; spawning in Yampa River and Green River	Rivers
Bonytail pahranagut	*Gila robusta jordoni*	Lincoln Co., Nevada	Spring outflow
Kendal Warm Springs dace	*Rhinichthys osculus thermalis*	Kendal Warm Springs, tributary to the Green River in Wyoming	Warm springs
Moapa dace	*Moapa coriacea*	Near source of Moapa (Muddy) River, Clark County, Nevada	Warm springs and outlets
Cui-ui (sucker)	*Chasmistes cujus*	Pyramid Lake, Washoe County, Nevada	Lakes

Table 10-9 , continued

Common Name	Scientific Name	Distribution	Habitat
Devil's Hole pupfish	*Cyprinodon diabolis*	Pool in Ash Meadows, Nye County, Nevada, east of Death Valley California	Spring-fed pool, warm water
Gila trout	*Salmo gilae*	Diamond, McKenna, and Spruce Creeks in the Black Primitive Area of the headwaters of Gila River, Gila National Forest, New Mexico	Clean, cold streams and rivers
Comanche Springs pupfish	*Cyprinodon elegans*	Phantom Lake Spring, near Toyahvale, Texas	Large springs and irrigation ditches
Tecopa pupfish	*Cyprinodon nevadensis calidae*	Reservoir and small creek, Tecopa Hot Springs, Inyo County, California	Outflow from well
Warm Springs pupfish	*Cyprinodon nevadensis pectoralis*	School, Spring and Scruggs Springs in northern part of Ash Meadows, Nye County, Nevada	Springs
Owens River pupfish	*Cyprinodon radiosus*	Fish Slough, Owens Valley, California; north of Big Pine, Owens Valley, California	Sloughs and ponds
Pahrump Killifish	*Empetrichthys latos*	Manse Ranch, Pahrump Valley, Nye County, Nevada	Spring fed pools
Big Bend gambusia	*Gambusia gaigei*	Big Bend National Park, Western Texas	Pools and warm springs
Gila topminnow	*Poeciliopsis occidentalis occidentalis*	Santa Cruz County, and San Carlos Indian Reservation, Arizona	Springs
Clear Creek gambusia	*Gambusia heterochir*	Clear Creek (10.4 miles west of Menard) Menard County, Texas	Headwater streams
Pecos gambusia	*Gambusia nobilis*	Toyahvale and Fort Stockton, Texas	Springs and spring-fed ditches
Unarmored threespine stickleback	*Gasterosteus aculeatus williamsoni*	Santa Clara River in Soledad Canyon, Los Angeles County, and Santa Maria River in San Luis Obispo County, California	Headwater streams

Common name	Scientific name	Location	Ecosystem
Fountain darter	*Etheostoma fonticola*	Coman and San Marcos Springs in Hays and Comal Counties, Texas	Spring outflow
Watercress darter	*Etheostoma nuchale*	Glen Springs at Bessemer, Jefferson County, Alabama (Black Warrior River drainage)	Springs with watercress
Okaloosa darter	*Etheostoma okaloosae*	Streams which originate on Eglin Air Force Base and empty into Choctawhatchee Bay, Okaloosa County, Florida	Small, clean streams
Maryland darter	*Etheostoma sellare*	Swan Creek near Havre de Grace, Maryland and another nearby stream	Small streams
Blue pike	*Stizostedion vitreum glaucum*	Lake Erie, possibly Lake Ontario	Deep, cold lakes
Scioto madtom	*Noturus trautmani*	Ohio, Scioto River (Pickaway Co.)	Rivers
Snail darter	*Percina tanasi*	Tennessee River	Cold, clean streams

Endangered Reptiles and Amphibians

Common name	Scientific name	Location	Ecosystem
Texas blind salamander	*Typhlomolge rathbuni*	Hays Co., Texas	Deep wells, caves, underground streams
Santa Cruz long-toed salamander	*Ambystoma macrodactylum croceum*	Santa Cruz Co., California	Ponds, wetlands
American crocodile	*Crocodylus acutus*	South Florida, and Keys	Salty wetlands, estuaries
Slender desert salamander	*Batrachoseps aridus*	California, Hidden Palm Canyon	Desert, under rock talus
American alligator[b]	*Alligator mississippiensis*	North Carolina, south to Texas, Florida Louisiana, Georgia, Arkansas, south-eastern Oklahoma	Fresh wetlands; slightly salty estuaries
San Francisco garter snake	*Thamnophis sirtalis tetrataenia*	San Francisco area, California	Near reservoirs' edges
Bluntnosed leopard lizard	*Crotaphytus silus*	Sacramento Valley area, California	Scrub/grassland
Houston toad	*Bufo houstonensis*	South-central Texas	Lablolly pine forests
Leatherback turtle	*Dermochelys coriacea*	Worldwide—tropical and temperate ocean and island beaches	Ocean and beaches
Hawksbill turtle	*Eretmochelys imbricata*	Tropical ocean and island beaches, worldwide	Oceans and beaches
Atlantic ridley sea turtle	*Lepidochelys kempii*	Tropical Mexican ocean and island beaches	Ocean and beaches

Table 10-9 , continued

Common Name	Scientific Name	Distribution	Habitat
Endangered Birds			
Eskimo curlew	*Numenius borealis*	Alaska, probably extinct	Grasslands and tundra
Yuma clapper rail	*Rallus longirostris yumanensis*	Lower Colorado River; California, Arizona	Marshes and sloughs
Light-footed clapper rail	*Rallus longirostris levipes*	Santa Barbara south to Mexico, California	Salt marshes
California clapper rail	*Rallus longirostris obsoletus*	San Francisco Bay, Tomales Bay, Humboldt Bay, Bollings and Morro Bay, California	Salt marshes and estuaries
Whooping crane	*Grus americana*	Winters Gulf coast Texas; migrates through central-western U.S. from Canada to Texas	Wetlands, coast, grain farmlands
Mississippi sandhill crane	*Grus canadensis pulla*	Jackson Co., Mississippi	Coastal plain, semi-open and wet pine savannah
Attwater's greater prairie chicken	*Tympanuchus cupido attwateri*	Coastal prairie counties Texas, primarily Refugia and Colorado Co.	Prairie, grasslands
Masked bobwhite	*Colinus virginianus ridgwayi*	Reintroduced into southern Arizona	grassland, mesquite, shrubs and cacti
Florida Everglade kite	*Rosthrhamus sociabilis plumbeus*	Southern Florida, resident	Fresh water marsh
American peregrine falcon	*Falco peregrinus anatum*	Breeds Alaska south to Baja Calif., Arizona to Rocky Mountains, most Western states	Coniferous forest and wetlands and along rivers
Arctic peregrine falcon	*Falco peregrinus tundrius*	Migrates through eastern and middle North America to Gulf	Breeds in treeless tundra; migrates along coasts and waterways, feeds in marshes
Southern bald eagle	*Haliaetus l. leucocephalus*	Atlantic and Gulf Coasts, resident of Florida south of 40th Parallel	Estuaries and freshwater lakes; wetlands cliffs, forests
California condor	*Gymnogyps californianus*	Santa Clara County California to Baja and Fresno Counties	Coastal ranges and foothills, cliffs
Mexican duck	*Anas diazi*	Southeastern Arizona, Southern New Mexico, West and Central Texas and Mexico	Shallow ponds, wetlands

Common name	Scientific name	Range	Habitat
Aleutian Canada goose	Branta canadensis leucopareia	Migrates through Oregon, California and Washington	Islands, wetlands
California brown pelican	Pelecanus occidentalis californicus	Islands (California), Ventura County to Baja	Islands, estuaries, ocean, coastal
Eastern brown pelican	Pelecanus occidentalis carolinensis	Florida, north to North Carolina, Texas, Louisiana (resident)	Ocean, estuaries, coast islands, mangroves, beaches
California least tern	Sterna albifrons	Mexico, California, western coast	Sandy beaches
Red-cockaded woodpecker	Dendrocopos borealis	Oklahoma, Arkansas, Western Kentucky, Southeastern Virginia south to Gulf and Florida	Mature pine forests
Ivory-billed woodpecker	Campephilus p. principalis	Southeastern Texas, South Louisiana and South Carolina	Mature bottomland hardwoods
Bachman's warbler	Vermivora bachmanii	Virginia, South Carolina, Alabama	Swamp forests and bottomlands
Kirtland's warbler	Dendroica kirtlandii	Lower Michigan (Au Sable watershed) (breeding area); migrates south to Bahamas	Jack pines, brushy undergrowth
Dusky seaside sparrow	Ammospiza nigrescens	Florida, east coast	Salt marshes (breeding)
Cape Sable sparrow	Ammospiza mirabilis	Florida, southwestern	Fresh and brackish marshes
Santa Barbara sparrow	Melospiza melodia graminea	California, Channel Islands	Scrub islands in Pacific Mountains
Thick-billed parrot	Rhynchopsitta pachyrhyncha	Arizona and New Mexico (former sporadic visitor)	
Endangered Mammals			
Sonoran pronghorn	Antilocapra americana sonoriensis	USA and Mexico - Arizona	Desert
Columbian white-tailed deer	Odocoileus virginianus leucurus	Oregon, Washington (Columbia river)	Lowland and bottomland forest
Key deer	Odocoileus virginianus clavium	Florida Keys	Surburban, open woodlands, brush
Southern sea otter	Enhydra lutris neresis	California coastal waters	Ocean, kelp beds

Table 10-9 , continued

Common Name	Scientific Name	Distribution	Habitat
West Indian (Florida) manatee	Trichechus manatus	Caribbean/adjacent Atlantic (Coastal) (Florida - southern)	Wetlands and rivers and estuaries
Delmarva fox squirrel	Sciurus niger cinereus	Delmarva Penninsula, Maryland	Woods
Gray bat	Myotis grisescens	Central and Southeastern states - Alabama, Arkansas, Florida, Illinois, Georgia, Virginia, Indiana, Kentucky, Mississippi, Missouri, and Tennessee	Limestone caves
Indiana bat	Myotis sodalis	Midwest and east (Oklahoma to Vermont to North Florida)	Limestone caves
Black-footed ferret	Mustela nigripes	Western USA and western Canada (North Dakota, Nebraska, Texas, Wyoming and California, South Dakota	Shortgrass prairie
Utah prairie dog	Cynomys parvidens	Utah	Grassland and cropland
Salt marsh harvest mouse	Reithrodontomys raviventris	California coast	Salt Marshes
Morro Bay kangaroo rat	Dipodomys heermanni morroensis	California (San Luis Obispo)	Sandy soils, open scrub
Eastern cougar	Felis concolor cougar	Eastern USA (Canada to Carolinas)	Remote woodlands, mountains
Florida panther	Felis concolor coryi	Florida (Everglades and Big Cypress) Georgia	Remote swamplands
San Joaquin kit fox	Vulpes macrotis mutica	California (San Joaquin Valley)	Foothills below 3000 ft
Red wolf	Canis rufus	Texas, Louisiana (Gulf regions)	Coastal prairie marshes, swamplands
Mexican wolf	Canis lupus baileyi	Southern Arizona, Texas and Mexico	Remote arid regions
Gray wolf	Canis lupus monstrabilis	Texas, New Mexico, Mexico	Remote arid regions
Northern Rocky Mountain wolf	Canis lupus irremotus	Wyoming, Montana, South Dakota (Black Hills), Idaho, Oregon and Washington	Remote mountain areas, forests and open lands

			Remote forested areas
Eastern timber wolf	*Canis lupus lycaon*	Northeastern USA - Minnesota, Michigan and Canada	
Blue whale	*Balaenoptera musculus*	Oceans (Atlantic and Pacific)	Oceans
Bowhead whale	*Balaena mysticetus*	Oceans (northern)	Oceans
Finback whale	*Balaenoptera physalus*	Oceans (Atlantic and Pacific)	Oceans
Gray whale	*Eschrichtius gibbosus*	Oceans (North Pacific)	Oceans
Humpback whale	*Megaptera novaeangliae*	Oceans (Atlantic and Pacific)	Oceans
Right whale	*Eugalaena spp.*	Oceans (Atlantic and Pacific)	Oceans
Sei whale	*Balaenoptera borealis*	Oceans (Atlantic and Pacific)	Oceans
Sperm whale	*Physeter catadon*	Oceans (Atlantic and Pacific)	Oceans
Endangered Clams and Snails			
Birdwing pearly mussel	*Conradilla caelata*	Powell and Clinch Rivers in Virginia and Tennessee, Duck River, Tennessee	River
Curtis' pearly mussel	*Epioblasma florentina curtisi*	Black River in Missouri	River
Sampson's pearly mussel	*Epioblasma sampsoni*	Wabash River in Indiana and Illinois	River
Green-blossom pearly mussel	*Epioblasma torulosa gubernaculum*	Clinch River in Virginia and Tennessee	River
Tuberculed-blossom pearly mussel	*Epioblasma torulosa torulosa*	Lower Ohio River in Kentucky and Illinois; Nolichucky River in Tennessee and Kanawha River in West Virginia	River
Fine-rayed pigtoe pearly mussel	*Fusconaia cuneolus*	Clinch River in Virginia and Tennessee, Powell River in Virginia and Tennessee, and Paint Rock River in northern Alabama	River
Shiny pigtoe pearly mussel	*Fusconaia edgariana*	Powell and Clinch Rivers in Virginia and Tennessee, Paint Rock River in Alabama, and Holston River in Virginia	River
Higgin's eye pearly mussel	*Lampsilis higginsi*	Mississippi River in Minnesota, Wisconsin, and Illinois; Meramec River in Missouri; St. Croix River in Wisconsin and Minnesota	River
Pink mucket pearly mussel	*Lampsilis orbiculata orbiculata*	Green River, Kentucky; Kanawha River in West Virginia, Tennessee River (Tennessee and Alabama); Muskingum River, Ohio	River

Table 10-9 , continued

Common Name	Scientific Name	Distribution	Habitat
Alabama lamp pearly mussel	*Lampsilis virescens*	Paint Rock River system in Alabama	River
White warty-back pearly mussel	*Plethobasis cicatricosus*	Tennessee River in Tennessee and Alabama	River
Orange-footed pimpleback mussel	*Plethobasis cooperianus*	Tennessee River in Tennessee and Alabama; Duck River in Tennessee	River
Rough pigtoe pearly mussel	*Pleurobema plenum*	Tennessee River, Tennessee; Green River, Kentucky; Clinch River, Virginia and Tennessee	River
Cumberland monkeyface pearly mussel	*Quadrula intermedia*	Powell and Clinch Rivers in Virginia and Tennessee; Duck River, Tennessee	River
Appalachian monkeyface pearly mussel	*Quadrula sparsa*	Powell and Clinch Rivers in Virginia and Tennessee; Duck River, Tennessee	River
Pale lilliput pearly mussel	*Toxolasma cylindrella*	Duck River, Tennessee; Paint Rock River, Alabama	River
Cumberland bean pearly mussel	*Villosa trabilis*	Cumberland and Rockcastle Rivers, Kentucky	River
Yellow- blossom pearly mussel	*Epioblasma florentina florentina*	Duck River in Tennessee	River
White cat's paw pearly mussel	*Epioblasma sulcata delicata* (including *perobliqua*)	Detroit River in Michigan; St. Joseph River in Ohio, Michigan and Indiana	River
Turgid-blossom pearly mussel	*Epioblasma turgidula*	Duck River in Tennessee	River
Fat pocketbook pearly mussel	*Potamilus capax*	White River, Arkansas; St. Francis River, Arkansas and Missouri	River
Dromedary pearly mussel	*Dromus dromas*	Powell and Clinch Rivers in Virginia and Tennessee	River
Manus Island tree snail	*Papustyla pulcherrina*	Admiralty Islands (Manus I.) (southwest Alaskan coast)	Island trees

Endangered Butterflies			
Lotis blue butterfly	*Lycaeides argyrognomon lotis*	California	
El Segundo blue butterfly	*Shijimiacoides battoides allyni*	California	
Smith's blue butterfly	*Shijimiacoides euopies smithi*	California	
Mission blue butterfly	*Icaricia icariodes missionensis*	California	
San Bruno Elfin butterfly	*Callophrys mossi bayensis*	California	
Lange's metalmark butterfly	*Apodemia mormo langei*	California	
Threatened Fishes			
Paiute cutthroat trout	*Salmo clarki seleniris*	California (Alpine County)	Tributaries and creeks
Lahontan cutthroat trout	*Salmo clarki henshawi*	California, Nevada	Lakes, reservoirs, and streams
Arizona trout	*Salmo apache*	Arizona	Streams
Bayou darter	*Etheostoma rubrum*	Mississippi (Bayou Pierre drainage)	Bayou
Threatened Reptiles and Amphibians			
American alligator	*Alligator mississippiensis*	Florida, Georgia, Louisiana, South Carolina, Texas (coastal), except Louisiana (Vermillion, Cameron, Calcasieu Parishes)	Coastal marshes
Red Hills salamander	*Phaeognathus hubrichti*	Alabama	Moist areas
Threatened Mammals			
Grizzly bear (brown)[c]	*Ursus arctos horribilis*	Montana, Idaho, Wyoming	Remote mountains
Jaguar	*Panthera onca*	In captivity in U.S.	Captive
Black lemur	*Lemur macaco*	In captivity in U.S.	Captive
Ring-tailed lemur	*Lemur catta*	In captivity in U.S.	Captive
Leopard	*Panthera pardus*	In captivity in U.S.	Captive
Tiger	*Panthera tigris*	In captivity in U.S.	Captive
Threatened Butterflies			
Bahama swallowtail	*Papilio andraemon bonhotei*	Florida	
Schaus swallowtail	*Papilio aristodemus ponceanus*	Florida	

Table 10-9 , continued

Common Name	Scientific Name	Distribution	Habitat
Rare Fishes[d]			
Deepwater cisco	*Coregonus johannae*	Once abundant in Lakes Michigan and Huron	Deep water, large lakes
Blackfin cisco	*Coregonus n. nigripinnis*	Lakes Michigan and Huron	Deep water, large lakes
Artic grayling	*Thymallus arcticus*	Montana, Utah, Wyoming, Washington, Colorado; and in Glacier and Yellowstone National Parks	Cold, gravel-bottomed lakes
Rio Grande cutthroat trout	*Salmo clarki virginalis*	Costilla County, Colorado; Sandoval and Taos Counties in northern New Mexico	Headwater streams and tributaries
Humboldt cutthroat trout	*Salmo clarki (subsp.)*	Humboldt River drainage of Lahontan Basin Nevada	Headwater tributaries
Little Kern golden trout	*Salmo aquabonita gilberti*	Little Kern River, tributary to main Kern River, Sequoia National Forest, California	Tributaries
Sunapee trout	*Salvelinus aureolus*	Flood's Pond, Hancock County, Maine	Lakes and ponds
Blueback trout	*Salvelinus alpinus oquassa*	St. John & Penobscot Rivers, Northwestern Maine	Lakes
Desert dace	*Eremichthys acros*	Soldier Meadows west of Black Rock Desert in Humboldt County, Nevada	Warm Springs
Little Colorado spinedace	*Lepidomeda vittata*	Upper part of Little Colorado River basin, eastern Arizona	Streams
White River (Mountain) sucker	*Catostomus clarki intermedius*	White River, White River Valley, Nevada	Cool springs and outflows
Modoc sucker	*Catostomus microps*	Rush Creek and Ash Creek, Modoc County, California; Pit River drainage of the Sacramento River basin	Streams
Ozark cavefish	*Amblyopsis rosae*	Southwestern Missouri and northwestern Arkansas	Caves and wells
Nevada pupfish	*Cyprinodon nevadensis*	Ash Meadows, southeastern Amargosa Desert, Nye County, Nevada	Springs

Olympic mudminnow	*Novumbra hubbsi*	Chehalis River watershed - from Satsop River and Deschutes River in the Olympic Penninsula in western Washington	Rivers
Rare Reptils and Amphibians			
Limestone salamander	*Hydromantes brunus*	Bear Creek, Briceburg, Mariposa County California	Limestone area near water
Shasta salamander	*Hydromantes shastae*	North of Lake Shasta in north-central California	Limestone area near water
Jemez Mountain salamander	*Pelthodon neomexicanus*	Jemez Mountains, New Mexico	Mountains, near water
Black toad (Inyo County toad)	*Bufo exsul*	Buckhorn Springs and Antelope Springs in Deep Springs Valley, and between White and Inyo Mountains, Inyo County, California	Springs, ditches and ponds
Vegas Valley leopard frog	*Rana pipiens fisheri*	Presently unknown; formerly in Vegas Valley, Clark County, Nevada	Springs and seepage areas
Pine Barrens tree frog	*Hyla andersoni*	Southern New Jersey; North Carolina; may also occur in Georgia	Pine barrens
Bog turtle	*Clemmys muhlengergi*	Connecticut to southwestern North Carolina	Freshwater marshes, meadows, and bogs
Green sea turtle	*Chelonia mydas*	Tropical oceans - U.S. coasts during the summer - Hawaii	Oceans and beaches
Loggerhead sea turtle	*Caretta caretta*	Ocean (Atlantic & Pacific)	Tropical and temperate seas and beaches
Pacific ridley sea turtle	*Lepidochelys olivacea*	Pacific ocean	Tropical and temperate seas and beaches
Gila monster	*Heloderma suspectum*	Desert southwest U.S. (Utah, Nevada, New Mexico)	Desert
Rare Birds			
Florida great white heron	*Ardea o. occidentalis*	Florida Keys to Biscayne Bay to central Florida	Mangrove estuaries

Table 10-9, continued

Common Name	Scientific Name	Distribution	Habitat
Prairie falcon	*Falco mexicanus*	Central British Columbia east to southern Saskatchewan and south to Baja California and northern Texas (western states)	Open country, canyons, mountains
Lesser prairie chicken	*Tympanuchus pallidicinctus*	Southwestern Kansas, southeastern Colorado eastern New Mexico, Texas panhandle and western Oklahoma	Brush-grassland prairies
California black rail	*Laterallus jamaicensis coturniculus*	Colorado River; and from Tomales Bay and San Francisco, south and casually inland	Alkali bulrush and salt-grass
Spotted owl	*Strix occidentalis*	Pacific coastal and Cascade Mountains, British Columbia to northwestern California; Sierra Nevada and mountains of Southern California; southern Rocky Mountains (Colorado, Arizona, New Mexico)	Mature coniferous forest
Golden-cheeked warbler	*Dendroica chrysoparia*	Texas; Edwards Plateau, Dallas and Palo-pinto Counties	Mature growth "cedar breaks"
California least tern	*Sterna albifrons browni*	Pacific coast from south San Francisco Bay, California, to southern Baja, California	Beaches
Wallowa gray-crowned rosy finch	*Leucosticte tephrocotis wallowa*	Wallowa Mountains, Oregon	Open, alpine habitats
Ipswich Sparrow	*Passerculus princeps*	Atlantic coast from Nova Scotia south to southern Georgia (breeding Sable Island)	Sand dunes
Golden eagle	*Aquila chrysaetos*	All over U.S. (eastern and western)	Mountains, canyons, plains
Florida sandhill crane	*Grus canadensis praensis*	South Florida and extreme southern Georgia (Okefenokee Swamp)	Wet prairies and dry sandy areas
Northern greater prairie chicken	*Tympanuchus cupido pinnatus*	From eastern North Dakota and northwest Minnesota south to northeastern Colorado, and southcentral Oklahoma east to central Michigan, northwest Indiana and south-central Illinois	Prairie and grassland

Trumpeter swan	Cygnus buccinator	Wyoming, Montana, Idaho, southern Alaska	Wetlands
Tule white-fronted goose	Anser albifrons gambelli	California, Arctic	Wetlands
Spoonbill	Platalea leucorodia	Florida	Shallow wetlands
Rare Mammals			
Ozark big-eared bat	Plecotus townsendii ingens	Northwestern Arkansas, Oklahoma and Missouri	Caves
Virginia big-eared bat	Plecotus townsendii virginianus	Pendelton County, West Virginia; Tazewell County, Virginia, and Lee County, Kentucky	Caves
Spotted bat	Euderma maculatum	All the Southwestern States	Cliffs
Kaibab squirrel	Sciurus kaibabensis	Kaibab plateau on north side of Grand Canyon, Arizona	Yellow pines

[a]Continental—list excludes Hawaii, Puerto Rico, Islands.

[b]Endangered in MS, AL, OK, NC and inland areas of SC, GA, TX, plus parts of LA.

[c]Lower 48 states.

[d]No legal protection.

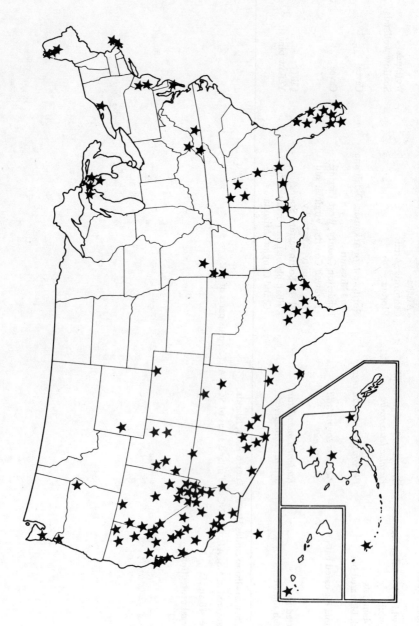

Figure 10-3. Distribution of endangered species that are geographically isolated

Table 10-10. Status of State Endangered Species Programs (Prance and Elias, 1976)

State	Committee Organized	Plant List	Animal List	Introduced	Legislation Passed	No./Code	Habitat	Program Species Research	Propagation	Administrative Office	Annual Budget
Alabama	X[a]	P[b]		1975						Department of Conservation; Department of Agriculture	
Alaska			P		X	16.20.180	X	X	X	Department of Fish and Game; Department of Natural Resources (DNR)	
Arizona	X	X			1975	S.B. 1334	X			Department of Natural and Cultural Heritage	
Arkansas											
California		X	X	X	X		X			Department of Fish and Game	$1 million
Colorado			X							Division of Wildlife	
Connecticut					1869	Acts 291					
Delaware	X	X	X				X				
Florida	X	X	X		1976		X		X	Game and Freshwater Fish Commission	$200[c] million
Georgia	X	X	X	X	Wild Flower Act–1973		X			Department of Natural Resources	
Hawaii											
Idaho	X	X	X							Department of Conservation	
Illinois		X			Endangered Species Act 1972		X				
Indiana	X	X					X			Natural Resources Commission	
Iowa		P			1975		X			Conservation Commission	
Kansas							X			Forestry, Fish and Game Commission	
Kentucky	X	X	X							Wildlife and Fisheries Commission; Forestry Commission	
Louisiana	X	P									
Maine											
Maryland	X	X	X	X	Endangered Species Conservation Act–1975; 1925; 1935 Plant Protection 1962	10-210C	X			Department of Natural Resources	
Massachusetts						266 MGLA-116A					
Michigan							X				

Table 10-10, continued

State	Committee Organized	Plant List	Animal List	Introduced	Legislation Passed	No./Code	Habitat	Program Species Research	Propagation	Administrative Office	Annual Budget
Minnesota					Protection of of Threatened and Endangered Species					Commissioner of Natural Resources Division of Fish and Wildlife	
Mississippi		P					X				
Missouri		X	X				X			Department of Conservation	
Montana		P					X			Department of Agriculture	
Nebraska					Endangered Species Conservation Act 1975						
Nevada	X	P			1969 d	Stat. 527.276				Division of Forestry	
New Hampshire	X		X	1971,1975							
New Jersey			X	1971	1975					Department of Environmental Protection	90,000[e]
New Mexico		X	X		1975	Art. 11, No. 563 Stat. 1953				State Game Commission	
New York		X[f]	X	1975	Conservation Law 1974	E.C.L. 9-1503			X	Department of Environmental Conservation	
North Carolina	X	X	X			E.C.L. 11-0535	X	X	X	Wildlife Resources Commission	
North Dakota											
Ohio	X	P	X	X	X		X			Division of Wildlife, DNR	
Oklahoma	X		X		f						
Oregon	X	X	X		Wildflowers		X			Land Conservation Development Commission; Department Agriculture	
Pennsylvania	X			X							
Rhode Island			X	X	1939						
South Carolina		X	X	X	Nongame Endangered Species Conservation Act–1974	Act 453-4	X		X	Wildlife and Marine Resources	$50,000[e]
South Dakota	X	X								Department of Agriculture Game Fish and Parks Department	

State				Year(s)	Statute	Agency	
Tennessee	P	X		1975, 1977	51-906	Wildlife Resources Commission	X
Texas	X	X		1977	127.70	Park and Wildlife Department	X
Utah	X						
Vermont	X			1921-1972	13 V.S.A. 3651-3	Environmental Conservation	
Virginia	X	X	X			Department of Natural Resources; Department of Wildlife	
Washington	X	X	X	1975			
West Virginia	P		X	1975		Heritage Trust Program, DNR	X
Wisconsin	X					Fish and Wildlife Management, DNR	X
Wyoming	d						

[a] X = Completed
[b] In preparation
[c] Bond issue
[d] Rare
[e] Proposed
[f] Protected native plants or animals

Table 10-11. Rare, Threatened or Endangered Plants and Animals
(U.S. Army, 1975; California Fish and Game Commission, 1976;
Florida Game and Freshwater Commission, 1976; McCollum, 1974;
Illinois Endangered Species Protection Board, 1977;   Kentucky Academy of
Science, 1975; Maryland State Code; Minnesota DNR, 1975;
Missouri DOC, 1974; New Jersey State Division of Fish, Game and
Shellfisheries, 1975; Berie, 1977; North Carolina Wildlife Resources Commission, 1977;
Smith *et al.*, 1975; Oklahoma Committee on Rare and Endangered Species, 1975;
Oregon State University, 1972; Russ, 1973)

Common Name	Scientific Name
California	
Rare or Endangered Mammals	
Guadalupe fur seal	*Arctocephalus townsendi*
Mohave ground squirrel	*Citellus mohavensis*
Morro Bay kangaroo rat	*Dipodomys heermanni morroensis*
Fresno kangaroo rat	*Dipodomys nitratoides exilis*
Stephen's kangaroo rat	*Dipodomys stephensi*
Wolverine	*Gulo luscus luteus*
California bighorn sheep	*Ovis canadensis californiana*
Peninsular bighorn sheep	*Ovis canadensis cremnobates*
Salt marsh harvest mouse	*Reithrodontomys raviventris*
Island fox	*Urocyon littoralis*
San Joaquin kit fox	*Vulpes macrotis mutica*
Rare or Endangered Birds	
California yellow-bellied cuckoo	*Coccyzus americanus occidentalis*
American peregrine falcon	*Falco peregrinus anatum*
California condor	*Gymnogyps californianus*
Southern bald eagle	*Haliaeetus leucocephalus leucocephalus*
California black rail	*Laterallus jamaicensis coturniculus*
Belding's savannah sparrow	*Passerculus sandwichensis beldingi*
California brown pelican	*Pelecanus occidentalis californicus*
Light-footed clapper rail	*Rallus longirostris levipes*
California clapper rail	*Rallus longirostris obsoletus*
Yuma clapper rail	*Rallus longirostris yumanensis*
California least tern	*Sterna albifrons browni*
Rare or Endangered Reptiles	
Southern rubber boa	*Charina bottae umbratica*
Blunt-nosed leopard lizard	*Crotaphytus silus*
Alameda striped racer	*Masticophis lateralis euryxanthus*
Giant garter snake	*Thamnophis couchi gigas*
San Francisco garter snake	*Thamnophis sirtalis tetrataenia*
Rare or Endangered Amphibians	
Santa Cruz long-toed salamander	*Ambystoma macrodactylum croceum*
Desert slender salamander	*Batrachoseps aridus*
Kern Canyon slender salamander	*Batrachoseps simatus*
Techachapi slender salamander	*Batrachoseps stebbinsi*
Black toad	*Bufo exsul*
Limestone salamander	*Hydromantes brunus*

Shasta salamander	*Hydromantes shastae*
Siskiyou Mountain salamander	*Plethodon stormi*

Endangered Fishes

Lost River sucker	*Catostomos luxatus*
Modoc sucker	*Catostomus microps*
Shortnose sucker	*Chasmistes brevirostris*
Rough Sculpin	*Cottus asperrimus*
Cottonball Marsh pupfish	*Cyprinodon milleri*
Tecopa pupfish	*Cyprinodon nevadenses calidae*
Owens River pupfish	*Cyprinodon radiosus*
Unarmored threespine stickleback	*Gasterosteus aculeatus williamsoni*
Owens tui chub	*Gila bicolor snyderi*
Thicktail chub	*Gila crassicauda*
Bonytail	*Gila elfgans*
Colorado River Squawfish	*Ptychocheilus lucius*
Mohave chub	*Siphateles mohavensis*
Humpback sucker	*Xyrauchen texanus*

Colorado

Endangered or Threatened Mammals

Lynx	*Lynx canadensis*
Wolverine	*Gulo luscus*
River otter	*Lutra canadensis*
Black-footed ferret	*Mustela nigripes*
Grizzly bear	*Ursus arctos*

Endangered or Threatened Birds

Bald eagle	*Haliaetus leucocephalus*
Peregrine falcon	*Falco peregrinus*
Whooping crane	*Grus americana*
Greater sandhill crane	*Grus canadensis tabida*
White pelican	*Pelecanus erythrorhynchos*
Sharptail grouse	*Pediocetes phasianellus*
Greater prairie chicken	*Tympanuchus cupido*
Lesser prairie chicken	*Tympanuchus pallidicinctus*

Endangered Fishes

Humpback chub	*Gila cypha*
Colorado River squawfish	*Ptychocheilus lucius*
Greenback cutthroat trout	*Salmo clarki stomias*
Bonytail chub	*Gila elegans*

Connecticut

Endangered Mammals

Atlantic right whale	*Euralaena glacialis*
Humpback whale	*Megaptera novaeangliae*
Blue whale	*Sibbaldus musculus*
Indiana bat	*Myotis sodalis*

Endangered Birds

American peregrine falcon	*Falco peregrinus anatum*
Bald eagle	*Haliaetus leucocephalus*
Ipswich sparrow	*Passerculus princeps*

Table 10-11 , continued

Common Name	Scientific Name
Florida	
Endangered Reptiles	
Pine barrens tree frog	*Hyla andersoni*
Atlantic green turtle	*Chelonia mydas mydas*
Atlantic hawksbill turtle	*Eretmochelys imbricata imbricata*
Atlantic ridley turtle	*Lepidochelys kempi*
Atlantic salt marsh snake	*Natrix faciata taeniata*
Short-tailed snake	*Stilosoma extenuatum*
Crocodile	*Crocodylus acutus*
Endangered Birds	
Wood stork	*Mycteria americana*
Florida everglades kite	*Rostrhamus sociabilis plumbeus*
Cuban snowy plover	*Charadrius alexandrinus tenuirostris*
Ivory-billed woodpecker	*Campephilus principalis*
American peregrine falcon	*Falco peregrinus*
Red-cockaded woodpecker	*Dendrocopus borealis hylonomus*
Bachman's warbler	*Vermvora bachmanii*
Kirtland's warbler	*Dendroica kirtlandii*
Florida grasshopper sparrow	*Ammodramus savannarum floridanus*
Dusky seaside sparrow	*Ammospiza maritima nigrescens*
Cape sable seaside sparrow	*Ammospiza maritima mirabilis*
Endangered Mammals	
Gray bat	*Myotis grisescens*
Indiana bat	*Myotis sodalis*
Mangrove fox squirrel	*Sciurus niger avicennia*
Goff's pocket gopher	*Geomys pinetis goffi*
Cudjoe Key rice rat	*Gryzomys spp.*
Pallid beach mouse	*Peromyscus polionotus decoloratus*
Key Largo cotton mouse	*Peromyscus gossypinus allapaticola*
Key Largo wood rat	*Neotoma floridana smalli*
Florida panther	*Felis concolor coryi*
Key deer	*Odocoileus virginianus clavium*
Threatened Fishes	
Okaloosa darter	*Etheostoma okaloosae*
Shortnose sturgeon	*Acipenser brevirostrum*
Suwannee bass	*Micropterus notius*
Threatened Amphibians	
Florida gopher frog	*Rana areolata aesopus*
Threatened Reptiles	
Key mud turtle	*Kinosternon bauri bauri*
Suwannee cooter	*Chrysemys cocinna suwanniensis*
Atlantic loggerhead turtle	*Caretta caretta caretta*
Gopher turtle	*Gopherus polyphemus*
Key mole skink	*Eumeces egregius egregius*
Blue-tailed mole skink	*Eumeces egregius lividus*

Sand skink	*Neoseps reynoldsi*
Big Pine Key ringneck snake	*Diadophis punctatus acricus*
Red rat snake	*Elaphe guttata guttata (Lower Keys only)*
Miami black-headed snake	*Tantilla oolitica*
Eastern indigo snake	*Drymarchon corais couperi*
Florida brown snake	*Storeria dekayi victa (Lower Keys only)*
Florida ribbon snake	*Thamnophis sauritus sackeni (Lower Keys only)*
American alligator	*Alligator mississippiensis*

Threatened Birds

Magnificent frigate bird	*Fregata magnificens rothschildi*
Osprey	*Pandion haliaetus carolinensis*
Southeast American kestrel	*Falco sparverius paulus*
American oystercatcher	*Haemotopus palliatus*
Roseate tern	*Sterna dougallii*
Least tern	*Sterna albifrons*
White-crowned pigeon	*Columba leucocephala*
Florida scrub jay	*Aphelocoma coerulescens coerulescens*
Louisiana seaside sparrow	*Ammospiza maritima fisheri*
Southern bald eagle	*Haliaetus leucocephalus leucocephalus*
Brown pelican	*Pelecanus occidentalis*
Audubon's caracara	*Caracara cheriway audubonii*
Arctic peregrine falcon	*Falco peregrinus tundrius*
Florida sandhill crane	*Grus canadensis pratensis*

Threatened Mammals

Sherman's fox squirrel	*Sciurus niger shermani*
Choctowatchee beach mouse	*Peromyscus polionotus allophrys*
Peridio Bay beach mouse	*Peromyscus polionotus trissyllepsis*
Florida mouse	*Peromyscus floridanus*
Keys cotton rat	*Sigmodon hispidus exsputus*
Key Vaca raccoon	*Procyon lotor auspicatus*
Manatee	*Trichechus manatus latirostris*
Everglades mink	*Mustela vison evergladensis*
Florida black bear	*Ursus americanus floridanus*

Georgia

Endangered Amphibians

Georgia blind cave salamander	*Haideotriton wallacei*
Tennessee cave salamander	*Gyrinophilus palleucus*
Pine barrens tree frog	*Hyla andersoni*

Endangered Reptiles

Bog turtle	*Clemmys muhlenbergi*
Atlantic ridley sea turtle	*Lepidochelys olinacea kempi*
Atlantic hawksbill turtle	*Eretmochelys imbricata imbricata*
Atlantic green turtle	*Chelonia mydas mydas*
Atlantic leatherback turtle	*Dermochelys coriacea coriacea*
Atlantic loggerhead turtle	*Caretta caretta caretta*
American alligator	*Alligator mississippiensis*
Eastern indigo snake	*Drymarchon carais couperi*

Table 10-11, continued

Common Name	Scientific Name
Endangered Birds	
Eastern brown pelican	*Pelecanus occidentalis*
Swallow-tailed kite	*Elanoides forficatus*
Bald eagle (southern)	*Haliaetus leucocephalus*
Peregrine falcon	*Falco peregrinus*
Ivory-billed woodpecker	*Campephilus principalis*
Red-cockaded woodpecker	*Dendrocopus borealis*
Kirtland's warbler	*Dendroica kirtlandii*
Bachman's warbler	*Vermivora bachmanii*
Endangered Fish	
Southern cavefish	*Typhlichthys subterraneus*
Endangered Mammals	
Indiana bat	*Myotis sodalis*
Cumberland Island pocker gopher	*Geomys cumberlandius (probably extinct)*
Anastasia Island cotton mouse	*Peromyscus gossypinus anastasae*
All marine mammals	Catacea
Couger	*Felis concolor*
Manatee	*Trichechus manatus*
Round-tailed muskrat	*Neofiber alleni*
Endangered Invertebrates	
Snail	*Somatogyrus cromax* (Flint River)
Snail	*Somatogyrus catostomus* (Flint River)
Snail	*Somatogyrus torrens* (Flint River)
Snail	*Somatogyrus rheophilus* (Flint River)
Snail	*Somatogyrus tenax* (Flint River)
Snail	*Goniobasis catenoides* (Mulberry Creek)
Snail	*Goniobasis baykiniana* (Chattahoochee River)
Clam	*Alasmidonta arcula* (Altamaha River)
Clam	*Elliptis hopetonensis* (Altamaha River)
Clam	*Elliptis dariensis* (Altamaha River)
Clam	*Elliptis shepardianus* (Altamaha River)
Clam	*Canthyria spinosa* (Altamaha River)
Clam	*Lampsilis dolabraeformis* (Altamaha River)
Clam	*Lampsilis binominata* (Flint River)
Clam	*Andontoa gibbosa* (Altamaha River)
Endangered Plants	
Hypnum	*Hypnum spp.*
Red algae	*Batrachospermum spp.*
Horsetail	*Equisetum arvense*
Shiny clubmoss	*Lycopodium lucidulum*
Rock clubmoss	*Lycopodium porophilum*
Fir clubmoss	*Lycopodium selago*
Ground pine	*Lycopodium obscurum*
Ground cedar	*Lycopodium tristachyum*

Spikemoss	*Selaginella ludoniciana*
Florida quillwort	*Isoetes flaccida*
Quillwort	*Isoetes melanopoda*
Winter grape fern	*Botrychium lunarioides*
Adder's tongue fern	*Ophioglossum engelmanni*
Climbing fern	*Lygodium palmatum*
Bristle fern	*Trichomanes boschianum*
Bristle fern	*Trichomanes petersii*
Smooth lipfern	*Cheilanthes alabamensis*
Glade fern	*Athyrium pycnocarpon*
Bulb fern	*Crytopteris bulbifera*
Mannagrass	*Glyceria acutiflora*
Mannagrass	*Glyceria melicaria*
Mannagrass	*Glyceria pallida*
Hillebore	*Veratrum viride*
Painted trillium	*Trillium undulatum*
Turk's-cap lily	*Lilium superbum*
Carolina lily	*Lilium michauxii*
Wood-featherling	*Tofieldia glutinosa*
Turkey-beard	*Xerophyllum asphodeloides*
Bellwort	*Uvularia grandiflora*
Swamp-pink	*Helonias bullata*
Wild canna	*Canna flaccida*
Spider-lily	*Hymenocallis caroliniana*
Gold-crest	*Lophiola americana*
Green-fly orchid	*Epidendrum conopseum*
Pink ladies slipper	*Cypripedium acaule*
Showy ladies slipper	*Cypripedium reginae*
Yellow ladies slipper	*Cypripedium calceolus*
Purple-fringed orchid	*Habenaria psycodes*
Orange rein orchid	*Habenaria integra*
Kidney-leaf tway blade	*Listera smallii*
Rosebud orchid	*Cleistes divaricata*
Showy orchis	*Orchis spectabilis*
Sweet fern	*Comptonia peregrina*
Corkwood	*Leitneria floridana*
White campion	*Silene ovata*
Pink campion	*Silene polypetala*
Goldenseal	*Hydrastis canadensis*
Dwarf larkspur	*Delphinium tricorne*
Monkshood	*Aconitum uncinatum*
Wolfsbane	*Aconitum reclinatum*
Twin leaf	*Jeffersonia diphylla*
Squirrel-corn	*Dicentra canadensis*
Dutchman's breeches	*Dicentra cucullaria*
Leavenworthia	*Leavenworthia exigua*
Leavenworthia	*Leavenworthia uniflora*
Sweet pitcher plant	*Sarracenia rubra*
Pitcher plant	*Sarracenia purpurea*
Stonecrop	*Sedum vigilmontis*
Grass-of-Parnassus	*Parnassia grandifolia*

Table 10-11, continued

Common Name	Scientific Name
Blue haw	*Crataegus brachyacantha*
Harbison's haw	*Crataegus harbisonii*
Big-fruited haw	*Crataegus ravenellii*
Yellow-wood	*Cladrastis lutea*
Perrenial partridge-pea	*Cassis fasciculata*
Buck-nuts	*Psoralea subacaulis*
Purple tassels	*Petalostemum gattingeri*
Fringed polygala	*Polygala paucifolia*
Allegheny-spurge	*Pachysandra procumbens*
Perpetual begonia	*Begonia semperflorens*
Edgeworthia	*Edgeworthia papyfera*
American ginseng	*Panax guinquefolia*
Wild sasparilla	*Aralia nudicaulis*
Cumberland azalea	*Rhododendron bakeri*
Plumleaf azalea	*Rhododendron prunifolium*
Purple-laurel	*Rhododendron catawbiense*
Sand myrtle	*Leiophyllum buxifolium*
Sheep-kill	*Kalmia caroliniana*
Shortia	*Shortia galacifolia*
Blue ash	*Fraxinus quadrangulata*
Large-flowered sabatia	*Sabatia capitata*
Dwarf ruellia	*Ruellia humilis*
Fly honeysuckle	*Lonicera canadensis*
Arrow-wood	*Viburnum bracteatum*
Stokesia	*Stokesia laevis*
Threatened Reptiles	
Barbour's map turtle	*Graptemys barbouri*
Spotted turtle	*Clemmys guttata*
Gopher tortoise	*Gopherus phlyphemus*
Threatened Birds	
Wood ibis	*Mycteria americana*
Mississippi kite	*Ictinia misisippiensis*
Sharp-shinned hawk	*Accipiter striatus*
Sparrow hawk	*Falco sparverius*
Florida sandhill crane	*Grus canadensis*
Threatened Fish	
Flame chub	*Hemitremia flammea*
Bluestripe shiner	*Notropis callitaenia*
Broadstripe shiner	*Notropis euryzonus*
Shoal bass	*Micropterus coosae*
Log perch	*Percina caprodes*
Darter	*Percina uranidea*
Goldline darter	*Percina aurolineata*
Trispot darter	*Etheostoma trisella*
Threatened Mammals	
Colonial pocket gopher	*Geomys colonus*
Sherman's pocket gopher	*Geomys fontanlus*

Threatened Invertebrates

Snail	*Marstonia castor* (Cedar Creek)
Snail	*Marstonia agarhecta* (Ocmulgee River)
Snail	*Notogillia sathon* (Ocmulgee River)
Snail	*Spilochlamys furgida* (Ocmulgee River)
Clam	*Amblema boykiniana* (Chattahoochee and Flint Rivers)

Threatened Plants

Green dragon	*Arisaema dracontium*
Sweet trillium	*Trillium vaseyi*
Yellow-mandarin	*Disporum lanuginosum*
Calesby's lily	*Lilium catesbaei*
Trumpet pitcher plant	*Sarracenia flava*
Parrot pitcher plant	*Sarracenia psittacina*
Dew threads	*Drosera filiformis*
Brook parnessia	*Parnassia asarifolia*
Leaf-cup	*Polymnia canadensis*
Coneflower	*Rudbeckia serecia*

Illinois

Endangered Fishes

Bluehead shiner	*Notropis* sp.
Harlequin darter	*Etheostoma histrio*
Longjaw cisco	*Coregonus alpenae*
Bigeye chub	*Hybopsis amblops*
Bluebreast darter	*Etheostoma camurum*

Threatened Fishes

Cisco	*Coregonus artedii*
Longnose sucker	*Catostomus catostomus*
Alligator gar	*Lepisosteus spatula*
Pugnose shiner	*Notropis anogenus*
Blacknose shiner	*Notropus heterolepus*
Lake whitefish	*Coregonus clupeaformis*
Lake sturgeon	*Acipenser fulvescens*
Bantam sunfish	*Lepomis symmetricus*

Endangered Amphibians and Reptiles

Silvery salamander	*Ambystoma platineum*
Spotted turtle	*Clemmys guttata*
Slider	*Pseudemys concinna*
Broad-banded water snake	*Natrix fasciata*
Eastern ribbon snake	*Thamnophis sauritus*
Dusky salamander	*Desmognathus fuscus*
Illinois mud turtle	*Kinosternen flavescens*

Threatened Amphibians and Reptiles

Illinois chorus frog	*Pseudacris streckeri*
Western hognose snake	*Heterodon nasicus*
Whip snake	*Masticophis flagellum*
Great Plains rat snake	*Elaphe guttata*

Endangered Breeding Populations—Birds

Double-crested cormorant	*Phalacrocorax auritus*
Snowy egret	*Leucopoyx thula*

Table 10-11, continued

Common Name	Scientific Name
Great egret	*Casmerodius albus* (Southern half of Illinois)
Little blue heron	*Florida caerulea*
American bittern	*Botaurus lentiginosus*
Black-crowned night heron	*Nycticorax nycticorax*
Mississippi kite	*Ictinia mississippiensis*
Sharp-shinned hawk	*Accipiter striatus*
Cooper's hawk	*Accipiter cooperii*
Red-shouldered hawk	*Buteo lineatus* (Northern 2/3 of Illinois)
Broad-winged hawk	*Buteo platypterus*
Swainson's hawk	*Buteo swainsoni*
Bald eagle	*Haliaetus leucocephalus*
Osprey	*Pandion haliaetus*
Marsh hawk	*Circus cyaneus*
Greater prairie chicken	*Tympanuchus cupido*
Yellow rail	*Coturnicops noveboracensis*
Black rail	*Laterallus jamaicensis*
Purple gallinule	*Prophyrula martinica*
Piping plover	*Charardrius melodus*
Upland snadpiper	*Bartramia longicauda*
Wilson's phalarope	*Steganopus tribolor*
Forster's tern	*Sterna forsteri*
Common tern	*Sterna hirundo*
Least tern	*Sterna albifrons*
Barn owl	*Tyto alba*
Long-eared owl	*Asio otus*
Short-eared owl	*Asio flammeus*
Saw-whet owl	*Aegolius acadicus*
Yellow-bellied sapsucker	*Sphyrapicus varius*
Western kingbird	*Tyrannus verticalis*
Red-breasted nuthatch	*Sitta canadensis*
Brown creeper	*Certhia familiaris*
Black tern	*Childonias niger*
Golden-winged warbler	*Vermivora chrysoptera*
Nashville warbler	*Vermivora ruficapilla*
Mourning warbler	*Oporornis philadelphia*
Yellow-headed blackbird	*Xanthocephalus xanthocephalus*
Bachman's sparrow	*Aimophila aestivalis*
Clay-colored sparrow	*Spizella pallida*

Threatened Breeding Populations—Birds

Veery	*Catharus fuscescens*
Loggerhead shrike	*Lanius ludovicianus* (Northern 1/2 of Illinois
Brewer's blackbird	*Euphagus cyanocephalus*
Common gallinule	*Gallinula chloropus*
Bewick's wren	*Thryomanes bewickii*
Swainson's warbler	*Limnothlypis swainsonii*
Henslow's sparrow	*Passerherbulus henslowii*

Endangered Mammals
- Eastern wood rat   *Neotoma floridana*
- Gray bat   *Myotis grisescens*
- Indiana bat   *Myotis sodalis*
- White-tailed jackrabbit   *Lepus townsendii*

Kentucky

Endangered Fishes
- Mud darter   *Etheostoma asprigene*
- Harlequin darter   *Etheostoma histrio*
- Tippecanoe darter   *Etheostoma tippecanoe*
- Longhead darter   *Percina macrocephala*
- Trout-perch   *Percopsis omiscomaycus*

Endangered Amphibians
- Tripoloid Jefferson's salamander   *Ambystoma platineum*
- Mole salamander[a]   *Ambystoma talpoideum*
- Red-backed salamander[a]   *Plethodon cinereus cinereus*
- Barking tree frog[a]   *Hyla gratiosa*

Endangered Reptiles
- Eastern ribbon snake   *Thamnophis sauritus*
- Western mud snake   *Farancia abacura reinwardti*
- Prairie king snake   *Lampropeltos calligaster calligaster*
- Southeastern crowned snake   *Tantilla coronata coronata*
- Green water snake[a]   *Natrix cyclopion cyclopion*
- Broad-banded water snake[a]   *Natrix fasciata confluens*
- Northern coal skink[a]   *Eumeces anthracinus anthracinus*

Endangered Birds
- Arctic peregrine falcon   *Falco peregrinus tundrius*
- Kirtland's warbler   *Dendroica kirtlandii*
- Red-cockaded woodpecker   *Dendrocopus borealis*
- Southern bald eagle   *Haliaetus leucocephalus leucocephalus*
- Common raven[a]   *Corvus corax*

Endangered Mammals
- Indiana bat   *Myotis sodalis*
- Virginia (Townsend's) big-eared bat   *Plecotus townsendii virginianus*
- Gray bat   *Myotis grisescens*
- Cougar   *Felis concolor*
- Cotton rat   *Sigmodon hispidus*
- Coyote   *Canis latrans*
- Meadow jumping mouse[a]   *Zapus hudsonius*
- River otter[a]   *Lutra canadensis*
- Black bear[a]   *Ursus americana*

Endangered Plants
- Kentuckiense fern   *Eupatorium resinosum kentuckiense*
- Sunflower   *Helianthus eggertii*
- Goldenrod   *Solidago albopilosa*
- Goldenrod   *Solidago shortii*
- Rock-cress   *Arabis perstellata perstellata*
- Leavenworthia   *Leavenworthia exigua laciniata*
- Conradina   *Conradina verticillata*

Table 10-11, continued

Common Name	Scientific Name
Threatened Plants	
Hog-fennel	*Oxypolis canbyi*
Chickering	*Prenanthes roanensis*
Leavenworthis	*Leavenworthis torulosa*
Lesquerella	*Lesquerella globosa*
Sandwort	*Arenaria fontinalis*
Sedge	*Carex purpurifera*
Rhododendron	*Rhododendron bakeri*
Groundnut	*Apios priceana*
St. John's-wort	*Hypericum sphaerocarpum turgidum*
Lady's slipper	*Cypripedium candidum*
Plae green orchis	*Platanthera flava*
Purple fringeless orchis	*Platanthera peramoena*
Muhly	*Muhlenbergia torreyana*
Phlox	*Phlox bifida stellaria*
Jacob's-ladder	*Polemonium reptans villosum*
Shooting-star	*Dodecatheon media frenchii*
Saxifrage	*Saxifraga caroliniana*
Sullivantia	*Sullivantia ohionis*
Sullivantia	*Sullivantia sullivantia*
Gerardia	*Aureolaria patula*
Violet	*Viola egglestonii*

Louisiana

Common Name	Scientific Name
Endangered Mammals	
Red wolf	*Canis rufus*
Cougar or Mountain lion	*Felis concolor*
Endangered Birds	
Ivory-billed woodpecker	*Campephilus principalis*
Red-cockaded woodpecker	*Dendrocopos borealis*
Peregrine falcon	*Falco peregrinus*
Southern bald eagle	*Haliaetus leucocephalus leucocephalus*
Brown pelican	*Pelecanus occidentalis*
Endangered Reptiles	
American alligator[b]	*Alligator mississippiensis*

Maryland

Common Name	Scientific Name
Endangered Mammals	
Delmarva Peninsula fox squirrel	*Sciurus niger cinereus*
Coyote	*Canis latrans*
Bobcat	*Lynx rufus rufus*
Porcupine	*Erethizon dorsatum*
Least weasel	*Mustela nivalis allegheniensis*
Mountain lion	*Felis concolor*
Black bear	*Ursus americanus*
Endangered Amphibians	
Hellbender	*Cryptobranchus alleganiensis alleganiensis*

Jefferson salamander	*Ambystoma jeffersonianum*
Eastern tiger salamander	*Ambystoma tigrinum tigrinum*
Green salamander	*Aneides aeneus*
Eastern narrow-mouthed toad	*Gastrophryne carolinensis*

Endangered Reptiles

Coal skink	*Eumeces anthracinus anthracinus*
Rainbow snake	*Farancia erytrogramma erytrogramma*
Mountain earth snake	*Virginia valeriae pulchra*
Bog turtle	*Clemmys muhlenbergi*
Atlantic green turtle	*Chelonia mydas mydas*
Atlantic hawksbill turtle	*Eretmochelys imbricata imbricata*
Atlantic loggerhead	*Caretta caretta caretta*
Atlantic ridley	*Lepidochelys kempi*
Atlantic leatherback	*Dermochelys coriacea coriacea*

Michigan

Endangered Mammals

Eastern timber wolf	*Canis lupus lycaon*
Cougar or mountain lion	*Felis concolor*
Indiana Bat	*Myotis sodalis*

Endangered Birds

Kirtland's warbler	*Dendroica kirtlandii*
American peregrine falcon	*Falco peregrinus anatum*
Artic peregrine falcon	*Falco peregrinus tundrius*

Endangered Fishes

Longjaw cisco	*Coregonus alpenae*
Blue pike	*Stizostedion vitreum glaucum*

Minnesota

Endangered Birds

American peregrine falcon	*Falco peregrinus*
Whooping crane	*Grus americanus*

Endangered Plants

Minnesota trout lily	*Erythronium propullans*

Threatened Mammals

Pine marten	*Martes americana*

Threatened Birds

Bobwhite quail	*Colinus virginianus*
Burrowing owl	*Speotyto cunicularia hypugea*
Greater sandhill crane	*Grus canadensis tabida*
Greater prairie chicken	*Tympanuchus cupida*

Threatened Reptiles and Amphibians

Blue-tailed skink	*Eumeces fascinatus*
Massasauga	*Sisturus catenatus*
Cricket frog	*Acris crepitans*

Missouri

Endangered Fishes

Lake sturgeon	*Acipenser fulvescens*
Pallid sturgeon	*Scaphirhynchus albus*
Sturgeon chub	*Hybopsis gelida*

Table 10-11, continued

Common Name	Scientific Name
Sicklefin chub	*Hybopsis meeki*
Blacknose shiner	*Notropis heterolepsis*
Pugnose minnow	*Opsopoeodus emiliae*
Eastern slim minnow	*Pimephales tenellus parviceps*
Neosho madtom	*Noturus placidus*
Pumpkinseed	*Lepomis gibbosus*
Harlequin darter	*Etheostoma histrio*
Goldstripe darter	*Etheostoma parvipinne*
Longnose darter	*Percina nasuta*
Endangered Amphibians	
Dwarf salamander	*Manculus quadridigitatus*
Wood frog	*Rana sylvatica*
Endangered Reptiles	
Western hognose snake	*Heterodon nasicus*
Endangered Birds	
Double-crested cormorant	*Phalacrocorax auritus*
Shart-shinned hawk	*Accipiter striatus*
Cooper's hawk	*Accipiter cooperii*
Osprey	*Pandion haliaetus*
Peregrine falcon	*Falco peregrinus*
Greater prairie chicken	*Tympanachus eupido*
Upland plover	*Bartramia longicauda*
Bachman's sparrow	*Aimophila aestivalis*
Golden eagle	*Aquila chrysaetos*
Bald eagle	*Haliaetus leucocephalus*
Endangered Mammals	
Indiana bat	*Myotis sodalis*
Small-footed bat	*Myotis leibii*
Gray bat	*Myotis grisescens*
Western big-eared bat	*Plecotus townsendii*
Eastern big-eared bat	*Plecotus rafinesquii*
Black bear	*Ursus americanus*
River otter	*Lutra canadensis*
Mountain lion	*Felis concolor*
White tailed jackrabbit	*Lepus townsendii*
Endangered Plants	
Liverwort	*Notothylas orbicularis*
Liverwort	*Riccia ozarkaniana*
Liverwort	*Riccardia palmata*
Liverwort	*Microlepidozia setacea*
Liverwort	*Microlepidozia sylvatica*
Liverwort	*Bassania trilobata*
Liverwort	*Nowellia curvifolia*
Liverwort	*Marsupella sullivantii*
Liverwort	*Ptilidium pulcherrimum*

Moss	*Archidium ohioense*
Sword moss	*Bryoxiphium norvegicum*
Moss	*Rhabdoweisia denticulata*
Moss	*Trematodon longicollis*
Moss	*Syrrhopodon texanus*
Moss	*Encalypta procera*
Moss	*Acaulon muticum*
Moss	*Barbula acuta*
Moss	*Barbula bescherellei*
Moss	*Barbula convoluta*
Moss	*Didymodon rigidulus*
Moss	*Tortula papillosa*
Moss	*Dicranum polysetum*
Moss	*Trichostomum mollissimum*
Moss	*Trichostomum tenuirostre*
Moss	*Grimmia ovalis*
Moss	*Grimmia teretinervis*
Moss	*Ptychomitrium leibergii*
Moss	*Ephemerum coharens*
Moss	*Ephemerum spinulosum*
Moss	*Orthotrichum diaphanum*
Moss	*Zygodon apiculatus*
Moss	*Philonotis capillaris*
Moss	*Bryum angustirete*
Moss	*Bryum minatum*
Moss	*Rhytidium rugosum*
Moss	*Rhytidiadelphus triquetrus*
Moss	*Isopterygium dischaceum*
Moss	*Isopterygium muellerianum*
Moss	*Leskea arenicola*
Moss	*Leskea australis*
Moss	*Homalia trichomanoides*
Moss	*Homaliadelphus sharpii*
Moss	*Thamnobryum alleghaniense*
Moss	*Leucodon brachypus*
Moss	*Brachelyma subulatum*
Moss	*Dichelyma capillaceum*
Moss	*Fontinalis biformis*
Moss	*Fontinalis disticha*
Moss	*Fontinalis hyphoides*
Sphagnum moss	*Sphagnum capillaceum tenerum*
Sphagnum moss	*Sphagnum cuspidatum*
Sphagnum moss	*Sphagnum recurvum tenue*
Round-branched ground pine	*Lycopodium obscurum dendroideum*
Seashore salt grass	*Distichlis spicata*
Spike grass	*Uniola laxa*
Swamp oats	*Trisetum pensylvanicum*
Narrow plume grass	*Erianthus strictus*
Many-spiked cyperus	*Cyperus polystachyos texansis*
Horsetail spike-rush	*Eleocharis equisetoides*

Table 10-11, continued

Common Name	Scientific Name
Wolf's spike-rush	*Eleocharis wolfii*
Hall's bulrush	*Scirpus hallii*
Swaying rush	*Scirpus subterminalis*
Torrey's bulrush	*Scirpus torreyi*
Canby's bulrush	*Scirpus etuberculatus*
Bayonet grass	*Scirpus paludosus*
Douglas' sedge	*Carex douglasii*
Straw sedge	*Carex straminea*
Bellows-beaked sedge	*Carex physorhyncha*
Shaved sedge	*Carex tonsa*
Wood's sedge	*Carex woodii*
Field sedge	*Carex conoidea*
Water sedge	*Carex aquatilis altior*
Tussock sedge	*Carex stricta strictior*
Schweinitz's sedge	*Carex schweinitzii*
Spiderwort	*Tradescantia ozarkana*
Canada rush	*Juncus canadensis canadensis*
Weak rush	*Juncus debilis*
Loesel's twayblade	*Liparis loeselii*
Large-toothed aspen	*Populus grandidentata*
Cordwood	*Leitneria floridana*
Ozark chinquapin	*Castanea ozarkensis*
Umbrella plant	*Eriogonum longifolium*
Halberd-leaved tear-thumb	*Polygonum arifolium*
Starwberry blite	*Chenopodium capitatum*
Bugseed	*Corispermum orientale emerginatum*
Pink	*Geocarpon minimum*
Cucumber tree	*Magnolia acuminata acuminata*
American barberry	*Berberis canadensis*
Fumitory	*Corydalis halei*
Whitlow grass	*Draba aprica*
Bladderpod	*Lesquerella filiformis*
Alum root	*Heuchera missouriensis*
Hardback, steeple bush	*Spiraea tomentosa rosea*
Queen of the prairie	*Filipendula rubra*
Red raspberry	*Rubus idaeus strigosus*
Prickly groundberry	*Rubus missouricus*
Snow wreath	*Neviusia alabamensis*
Spurge	*Euphorbia geyeri*
Flase mermaid	*Floerkea proserpinacoides*
American holly	*Ilex opaca*
Mallow	*Sida elliottii*
Waterwort	*Elatine triandra americana*
Swamp loosestrife	*Decodon verticillatus*
Evening primrose	*Stenosiphon linifolius*
Stagger bush	*Lyonia mariana*
Southern gooseberry	*Vaccinium stamineum malanocarpum*

Marsh pink	*Sabatia brachiata*
Screw-stem	*Bartonia paniculata*
Pennywort	*Obolaria virginica*
Buckbean	*Menyanthes trifoliata*
Waterleaf	*Hydrolea ovata*
Blue curls	*Trichostema setaceum*
Skullcap	*Scutellaria serrata montana*
Hedge hyssop	*Gratiola viscidula*
Mudwort	*Limosella aquatica*
Beard-tongue	*Penstemon grandiflorus*
Beard-tongue	*Penstemon cobaea cobaea*
American brooklime	*Veronica americana*
Gerardia	*Gerardia heterophylla*
Purple-painted cup	*Castelleja purpurea*
Broom-rape	*Orobanche ludoviciana*
Beech-drops	*Epifagus virginiana*
Northern bedstraw	*Galium boreale hyssopifolium*
Arrow-wood	*Viburnum recognitum*
Bluebell	*Campanula rotundifola*
Marsh bellflower	*Campanula aparinoides*
Bellflower	*Lobelia puberula mineolana*
Thoroughwort	***Eupatorium hyssopifolium calcaratum***
Horseweed	*Erigeron pusillus*
Marsh fleabane	*Pluchea foetida*
Leaf-cup	*Polymnia laevigata*
Purple coneflower	*Echinacea angustifolia*
Beggarticks	*Bidens laevis*
Flaveria	*Flaveria campestris*
Gaillardia	*Gaillardia lutea*
Lettuce	*Lactuca ludoviciana ludoviciana*
Rattlesnake-root	*Prenanthes racemosa*

Montana

Endangered Mammals
    Northern Rocky Mountain wolf   *Canis lupus irremotus*
    Black-footed ferret   *Mustela nigripes*
Endangered Birds
    American peregrine falcon   *Falcon peregrinus anatum*
    Whooping crane   *Grus americana*

Nebraska

Endangered Mammals
    Black-footed ferret   *Mustela nigripes*
    Swift fox   *Vulpes velox*
Endangered Birds
    American peregrine falcon   *Falco peregrinus anatum*
    Whooping crane   *Grus americana*
Endangered Fishes
    Lake sturgeon   *Acipenser fulvescens*

Table 10-11, continued

Common Name	Scientific Name
Nevada	
Protected Mammals	
Mountain beaver	*Aplodontia rufa*
Spotted bat	*Euderma maculatum*
Flying squirrel	*Glaucomys volans*
Pika	*Ochotona princeps*
Gray squirrel	*Sciurus carolinensis*
Douglas squirrel	*Tamiasciurus douglasi*
Kit (swift) fox	*Vulpes velox*
Protected Birds	
Cooper's hawk	*Accipiter cooperii*
Goshawk	*Accipiter gentilis*
Sharp-shinned hawk	*Accipiter striatus velox*
Short-eared owl	*Asio flammeus*
Long-eared owl	*Asio otus*
Great horned owl	*Bubo virgianus*
Red-tailed hawk	*Buteo jamaicensis*
Rough-legged hawk	*Buteo lagopus*
Ferruginous hawk	*buteo regalis*
Swainson hawk	*Buteo swainsoni*
Turkey vulture	*Cathartes aura*
Nighthawk	*Chordeiles minor*
Marsh hawk	*Circus cyaneus*
Merlin (pigeon hawk)	*Falco columbarius*
Prairie falcon	*Falco mexicanus*
Peregrine falcon	*Falco peregrinus*
Sparrow hawk	*Falco sparverius*
Road runner	*Geoccyx californianus*
Sparrow hawk	*Falco sparverius*
Roadrunner	*Geoccyx californianus*
Southern bald eagle	*Haliaetus leucocephalus leucocephalus*
Kingfisher	*Megacyrle alcyon*
Osprey	*Pandion haliaetus*
White pelican	*Pelecanus erythrorhynchos*
Brown pelican	*Pelecanus occidentalis*
White-faced glossy ibis	*Plegadis chihi*
Burrowing owl	*Speotyto cunicularia*
Barn owl	*Tyto alba*
Protected Reptiles	
Desert tortoise	*Gopherus agassizi*
Gila monster	*Heloderma suspectum*
Protected Fishes	
Spring cavefish	*Cholagaster agassizi*
White River springfish	*Crenichthys baileyi*
Railroad valley springfish	*Crenichthys nevadae*
Devil's Hole pupfish	*Cyprinodon diabolis*

Tecopa pupfish	*Cyprinodon nevadensis calidae*
Pahrump killifish	*Empetrichythys latos*
Desert dace	*Eremichthys acros*
Colorado bonytail	*Gila robusta elegans*
Pahranagat bonytail	*Gila robusta jordani*
White River spindace	*Lepidomeda albivallis*
Virgin River spindace	*Lepidomeda mollispinis mollispinis*
White River sucker	*Pantosieus intermedius*
Woundfin	*Plagopterus argentissimus*
Colorado River squawfish	*Ptychocheilus lucius*
Steptoe dace	*Relictus solitarius*
Utah cutthroat trout	*Salmo clarki utah*
Humpback sucker	*Xyrauchen taxanus*

New Jersey

Endangered Mammals
Indiana bat	*Myotis sodalis*
Sperm whale	*Physeter catodon*
Blue whale	*Balaenoptera musculus*
Finback whale	*Balaenoptera physalus*
Sei whale	*Balaenoptera borealis*
Humpback whale	*Megaptera novaeangliae*
Right whale	*Eubalaena* spp.

Endangered Fish
Shortnose sturgeon	*Acipenser brevirostrum*

Endangered Amphibians and Reptiles
Blue-spotted salamander	*Ambystoma laterale*
Eastern tiger salamander	*Ambystoma tigrinum*
Bog turtle	*Clemmys muhlenbergi*
Atlantic green turtle	*Chelonia mydas*
Atlantic hawksbill	*Eretmochelys imbricata*
Atlantic ridley	*Lepidochelys kempi*
Atlantic leatherback	*Dermochelys coriacea*

Endangered Birds
Bald eagle	*Haliaetus leucocephalus*
Peregrine falcon	*Falco peregrinus*
Osprey	*Pandion haliaetus*
Cooper's hawk	*Accipiter cooperii*

Threatened Fish
Atlantic tomcod	*Microgadus tomcod*

Threatened Amphibians and Reptiles
Pine barrens treefrog	*Hyla andersoni*
Eastern earth snake	*Virginia valeriae*
Timber rattlesnake	*Crotalus horridus*

Threatened Birds
Yellow-crowned night heron	*Nyctanassa violacea*
Least bittern	*Ixobrychus exilis*
Short-eared owl	*Asio glammeus*
Barred owl	*Strix varia*
Red-shouldered hawk	*Buteo lineatus*

Table 10-11, continued

Common Name	Scientific Name
Marsh hawk	*Circus cyaneus*
Sharp-shinned hawk	*Accipiter striatus*
Merlin (pigeon hawk)	*Falco columbarius*
King rail	*Laterallus jamaicensis*
Roseate tern	*Sterna dougallii*
Piping plover	*Charadrius melodus*
Upland plover	*Bartramia americana*
Short-billed marsh wren	*Cistothorus platensis*
Henslow's sparrow	*Passerherbulus henslowii*
Grasshopper sparrow	*Ammodramus savannarum*
Vesper sparrow	*Poaecetes gramineus*
Bobolink	*Dolichonyx oryzivorus*
Ipswich sparrow	*Passerculus sandwichensis princeps*
Red-headed woodpecker	*Melanerpes erythrocephalus*
Threatened Mammals	
Keen's bat	*Myotis keenii*
Small-footed bat	*Myotis subulatus*
Southern bog lemming	*Synaptomys cooperi*
Blainville's beaked whale	*Mesoplodon densirostris*
Gulf stream beaked whale	*Mesoplodon gervaisi*
True's beaked whale	*Mesoplodon mirus*
Goose-beaked whale	*Ziphius cavirostris*
Pigmy sperm whale	*Kogia breviceps*

New York

Endangered Mammals	
Indiana bat	*Myotis sodalis*
Eastern cougar	*Felis concolor cougar*
Eastern timber wolf	*Canis lupus lycaon*
Endangered Birds	
Northern bald eagle	*Haliaetus leucocephalus alascanus*
Southern bald eagle	*Haliaetus leucocephalus leucocephalus*
American peregrine falcon	*Falco peregrinus anatum*
Arctic peregrine falcon	*Falco peregrinus tundrius*
American osprey	*Pandion haliaetus carolinensis*
Endangered Reptiles	
Bog turtle	*Clemmys muhlenbergi*
Endangered Fishes	
Longjaw cisco	*Coregonus alpenae*
Blue pike	*Stizostedion vitreum glaucum*
Shortnose sturgeon	*Acipenser brevirostrum*
Endangered Invertebrates	
Karner blue butterfly	*Lycaeides melissa samuelis*
Chittenango ovate amber snail	*Succinea ovalis chittenangoensis*

North Carolina

Endangered Birds
Southern bald eagle — *Haliaetus leucocephalus*
Brown pelican — *Pelecanus occidentalis*
Red-cockaded woodpecker — *Dendrocopus borealis*
American peregrine falcon — *Falco peregrinus anatum*
Arctic peregrine falcon — *Falco peregrinus tundrius*

Endangered Mammals
Eastern cougar — *Felis concolor cougar*
Indiana bat — *Myotis sodalis*
Manatee — *Trichechus manatus*

Endangered Reptiles
American alligator — *Alligator mississippiensis*
Leatherback turtle — *Dermochelys coriacea*

Endangered Fish
Mooneye — *Hiodon tergisus*
Longhead darter — *Percina macrocephala*
Spotfin chub — *Hybopsis monacha*
Waccamaw killifish — *Fundulus waccamensis*
Waccamaw silverside — *Menidia extensa*

North Dakota

Endangered Mammals
Black-footed ferret — *Mustela nigripes*

Endangered Birds
American peregrine falcon — *Falco peregrinus anatum*
Arctic peregrine falcon — *Falco peregrinus tundrius*
Whooping crane — *Grus americana*
Southern bald eagle — *Haliaetus leucocephalus leucocephalus*

Ohio

Endangered Fishes
Lake sturgeon — *Acipenser fulvescens*
Rosyside dace — *Clinostomus funduloides*
Tonguetied minnow — *Exoglossum laurae*
Pugnose minnow — *Notropis emiliae*
Lake chubsucker — *Erimyzon sucetta*
Greater redhorse — *Moxostoma valenciennesi*
Scioto madtom — *Noturus trautmani*
Pirate perch — *Aphredoderus sayanus*
Eastern sand darter — *Ammocrypta pellucida*
Iowa darter — *Etheostoma exile*
Channel darter — *Percina copelandi*
Blue pike — *Stizostedion vitreum glaucum*
Blue sucker — *Cycleptus elongatus*
Great Lakes muskellunge — *Esox masquinongy masquinongy*
Banded killifish — *Fundulus diaphanus*
Silver chub — *Hybopsis storeiana*
Ohio lamprey — *Ichthyomyzon bdellium*

Table 10-11, continued

Common Name	Scientific Name
Northern brook lamprey	*Ichthyomyzon fosser*
Allegheny brook lamprey	*Ichthyomyzon grefleyi*
Silver lamprey	*Ichthyomyzon unicuspis*
American brook lamprey	*Lampetra lamottei*
River redhorse	*Moxostoma carinatum*
Blacknose shiner	*Notropis heterolepsis*
Mountain madtom	*Noturus eleutherus*
Northern madtom	*Noturus stigmosus*
Longhead darter	*Percina macrocephala*
River darter	*Percina shumardi*
Paddlefish	*Polyodon spathula*
Endangered Reptiles[c]	
Northern copperbelly (Red-bellied water snake)	*Natrix erythrogaster neglecta*
Endangered Birds[c]	
Northern bald eagle	*Haliaetus leucocephalus alascanus*
Kirtland's warbler	*Dendroica kirtlandii*
American peregrine falcon	*Falco peregrinus anatum*
Endangered Mammals[c]	
Indiana bat	*Myotis sodalis*

Oklahoma

Endangered Fishes	
Shovelnose sturgeon	*Scaphirhynchus platorynchus*
Ironcolor shiner	*Notropis chalybaeus*
Arkansas darter	*Etheostoma cragini*
Scaleyhead darter	*Etheostoma fusiforme barratti*
Leopard darter	*Percina pantherina*
Chain pickerel	*Esox niger*
Endangered Reptiles	
American alligator	*Alligator mississippiensis*
Endangered Birds	
Eskimo curlew	*Numenius borealis*
Southern bald eagle	*Haliaetus leucocephalus*
Whooping crane	*Grus americana*
Ivory-billed woodpecker	*Campephilus principalis*
Bachman's warbler	*Vermivora bachmanii*
Peregrine falcon	*Falco peregrinus*
Red-cockaded woodpecker	*Dendrocopos borealis*
Endangered Mammals	
Indiana bat	*Myotis sodalis*
Black-footed ferret	*Mustela nigripes*
Red wolf	*Canis niger*

Oregon

Endangered Mammals
    Richardson ground squirrel   *Spermophilus richardsoni*
    Kit fox   *Vulpes macrotis*
    Sea otter   *Enhydra lutris*
    Lynx   *Lynx canadensis*
    Columbian white-tailed deer   *Odocoileus virginianus leucurus*

Endangered Birds
    Aleutian Canada goose   *Branta canadensis leucopareia*
    Tule white-fronted goose   *Anser albifrons gambelli*
    American peregrine falcon   *Falco peregrinus anatum*
    Prairie falcon   *Falco mexicanus*
    Greater sandhill crane   *Grus canadensis tabida*
    Trumpeter swan   *Cygnus buccinator*
    Northern bald eagle   *Haliaetus leucocephalus alascanus*
    Western pigeon hawk   *Falco columbarius*
    Franklin's spruce grouse   *Canachites canadensis franklinii*
    Northern spotted owl   *Strix occidentalis caurina*

Endangered Fishes
    Warner sucker   *Catostomus warnerensis*
    Shortnose sucker   *Chasmistes brevirostris*

Pennsylvania

Endangered Reptiles
    Bog turtle   *Clemmys muhlenbergi*
    Blanding's turtle   *Emydoidea blandingii*
    Eastern mud turtle   *Kinosternon subrubrum*
    Red-bellied turtle   *Pseudemys rubriventris*
    Smooth softshell turtle   *Trionyx muticas*

Endangered Fishes
    Shortnose sturgeon   *Acipenser brevirostrum*
    Lake sturgeon   *Acipenser fulvescens*
    Unarmored threespine stickleback   *Gasterosteus aculeatus williamsoni*
    Blue pike   *Stizostedion vitreum glaucum*

Rhode Island

Mammals
    Sei whale   *Balaenoptera borealis*
    Blue whale   *Balaenoptera musculus*
    Fin whale   *Balaenoptera physalus*
    Eastern cougar   *Felis concolor cougar*
    Humpback whale   *Megaptera novaeangliae*
    Indiana bat   *Myotis sodalis*
    Sperm whale   *Physeter catodon*

Birds
    Arctic peregrine falcon   *Falco peregrinus tundrius*
    Southern bald eagle   *Haliaetus leucocephalus leucocephalus*

Fishes
    Shortnose sturgeon   *Acipenser brevirostrum*

Table 10-11, continued

Common Name	Scientific Name

South Dakota

Endangered Mammals
Black-footed ferret — *Mustela nigripes*

Texas

Endangered Mammals

Common Name	Scientific Name
Bat, lesser yellow	*Lasiurus ega xanthinus*
Bat, Rafinesque's big-eared	*Plecotus rafinesquii*
Bat, southeastern	*Myotis austroriparius mumfordi*
Bat, spotted	*Euderma maculatum*
Dolphin, bridled	*Stenella frontalis*
Dolphin, rough-toothed	*Steno bredanensis*
Dolphin, spotted	*Stenella plagiodon*
Mouse, Palo Duro	*Peromyscus comanche*
Rat, Texas kangaroo	*Dipodomys elator*
Whale, drawf sperm	*Kogia simus*
Whale, false killer	*Pseudorca crassidens*
Whale, goose-beaked	*Ziphius cavirostris*
Whale, Gulf Stream beaked	*Mesoplodon europaeus*
Whale, killer	*Orcinus orca*
Whale, short-finned pilot	*Globicephala macrorhyncha*
Whale, pygmy killer	*Feresa attenuata*
Whale, pygmy sperm	*Kogia breviceps*
Blue whale	*Balaenoptera musculus*
Finback whale	*Balaenoptera physalus*
Right whale	*Eubalaena* spp. (all species)
Sperm whale	*Physeter catodon*
Black-footed ferret	*Mustela nigripes*
Jaquar	*Panthera onca*
Jaguarundi	*Felis yagouaroundi cacomitli*
Margay	*Felis wiedii*
Ocelot	*Felis pardalis*
Red wolf	*Canis rufus*
Gray wolf	*Canis lupus monstrabilis*
Mexican wolf	*Canis lupus baileyi*
West Indian manatee	*Trichechus manatus*
Bighorn sheep	*Ovis canadensis*

Endangered Birds

Common Name	Scientific Name
Brown pelican	*Pelecanus occidentalis*
Mexican duck	*Anas diazi*
Southern bald eagle	*Haliaeetus l. leucocephalus*
American peregrine falcon	*Falco peregrinus anatum*
Arctic peregrine falcon	*Falco peregrinus tundrius*
Attwater's greater prairie chicken	*Tympanuchus cupido attwateri*
Whooping crane	*Grus americana*
Eskimo curlew	*Numenius borealis*

Interior least tern	*Sterna albifrons athalassos*
Ivory-billed woodpecker	*Campephilus principalis*
Red-cockaded woodpecker	*Dendrocopos borealis*
Bachman's warbler	*Vermivora bachmanii*
Egret, reddish	*Dichromanassa r. rufescens*
Falcon, aplomado	*Falco femoralis septentrionalis*
Hawk, black	*Buteogallus a. anthracinus*
Hawk, gray	*Buteo nitidus maximus*
Hawk, white-tailed	*Buteo albicaudatus hypospodius*
Hawk, zone-tailed	*Buteo albonotatus*
Ibis, white-faced	*Plegadis chihi*
Kite, swallow-tailed	*Elanoides f. forficatus*
Osprey	*Pandion haliaetus carolinensis*
Owl, ferruginous	*Glaucidium brasilianum cactorum*
Stork, wood	*Mycteria americana*
Tern, least	*Sterna albifrons antillarum*
Warbler, golden-cheeked	*Dendroica chrysoparia*

Endangered Reptiles

Speckled racer	*Drymobius m. margaritiferus*
Harter's water snake	*Natrix harteri*
Atlantic ridley turtle	*Lepidochelys kempii*
Hawksbill turtle	*Eretmochelys imbricata*
Leatherback turtle	*Dermochelys coriacea*
American alligator	*Alligator mississipiensis*
Loggerhead, Atlantic	*Caretta c. caretta*
Tortoise, Texas	*Gopherus berlandieri*
Turtle, Atlantic green	*Chelonia m. mydas*
Turtle, Big Bend mud	*Kinosternon hirtipes murrayi*
Gecko, Big Bend	*Coleonyx reticulatus*
Lizard, Big Bend canyon	*Sceloporus merriami annulatus*
Lizard, Presidio canyon	*Sceloporus merriami longipunctatus*
Lizard, reticulate collared	*Crotaphytus reticulatus*
Lizard, Texas horned	*Phrynosoma cornutum*
Lizard, mountain short-horned	*Phrynosoma douglassi hernandesi*
Copperhead, Trans-Pecos	*Agkistrodon contortrix pictigaster*
Kingsnake, gray-banded	*Lampropeltis mexicana alterna*
Rattlesnake, rock	*Crotalus lepidus*
Snake, black-striped	*Coniophanes i. imperialis*
Snake, northern cat-eyed	*Leptodeira s. septentrionalis*
Snake, Texas indigo	*Drymarchon corais erebennus*
Snake, Texas lyre	*Trimorphodon biscutatus vilkinsoni*
Snake, Big Bend milk	*Lampropeltis triangulum celaenops*
Snake, central plains milk	*Lampropeltis triangulum gentilis*
Snake, Louisiana milk	*Lampropeltis triangulum amaura*
Snake, Mexican milk	*Lampropeltis triangulum annulata*
Snake, Louisiana pine	*Pituophis melanoleucus ruthveni*
Snake, Baird's rat	*Elaphe obsoleta bairdi*
Snake, Trans-Pecos rat	*Elaphe subocularis*

Table 10-11, continued

Common Name	Scientific Name
Endangered Amphibians	
Cascade Cavern salamander	*Eurycea latitans*
Texas blind salamander	*Typhlomolge rathbuni*
Houston toad	*Bufo houstonensis*
Frog, Mexican cliff	*Syrrhophus guttilatus*
Frog, Mexican tree	*Smilisca baudini*
Frog, Rio Grande	*Syrrhophus cystignathoides campi*
Frog, white-lipped	*Leptodactylus labialis*
Newt, black-spotted	*Notophthalmus m. meridionalis*
Salamander, Fern Bank	*Eurycea neotenes pterophila*
Salamander, Honey Creek	*Eurycea tridentifera*
Salamander, mole	*Ambystoma talpoideum*
Salamander, San Marcos	*Eurycea nana*
Salamander, Valdina Farms	*Eurycea troglodytes*
Siren, Rio Grande	*Siren intermedia texana*
Toad, giant	*Bufo marinus*
Toad, Mexican burrowing	*Rhinophrynus dorsalis*
Endangered Fishes	
Blindcat, toothless	*Trogloglanis pattersoni*
Blindcat, widemouth	*Satan eurystomus*
Chub, Rio Grande	*Gila pandora*
Darter, Rio Grande	*Etheostoma grahami*
Darter, river	*Hadropterus shumardi*
Darter, Western sand	*Ammocrypta clara*
Gambusia blotched	*Gambusia senilis*
Paddlefish	*Polyodon spathula*
Shovelnose sturgeon	*Scaphirhynchus platorynchus*
Amistad gambusia	*Gambusia amistadensis*
San Marcos gambusia	*Gambusia georgei*
Big Bend gambusia	*Gambusia gaigei*
Clear Creek gambusia	*Gambusia heterochir*
Pecos gambusia	*Gambusia nobilis*
Comanche Springs pupfish	*Cyprinodon elegans*
Leon Springs pupfish	*Cyprinodon bovinus*
Fountain darter	*Etheostoma fonticola*
Bluntnose shiner	*Notropis simus*
Minnow, Devils River	*Dionda diaboli*
Pupfish, Conchos	*Cyprinodon eximius*
Shiner, Chihuahua	*Notropis chihuahua*
Shiner, Kiamichi	*Notropis ortenburgeri*
Shiner, proserpine	*Notropis proserpinus*
Stoneroller, Mexican	*Campostoma ornatum*
Sucker, blue	*Cycleptus elongatus*

Virginia

Endangered Reptiles

Wood turtle	*Clemmys insculpta*
Bog turtle	*Clemmys muhlenbergi*
Northern pine snake	*Pituophis malenoleucus*
Scarlet king snake	*Lampropeltis triangulum elapsoides*
Canebrake rattlesnake	*Crotelus horridus atricaudatus*

Endangered Amphibians

Mudpuppy	*Necturus maculosus*
Dwarf waterdog	*Necturus punctatus*
Greater siren	*Siren lacartina*
Carpenter frog	*Rana virgatipes*

Endangered Birds

Bachman's warbler	*Vermivora bachmanii*
Southern bald eagle	*Haliaetus leucocephalus*
Red-cockaded woodpecker	*Dendrocopos borealis*
Ipswich sparrow	*Passerculus princeps*

Endangered Mammals

Dismal Swamp lemming mouse	*Synaptomys cooperi helaletes*
Virginia big-eared bat	*Plecotus townsendii virginianus*
Rafinesque's big-eared bat	*Plecotus townsendii rafinesquii*
Indiana bat	*Myotis sodalis*
Northern flying squirrel	*Glaucomys sabrinus fuscus*
Delmarva fox squirrel	*Sciurus niger neglecus*
Eastern panther	*Felis concolor couguar*

Washington

Protected Mammals

Northern fur seal	*Callorhinus ursinus*
Whales, dolphins and porpoises	Catacea
Sea otter	*Enhydra lutris*
Flying squirrel	*Glaucomys volans*
Wolverine	*Gulo gulo*
White-tailed jackrabbit	*Lepus townsendii*
Hoary marmot	*Mormota caligata*
Fisher	*Martes pennanti*
Pikas	Ochotonidae
Sea lions	Otariidae
Seals	Phocidae
Gray squirrel	*Sciurus carolinensis*
Fox squirrel	*Sciurus niger*
Golden-mantled ground squirrel	*Spermophilus lateralis*
Pigmy rabbit	*Sylvilagus idahoensis*
Douglass (chickaree) squirrel	*Tamiasciurus douglasii*
Red squirrel	*Tamiasciurus hudsonicus*

Amphibians

Western Washington turtle	*Tesudinata sp.*

Table 10-11, continued

Common Name	Scientific Name
Wisconsin	
Protected Mammals	
Canada lynx	*Lynx canadensis*
Pine marten	*Martes americana*
Protected Birds	
Bald eagle	*Haliaetus leucocephalus*
Osprey	*Pandion haliaetus*
Double-crested comorant	*Phalacrocorax auritus*
Protected Reptiles	
Queen snake	*Natrix septemvittata*
Ornate box turtle	*Terrapene ornata ornata*
Protected Fishes	
Longjaw cisco	*Coregonus alpenae*
Kiyi	*Coregonus kiyi*
Shortnose cisco	*Coregonus reighardi*
Shortjaw cisco	*Coregonus zenithicus*
Ozark minnow	*Dionda nubila*
Greater redhorse	*Moxostoma valenciennesi*
Pugnose shiner	*Notropis anogenus*
Wyoming	
Mammals	
Wolverine	*Gulo luscus*
River otter	*Lutra canadensis*
Canada lynx	*Lynx canadensis*
Fisher	*Martes pennanti*
Black-footed ferret	*Mustela nigripes*
Pika	*Ochotona princeps*
Birds	
Kingfisher	*Megaceryle alcyon*
Trumpeter swan	*Olor buccinator*
Whistling swan	*Olor columbianus*
White pelican	*Pelecanus erythrorhynchos*

[a]Recommended addition by the Kentucky Academy of Science.
[b]Declassified to threatened on federal list, except in three parishes.
[c]Incomplete list.

REFERENCES

Agriculture, U.S. Department of, "Agricultural Statistics," U.S. Government Printing Office, Washington, D.C. (1975).

Alaska, Department of Fish and Game. "Survey-Inventory Progress Report" (1976).

Allen, D. L. *Our Wildlife Legacy,* revised ed. (New York: Funk and Wagnalls Co., 1962).

Army Engineer Waterways Experiment Station, U.S. "Selected Legally Protected Animals," Report 2, NTIS-AD-A015–578 (1975).

Arner, D. H., J. Baker and D. Wesley. "The Management of Beaver and Beaver Ponds in the Southeastern United States," Mississippi State University, State College, Mississippi (1966).

Beard, E. B. "The Importance of Beaver in Waterfowl Management at the Seney National Wildlife Refuge," *J. Wildlife Managemt.* 17:398-436 (1953).

Berle, P. A. A. Commissioner of Environmental Conservation, New York State, Albany. Section 11-0535, Environmental Conservation Law, 1977.

California Fish and Game Commission. "At the Crossroads," A Report on California's Endangered and Rare Fish and Wildlife (1976).

Carlander, K. S. "The Standing Crop of Fish in Lakes," *J. Fish Res. B. Can.* 12:543-570 (1955).

Cole, G. F. "Management Involving Grizzly Bears in Yellowstone," *Proc. 26th Ann. AIBS Meeting* (1976).

Ernest, J. "Snowshoe Hare Studies," Alaska Department of Fish and Game, Final Report (1974).

Errington, P.L. *Of Predation and Life* (Ames, IA: Iowa State University Press, 1967).

Florida Game and Freshwater Fish Commission, Wildlife Management Division. "Endangered and Threatened Species Included in Wildlife Code," Tallahassee, Florida (1976).

Gier, H. T. "Coyotes in Kansas," Bulletin 393, Agriculture Experiment Station, Kansas State University, Manhattan, Kansas (1968).

Illinois Endangered Species Protection Board. "Official List Being Recommended," Unpublished, 1977.

Interior, U.S. Department of, Fish and Wildlife Service. "Threatened Wildlife of the United States" (1973).

Interior, U.S. Department of, Fish and Wildlife Service. "United States List of Endangered Fauna" (May 1974).

Interior, U.S. Department of, Fish and Wildlife Service, "Endangered and Threatened Wildlife," CFR, Title 50 (1975).

Interior, U.S. Department of, Fish and Wildlife Service. "Endangered and Threatened Wildlife," 41FR 106:22041 (1976a).

Interior, U.S. Department of, Fish and Wildlife Service. "Endangered and Threatened Wildlife," 41FR 115:24062 (1976b).

Interior, U.S. Department of, Fish and Wildlife Service. "Convention on International Trade," 41FR 117:24367 (1976c).

Interior, U.S. Department of, Fish and Wildlife Service."Endangered and Threatened Wildlife," 42FR 105:28056 (1977a).

Interior, U.S. Department of, Fish and Wildlife Service. "Endangered and Threatened Wildlife," 42FR:135:36420 (1977b).

Kendeigh, S. C. *Animal Ecology* (Englewood Cliffs, NJ: Prentice Hall, Inc, 1961).

Kentucky Academy of Science ad hoc Committee on Rare and Endangered Species. "Kentucky's Rare and Endangered Species," (1975).

Küchler, A. W. Potential Natural Vegetation (map), *The National Atlas* (1966).

Martin, A. C., H. S. Zim and A. L. Nelson. *American Wildlife and Plants: A Guide to Wildlife Food Habits* (New York: Dover Publications, 1961).

Maryland State Code. "Maryland State Endangered Species List," Title 10 Section 210C.

McCollum, J. L., Ed. "Endangered Species of Georgia," *Proc. 1974 Conf,* Georgia Department of Natural Resources. Atlanta, Georgia (1974).

Minnesota Department of Natural Resources. "The Uncommon Ones" (1975).

Missouri Department of Conservation. "Rare and Endangered Species of Missouri" (1974).

New Jersey State, Division of Fish, Game, and Shellfisheries. Endangered and Nongame Species Project, Department of Environmental Protection, 1975.

North Carolina Wildlife Resources Commission. "Endangered Species of North Carolina" (1977).

Odum, E. P. *Fundamentals of Ecology,* 3rd ed. (Philadelphia: W. B. Saunders Co., 1971).

Oklahoma Committee on Rare and Endangered Species and U.S. Department o of Agriculture. Rare and Endangered Vertebrates and Plants of Oklahoma (1975).

Olson, J. S. "Productivity of Forest Ecosystems," *Productivity of World Ecosystems* (Washington, D.C.: National Academy of Sciences, 1975).

Oregon State University, Agriculture Experiment Station. "Endangered Plants and Animals of Oregon," I Fishes (1974); III Birds (1969); and IV Mammals (1972).

Prana, G. T., and T. S. Elias, Eds. *Extinction is Forever* (Millbrook, NY: New York Botanical Garden, 1976).

Rodin, L. E., N. I. Bazilevich and N. N. Rozov. "Productivity of the World's Main Ecosystems," *Productivity of World Ecosystems* (Washington, D.C.: National Academy of Sciences, 1975).

Russ, W. P. "The Rare and Endangered Terrestrial Vertebrates of Virginia," M.S. Thesis, Virginia Polytechnical Institute, Blacksburg, Virginia, 1973, unpublished.

Seton, E. T. *Life Histories of Northern Animals* (New York: Charles Scribner's Sons, 1909).

Smith, H. G., R. K. Burnard, E. E. Good and J. M. Keener. "Rare and Endangered Vertebrates of Ohio," *Ohio J. Sci.* 73(5):257-271 (1973).

Stephenson, R. O. "Wolf Report," Alaska Department of Fish and Game, Vol. XIV (1975).

Taylor, W. P., Ed. *The Deer of North America* (Harrisburg, PA: Stackpole Co., 1965).

Weeden, R. B. "Management of Ptarmigan in North America," *J. Wildlife Managemt.* 27:673-683 (1963).

Young, S. P. *The Bobcat of North America* (Harrisburg, PA: Stackpole Co., 1958).

CHAPTER 11

ECOSYSTEMS–EXAMPLES

INTRODUCTION

The following section presents a wide range of ecosystem examples one might encounter on site visits and should prove useful to those preparing an EIS. Its use should be of considerable value to those who have not had first-hand experience with specific site types.

BEACH AND DUNE SUCCESSION

Figures 11-1 to 11-9 present a variety of ecosystem types that can be found on beaches and dunes.

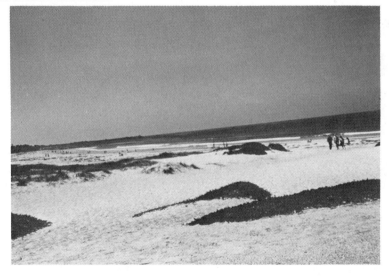

Figure 11-1. Beach and primary dune (severely disturbed) (photo by Sharon Saari).

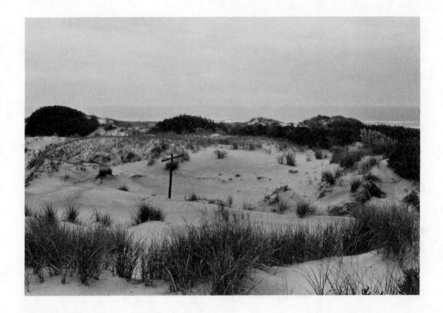

Figure 11-2. Primary dune, trough and secondary dune (drifting) (photo by Sharon Saari).

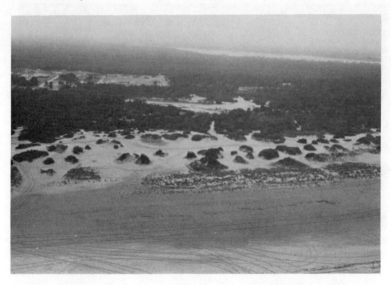

Figure 11-3. Beach (foreground); primary dune and trough (impacted by off-road vehicles); and backdune and bayshore (background) (photo by Sharon Saari).

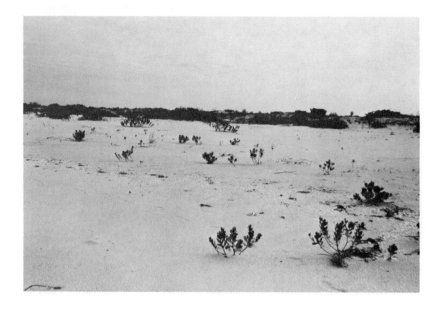

Figure 11-4. Beach colonization (first step in succession) (photo by Sharon Saari).

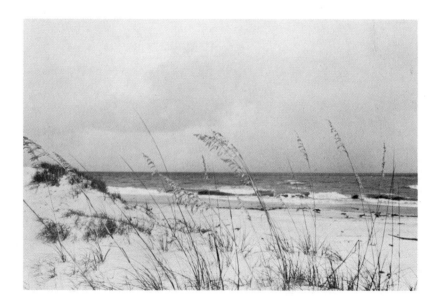

Figure 11-5. Primary dune building (early seral stage) (photo by Sharon Saari).

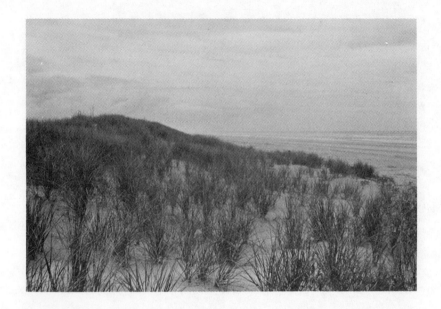

Figure 11-6. Dune stabilization (beachgrass planted) (photo by Sharon Saari).

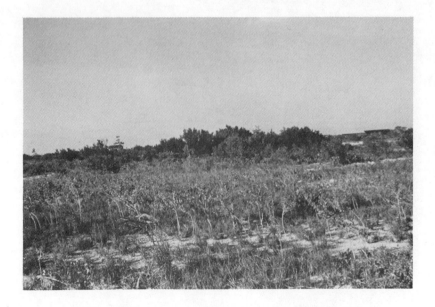

Figure 11-7. Beach trough (behind duneline) (photo by Sharon Saari).

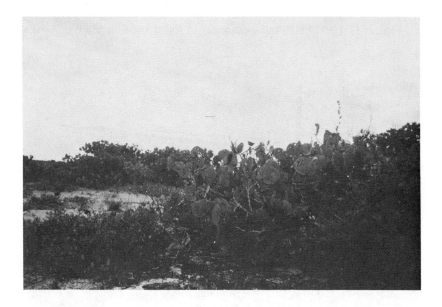

Figure 11-8. Secondary dune (stabilized with shrubs) (photo by Sharon Saari).

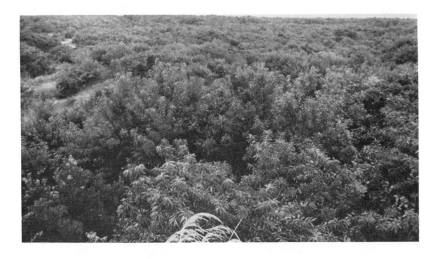

Figure 11-9. Backdune (relatively stable behind primary and secondary dunes) (photo by Sharon Saari).

FOREST FIRE SUCCESSION

Figures 11-10 to 11-16 show examples of forest fire succession in Alaska.

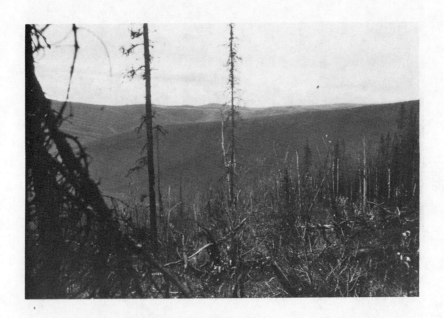

Figure 11-10. Northern spruce forest fire (Alaska) (photo by Sharon Saari).

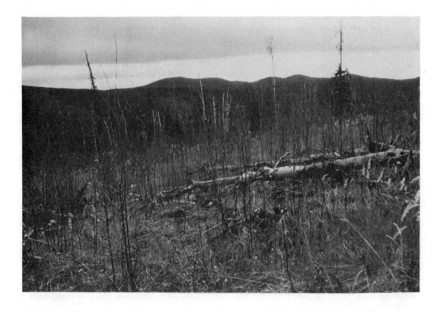

Figure 11-11. First seral stage after fire—high brush regrowth (photo by Sharon Saari).

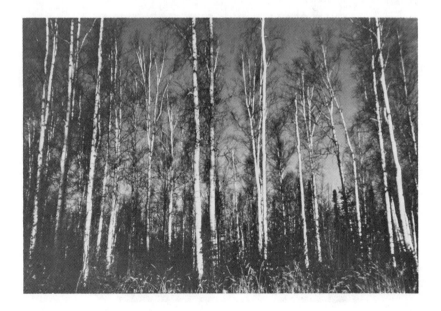

Figure 11-12. Second seral stage after fire—hardwood (birch) (photo by Sharon Saari).

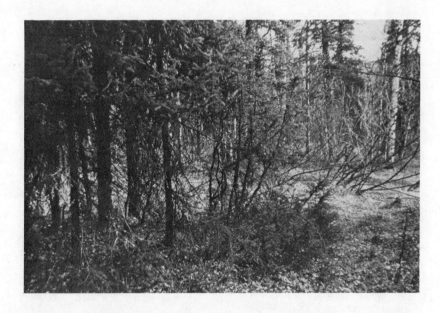

Figure 11-13. Spruce/hardwood ecotone (intermediate stage after fire) (photo by Sharon Saari).

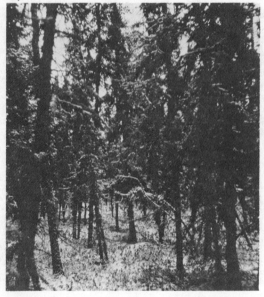

Figure 11-14. Black spruce forest (mature stage) (photo by Sharon Saari).

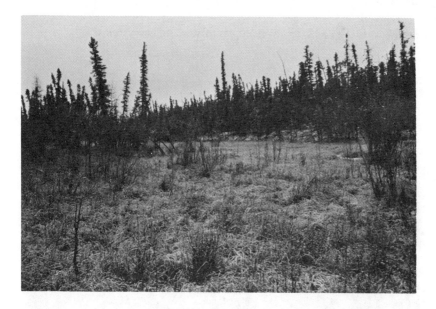

Figure 11-15. Tundra biome; black spruce/muskeg (Alaska) (photo by Sharon Saari).

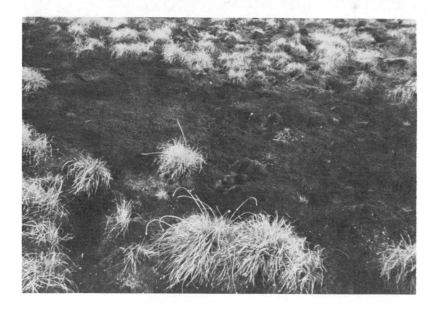

Figure 11-16. Tundra biome (Alaska); moist tundra (photo by Sharon Saari).

WETLANDS

Figures 11-17 to 11-23 are examples of wetland ecosystems.

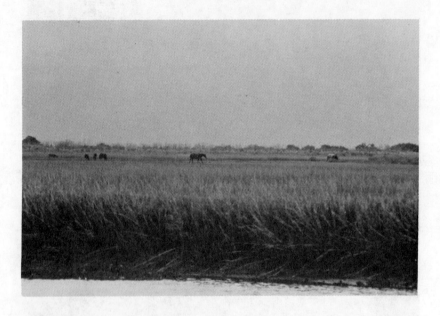

Figure 11-17. Wetland type: coastal salt meadow (*Spartina*) (photo by Sharon Saari)

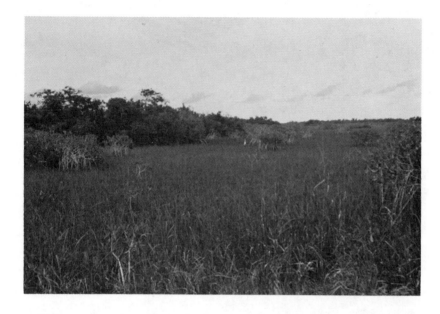

Figure 11-18. Wetland type: inland fresh meadow (Everglades) (photo by Sharon Saari).

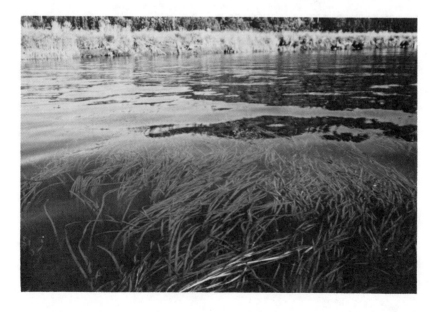

Figure 11-19. Wetland type: coastal open brackish (eelgrass floating) (photo by Sharon Saari).

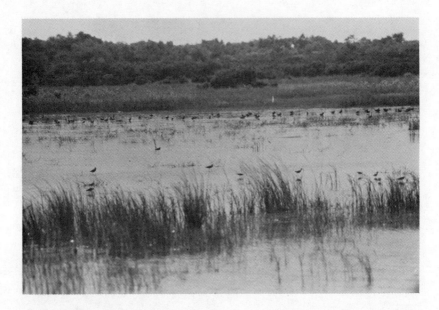

Figure 11-20. Wetland type: coastal shallow fresh marsh (emergent) (photo by Sharon Saari).

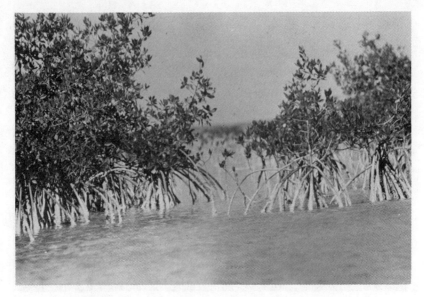

Figure 11-21. Wetland type and tropical biome: mangrove swamp (photo by Sharon Saari).

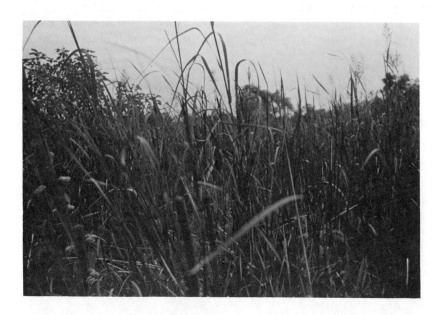

Figure 11-22. Wetland type: inland shallow fresh marsh (Cattail) (photo by Sharon Saari).

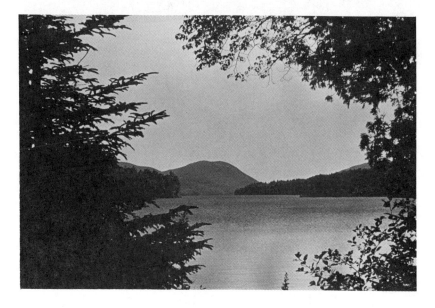

Figure 11-23. Wetland type: inland open fresh water (photo by John Bendall).

BIOME REPRESENTATIVES

Figures 11-24 to 11-30 are tropical biome representatives of ecosystems.

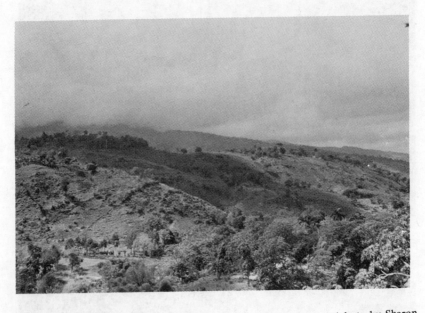

Figure 11-24.   Tropical biome (Caribbean); cleared hardwood forest (photo by Sharon Saari).

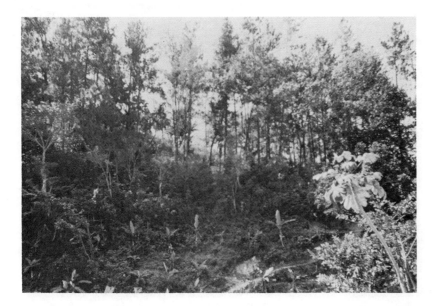

Figure 11-25. Tropical biome (Caribbean); early seral stage of hardwood forest (photo by Sharon Saari).

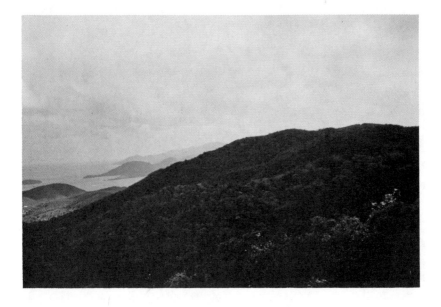

Figure 11-26. Tropical biome (Caribbean); hardwood forest climax (photo by Sharon Saari).

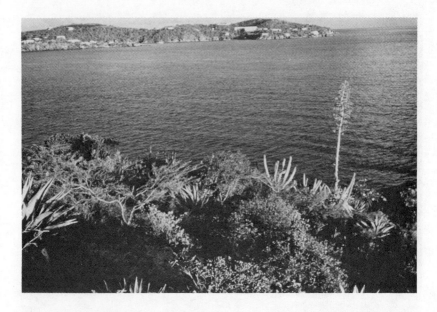

Figure 11-27. Tropical biome (Caribbean); cactus/agave coastal shrub (photo by Sharon Saari).

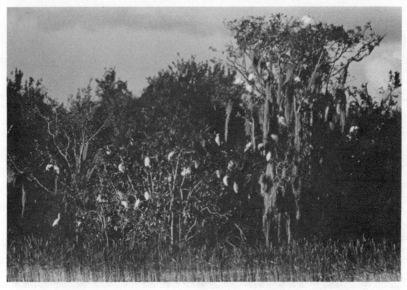

Figure 11-28. Tropical biome; Everglades hammock (photo by Sharon Saari).

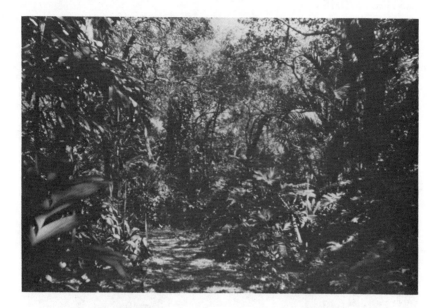

Figure 11-29. Tropical biome; hardwood forest (mature stage) (photo by Sharon Saari).

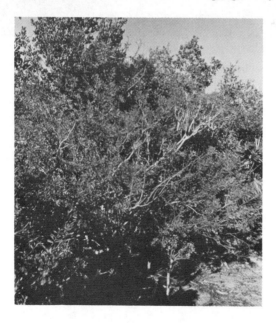

Figure 11-30. Tropical biome; mangrove forest (photo by Sharon Saari).

EASTERN BIOMES

Figures 11-31 to 11-41 show examples of eastern biomes.

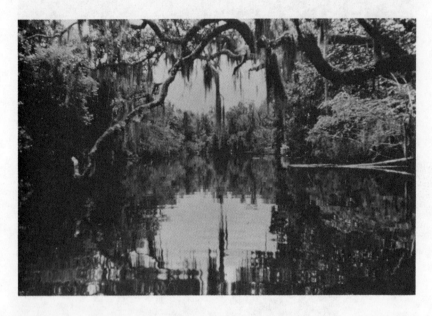

Figure 11-31. Southern mixed forest biome; southern floodplain forest/swamp (mature) (photo by Sharon Saari).

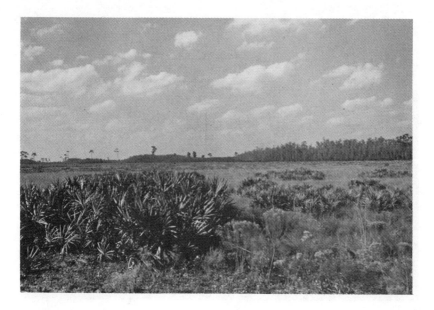

Figure 11-32. Southern mixed forest biome; palmetto prairie (photo by Sharon Saari).

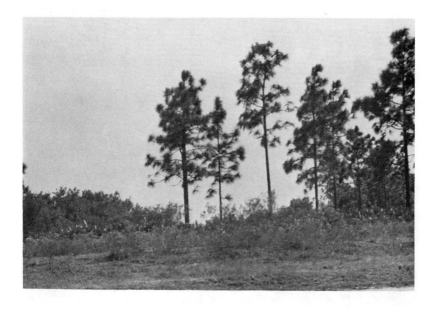

Figure 11-33. Southern mixed forest biome; sand pine scrub (photo by Sharon Saari).

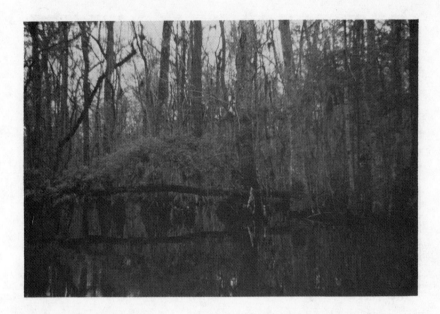

Figure 11-34. Southern mixed forest biome; cypress swamp (immature stage) (photo by (Sharon Saari).

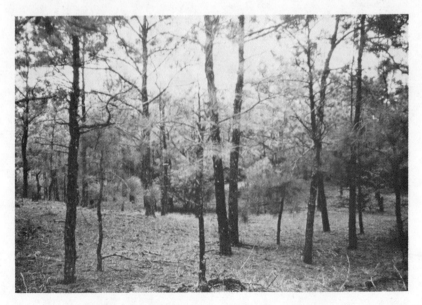

Figure 11-35. Southern mixed forest biome; southeastern pine forest (immature stage) (photo by Sharon Saari).

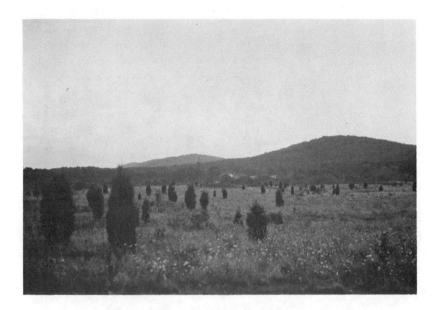

Figure 11-36. Deciduous forest biome; old field prairie/red cedar (first seral stage) (photo by Sharon Saari).

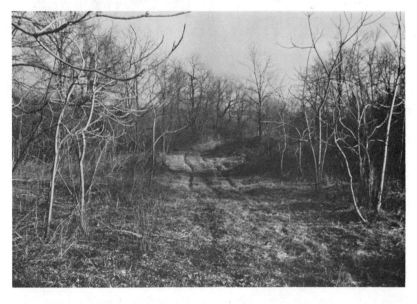

Figure 11-37. Deciduous forest biome; immature hardwood brush (early seral stage) (photo by Sharon Saari).

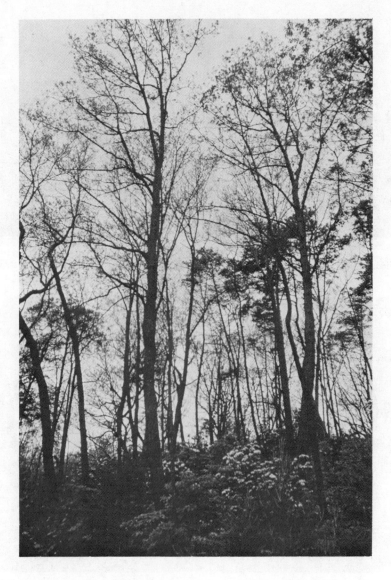

Figure 11-38. Deciduous forest biome; mixed mesophytic forest (immature stage) (photo by Sharon Saari).

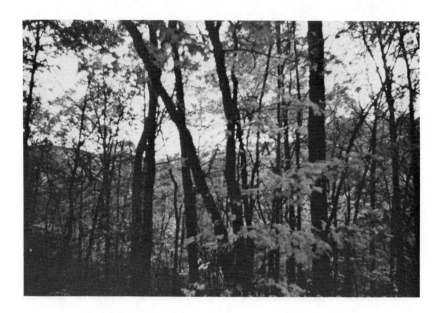

Figure 11-39. Deciduous forest biome; oak/hickory/maple (immature stage) (photo by (Sharon Saari).

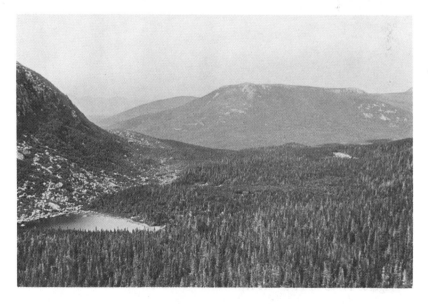

Figure 11-40. Northern coniferous biome: northeastern spruce/fir (photo by John Bendall).

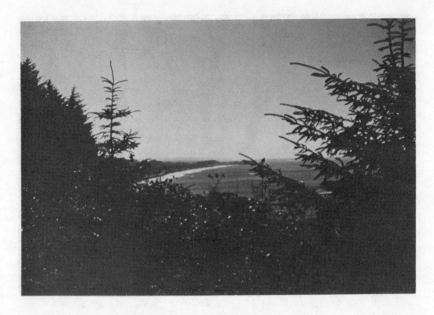

Figure 11-41. Northern coniferous forest biome; Great Lakes spruce/fir (mature stage) (photo by Sharon Saari).

WESTERN BIOMES

Figures 11-42 to 11-59 are representative of western biomes.

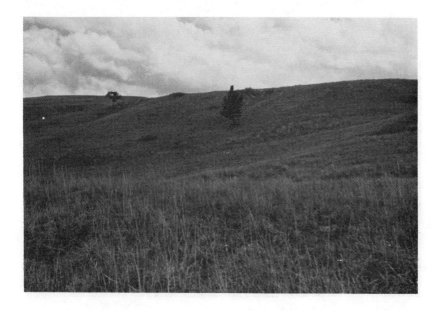

Figure 11-42. Grassland biome; shortgrass (wheatgrass/grama)/prairie (mature stage) (photo by Sharon Saari).

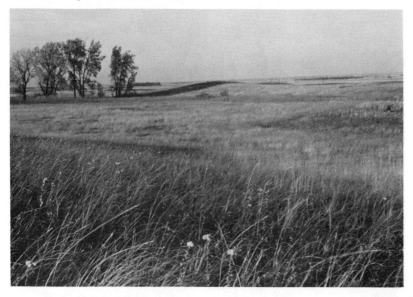

Figure 11-43. Grassland biome; tallgrass (bluestem) prairie (mature stage) (photo by Sharon Saari).

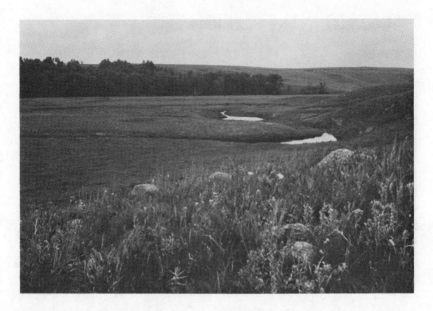

Figure 11-44. Deciduous forest ecotone with grassland biome; bluestem (tallgrass) prairie (mature stage) (photo by Sharon Saari).

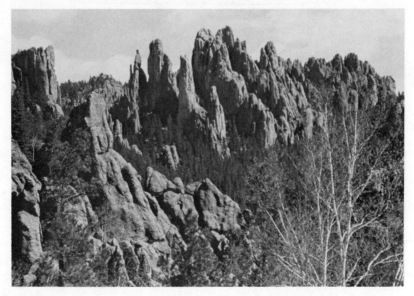

Figure 11-45. Grassland biome; eastern ponderosa forest and northern badlands (photo by Sharon Saari).

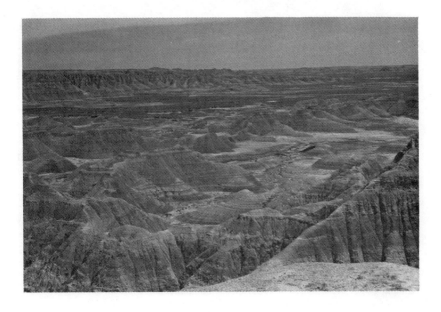

Figure 11-46. Grassland biome; southern badlands (South Dakota) (photo by Sharon Saari).

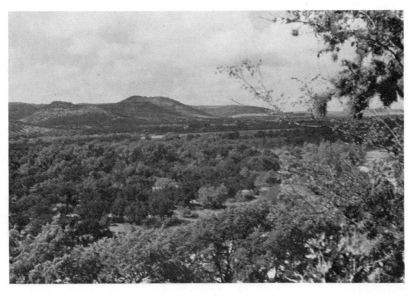

Figure 11-47. Grassland biome: live oak savanna (photo by John Bendall).

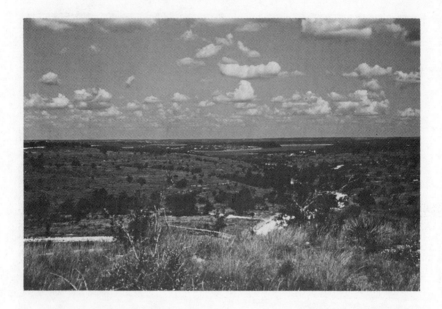

Figure 11-48. Grassland biome: juniper oak savanna (photo by John Bendall).

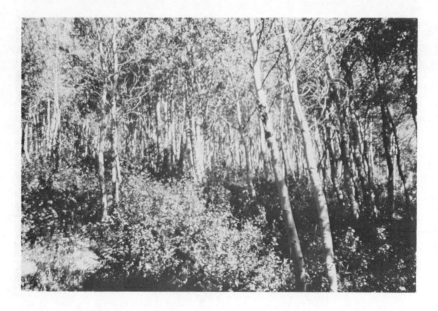

Figure 11-49. Western coniferous forest biome; aspen (intermediate seral stage) (photo by Sharon Saari).

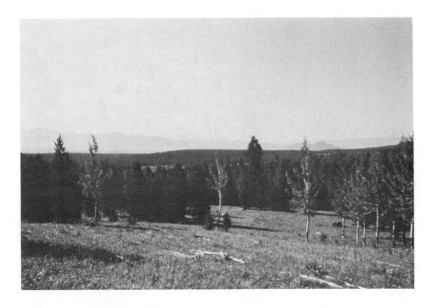

Figure 11-50. Western coniferous biome; western spruce/fir forest (aspen in foreground) (photo by Sharon Saari).

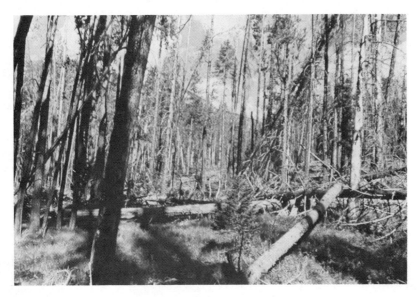

Figure 11-51. Western coniferous forest biome; douglas fir/ponderosa pine (mature stage)(photo by Sharon Saari).

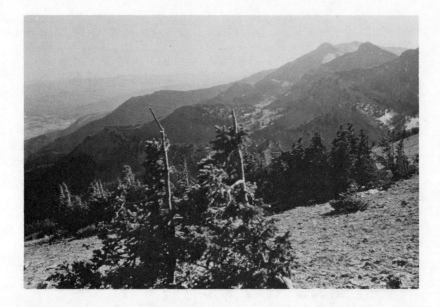

Figure 11-52. Western coniferous forest; petran subalpine forest (mature stage) (photo by Sharon Saari).

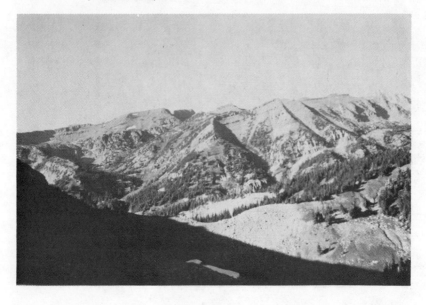

Figure 11-53. Western coniferous forest; alpine (above treeline) (photo by Sharon Saari).

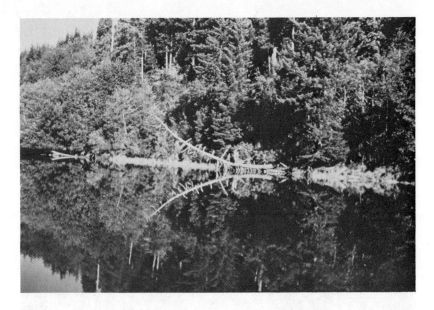

Figure 11-54.   Western coniferous forest biome; spruce/cedar/hemlock forest (immature stage)(photo by Sharon Saari).

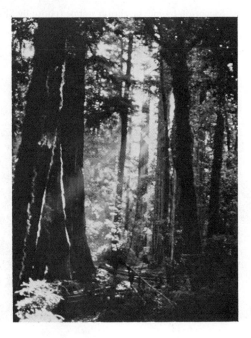

Figure 11-55.   Western coniferous forest biome; redwood forest (mature stage) (photo by John Bendall).

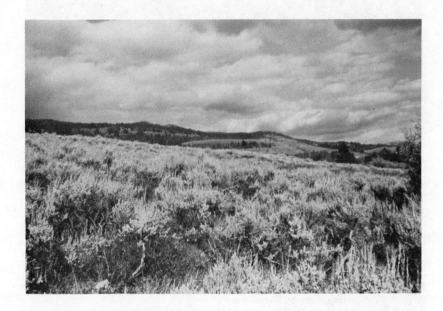

Figure 11-56. Sagebrush biome; sagebrush steppe (photo by Sharon Saari).

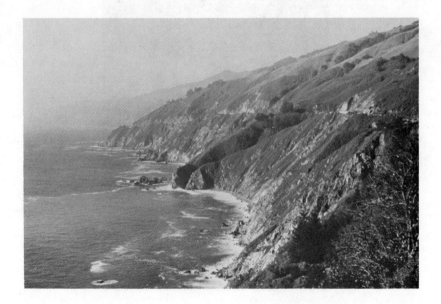

Figure 11-57. Steppe biome; coastal sagebrush and rocky coast (photo by John Bendall).

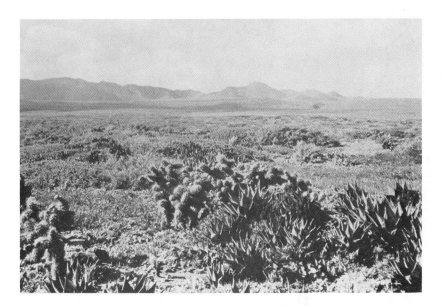

Figure 11-58. Desert scrub pine (mature stage) (photo by John Bendall).

Figure 11-59. Western coniferous biome: California mixed evergreen (photo by John Bendall).

CHAPTER 12

TOXIC CHEMICALS

THE SCOPE OF THE PROBLEM

The Chemical Abstract Service recognizes two million different chemical entities. Some 250,000 new chemicals are added each year to the computerized file. About 20,000 chemical products are currently in commerce with some 300 to 500 new compounds being added to commercial use annually (Howard, 1975).

Some 6,000 compounds have been investigated in the National Cancer Institute Bioassay Program (HEW, 1971). The National Institute of Occupational Health and Safety (NIOSH) has listed some 42,000 compounds in the working environment that are in need of review (Demkovich, 1974). NIOSH has also initiated the necessary studies for OSHA to define occupational standards for 400 compounds under its Standards Completion Project (Clack, 1975). In its latest edition, the catalog of known toxic substances exceeds 15,000 (HEW, 1973; 1975).

Numerous lists of chemicals potentially adversely affecting man's health and the quality of our environment have been produced by individuals, panels of experts, government agencies and industrial groups identifying compounds of concern according to their mission, interest and perception (EPA, 1975; Chemical Engineering News, 1974; NSF, unpublished).

Synthetic Organic Chemical production in the United States increased from 10 billion pounds in 1943 to 140 billion pounds in 1972. This growth rate approximates 10%/yr.

Chemicals are used as intermediates in chemical synthesis, as fuel additives, in plastics, in rubbers, in paints and lacquers, as solvents, as fire retardants in fabric, as brighteners in detergent, in cooling systems, as pesticides, fertilizers, food additives and in pharmaceutical preparations. The legislative authority covering chemicals in the environment is spread across numerous federal agencies (Table 12-1).

699

Table 12-1. Legislative Responsibilities of Agencies in the Control of Chemicals (Bracken et al., 1977)

Agencies	Types of Chemicals						
	Foods	Drugs	Cosmetics	Pesticides	Other Consumer Products	Industrial	Research
Food and Drug Administration (FDA)	X	X	X				
Consumer Protection Safety Commission (CPSC)		X[a]			X		
Occupational Safety & Health Administration/National Institute of Occupational Safety & Health (OSHA/NIOSH)	X	X	X	X	X	X	X
Energy Research & Development Administration (ERDA)							X
Department of Transportation (DOT)[b]				X	X	X	X
Environmental Protection Agency (EPA)[c]				X		X	
U.S. Department of Agriculture (USDA)	X						
Department of Defense (DOD)							X

[a]Child resistant packaging regulations.
[b]Transportation regulations.
[c]Also responsible in terms of plant emissions and effluents for all types of chemicals.

The super-industrial society, epitomized by the United States, could not have been born and evolved so rapidly without the use of chemicals. This growth is welcomed as essential to the well-being of the nation and the world. The fundamental issue facing the responsible scientist is one of balancing benefits and damages associated with the expanded usage of an ever-wider spectrum of chemicals.

PARAMETERS OF ENVIRONMENTAL ASSESSMENT

Under what conditions is a chemical a health or environmental hazard? Five parameters are essential to answer this question. They are: rate of entry in the environment, stability, movement, bioconcentration and toxicity (Moolenaar, 1975). Table 12-2 provides a summary of primary and secondary indicators suggested as necessary, although not necessarily sufficient, to adequately document each aspect of chemical pathways, fate and effects on the environment.

Table 12-2. Major Indicators

Parameter	Primary Indicators	Secondary Indicators
Entry	Production Release rate Dispersive use	Import/export Impurities Spills/accidents Emission/effluent factors
Movement	Water solubility Vapor pressure	Lipid solubility Heat of vaporization
Stability	Hydrolysis in water Photodegradation Microbial degradation	Autooxidation Reactivity toward OH, O_2 Oxydoreduction potential
Bioconcentration	Bioaccumulation Biomagnification Partition coefficient (octanol/water)	Biological half-life
Toxicity	LD_{50} Carcinogenicity	TLV 96 TLC_{50} Teratogenicity Mutagenicity Feeding studies Metabolic studies

Entry

This is a measure of the quantity and rate of introduction of chemicals in the general environment. Traditionally, measures of production and consumption have been used as a rough indication of possible contamination. An interesting index recently developed (NSF, 1975) is the release rate, R, defined as follows:

$$R = (P)L + (P + I) D$$

where　　P = overall annual U.S. production
I = annual quantity imported
L = fraction of the production lost during manufacturing, conversion and formulation and which escapes at the plant site
D = fraction of the material which goes to nonintermediate, dispersive uses

Admittedly, it is a very limited definition and some of the parameters are difficult to quantify. If they are significant, export quantities should be added to the production in the first term, and the second term should really be redefined as consumption. Losses in transportation and storage should also be included.

Other parameters of interest are the location of the production facilities (concentrated or dispersed), the type and quantities of waste and by-product and their methods of disposal (deep well, incineration, air, water, soil). Also of increasing importance are impurities and contaminants in the original product.

Movement

The behavior of a chemical once introduced in the environment depends on the characteristics of the surrounding environment and the physical-chemical properties of the substance. A number of indicators of movement in the environment are available. Besides indicating the propensity for movement and dispersion, they indicate the media of choice. Vapor pressure and water solubility are the traditional indicators. Vapor pressure primarily defines: (1) whether a compound will be transported in the air phase, (2) water solubility and (3) heat of solution control transport in the hydrosphere. Most chemicals come in contact with a solid surface (plant, soil particle) when they are released (intentionally or not) in the environment. The heterogeneous surface offered for example by soil particles provides interaction sites for absorption and binding to macromolecules. Over time, such chemicals are desorbed and leached into the general environment.

Since most chemicals come into contact with surfaces in the environment, the above indicators are not sufficient to cover all possible conditions. The soil organic carbon/water concentration ratio is a good indicator of soil sorption and leaching potential. Other derived parameters such as water/air concentration and wet soil/air concentration ratios allow inference

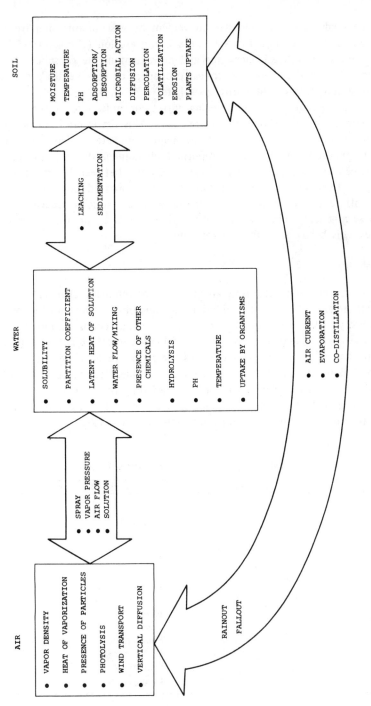

Figure 12-1. Movement of chemicals.

to be made as to the potential movement by gaseous diffusion from soil to air, and percolation through the soil and erosion (Goring, 1975).

Concentration, residence time and movement in the geosphere are functions of both the physical-chemical properties of the chemicals and of the nature and state of the entire geosphere.

A number of factors influencing entry, concentration, movement and residence time are shown in Figure 12-1. This list is far from being exhaustive but is representative of the major parameters. The diagrams document the concept that many important phenomena occur at the interface between media (*e.g.,* air/water, water/soil) and between layers within media (*e.g.,* oil/water). Reactions occurring at such phase discontinuities tend to be different in type and rate from those same reactions occurring in the phase matrices. These boundary reactions are often limiting in defining chemicals behavior in the environment.

Stability

A number of mechanisms are possible for removing chemicals from the environment. Photolysis, oxidation and microbial action are the major pathways. If a chemical degrades rapidly to innocuous compounds already in the environment, the probability of long-term effect is much diminished. Unfortunately, in a number of cases the by-products of degradation are as toxic, if not more so, than the parent molecule. The degradation of chemicals in the environment is the rule rather than the exception. Degradation can take place by chemical, biological and photochemical processes. Some of the most common reactions are listed in Table 12-3.

Table 12-3. Common Degradation Reactions

Processes	Some of the Reactions
Chemical	Hydrolysis
	Dealkylation
	Decarboxylation
	Demethylation
Biological	Epoxidation
	Hydroxylation
	Dechlorination
Photochemical	Hydrogenation
	Isomerization
	Desulfuration
	Sulfoxidation
	Cyclic cleavage
	Oxidation
	Conjugation

Autooxidation Propensity

Autooxidation denotes the reactions of initiation, propagation, peroxide decomposition, self-termination and chain-breaking inhibition of organic substances under environmental conditions of temperature and pressure. Autooxidation processes are characterized by oxygen uptake. The more easily a compound undergoes autooxidation, the less likely it is to persist in the environment.

Redox Potential

Oxidation is the withdrawal of electrons. Conversely, reduction is the addition of electrons. Redox potential then refers to the comparison of the total energy change of any chemical reaction relative to the decomposition of hydrogen. This is a useful parameter to assess the persistence of a pollutant in the environment.

Partition Coefficient

The partition coefficient is a measure of the distribution of a solute between two liquid phases in which it is soluble. The most commonly used system is the water-octanol system. Essentially, it is a measure of solubility in an aqueous or polar solution or an organic nonpolar solution.

Since the transfer of organic molecules across biological membranes is related to hydrophobic properties of the chemical, the partition coefficient is a useful parameter to characterize a compound in terms of its persistence in the environment, its removal from the environment by living organisms and its storage or concentration by fatty materials.

Solubility

Solubility is the concentration of the ions of a chemical in a saturated solution. It is an important parameter defining the major mode of transport in the environment. It also reflects several properties concerning persistence in the environment.

Acid-Base Characteristics

The PK_a and PK_b are measures of ionization of the compound. PKs of compounds greatly influence absorption and transportation in living systems. Biological membranes are relatively impermeable to ionized forms. Acid-base characteristics are illuminating on issues of persistence, bioabsorption and transformation.

Hydrolysis

Hydrolysis is a process in which a compound is cleaved and the products of the reaction take up the elements of water. Of major interest are the rate of hydrolysis as a function of pH and the by-products of the reaction. The rate of hydrolysis indicates whether a compound will remain in the environment for a shorter or longer period of time.

Photolysis

Photolysis is a process of molecular modification under the influence of solar radiation. The parameters of interest here are photolysis rate, quantum yield, by-products and effective wavelengths. This parameter measures persistence in the air environment.

Bioconcentration

Bioconcentration, to a large extent, defines persistence and availability. On the other hand, this phenomenon cannot be explained solely as a mass transfer phenomenon through a food web. The acquisition and especially the retention of material by organisms depends primarily on physical-chemical properties of the material itself. For instance, pesticides are excreted by fish in the order of their water solubility but biomagnified in the inverse order to their water solubility. The situation is rendered even more complex in a marine environment in which the introduced contaminant can be lost to a sink, transformed or recycled, decomposed or adsorbed on other particles. For example, most organic compounds are unstable in an oxidizing surface water environment and tend to be degraded to lower-molecular-weight compounds and CO_2.

Nevertheless, under the heading of bioconcentration we can define two useful concepts: bioaccumulation, or the concentration (usually according to the lipid solubility scale) of material in living tissues of a single organism, and biomagnification, or the active concentration in living tissue in excess of the prevailing media concentrations, throughout a trophic web.

From an environmental viewpoint, bioconcentration becomes most important when acute toxicity is low. Often, under conditions of bioconcentration of low-toxicity compounds, physiological effects go unnoticed until chronic effects have taken place. Under these conditions, standard control techniques are ineffective in alleviating biological damages. Hence, it is most important to predict bioconcentration in the laboratory. The best tool currently available is the correlation of bioconcentration with partition coefficient and the ability to predict biological effect from a study of the effect of substitution groups on the partition coefficient.

Partition coefficient is the ratio of the equilibrium concentration of a chemical in a polar or nonpolar solvent. It has been shown that log

partition coefficients correlate well with log bioconcentration for a variety
of diverse chemicals (Figure 12-2).

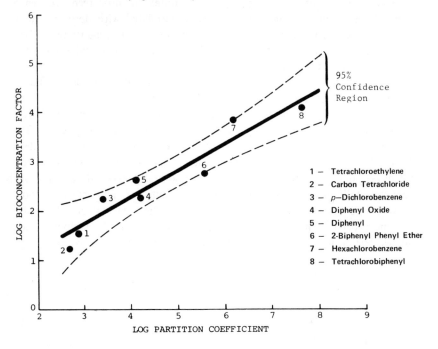

Figure 12-2. The linear regression between the logarithms of the partition coefficient
and the bioconcentration of various chemicals in trout muscle (Neeley *et al.,* 1975).

Using data from Leo (1971) and the chemical additivity principle as
described by Hansch (1972), the effect of chemical substituents can be
used to predict the bioconcentration factor when the partition coefficient
of the parent structure is known.

$$\text{Log } P_X = \text{substituent constants} + \text{Log pH}$$

where Log P_X = log partition coefficient of the chemical of interest
    Log pH = log partition coefficient of the parent structure

The new bioconcentration factor can be derived by regression. Using the
data presented in the figure:

$$\text{Log (Bioconcentration factor)} = 0.542 \text{ log (Partition Coefficient)} + 0.124$$

The above equation is based on the data of Neely *et al.* (1975).

Toxicity

Toxicology is often investigated in the context of dose response—where a physiological or toxicological response is correlated with dose, a product of time of exposure and effective concentration. This construction allows one to incorporate such issues as threshold level, lag time and limits of adaptability (Figure 12-3).

It is important to distinguish toxicity from hazard. Toxicity is the capacity of a substance to produce injury. Hazard is a measure of potential risk and must, of necessity, incorporate information on intended use, anticipated route of entry, and frequency and duration of exposure. Toxicity tests are categorized according to the duration of exposure as follows (NAS, 1975): (1) acute (24 hours or less); (2) subchronic (few days to 90 days); and (3) chronic (few months to several years). More importantly, each test tells us something different. The acute test is a screening tool as well as a first method to delineate the specific toxic effect. The subchronic procedure usually does not use lethal effect as the endpoint and shows deleterious effects only after prolonged and repeated exposure.

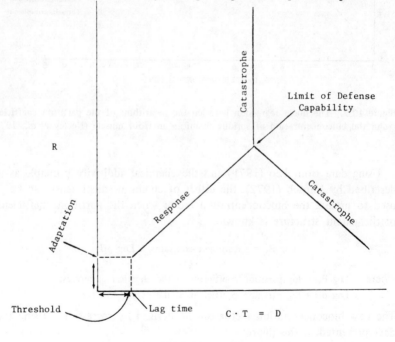

(C = Concentration, T = Time)

Figure 12-3. Dose (D) response (R) relationship.

Chronic studies are measures of the systematic effects due to cumulative exposure.

Toxicity is primarily evaluated in terms of acute toxicity (LD_{50} or other parameters), carcinogenicity, mutagenicity and teratogenicity. Each will be defined in general terms below. When information is readily available, additional information is also collected on long-term chronic exposure studies such as feeding and painting studies.

The widely accepted yardstick for measuring acute toxicity is the LD_{50}. This is defined as the single dose (expressed as a fraction of the animal's live body weight) that will kill 50% of the experimental population of animals. Species, sex, age, route of administration, period of observation, solvent, etc., are all important variables responsible for much variation in the results.

Typically, an LD_{50} of less than 1 mg kg^{-1} represents an extremely toxic substance. Any compound with an LD_{50} of less than 50 mg kg^{-1} indicates high toxicity. The actual LD_{50} numbers are sometimes over-emphasized. It should be recalled that most industrial poisonings result from repeated chronic exposures. The most important value of the LD_{50} is the qualitative information regarding the nature of the effect, and the center of action.

A commonly used parameter is the threshold limit value (TLV), which is defined as the atmospheric level in the workroom air of a potentially hazardous gas, dust or aerosol to which workers cannot be exposed for more than eight hours a day, five days a week. It is important to realize that this parameter is not a measure of toxicity.

Aquatic biota and plants are potentially sensitive to chemical insults. Compilation of effects have been made and sample tables from the compilations are presented as Tables 12-4, 12-5 and 12-6. The analyst should consult the references for the chemical or affected section of interest (Becker, 1973; Yupp, 1974; McKim, 1976).

Complex associations and relationships have been proposed between carcinogenicity, mutagenicity and teratogenicity. While the three phenomena share characteristics in terms of susceptibility, etiological factors, lag time, effect and irreversibility of the disease, the differences are also striking (Table 12-7).

Carcinogenesis results when cells proliferate out of control, having lost the original restraint built in the nuclear message of the parent or host tissue. Mutagenesis takes place when a change occurs in sequence or type of nucleotide in strands of chromosomal DNA. It is a transmissable effect, through the germinal tissues. Teratogenesis is a significant change during the development resulting in structural or functional anomalies.

In the final analysis, the three phenomena will be explained in terms of molecular biology and chemistry.

Table 12-4. Toxicity of Acids to Aquatic Biota

Chemical Compound	Test Organism[a]	Test Conditions	Concentration (ppm)	Remarks	Reference
Arsenic Acid	See: Arsenates & Arsenites				
Boric Acid	See: Boron				
Citric Acid	Salmo gairdneri	SB,FW,LS	5.0	No effect in 24 hr; 12.8°C	Applegate et al, 1957
Citric Acid	Carassius auratus	SB,FW,LS	625	Not lethal; hard water	Ellis (1937)
			894	Killed in 4-28 hr	
			1,433		
	Daphnia magna (cladocera)		120	Lethal in 24-72 hr; soft water	
			185	Lethal in 10-17 hr	
			248	Lethal in 2-17 hr	
Citric Acid	Daphnia magna (cladocera)	SB,FW,LS	153	Highest concentration not immobilizing under prolonged exposure, 25°C	Anderson (1944)
Citric Acid	Lymnaea caillaudi (snail)	SB,FW,LS	800	Lethal concentration, 24 hr; 28°C	Gohar & El-Gindy (1961)
	Biomphalaria alexandrina (snail)		1,200	Lethal concentration, 24 hr; 27°C	
	Bulinus truncatus (snail)		1,000	Lethal concentration, 24 hr; 27°C	
Citric Acid	"Fish"	——	——	Citric acid is directly lethal to fully developed fish only when it lowers the pH value to 5.0 or below.	Doudoroff & Katz (1950)
Ethylenediamine Tetraacetic Acid (EDT)	Ictalurus punctatus	SB,FW,LS	167	24 hr-tlm; 25°C, tap water	Clemens & Sneed (1959)
			133	48 hr-tlm; 25°C, tap water	
			129	96 hr-tlm; 25°C, tap water	
			100	No mortality in 96 hr	
			316	Total mortality in 96 hr	

Chemical	Species	Test	Conc.	Effect	Reference
Ethylenediamine Tetraacetic Acid (EDTA)	"Tubificid worms"	SB,FW&SW,LS	380	24-hr lethal dose; freshwater, 18-21°C	Jancovic & Mann (1969)
	Artemia salina (brine shrimp)		280	24-hr lethal dose; freshwater, 18-21°C	
			200	24-hr lethal dose; seawater, 20-21°C	
	Salmo gairdneri		340	24-hr lethal dose; freshwater, 18-21°C	
Ethylenediamine Acetate (sodium salt)	"Tubificid worms"	SB,FW&SW,LS	2,000	24-hr lethal dose; freshwater, 18-21°C	Jancovic & Mann (1969)
	Artemia salina (brine shrimp)		660	24-hr lethal dose; freshwater, 18-21°C	
			550	24-hr lethal dose; seawater, 20-21°C	
	Salmo gairdneri		860	24-hr lethal dose; freshwater, 18-21°C	
Nitrilotriacetic acid (NTA)	Cyclotella nana (algae)	SB,SW,LS	0.25-0.5	Slight increase in growth in 24 hr; (all data from lab cultures without copper trace)	Erickson et al. (1970)
			1.0	Slight decrease in growth in 24 hr	
			5.0	About 25% average decrease in growth in 24 hr	
			0.25-0.5	Slight increase in growth in 72 hr	
			1.0	Slight decrease in growth in 72 hr	
			5.0	About 45% decrease in growth in 72 hr; (additional experiments showed that NTA counteracts copper toxicity).	
Nitrilotriacetic acid (NTA)	"Tubificid worms"	SB,FW&SW,LS	400	24-hr lethal dose; freshwater, 18-21°C	Jancovic & Mann (1969)
	Crangon allmanni (shrimp)		240	24-hr lethal dose; seawater, 20-21°C	
	Artemia salina (brine shrimp)		290	24-hr lethal dose; freshwater, 18-21°C	
			240	24-hr lethal dose; brackish water, 20-21°C	
			230	24-hr lethal dose; seawater, 20-21°C	

Table 12-4. Continued

Chemical Compound	Test Organism[a]	Test Conditions	Concentration (ppm)	Remarks	Reference
Nitrilotriacetic acid (NTA)	*Gammarus locusta* (amphipod)		240	24-hr lethal dose; seawater, 20-21°C	
	"Capepods"		120	24-hr lethal dose; seawater, 20-21°C	
	Lebistes reticulatus		340	24-hr lethal dose; freshwater, 18-21°C	
	Anquilla rostrata		320	24-hr lethal dose; freshwater, 18-21°C	
			300	24-hr lethal dose; brackish water, 20-21°C	
			250-260	24-hr lethal dose; seawater, 20-21°C	
	Salmo gairdneri		260	24-hr lethal dose; freshwater, 18-21°C	Woelke (1972)
Nitrilotriacetate (NTA)	*Crassostrea gigas* (oyster)	SW,LS	100	0.6% abnormal embryos in 48 hr	
			400	4.4% abnormal embryos in 48 hr	
			600	10.0% abnormal embryos in 48 hr	
			800	34.2% abnormal embryos in 48 hr	
			1,000	92% abnormal embryos in 48 hr	
	Tresus capax (horse clam)		100	2.6% abnormal embryos in 48 hr	
			400	61.2% abnormal embryos in 48 hr	
			600	99.0% abnormal embryos in 48 hr	

[a]SB: Static Bioassay; CB: Constant-flow Bioassay; FW: Freshwater; SW: Sea (Salt) Water; LS: Lab Study; FS: Field Study.

Table 12-5. Summary of the Acute and Chronic Toxicity of Inorganic and Organic Pollutants to Freshwater Fish (McKim et al., 1976)

Pollutant	Species	Exposure Time	Exposure Type	Temperature (°C)	Effect Endpoint	Concentration	Remarks
Inorganics							
Metals							
Barium chloride	Brown trout (*Salmo trutta*)	48 hr	S	15	LC_{50}	150 mg/l	pH=7.8 ALK=165-200 HD=210-290
Cadmium chloride	Flagfish juveniles (*Jordanella floridae*)	96 hr	FT	25	LC_{50}	2.5 mg/l	pH=7.4 HD=43 ALK=42 DO=7-8
	Flagfish	100 days	FT	25	No effect on survival, growth, or reproduction	0.0041 mg/l	A=2.8
Cadmium sulfate	Stone loach (*Noemacheilus barbatulus*)	>66 days	S	12	Median period of survival days	0.7 mg/l	pH=7.2-7.4 HD=240-290 mg/l as $CaCO_3$
	Stone loach	>66 days	S	12	Median period of survival days	1.2 mg/l	
	Stone loach	34 days	S	12	Median period of survival days	3.4 mg/l	
	Stone loach	35 days	S	12	Median period of survival days	5.2 mg/l	
Copper chloride	Blue gourami adults (*Trichogaster trichopterus*)	24 hr	S	27	LC_{50}	0.209 mg/l	pH=7.4 DO=10
	Blue gourami adults	48 hr	S	27	LC_{50}	0.123 mg/l	
	Blue gourami adults	96 hr	S	27	LC_{50}	0.091 mg/l	

Table 12-5. Continued

Pollutant	Species	Exposure Time	Exposure Type	Temperature (°C)	Effect Endpoint	Concentration	Remarks
Copper sulfate	Bluegill (Lepomis macrochirus)	96 hr	FT	20-28	LC$_{50}$	1.1 mg/l	pH=7 ALK=43
	Bluegill larvae-juveniles	90 days	FT	20-28	Reduced survival	0.04 mg/l	HD=45
	Bluegill	22 mo	FT	20	No effect on survival, growth or reproduction	0.021 mg/l	
Copper sulfate	Guppy (Poecilia mexicana)	24 hr	S	24	LC$_{50}$	1.42 mg/l	pH=6.8 HD=32
Copper sulfate	Ophicephalus punctatus	48 hr	S	25-28	LC$_{50}$	70 mg/l	pH=7.5 HD=160 ALK=87 Test solution renewed after 24 hr

Table 12-6. Phytotoxic Effects Exerted by Lead on Plants of Economic Importance in Illinois (Yupp et al., 1971)

Plants by Economic Class	Growing Medium	Minimum Phyto-toxic Concentration (ppm)	Plant Part Affected	Developmental Status	Symptomology
Corn	Defined nutrient medium	2.0	Roots	Seedling	Retardation of root growth
Corn	Defined nutrient medium	0.4	Roots	Seedling	Root and shoot retardation
Fescue, Sheep	Defined nutrient medium	3.0	Roots	Seedling	Root and shoot retardation
Bean, Dwarf French, var. Carteis	Defined nutrient medium	30.0	Roots	Seedling	Root and shoot retardation
Onion	Defined nutrient medium	24.0	Roots	Seedling	Root and shoot retardation
Bean, Dwarf	Defined nutrient medium	24.0	Roots	Seedling	Root and shoot retardation
Beet, Sugar	Medium in sand culture	51.0	Roots	Seedling	Interveinal chlorosis
Lettuce, var. Salad Bowl	Defined soil type	1000.0	Roots and shoots	Seedling	30% yield
Lupine	Defined nutrient solution	40.0	Roots and shoots	Seedling	Root and shoot reduction
Pine, Loblolly	Defined soil type	207.0	Roots and shoots	Seedling	Smaller milky-green needles, reduced root growth
Maple, Red	Defined soil type	207.0	Roots and shoots	Seedling	Increased anthocyanin production; increased leaf abscission

Table 12-7. Comparison of Carcinogenicity, Mutagenicity and Teratogenicity

Phenomenon		Level of Action	Susceptible Tissues	Optimal Time of Exposure	Effective Exposure and Dosage
Carcinogen	Uncontrolled proliferation	Cellular	Profilerating tissues	Probably all stages capable of mitosis	Usually chronic, possibly all doses
Mutagen	Altered nucleotide sequence or number	Molecular	Germinal tissues	All stages of gametogenesis	Acute and chronic, possibly all doses
Teratogen	Change in development pattern	Tissue or organ	Immature tissues	Early differentiation	Acute

A CLASSIFICATION OF EFFECTS

Chemical effects are usually perceived as biological or health related, and essentially in terms of toxicity. While toxic health effects are important because of their devastating and sometimes definitive consequences, other slower-acting and more insidious effects cannot be ignored. A general classification of effects is presented in Table 12-8 and described below (NSF, 1975).

Table 12-8. Effects

Type	Example
Remote	Chlorofluorocarbons
Geochemical	Sulfur dioxide
Meteorological	Carbon dioxide
Secondary	
By-product	Endrin $\overset{h\mu}{\rightarrow}$ Dieldrin
Reaction	smog
Transport Interference	
or Facilitation	EDTA
Bulk	Ethylene glycol
Physico-Chemical	Surfactant
	chelating agents
Biological	
Acute	Carbon Tetrachloride
Chronic	DDT
Sporadic	Chlorine

Remote Effects

Substances introduced in the environment may move over long distances and over considerable periods of time. In such cases, any inert substance (or relatively inactive) at the point of entry can have deleterious and sometimes dramatic effects at a remote site or upon transfer to a different media or upon accumulation in a "sink". A current example is the chlorofluorocarbons that yield chlorine atoms in the upper atmosphere from the effect of ultraviolet radiation. Such chlorine atoms have been implicated in the destruction of the protective ozone layer.

Meteorological Effects

Certain chemicals produced in large quantity over the years can possibly affect our climate. The impact of carbon dioxide increasing the average temperature of the earth (the so-called greenhouse effect), the cooling effect of loading the atmosphere with particulate, the impact of fine particulate on visibility and precipitation, the formation of heat islands over major cities are but a few examples.

Effect on Geochemical Cycles

The great geochemical cycles of our planet, especially sulfur, phosphorous and nitrogen, are also subject to interference. The pool associated with such cycles are very large, but every compound, regardless of its form, eventually moves through these cycles. Obviously, massive releases would be required to affect the proper functioning of such cycles. The release of ammonia resulting in increased nitrate and the phosphate-promoted eutrophication of lakes are evidence of early disturbances.

Transport Interference or Facilitation

To perform their intended function, most chemicals must be transported in the environment and translocated within living systems. This is especially critical for micronutrients essential for plant growth. Certain contaminating chemicals impede and, in rare cases, facilitate such movement. Cases in point include the impact of EDTA and NTA on trace metals on one hand and the solubility increases associated with binding metals to amino acids and proteins.

Bulk Effect

Certain persistent chemicals in the environment do not appear to have any significant effect. Their accumulation in large quantities and their indefinite persistence might be more damaging in the very long term than their limited toxic effect. Compounds in this class include plastics and polyethylene glycols.

Secondary Effect

Certain substances, not very toxic by themselves, see their activity greatly enhanced by slight molecular rearrangements or by partial degradation. An example is the conversion of endrin to dieldrin by light. Other compounds, relatively nondeleterious, become very toxic on reacting with other compounds in the general milieu. Smog is the best known example.

Physical Effect

Many chemicals when added to the natural environment change the properties of the water, air or soil. Changes in surface tension caused by surfactants, in freezing point by salts, solubility by addition of protein, pH by acid and bases, and oxygen depletion by organic chemicals, are but a few examples.

Sporadic Effect

Accidental or intended short-term releases ranging from industrial spills, transportation accidents resulting in spills to system purging and dumping are difficult to detect and may escape most monitoring systems. Chlorine gas escaping from a ruptured tank is an example. Table 12-9 summarizes some of the most useful literature items for conducting an assessment of toxic chemicals in the environment.

Table 12-9. Sources of Information

Parameter	Source
General References	National Research Council, Committee on Toxicology. *Principles and Procedures for Evaluating the Toxicity of Household Substances,* National Academy of Sciences, (Washington, D.C.: 1964).
	Coolston, F. and F. Korte, Eds. *Environmental Quality: Global Aspects of Chemistry, Toxicology and Technology as Applied to the Environment,* Vol. 1 (New York: Academic Press, 1972).
	Encyclopedia of Chemical Technology (New York: John Wiley & Sons, Inc.).
	Principles for Evaluating Chemicals in the Environment. National Academy of Sciences, (Washington, D.C.: 1975).
	Fishbein, L. and W. G. Flamm. "Potential Environmental Chemical Hazards," Part I, "Drugs," Part II, "Feed Additives and Pesticides," *Sci. Total Environ.* 1:15-63 (1972).
	Chemical Economic Newsletter, SRI.
	Bretherick, L. *Handbook of Reactive Chemical Hazards* (London: The Butterworth Group, 1975).
	Kirk, R. E., and D. E. Othmer. *Encyclopedia of Chemical Technology* (New York: John Wiley & Sons, Inc., 1968-70).
	Industrial Chemicals (New York: John Wiley & Sons, Inc.)
	Modern Plastics Encyclopedia (New York: McGraw Hill Book Co.)
	Perry, R. H., and C. H. Chilton. *Chemical Engineers Handbook,* 5th ed. (New York: McGraw Hill Book Co., 1973).
	Council on Environmental Quality. "Toxic Substances," Washington, D.C. (1971).

Table 12-9. Continued

Parameter	Source
General References (cont.)	Rose, A., and E. Rose. *The Condensed Chemical Dictionary.* (New York: Van Nostrand Reinhold, 1966).
	Chemical Technology: An Encyclopedic Treatment, Vol. 1 - Vol. 8 (Barnes & Noble, 1968).
	Office of Management and Budget. "Standard Industrial Classification," U.S. Government Printing Office (1972).
Production	"Chemical Profiles," Chemical Marketing Reports.
	"Synthetic Organic Chemicals," U.S. Tariff Commission Reports.
	Chemical Statistic Handbook (Manufacturing Chemist Association).
	Faith, W. L., D. B. Keyes and R. L. Clark. *Industrial Chemicals,* 4th ed. (New York: John Wiley & Sons, Inc., 1976).
Import/Export	"Imports – Commodity by Country," U.S. Department of Commerce.
	"Exports – Commodity by Country," U.S. Department of Commerce.
Location of Producer	*Directory of Chemical Producers,* SRI.
	Chemical Marketing Reporter. *Chemical Buyers Directory,* (New York: Schnell Publishing Co., Inc., 1975).
Uses	*Chemical Economic Handbook,* SRI.
	Kirk, R. E., and D. E. Othmer. *Encyclopedia of Chemical Technology* (New York: John Wiley & Sons, Inc., 1968-1970).
	Chemical Technology: An Encyclopedia Treatment. The Application of Modern Technological Developments Based Upon Work Originally Devised by the Late Dr. J. V. Van Oss With Special Introduction by John J. McKetta, Jr. (New York: Harper & Row [Barnes & Noble], 1968-1976).

> Vol. 1 - Air, Water, Inorganic Chemicals and Nucleonics (1968)
> Vol. 2 - Non-Metallic Ores, Silicate Industries and Solid Mineral Fuels (1971)
> Vol. 3 - Metals and Ores (1970)
> Vol. 4 - Petroleum and Organic Chemicals (1972)
> Vol. 5 - Natural Organic Materials and Related Synthetic Products (1972)
> Vol. 6 - Wood, Paper, Textiles, Plastics and Photographic Materials (1973)
> Vol. 7 - Vegetable Food Products and Luxuries (1975)

Table 12-9.   Continued

Parameter	Source
Uses	Vol. 8 - Edible Oils and Fats and Animal Food Products (1975)
	Waddams, A. L. *Chemicals from Petroleum,* 3rd ed. (New York: John Wiley & Sons, Inc., 1973).
	Modern Plastic Encyclopedia 1975/1976, Vol. 52, No. 10A (New York: McGraw-Hill Book Co., 1976).
	Farm Chemicals Handbook, 1976 (Pennsylvania: Meister Publishing Co., 1976).
	Herbicide Handbook, 3rd ed. (Illinois: Weed Science Society of America, 1974).
	"Guide to the Chemicals Used in Crop Production," Pub. 1093, 6th ed., Agriculture Canada (1973).
	Lubs, H. A., Ed. *The Chemistry of Synthetic Dyes and Pigments* (New York: R. E. Krieger Publishing Co., 1972).
List of Toxic Substances	Office of Solid Waste Management Programs. Report to Congress; "Disposal of Hazardous Wastes," EPA, Pub. No. SW115, Washington, D.C. (1974).
	Winell, M. "An International Comparison of Hygienic Standards for Chemicals in the Work Environment," *AMBIO* 4(1): 33-36 (1975).
	"EPA Toxic Substances, SW311," Federal Water Pollution Control Act, FR (August 22, 1974).
	Austin, G. T. "The Industrially Significant Organic Chemicals,"

PART 1   *CHEM ENG*   127-132   (January 21, 1974)
     2   125-128   (February 18, 1974)
     3   87-92   (March 18, 1974)
     4   86-90   (April 15, 1974)
     5   143-150   (April 29, 1974)
     6   101-106   (May 27, 1974)
     7   149-156   (June 24, 1974)
     8   107-116   (July 22, 1974)
     9   96-100   (August 5, 1974)

	HEW/NIOSH. "Registry of Toxic Effects of Chemical Substances," (1975).
	NAS. "Principles for Evaluating Chemicals in the Environment," (1975).
Toxicity	Little, A. D. "Water Pollution Potential of Manufactured Products," EPA.

Table 12-9. Continued

Parameter	Source
Toxicity (cont.)	Battelle Northwest Laboratories. "Toxicity of Power Plant Chemicals to Aquatic Life," AEC.
	Office of Science and Technology. "Effect of Pesticides on Non-Target Species."
	Critical Toxicity of Commercial Products (Baltimore: Williams & Wilkins Co.).
	National Academy of Sciences. *Handbook of Toxicology.*
	Dangerous Properties of Industrial Materials (Van Nostrand Reinhold).
	Toxicity and Metabolism of Industrial Solvents (Amsterdam: Elsevier Publ. Co.).
	Matsumura, F., G. M. Boush and T. Misato, Eds. *Environmental Toxicology of Pesticides* (New York: Academic Press, 1972).
	Irvine, D. E. G., and B. Knight, Eds. *Pollution and the Use of Chemicals in Agriculture* (Ann Arbor, MI: Ann Arbor Science Publishers, Inc., 1974).
	Hawley, G. G. *The Condensed Chemical Dictionary* (New York: Van Nostrand Reinhold Co., 1971).
	Sunshine, I., Ed. *CRC Handbook of Analytical Toxicology,* (Cleveland, Oh: The Chemical Rubber Co., 1969).
	Fassett, D. W., and D. I. Irish, Eds. *Industrial Hygiene and Toxicology* 2nd rev. ed., Vol. II, Toxicology (New York: Wiley-Interscience, 1963).
	MacKenzie, C. A. *Unified Organic Chemistry* (New York: Harper & Row, 1962).
	Gerarde, H. W. *Toxicology and Biochemistry of Aromatic Hydrocarbons* (New York: American Elsevier, 1965).
	Browning, E. *Toxicity and Metabolism of Industrial Solvents* (New York: American Elsevier, 1965).
	Williams, R. T. *Detoxification Mechanisms* (New York: John Wiley & Sons, Inc., 1959).
	Dawson, G. W., *et al.* "Control of Spillage of Hazardous Polluting Substances," Battelle Memorial Institute, PB197-596, (1970).
	Beynon, L. R., and E. B. Cowell, Eds. *Ecological Aspects of Toxicity of Testing Oils and Dispersants,* Proceedings of a Workshop (New York: John Wiley & Sons, Inc., 1974).

Table 12-9. Continued

Parameter	Source
Toxicity (cont.)	Becker, C. D., and T. O. Thatcher. "Toxicity of Power Plant Chemicals to Aquatic Life," Battelle for AEC, Washington, D.C. (1973).
	Coulston, F., and F. Korte, Eds. *Global Aspects of Chemistry, Toxicology and Technology as Applied to the Environment,* Vol. 1 (New York: Academic Press, 1972).
	Toody, T. E., and P. A. Hursey. The Acute Toxicity of 102 Pesticides and Miscellaneous Substances to Fish, *Chem. Industry* (June):523-576; 1975.
	Alabaster, J. S. "The Survival of Fish to 164 Herbicides, Insecticides, Fungicides, Wetting Agents and Miscellaneous Substances," *Int. Pest Control* (March/April, 1969).
	Gleason, *et al.* "Clinical Toxicology of Commercial Products," (1969).
	Patty, F. A. *Industrial Hygiene and Toxicology,* 2nd ed. (New York: Wiley-Interscience, 1967).
	Suffet, I. H. "Organics," *J. Water Poll. Control Fed.* 47(6): 1169-1241 (1975).
Carcinogenicity	National Cancer Institute. "Survey of Compounds Which Have Been Tested for Carcinogentic Activity."
	International Agency for Research on Cancer, WHO. "IARC Monographs on the Evaluation of Carcinogenic Risk of Chemicals to Man."
	NCI. "A Research Program to Acquire and Analyze Information on Chemicals that Impact on Man and his Environment."
	NCI. "Surveillance, Epidemiology and End-Results Reporting (SEER)."
Mutagenicity	Sutton, H. E., and M. I. Harris, Eds. *Mutagenic Effects of Environmental Contaminants* (New York: Academic Press, 1972).
	Epstein, S. S. "Chemical Mutagens in the Human Environment." *Nature* 219:385-386 (1968).
	Malling, H. V. "Chemical Mutagens as a Possible Genetic Hazard in Human Populations," *Am. Ind., Hyg. Assoc. J.* 31:657-666 (1970).

Table 12-9. Continued

Parameter	Source
Mutagenicity	Fishbein, L., W. G. Flamm and H. L. Falk. *Chemical Mutagens: Environmental Effects on Biological Systems* (New York: Academic Press, 1970).
	Hollaender, A. *Chemical Mutagens, Principles and Methods For Their Detection,* Vol. 1, 2 (New York: Plenum Press, 1971).
	"The Evaluation of Chemical Mutagenicity Data in Relation To Population Risk," *Environmental Health Perspective* (November 1973).
	Epstein, S. S., and M. S. Legator. *The Mutagenicity of Pesticides Concepts and Evaluation* (Cambridge, Ma: The MIT Press, 1971).
	Adler, I. D., J. S. Wasson and H. V. Malling. "A Bibliography on the Genetic Effects of Caffeine," *Environ. Mutagen Soc. Newsletter,* 4:44 (1971).
	Generoso, W. M. "Literature Citation on Chemical Mutagenesis in Mammals," Environmental Mutagen Information Center Pamphlet #1 (1969).
	Legator, M. S., J. S. Wassom and H. V. Malling. "General Literature Collection on Cyclamates." Environmental Mutagen Information Center Pamphlet #3 (1970).
	Malling, H. V., and J. S. Wassom. "Literature Survey on Pesticides with Special Reference to Their Mutagenic Activity," *Environ. Mutagen Soc. Newsletter* 2:34 (1969).
	Malling H. V., and J. S. Wassom. "Environmental Mutagen Information Center (EMIC). I. Initial Organization," *Environ. Mutagen Soc. Newsletter* 1:16 (1969).
	Malling, H. V., and J. S. Wassom. "Tabulation of the Mutagenic Effect of Certain Pesticides With Supporting Bibliographical References. Report of the Secretary's Commission on Pesticides and Their Relationship to Environmental Health," Parts I and II, U.S. Department of Health, Education and Welfare (1969).
	Malling, H. V., J. S. Wassom and E. S. Von Halle. "A Survey of the 1969 Literature on Chemical Mutagenesis," *Environ. Mutagen Soc. Newsletter* 3 (Suppl. 1):1 (1970).
	Malling, H. V., J. S. Wassom and S. S. Epstein. "Mercury in Our Environment," *Environ. Mutagen Soc. Newsletter* 3:7 (1970).

Table 12-9. Continued

Parameter	Source
Mutagenicity	Malling, H. V. "Environmental Mutagen Information Center (EMIC). II. Development for the Future," *Environ. Mutagen Soc. Newsletter* 4:11 (1971). Wassom, J. S., E. Zeiger and H. V. Malling. "A Bibliography on the Mutagenicity of Nitroso Compounds and Related Chemicals," Environmental Mutagen Information Center Pamphlet #5. Wassom, J. S., and H. V. Malling. "The Environmental Mutagen Information Center During FY 1971," Abstract of a Paper Delivered at the 2nd Annual Meeting of the Environmental Mutagen Society, Washington, D.C., March 21-24, 1971. Wassom, J. S., and H. V. Malling. "Literature Citations on Chemical Mutagenesis, January 1 to April 30, 1969," Environmental Mutagen Information Center Pamphlet #2. Wassom, J. W., H. V. Malling and F. J. De Serres. "Literature Citations on Drugs of Abuse, 1. The Genetic Effects of LSD and Related Psychotic Compounds," Environmental Mutagen Information Center Pamphlet #4.
Teratogenicity	Wilson, J. G. *Environment and Birth Defects* (New York: Academic Press, 1973). World Health Organization. "Principles for the Testing of Drugs for Teratogenicity," ITS Tech. Report, Ser. No. 364, GENEVA (1957).
Threshold Limit Values (TLVs)	Threshold Limit Values for Chemical Substitutes in Workroom Air Adopted by American Conference of Government Industrial Hygienists (ACGIH).

Properties
General
	Consumer Product Safety Commission
	
	Patte, F., M. Etcheto and P. Laffort. "Selected and Standardized Values of Supra Threshold Odor Intensities for 110 Substances," *Chem. Senses Flavor* 1:283-305 (1975).
	
	Dreisbach, R. R. Physical Properties of Chemical Compounds, ACS.
	
	    Vol. 1 - Organic Cyclic (1955)
	    Vol. 2 - Alkanes, Haloalkanes, Alkenes and Haloalkenes (1959)
	    Vol. 3 - Alphatic
	           Miscellaneous (1961)
	
	Oxidation of Organic Compounds, Vols. 1, 2, 3 (Washington, D.C.: American Chemical Society, 1968).

Table 12-9. Continued

Parameter	Source
Properties *General* (cont.)	Werst, R. C. *Handbook of Chemistry and Physics,* 54th ed. (Cleveland, Oh: CRC Press, 1973).
	Stecher, P. G., Ed. *The Merck Index,* Merck and Co.
	Sax, N. I. *Dangerous Properties of Industrial Chemicals,* 4th ed. (New York: Van Nostrand Reinhold Co., 1975).
	Physical Properties of Chemical Compounds (Washington, D.C.: American Chemical Society, 1955).
	Garrett, H. E. Surface Active Chemicals (New York: Pergamon Press, 1972).
	Handbook of Environmental Control (Cleveland, Oh: CRC Press).
	Vol. 1 - Air Pollution
	Vol. 2 - Solid Waste
	Vol. 3 - Water Supply and Treatment
	Vol. 4 - Wastewater: Treatment and Disposal
	Clark, W. M. *Oxidation-Reduction Potential of Organic Systems* (Robert E. Krieger Publications, 1972).
Specific Autooxidation	Betts, J. *Quart. Rev.* 25:265 (1971).
Retox Potential	Clarke, W. Oxidation-Reduction Potentials of Organic Systems (Baltimore, Md: Williams & Wilkins, 1960).
Partition Coefficient	Leo, A., C. Hansch and D. Elkins. "Partition Coefficients and Their Use," *Chem. Rev.* 71(6):525-617 (1971).
	Franzen, K. L., and J. E. Kinsella. "Physico-Chemical Aspects of Food Flavoring," *Chem. & Ind.* 505-508 (1975).
Solubility	Seidell, A. *Solubilities of Inorganic and Organic Compounds,* Vol. 1 & 2 (New York: Van Nostrand Co., 1928).
	Seidell, A. *Solubilities of Inorganic and Organic Compounds,* 3rd ed., Vol. 1 & 2 (New York: Van Nostrand, Reinhold, 1941).
	Seidell, A., and W. Linke. *Solubilities of Inorganic and Organic Compounds,* Supplement to 3rd ed. (New York: Van Nostrand, Reinhold, 1952).
	Seidell, A., and W. Linke. *Solubilities of Inorganic and Organic Compounds,* 4th ed. (Washington, D.C.: American Chemical Society, 1958).

Table 12-9. Continued

Parameter	Source
Properties *Specific* Solubility	Weast, R. *Handbook of Chemistry and Physics,* 51st ed. (Cleveland, Oh: Chemical Rubber Handbooks Co., 1970).
	Lange, N. *Handbook of Chemistry,* 10th ed. (New York: McGraw-Hill Book Co., 1961).
	Linke, W. F. *Seidell's Solubilities: Inorganic and Metal Organic Compounds,* 4th ed., Vol. 2, American Chemical Society, 1969.
Acid-Base Characteristics	Kortum, G., *et al. Dissociation Constants of Organic Acids in Aqueous Solutions* (London: Butterworths, 1961).
	Lange, N. *Handbook of Chemistry,* 10th ed. (New York: McGraw-Hill Book Co., 1961).
	Weast, R. *Handbook of Chemistry and Physics,* 50th ed. (Cleveland, Oh: Chemical Rubber Co., 1970).
Hydrolysis/ Photolysis	Streitweiser, A., Jr. *Chem. Rev.* 50:571 (1950).
	NAS. "Degradation of Synthetic Organic Molecules in the Biosphere," Washington, D.C. (1972).
	Degradation of Herbicides (New York: Marcel Dekker, Inc.).
	Swisher, R. D. *Surfactant Biodegradation* (New York: Marcel Dekker, Inc., 1970).
	Birks, J. B. *Photophysics of Aromatic Molecules* (New York: Wiley–Interscience, 1970).
	Howard, P. H., *et al.* "Review and Evaluation of Available Techniques for Determining Persistence and Routes of Degradation of Chemical Substances in the Environment," EPA, PB243-825 (1975).
Transportation	Manufacturing Chemists Association. Chemtrec: Chemical Transportation Emergency Center, MCA, Washington, D.C., 1971.
	Cheremisinoff, P. N. "Disposal of Hazardous Wastes: Treat or Truck," *Poll. Eng.,* 52-53 (May 1975).
	Chris: A Condensed Guide to Chemical Hazards, U.S. Coast Guard, AD-A002 390, Washington, D.C. (1974).
	Department of Transportation. Emergency Services Guide for Selected Hazardous Materials, Washington, D.C. (1974).
	DOT. "4th Annual Report of the Secretary of Transportation on Hazardous Materials Control," Washington, D.C. (1974).

Table 12-9. Continued

Parameter	Source
Transportation	Philipson, L. M., and M. S. Schaeffer. "Predictions of Risk in the Transportation of Hazardous Materials Employing Statistical Data." 47th National ORSA Meeting Tims, 1975, North American Meeting, Chicago, Illinois.
Control	"Control of Spillage of Hazardous Polluting Substances." Battelle Northwest for FWQA. "Organic Chemicals Manufacturing Point Source Category Final Regulations," Effective 5/13/74 39 FR 81, Part II Development Document, EPA 440/1474-009-a (April 25, 1974). Ethylene, Propylene, Ethylene Dichloride, Methanol, Ethylbenzene, Formaldehyde, Styrene, Vinyl Chloride, Ethylene Oxide, Butadiene, Ethylene Glycol, Dimethyl Terephthalate, Terephthalic Acid, Acetic Acid, Cyclohexane, Phenol, Acetone, Vinyl Acetate, Acetaldehyde. "Inorganic Chemicals Manufacturing Point Source Category Final Regulations," Effective 5/13/74 39 FR 49, Part II, Development Document, EPA 440/1-74-007-a (March 12, 1974). Sulfuric Acid, Sodium Hydroxide, Chlorine, Sodium Carbonate, Nitric Acid, Hydrochloric Acid, Sodium Sulfate, Calcium Chloride, Aluminum Sulfate, Titanium Dioxide, Sodium Silicate. "Plastics and Synthetics Point Source Category Final Regulations," Effective 6/4/74 39 FR 67, Part II, Development Document, EPA 440/1-74-010-a (April 5, 1974). Styrene, Butadiene, Acrylonitrile. "Fertilizer Manufacturing Point Source Category Final Regulations," Effective 6/7/74 39 FR 68, Part III, Development Document, EPA 440/1-74-001-b (April 8, 1974). Sulfuric Acid, Phosphoric Acid, Nitric Acid, Urea, Ammonium Nitrate, Ammonia. "Soap and Detergent Manufacturing Point Source Category Final Regulations," Effective 6/11/74 39 FR 72, Part II, Development Document, EPA 440/1-74-018-a (April 12, 1974). Sodium Hydroxide, Sodium Tripolyphosphate, Methanol, Sulfuric Acid, Urea, Ethanol, Phenol. "Rubber Processing Point Source Category Final Regulations," Effective 4/22/74 39 FR 36, Part II, Development Document, EPA 440/1-74-013-a (February 21, 1974). Carbon Black, Styrene, Butadiene, Acrylonitrile, Ethylene, Propylene, Sodium Hydroxide.

Table 12-9. Continued

Parameter	Source
Control	"Phosphate Manufacturing Point Source Category Final Regulations," Effective 4/22/74 39 FR 35, Part II, Development Document, EPA 440/1-74-006-a (February 20, 1974).
	Phosphoric Acid, Sodium Tripolyphosphate.
	Sittig, M. "Pollution Control in the Organic Chemical Industry." Noyes Data Corporation, N.J. (1974).
	Saxton, J. C., and M. Narkus-Kramer. "EPA Findings on Solid Wastes From Industrial Chemicals," *Chem. Eng.*, 107-112 (April 1975).
Literature Sources	"Literature Resources for Chemical Process Industries," American Chemical Society (1954).
	"Searching the Chemical Literature," American Chemical Society (1961).
	Smith, J. F. (Symposium Chairman). "Literature of Chemical Technology," American Chemical Society (1968).
	Lawrence, B. "Preliminary Project Evaluation – Any Technology Can Do It. Guide to Chemical Business Information Sources," *Chemtech,* 678-681 (November 1975).

REFERENCES

Becker, C. D., and J. O. Tatcher. "Toxicity of Power Plant Chemicals to Aquatic Life," U.S. Atomic Energy Commission, WASH – 1347-UC-11 (June 1973).

Bracken, M., J. Dorigan, J. Hushon and J. Overbey. *Chemical Substances Information Network,* MTR-7558 (McLean, Va: The MITRE Corporation, 1977).

Chem. Eng. News 52(18):11 (1974).

Clack, G. "The First of 400," *Job Safety Hlth* 3(6):4-10 (1975).

Demkovich, L. E. "Labor Report/OSHA Launches Dual Effort to Reduce Job Health Hazards," *Nat. J. Rep.* 6(9):1831-1839 (1974).

Environmental Protection Agency. "Activities of Federal Agencies Concerning Selected High Volume Chemicals," EPA-560/4-75-001 (February 1975).

Goring, C. A. I., J. W. Hamaker and D. A. Laskowski. "A Proposed Approach to PR70-15 Guidelines," in *Chemicals, Human Health and the Environment,* Dow Chemicals, Midland, Mi. (1975).

Hansch, C., A. Leo and D. Nikaitani. *J. Org. Chem.* 37:3090 (1972).

Health, Education and Welfare, U.S. Department of. "Survey of Compounds Which Have Been Tested for Carcinogenic Activity," Public Health Service Publication 149 (1971).

Howard, P. H. "Establishing Environmental Priorities for Synthetic Organic Chemicals: Focusing on the Next PCB's," Papers of a Seminar on Early Warning Systems for Toxic Substances, EPA-560/1-75-003 (July 1975).

Leo, A., C. Hansch and D. Elkins. *Chem. Rev.* 71:525 (1971).

McKim, J. M., *et al.* "Effects of Pollution on Freshwater Fish," *J. Water Poll. Control Fed.* 1544-1580 (June 1976).

Moolenaar, R. J. "Environmental Impact of Chemicals," Papers of a Seminar on Early Warning Systems for Toxic Substances, EPA-560/1-75-003 pp. 167-174 (July 1975).

National Science Foundation. "Final Report of the NSF Workshop Panel to Select Organic Compounds Hazardous to the Environment," Unpublished.

Neely, W., D. R. Branson and G. E. Blau. "Predicting Bioconcentration Potential," in *Chemicals, Human Health and the Environment,* Vol. 1, Dow Chemicals, Midland, MI (1975).

Ouellette, R. P. *Waste or Resource,* M74-60, The MITRE Corporation (1974).

Christensen, H. E., Ed. *Suspected Carcinogens – A Subfile of the NIOSH Toxic Substances List* (Washington, D.C.: Department of Health, Education and Welfare, 1975).

Christensen, H. E., Ed. *The Toxic Substances List,* 1973 ed. (Washington, D.C.: Department of Health, Education and Welfare, 1973).

Yupp, J. H., W. E. Schmid and R. W. Holst. "Determination of Maximum Permissible Levels of Selected Chemicals that Exert Toxic Effects on Plants of Economic Importance in Illinois," PB-237-654, Illinois Institute for Environmental Quality (August 1971).

CHAPTER 13

CULTURAL

INTRODUCTION

The cultural impacts caused by a specific action often affects the socio-cultural aspect of a community and/or region far more than the physical or biological changes that may occur. For those actions involving construction, where large numbers of people are needed over a relatively short period of time—*e.g.*, up to two or three years—major cultural impacts are observed. The first sector to be affected is usually housing. The second sector of the community service base to be broken is the urban infrastructure—*e.g.*, sewers, water lines, etc. are overloaded. The third threshold to be broken is the human resources, *e.g.*, police, fire, health services, etc. become overloaded. The ability to finance the capital costs associated with growth is the clearest indicator of the community's ability to absorb that growth. The typical lag times for Federal funds to become available for capital items is about two to three years. A typical factor in the impact analysis of construction activities is the true construction force to be employed. Due to the high turnover rate experienced in large projects, the number of individuals actually used on the project can be underestimated by 100%. Table 13-1 gives the estimated work force required for various energy technologies. These numbers represent approximate jobs and not individual people.

Another important factor is the multiplier impact. The figures shown in Table 13-2 reflect the indirect and induced income effects in a particular state or region resulting from an increase in the demand for the output of the indicated sectors. As an example, if $1.00 were generated from the coal mining sector in the New England Region, an extra $2.15 would be generated throughout the economy of the region (in addition

731

Table 13-1. Estimated Work Force Requirements for Various Energy Technologies

Energy Technology	Representative Size	Work Force	Life Expectancy of Operation
Power Plant Construction[a]			
Nuclear	1000 MWe	1000	5 years
Fossil Fuel (coal)	1000 MWe	1000	5 years
Power Plant Operation[a]			
Nuclear	1000 MWe	100	25-30 years
Fossil Fuel (coal)	1000 MWe	100	25 years
Coal			
Extraction[b]-Western Surface Mine	6×10^6 T/yr	215	25 years
Extraction[b]-Eastern Surface Mine	5.32×10^6 T/yr	250	15 years
Extraction[b]-Eastern Underground	2.66×10^6 T/yr	640	
Gasification-High Btu[c] Construction[c]	2.5×10^8 SCF/day	2500-3000	3-4 years
Operation[b]		589	20 years
Gasification-Low Btu[c] Construction[c]	2.5×10^9 SCF/day	860	3-4 years
q Operation		325	20 years
Liquefaction-SRC Process[c]	3.5×10^4 bbl/day		5 years
Construction[c]		1300	
Operation[b,c]		180-600	20 years
Liquefaction-Other Direct[c]	5×10^4 bbl/day		
Construction		1300	
Operation		550	20 years
Oil Shale[c]			
Surface Processing	5×10^4 bbl/day		
Construction		1220-1470	3 years
Operation		1062-1430	20 years
Modified *In Situ* Processing	5×10^4 bbl/day		
Construction		1820	3 years
Operation		1150	20 years
Oil and Gas Production Land	Oil: 10.63×10^3 bbl/well/yr Gas: 249.5×10^6 SCF/well/yr	per 100 wells	
Exploration Services		250	3-7 years[d]
Development and Exploitation		33	15-20 years

Table 13-1. Continued

Energy Technology	Representative Size	Work Force	Life Expectancy of Operation
Offshore	Oil: 133.52×10^3 bbl/well/yr[e] Gas: 2.48×10^9 SCF/well/yr 24 wells	per platform handling 24 wells[e]	
Exploration and Services		175[e]	3-5 years
Development and Exploitation		75-90[e]	15 years
Oil Refineries	2×10^5 bbl/day		
Construction		2000-2200[a]	3-4 years
Production Operation		360-565[6]	30 or more years
Natural Gas Processing[e]	5×10^8 SCF/day		
Plant Construction		300-350[e]	2-3 years
Operation		47-55[e]	30 or more years
Uranium Production			
Mining[b,c]	1.600 MT/day of ore	240-416	10 years
Milling-Plant[f] Construction	960 MT/yr U_3O_8	1000	2-3 years
Milling-Plant[b] Operation	960 MT/yr U_3O_8	130	$\geqslant$20 years
Enrichment-Plant[f] Construction	8.75×10^6 SWU/yr	4000 (peak)	7 1/2 years
Enrichment-Plant[f]	8.75×10^6 SWU/yr	1200	$\geqslant$30 years
Fuel Fabrication Construction	600-800 MT/yr UO_2	1200	1 1/2 years
Operation and Maintenance	600-800 MT/yr UO_2	500	30 years
Fuel Reprocessing and Conversion			
Plant Construction	1500 MT/yr Uranium	2500	3-5 years
Plant Operation	1500 MT/yr Uranium	600-900	30-40 years

[a]DOI, 1976a.
[b]Bechtel, 1976.
[c]DOI, 1975.
[d]DOI, 1976b/d.
[e]Council of Environmental Quality, 1974.
[f]DOI, 1976c.

Table 13-2. Multipliers (Watson et al., 1977)

Indirect Multipliers Regions and States	Coal Mining	Crude Petroleum, Gas Mining	Power Plant Construction	Power Plant Operation (Electric Utilities)	Oil and Gas Well Construction	Oil and Gas Well Exploration	All Other Construction	Petroleum Refining
New England	2.149	1.002	2.753	1.160	2.243	1.550	2.188	0.772
Maine	—	—	1.353	0.793	1.000	0.921	1.130	—
New Hampshire	—	0.712	1.744	0.792	1.202	0.991	1.366	0.451
Vermont	—	—	1.310	0.705	0.887	0.860	1.093	—
Massachusetts	1.952	0.920	2.392	1.056	1.908	1.405	1.950	0.704
Rhode Island	—	—	1.903	0.813	1.589	1.082	1.540	0.524
Connecticut	1.883	0.926	2.361	0.980	2.120	1.380	1.933	0.727
Middle Atlantic	3.140	1.368	3.326	1.618	3.027	2.015	2.768	1.463
New York	2.324	1.224	2.600	1.254	2.392	1.769	2.250	1.265
New Jersey	2.126	1.089	2.628	1.157	2.289	1.646	2.227	1.006
Pennsylvania	2.617	1.045	2.848	1.381	2.535	1.676	2.356	1.269
South Atlantic	2.701	1.153	2.599	1.425	2.235	1.659	2.221	1.065
Florida	1.848	0.976	2.016	0.952	1.664	1.386	—	0.916
Delaware	1.388	0.723	1.271	0.826	1.268	1.097	1.221	0.833
Maryland	1.768	0.892	2.007	0.976	1.954	1.307	1.739	0.736
Virginia	2.086	0.885	1.914	1.001	1.597	1.275	1.652	0.665
West Virginia	1.867	0.730	1.952	1.065	1.761	1.183	1.639	1.933
North Carolina	1.589	0.743	1.827	0.875	1.457	1.130	1.566	0.576
South Carolina	—	0.725	1.713	0.834	1.324	1.070	1.483	0.646
Georgia	1.694	0.856	1.914	0.970	1.599	1.250	1.670	0.744
East North Central	2.808	1.082	3.179	1.491	2.805	1.838	2.627	1.429
Ohio	2.499	0.988	2.730	1.312	2.436	1.598	2.272	1.481
Indiana	2.044	0.755	2.271	1.094	2.021	1.319	1.912	0.863
Illinois	2.524	1.041	2.733	1.321	2.460	1.630	2.273	1.352

Michigan	1.913	0.772	2.513	1.072	2.115	1.390	2.075	0.938
Wisconsin	—	0.669	2.346	0.945	1.795	1.185	1.816	0.555
East South Central	2.291	0.880	2.570	1.177	2.189	1.421	2.095	1.422
Kentucky	1.939	0.671	2.125	0.999	1.713	1.196	1.752	1.180
Tennessee	1.953	0.748	2.313	0.869	1.779	1.280	1.873	0.624
Alabama	1.980	0.743	2.100	1.069	1.863	1.251	1.736	0.903
Mississippi	1.298	0.612	1.543	0.800	1.232	1.019	1.312	1.665
West North Central	1.702	0.776	1.865	0.958	1.598	1.201	1.611	1.115
Minnesota	1.499	0.645	1.749	0.865	1.437	1.090	2.437	0.599
Iowa	1.200	0.479	1.311	0.671	0.952	0.827	1.153	0.420
Missouri	1.849	0.847	2.058	1.021	1.726	1.268	1.743	0.734
North Dakota	0.885	0.303	0.616	0.461	0.621	0.595	0.621	0.877
South Dakota	—	0.277	0.720	0.486	0.644	0.589	0.683	—
Nebraska	1.111	0.508	1.163	0.598	0.996	0.818	1.032	0.526
Kansas	1.355	0.692	1.312	0.780	1.223	0.993	1.223	1.588
West South Central	2.024	1.193	2.382	1.168	2.030	1.581	2.069	2.493
Arkansas	1.275	0.719	1.502	0.709	1.223	0.957	1.269	1.295
Louisiana	—	0.800	1.672	0.926	1.545	1.316	1.554	2.086
Oklahoma	1.536	0.868	1.679	0.849	1.454	1.136	1.461	1.788
Texas	1.955	1.161	2.277	1.122	2.020	1.539	1.998	2.416
Mountain	2.137	1.066	2.077	1.183	1.828	1.358	1.737	2.163
Montana	1.216	0.516	0.919	0.703	0.826	0.797	0.847	1.348
Idaho	—	0.449	1.038	0.679	0.892	0.806	0.964	0.408
Wyoming	1.374	0.505	1.013	0.830	0.918	0.866	0.943	1.477
Colorado	1.998	0.994	1.765	1.079	1.710	1.229	1.519	1.900
New Mexico	1.590	0.766	1.141	0.873	1.138	1.019	1.067	1.669
Arizona	1.615	0.782	1.786	0.886	1.438	1.114	1.448	0.646
Utah	1.815	0.830	1.444	0.994	1.739	1.141	1.422	1.805
Pacific	2.250	1.277	2.757	1.241	2.268	1.749	2.272	2.192
Nevada	—	0.704	1.150	0.800	1.240	0.993	1.096	—
Alaska	1.315	0.627	0.953	0.754	0.902	0.876	0.931	1.509
Hawaii	—	0.682	1.140	0.779	1.137	1.047	1.087	0.554
Washington	1.640	0.795	1.760	0.839	1.667	1.204	1.508	0.650

to the original $1 stimulus). The direct and indirect income effect results from increased demands for the output of all sectors directly linked to the affected sector (*e.g.,* mining equipment manufacturers), and all subsequent indirect linkages (*e.g.,* iron and steel producers). The induced income effect is generated from increased consumption expenditures resulting from the extra labor needed to produce the additional output of all affected sectors. The multipliers also work in the reverse, indicating the total economic loss in an area caused by a $1.00 reduction in the demand for particular sector outputs. These income multipliers are sometimes used as employment multipliers, where it is assumed that the productivity of the workers (*i.e.,* value added per employee) remains the same throughout the economy.

Table 13-3 presents environmental loadings from typical community expansion—per 1,000 population. Again, these values should be used as approximate values in evaluating the impact of increased population on the existing structure.

Table 13-4 presents the approximate area requirements for community development; again per 1,000 population expansion. Table 13-5 gives average dollars (1974) spent for community expansion. A differentiation is made between low-density sprawl, high density and a mix of the two. Table 13-6 presents the service factors for expanding populations with Table 13-7 giving factors for these expanding populations. It is not unusual for construction personnel to travel more than 50 miles (one-way) to get to the job. Table 13-8 presents general standards for park lands for local recreational needs with Table 13-9 presenting the recreational activities needs of various sports activities. Following Table 13-9 is a list of the steps taken in determining if a proposed project (or action) has the potential to affect any historic site within the area. Also given is a list of the individual state historic presentation officers.

One of the most difficult and least quantitative impact assessments deals with the esthetic nature of an area. In an effort to evaluate the esthetic uniqueness of the Hell's Canyon area of the Snake River, Leopold (1973) developed a group of factors to be considered in such a determination. These factors are given in Table 13-10. Each of these factors are related to five evaluation categories. During Leopold's evaluation each site was described by numerical means according to its physical, biological and human interest characteristics. The "evaluation numbers" serve as a descriptive function only, *e.g.,* evaluation number 5 is not interpreted as "superior" to number 1, or vice versa.

To calculate the relative uniqueness of a particular site among many, the following example from Leopold (1973) is given: After obtaining the checklist data (Table 13-10) for 12 river sites in the Idaho region, each

Table 13-3. Environmental Loadings from Community Expansion
(per 1000 population)

Loading	Value	Reference	Comment
Air Quality			
SO	315		Units in ton/yr/1,000
NO^x	124		population
CO^x	1585	Littman et al., 1974	
Hydrocarbons	118		
Particulates	145		
Water Quality			Units in lb/ac/yr
Sediment	70.25	Colston, 1975	
pH	13.3		
Metals	12.0		
Water Required	166,000	Murray and Reeves, 1975	Gal/1,000 population/day
Land Required	220	Hittman Assoc., 1976	Ac/1,000 population
Population			
Workers	364	TRW, 1975	
Associated	1000		Association includes
Service	510		workers and families
Fiscal			
Payroll	$5.8 million		$ million/yr based on
Total Income Generated	$11.1 million	Department of Labor, 1976	$16,000 salary
Community Costs			
Education	$0.3 million	EPA, 1976	$/1,000 expenditure/255
Sewerage	$0.1 million/day	EPA, 1975	children
Solid Waste	$50000 collection	EPA, 1976	
Planning & Other Advanced Costs	$207,000	Hittman Assoc., 1976	
Infrastructure	$1,678,000	Hittman Assoc., 1976	

Table 13-3. Continued

Loading	Value	Reference	Comment
Housing	$3,386,000	Hittman Assoc., 1976	
Public Facilities	$1,301,000	Hittman Assoc., 1976	
Commercial	$740,000	Hittman Assoc., 1976	
Social Services			
Doctors			
Primary	0.7/1000	HEW, 1976	Metropolitan Counties
Specialists	1/1000	HEW, 1976	Metropolitan Counties
Registered Nurses	4/1000	HEW, 1976	
Hospital Beds	5/1000	HEW, 1976	
Dentists	0.45/1000	HEW, 1975	
Pharmacists	0.54/1000	HEW, 1975	
Optometrists	0.085/1000	HEW, 1975	
Educator/pupils	1/18.6		Includes all teaching staff
Classroom/pupils	1/20.9		land on teachers/pupil
Police Officers	2.1/1000	Hindelang et al., 1975	
Full-Time Law Enforcement Employees	1.9/1000	Hindelang et al., 1975	
Firemen	2/1000	National Fire Protection Assoc., 1967	

Table 13-4. Area Required for Community Development
(Hittman Associates, 1976)

Land Use	Area[a]
Residential	55[b]
Manufacturing	3
Retail Trade	1
Services	6
Schools	3
Miscellaneous	1
Health	0.5
Roads, Recreation, Parks, Open Space	149

[a]Acres per 1,000 population.
[b]Approximately five housing units per acre.

Table 13-5. Community Cost Analysis
(1974 dollars) (CEQ, 1974)

Costs[a] and Community Type	Low-Density Sprawl	Combination Mix	High-Density Planned
Capital Costs			
Land	$3,000	$2,500	$2,000
Schools, public facilities, and public open space	$6,000	$6,000	$6,000
Transportation	$4,000	$3,000	$6,000
Utilities	$6,000	$4,000	$2,000
Residential	$31,000	$21,000	$17,000
Government	$9,000	$7,000	$5,000
Private	$39,000	$27,500	$22,000
Annual Operating and Maintenance Costs			
Schools and open space	$1,000	$1,000	$1,000
Public facilities including transportation	$600	$600	$500
Utilities	$600	$400	$300
Government	$1,200	$1,200	$1,000
Private	$1,000	$800	$800

[a]Units: Average dollars per dwelling unit.

Table 13-6. Service Factors for Expanding Populations

Item	Value
Doctors	
Primary	1 per 1390 population (HEW, 1976)
Specialists	1 per 1042 population (HEW, 1976)
Registered Nurses	1 per 255 population (HEW, 1976)
Hospital Beds	1 per 200 population (HEW, 1976)
Dentists	0.9 per 2000 population (HEW, 1975)
Pharmacists	0.54 per 1000 population (HEW, 1975)
Optometrists	0.085 per 1000 population (HEW, 1975)
Classrooms	1 per 21 pupils (Foster, 1975)
Educators	1 per 18.6 pupils (Foster, 1975)
Police Officers	2.1 per 1000 population (FBI, 1975)
Firemen	2 per 1000 population (NFPA, 1967)
Sanitary Fill	0.1 acres/1000 population/year (EPA, 1975)
Wastewater Treatment	166 gallons per day per person (Murray and Reeves, 1975)
Sewage Treatment	100 gallons per day per person

Table 13-7. Factors for Expanding Populations

Item	Value
Percent of Married Workers (aged 18-54)	75 (Bureau of the Census, 1975)
Percent Married Workers Bringing Family	
Construction	40 (Gilmore et al, 1973)
Operation	100[a]
Average Family Size	3.5 (Bureau of the Census, 1975)
Average Number of Dependents per Married Worker	2.5 (Bureau of the Census, 1975)
Number of School-aged Children	1 (Bureau of the Census, 1975)
Percentage of school-age children	
Elementary	52 (Foster, 1975)
Junior High	25 (Foster, 1975)
Senior High	23 (Foster, 1975)
Number of Indirect Jobs Created	1.4[b] (Bureau of the Census, 1975)

[a]Assumes all operational workers settle in site area for duration of employment.
[b]Based on comparison of service sector workers and basic sector workers.

Table 13-8. Typical Parkland and Recreation Area Needs

Item	Value [a]
Neighborhood Park	1-5
City Park	4-20
State Park	45
Regional Park	2-14
Urban Recreation Area	10-15
Statewide Recreation Area	30
Regional Recreation Area	20-120

[a]Acres per 1000 population

Table 13-9. Recreation Activities Needs

Facility	Value
Ski Slope	1 acre per 20/30 skiers
9-hole Gulf Course	1 per 25,000 persons (minimum acres, 45-75)
18-hole Golf Course	1 per 50,000 persons (minimum acres 120-140)
Tennis Court	1 per 2,000/10,000 persons (2 acres)
Boating	20 acres per power boat; 1 acre per canoe; 1 ramp per 150 acres water
Water Skiing	5-40 acres per boat

Table 13-10. Measurement of Aesthetics on Rivers (Leopold, 1973)

Descriptive Categories	Evaluation Number				
	1	2	3	4	5[a]
Physical Factors					
River Width (ft)	<3	3-10	10-30	30-100	>100
Depth ft.	<0.5	0.5-1.0	1-2	2-5	>5
Velocity ft/sec	<0.5	0.5-1	1-2	3-5	>5
Stream depth, ft	<1	1-2	2-4	4-8	>8
Flow variability	Little variation		Normal	Ephemeral or large variation	
River pattern	Torrent	Pool and riffle	Without riffles	Meander	Braided
Valley height/width	≤1	2-5	5-10	11-14	≥15
Stream bed material	Clay or silt	Sand	Sand and gravel	Gravel	Cobbles or larger
Bed slope, ft/ft	<0.0005	0.0005-.001	0.001-.005	0.005-0.01	>0.01
Drainage area, mi²	<1	1-10	10-100	100-1000	>1000
Stream order	≤2	3	4	5	≥6
Erosion of banks	Stable	--	Slumping	--	Eroding large-scale deposition
Sediment deposition in bed	Stable	--	--	--	--
Width of valley flat, ft	<100	100-300	300-500	500-1000	>1000
Biologic and Water Quality Factors					
Water color	Clear, colorless	--	Green tints	--	Brown
Turbidity, ppm	<25	25-150	150-1000	1000-5000	>5000
Floating material	None	Vegetation	Foamy	Oily	Variety
Water condition (general)	Excellent	--	Good	--	Poor
Algae					
Amount	Absent	--	--	--	Infested
Type	Green	Blue-green	Diatom	Floating green	None

Larger plants					
Amount	Absent	--	--	--	Infested
Type	None	Unknown rooted	Elodea, duck weed	Water lily	Cattail
River fauna	None	--	--	--	Large variety
Pollution evidence	None	--	--	--	Evident
Land flora					
Valley	Open	Open with grass, trees	Brushy	Wooded	Trees and brush
Hillside	Open	Open with grass, trees	Brushy	Wooded	Trees and brush
Diversity	Small	--	--	--	Great
Condition	Good	--	--	--	Overused
Human Use and Interest Factors					
Trash and little					
Metal	<2	2-5	5-10	10-50	>50
Paper	<2	2-5	5-10	10-50	>50
Other	<2	2-5	5-10	10-50	>50
Material removable	Easily removed	--	--	--	Difficult removal
Artificial controls (dams, etc.)	Free and natural	--	--	--	Controlled
Accessibility					
Individual	Wilderness	--	--	--	Urban or paved access
Mass use	Wilderness	--	--	--	Urban or paved access
Local scene	Diverse views and scenes	--	--	--	Closed or without diversity
Vistas	Vistas of far places	--	--	--	Closed or no vistas
View confinement	Open or no obstructions	--	--	--	Closed by hills, cliffs or trees
Land use	Wilderness	Grazed	Lumbering	Forest, mixed recreation	Urbanized
Utilities	Scene unobstructed by power lines	--	--	--	Scene obstructed by utilities

Table 13-10. Continued

Descriptive Categories	1	2	3	4	5[a]
Degree of change	Original	—	—		Materially altered
Recovery potential	Natural recovery	—	—		Natural recovery unlikely
Urbanization	No buildings	—	—		Many buildings
Special views	None	—	—		Unusual interest
Historic features	None	—	—		Many
Misfits	None	—	—		Many

[a]Higher value = less desirable character.

site was compared factor by factor in order to determine the relative uniqueness of each factor at each site. For the "river width" category a determination was made on how many sites fall within each evaluation number. If there was only one river, say, more than 100 feet wide, no other sites would share the 5 category. The uniqueness ratio is equivalent to the reciprocal of the number of sites sharing the category value. In the above case the uniqueness ratio for that site is 1. If 2 rivers shared category 5, then each would be assigned a value of 0.5 for that category. By this method each site is evaluated for each of the 46 factors in the table. Adding each uniqueness ratio gives the "total uniqueness ratio." In this manner to total uniqueness of many sites can be evaluated and compared, with the higher the ratio, the more unique the site.

HISTORICAL SIGNIFICANCE

This section outlines the steps taken in determining whether a proposed project (or action) has any effect on any historical site within the project area. The evaluation is comprised of the following three steps: (1) historic site identification; (2) determination of any potential project effects on the sites identified in (1); and (3) mechanism for addressing effects.

Historic Site Determination

In evaluating the possibility that a proposed action, if implemented, would affect any historic site in an area, the National Register of Historic Places (DOI, 1977) is used as the primary source for determining sites of historical significance for the area. This document is a listing compiled and updated by the National Park Service of the U.S. Department of the Interior. Additionally, the State Historic Preservation Officers responsible for state activities under the National Historic Preservation Act can serve as the second source for historical data. They will have information on sites which the states are nominating for inclusion or which the states may consider eligible for inclusion in the *National Register.*

The criteria for listing a site in the National Register are found in the Advisory Council on Historic Preservation's Procedures for the Protection of Historic and Cultural Properties (36 CFR 800.10) and are as follows:

> The quality of the site with respect to significance in American history, architecture, archaeology, and culture is present in districts, sites, buildings, structures and objects of State and local importance that possess integrity of location, design, setting, materials, workmanship, feeling and association and:

1. that are associated with events that have made a significant contribution to the broad patterns of our history; or

2. that are associated with the lives of persons significant in our past; or

3. that embody the distinctive characteristics of a type, period, or method of construction, or that represent the work of a master, or that possess high artistic values, or that represent a significant and distinguishable entity whose components may lack individual distinction; or

4. that have yielded, or may be likely to yield, information important in prehistory or history.

Criteria Considerations

Ordinarily, cemeteries, birthplaces or graves of historical figures, properties owned by religious institutions or used for religious purposes, structures that have been moved from their original locations, reconstructed historic buildings, properties primarily commemorative in nature, and properties that have achieved significance within the past 50 years shall not be considered eligible for the *National Register*. However, such properties will qualify if they are integral parts of districts that do meet the criteria or if they fall within the following categories:

1. a religious property deriving primary significance from architectural or artistic distinction or historical importance;

2. a building or structure removed from its original location but which is significant primarily for architectural value, or which is the surviving structure most importantly associated with a historic person or event;

3. a birthplace or grave of an historical figure of outstanding importance if there is no appropriate site or building directly associated with his productive life;

4. a cemetary which derives its primary significance from graves of persons of transcendent importance, from age, from distinctive design features, or from association with historic events.

5. a reconstructed building when accurately executed in a suitable environment and presented in a dignified manner as part of a restoration master plan, and when no other building or structure with the same association has survived;

6. a property primarily commemorative in intent if design, age, tradition, or symbolic value has invested it with its own historical significance; or

7. a property achieving significance within the past 50 years if it is of exceptional importance.

Project Effect

Once sites, building, etc. have been identified as being in the project area, the criteria used to define effect as outlined in the Advisory Council's Procedures are used. These criteria of effect are as follows:

Criteria of Effect (36 CFR 800.8)

A federal, federally assited, or federally licensed undertaking shall be considered to have an effect on a *National Register* property or property eligible for inclusion in the *National Register* (districts, sites, buildings, structures, and objects, including their setting) when any conditions of the undertaking causes or may cause any change, beneficial or adverse, in the quality of the historical, architectural, archeological, or cultural character that qualified the property under the *National Register* Criteria.

Criteria of Adverse Effect (36 CFR 800.9)

Generally, adverse effects occur under conditions which include but are not limited to:

1. destruction or alteration of all or part of a property;
2. isolation from or alteration of its surrounding environment;
3. introduction of visual, audible, or atmospheric elements that are out of character with the property or alter its settings;
4. transfer or sale of a federally owned property without adequate conditions or restrictions regarding preservation, maintenance, or use; and
5. neglect of a property resulting in its deterioration or destruction.

These criteria of effect and adverse effect can be used as guidelines in determining whether a proposed action, if implemented, will affect any site.

Mechanism for Addressing Potential Effect

No Adverse Effect

If there is an effect on any of the sites uncovered and it is not considered adverse, a memorandum of understanding (including description of action, statement of consultation with State Historic Preservation Officer, and steps taken for mitigating measures) by the federal agency proposing the action, the Historical Council, and the State Liaison Officer is needed. This memorandum is also required if there is an adverse effect but it can be removed, or if there is an adverse effect but it can be mitigated.

Adverse Effect

On finding the effect to be adverse or on notification that the Executive Director of the Advisory Council on Historic Preservation does not accept a determination of no adverse effect, the agency official must proceed in the following manner:

1. request, in writing, the comments of the Advisory Council;
2. notify the State Historic Preservation Officer of this request;
3. prepare a preliminary case report; and
4. proceed with the consultation process.

The consultation process essentially provides for an onsite inspection by the Executive Director, the State Historic Preservation Officer and agency official, a public meeting (optional) and consideration of alternatives. If the parties can unanimously agree on an appropriate alternative, a memorandum of agreement is formulated. If a unanimous decision cannot be reached, the matter is referred to the full council. The comments of the Advisory Council are based on the report of the Executive Director. This report consists of:

1. verification of legal historical status;
2. the agency EIS (where appropriate);
3. reports from other federal agencies involved in the project;
4. report from State Historic Preservation Officer;
5. report from beneficiary of the action (if any);
6. other pertinent information (*i.e.,* transcript of public meeting); and
7. agency coordination with other federal agencies.

Having complied with this procedural requirement, the federal agency may adopt any course of action it may feel appropriate. While the Advisory Council comments must be taken into account and integrated into the decision-making, the program decision rests with the agency implementing the undertaking.

In addition to requirements of the Historic Preservation Act, agencies must also meet the requirements of the Antiquities Act of 1906 (74 Stat. 220; 16 U.S.C. 469-469c), Executive Order 11593, Archaeological and Historic Preservation Act of 1974 (88 Stat, 174) and any statutes that relate to historic preservation in a particular locality. To meet responsibilities under these laws and the Executive Order, the agency proposing the project must include in the project plans, a program for historic inventory, evaluation and nomination of sites, in cooperation and consultation with the appropriate state authorities. For example, in Executive Order 11593 Section 2 paragraph (c) the heads of Federal agencies shall:

> ". . .initiate measures to assure that where as a result of Federal action or assistance a property listed on the National Register of Historic Places is to be substantially altered or demolished, timely steps be taken to make or have made records, including measured drawings, photographs and maps, of the property, and that copy of such records then be deposited in the Library of Congress as part of the Historic American Buildings Survey or Historic American Engineering Record for future use and reference."

State Historic Preservation Officers

ALABAMA
Chairman, Alabama Historical Commission, Alabama Department of Archives and History, Archives and History Building, Montgomery, AL 36104

ALASKA
Director, Department of Natural Resources, Division of Parks, 323 East Fourth Avenue, Anchorage, AK 99501

ARIZONA
Director, State Parks Board, 1688 West Adams, Phoenix, AZ 85007

ARKANSAS
Director, Department of Natural and Cultural Heritage, 300 West Markham, Little Rock, AR 72201

CALIFORNIA
Director, Department of Parks and Recreation, State Resources Agency, P.O. Box 2390, Sacramento, CA 95811

COLORADO

Chairman, State Historical Society, Colorado State Museum, 200 14th Avenue, Denver, CO 80203

CONNECTICUT

Director, Connecticut Historical Commission, 59 South Prospect Street, Hartford, CT 06106

DELAWARE

Director, Division of Historical and Cultural Affairs, Department of State, Dover, DE 19901

FLORIDA

Director, Division of Archives, History and Records Management, Department of State, 401 East Gaines Street, Tallahassee, FL 32304

GEORGIA

Chief, Historic Preservation Section, Department of Natural Resources, 270 Washington Street, S.W., Atlanta, GA 30334

HAWAII

Chairman, Department of Land and Natural Resources, State of Hawaii, P.O. Box 621, Honolulu, HI 96809

IDAHO

Director, Idaho Histrical Society, 610 North Julia Davis Drive, Boise, ID 83706

ILLINOIS

Director, Department of Conservation, 602 State Office Building, 400 South Spring Street, Springfield, IL 62706

INDIANA

Director, Department of Natural Resources, State of Indiana, 608 State Office Building, Indianapolis, IN 46204

IOWA

Director, Division of Historic Preservation, B-13, MacLean Hall, Iowa City, IA 52242

KANSAS

Executive Director, Kansas State Historical Society, 120 West 10th Street, Topeka, KS 66612

KENTUCKY

Director, Kentucky Heritage Commission, 401 Wapping Street, Frankfort, KY 40601

LOUISIANA
Director, Department of Art, Historical and Cultural Preservation, Old State Capitol, Baton Rouge, LA 70801

MAINE
Director, Maine Historical Preservation Commission, 31 Western Avenue, Augusta, ME 04330

MARYLAND
Director, Maryland Historical Trust, 21 State Circle, Annapolis, MD 21401

MASSACHUSETTS
Director, Massachusetts Historical Commission, 40 Beacon Street, Boston, MA 02108

MICHIGAN
Director, Michigan History Division, Department of State, Lansing, MI 48918

MINNESOTA
Director, Minnesota Historical Society, 690 Cedar Street, St. Paul, MN 55101

MISSISSIPPI
Director, State of Mississippi, Department of Archives and History, P.O. Box 571, Jackson, MS 39205

MISSOURI
Director, Missouri Department of Natural Resources, P.O. Box 176, 1204 Jefferson Building, Jefferson City, MO 65101

MONTANA
Administrator, Recreation and Parks Division, Department of Fish and Game, State of Montana, Mitchell Building, Helena, MT 59601

NEBRASKA
Director, Nebraska State Historical Society, 1500 R Street, Lincoln, NE 68508

NEVADA
Administrator, Division of State Parks, 201 South Fall Street, Carson City, NV 89701

NEW HAMPSHIRE
Commissioner, Department of Resources and Economic Development, P. O. Box 856, Concord, NY 03301

NEW JERSEY
Commissioner, Department of Environmental Protection, P.O. Box 1420, Trenton, NJ 08625

NEW MEXICO
State Historic Preservation Officer, State Capitol, 403 Capitol Building, Santa Fe, NM 87503

NEW YORK
Commissioner, Parks and Recreation, Room 303, South Swan Street Building, Albany, NY 12238

NORTH CAROLINA
Director, Division of Archives and History, Department of Cultural Resources, 109 East Jones Street, Raleigh, NC 27611

NORTH DAKOTA
Superintendent, State Historical Society of North Dakota, Liberty Memorial Building, Bismarck, ND 58501

OHIO
Director, Ohio Historical Society, Interstate #71 at 17th Avenue, Columbus, OH 43211

OKLAHOMA
State Historic Preservation Officer, 1108 Colcord Building, Oklahoma, OK 73102

OREGON
State Parks Superintendent, 300 State Highway Building, Salem, OR 97310

PENNSYLVANIA
Executive Director, Pennsylvania Historical and Museum Commission, Box 1026, Harrisburg, PA 17120

RHODE ISLAND
Director, Rhode Island Department of Community Affairs, 150 Washington Street, Providence, RI 02903

SOUTH CAROLINA
Director, State Archives Department, 1430 Senate Street, Columbia, SC 29211

SOUTH DAKOTA
Director, Office of Cultural Preservation, Department of Education and Cultural Affairs, State Capitol, Pierre, SC 57501

TENNESSEE
Director, Tennessee Historical Commission, 170 Second Avenue North, Suite 100, Nashville, TN 37219

TEXAS
Executive Director, Texas State Historical Survey Committee, P.O. Box 12276, Capitol Station, Austin, TX 78711

UTAH
Director, Division of State History, 603 East South Temple, Salt Lake City, UT 84102

VERMONT
Director, Vermont Division of Historic Sites, Pavilion Building, Montpelier, VT 05602

VIRGINIA
Executive Director, Virginia Historic Landmarks Commission, 221 Governor Street, Richmond, VA 23219

WASHINGTON
Director, Washington State Parks and Recreation Commission, P.O. Box 1128, Olympia, WA 98504

WEST VIRGINIA
State Historic Preservation Officer, West Virginia Antiquities Commission, Post Office Box 937, Morgantwon, WV 26506

WISCONSIN
Director, State Historical Society of Wisconsin, 816 State Street, Madison, WI 53706

WYOMING
Director, Wyoming Recreation Commission, 604 East 25th Street, Box 309, Cheyenne, WY 82001

DISTRICT OF COLUMBIA
Director, Office of Housing and Community Development, Room 112-A, District Building, 14th and E Streets, N.W., Washington, D. C. 20004

AMERICAN SAMOA
Territorial Historic Preservation Officer, Department of Public Works, Government of American Samoa, Pago Pago, American Sanoa 96799

COMMONWEALTH OF PUERTO RICO
State Historic Preservation Officer, Institute of Puerto Rico Culture, Apartado 4184, San Juan, Puerto Rico 00905

GUAM
Director, Department of Parks and Recreation, Government of Guam,
P.O. Box 682, Agana, Guam 96910

TRUST TERRITORY
Chief, Land Resources Branch, Department of Resources and Development, Trust Territory of the Pacific Islands, Saipan, Marianas Islands
96950

VIRGIN ISLANDS
Planning Director, Virgin Islands Planning Board, Charlotte Amalie,
St. Thomas, Virgin Islands 00801

VISUAL MANAGEMENT SYSTEM

A system known as the Visual Management System,* allows for the
determination of the degree of acceptable alteration of the natural landscape (forests primarily). Figure 13-1, below, gives the relationship between the system elements.

Variety Classes are obtained by classifying the landscape into degrees
of variety. Three classes are used. Class A: distinctive, refers to those
areas whose features contain variety in form, line, color and texture but
tend to be common throughout the area; and Class C: minimal, refers
to those areas whose features have little change in form, line, color or
texture. Features such as land forms, water forms, rock formations and
vegetative patterns are compared singularly or in combination with those
commonly found in the character type. Class A features usually exhibit
a great deal of variety in form, line, color and texture. Ranking the
Class B features within the area should be done first as a means of establishing a benchmark from which distinctive and minimal can be judged.
Class C features have very little variety, if any, in form, line, color, and
texture. An example of a chart illustrating the Variety Classes is shown
in Table 13-11 (illustrative only; is appropriate for particular subtype—
steep mountain slope—only since descriptions for other character or
subtypes vary according to the characteristics of the land). From the
chart, the basic analytical tool is prepared—the variety class map. Information on the base map will be used for the visual management system.

---

*U.S. Department of Agriculture. Agriculture Handbook Number 462, 1974.

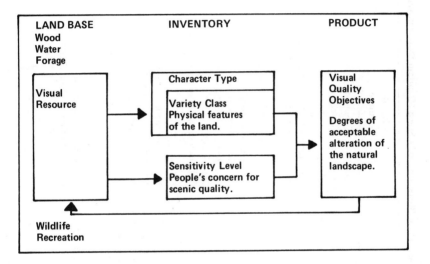

Figure 13-1. Relationship between system elements.

Therefore, other features besides variety classes should be shown. These include topographical data; landowndership boundaries, existing/proposed tract routes, existing and proposed used areas and water bodies.

The next step in the preparation of the system is the delineation of sensitivity levels. These levels are a measure of people's concern for the scenic quality of the national forests. Three sensitivity levels are used. Level 1—Highest Sensitivity; Level 2—Average Sensitivity; Level 3—Lowest Sensitivity. All travel routes, use areas, and water bodies are identified

Table 13-11. Illustration of Variety Class Breakdown of a Steep Mountain Slope Subtype

	Class A Distinctive	Class B Common	Class C Minimal
Land Form	Over 60% slopes which are dissected, uneven, sharp exposed ridges or large dominant features	30-60% slopes which are moderately dissected or rolling	0-30% slopes which have little variety; No dissection and no dominant features
Rock Form	Features stand out on land form. Unusual or outstanding, avalanche chutes, talus slopes, outcrops, etc., in size, shape, and location	Features obvious but do not stand out. Common but not outstanding avalanche chutes, talus slopes, boulders and rock outcrops	Small to nonexistent features; no avalanche chutes, talus slopes, boulders and rock outcrops
Vegetation	High degree of patterns in vegetation Large, old-growth timber Unusual or outstanding diversity in plant species	Continuous vegetative cover with interspersed patterns. Mature but not outstanding old-growth Common diversity in plant species	Continuous vegetative cover with little or no pattern No understory, overstory or ground cover
Water Forms, Lakes	50 acres or larger Those smaller than 50 acres with one or more of the following: (1) Unusual or outstanding shoreline configuration, (2) reflects major features, (3) islands, (4) Class A shoreline vegetation or rock forms.	5-50 acres Some shoreline irregularity; Minor reflections only; Class B shoreline vegetation	Less than 5 acres; No irregularity or reflection
Water Forms, Streams	Drainage with numerous or unusual changing flow characteristics, falls, rapids, pools and meanders or large volume	Drainage with common meandering and flow characteristics	Intermittent streams or small perennial streams with little or no fluctuation in flow or falls, rapids, or meandering

as being of either primary of secondary importance. The following list provides a general method for determining into which category each facility belongs.

	Primary Importance	Secondary Importance
Travel Route	National importance High-use volume Long-use duration Forest land access roads	Local importance Low-use volume Short-use duration Project roads
Use Areas	National importance High-use volume Long-use duration Large size	Local importance Low-use volume Short-use duration Small size
Water Bodies	National importance High fishing use High boating use High swimming use	Local importance Low fishing use Low boating use Low swimming use

The major/minor concern of "users" is identified next. Major concern for aesthetics is usually expressed by people who are driving for pleasure, hiking scenic trails, camping at primary use areas, using lakes and streams, along with other forms of recreational activities. Minor concern for aesthetics is usually expressed by these people involved with daily commuter driving, hauling forest products, employed in the woods and other commercial uses of forest. Sensitivity Level 1 includes all seen areas from primary travel routes, use areas and water bodies where, as a minimum, at least one-fourth of the forest visitors have a major concern for scenic qualities. Sensitivity Level 1 also includes all seen areas from secondary travel routes, use areas and water bodies where at least three-fourths of the forest visitors have a major concern for the scenic qualities. Sensitivity Level 2 and Level 3 are summarized below.

	Sensitivity Level		
Use	1	2	3
Primary Travel Routes, Use Areas, and Water Bodies	At least ¼ of users have major concern for scenic qualities	Less than ¼ of users have major concern for scenic qualities	
Secondary Travel Routes, Use Areas, and Water Bodies	At least ¾ of users have major concern for scenic qualities	At least ¼ and not more than ¾ of users have major concern for scenic qualities	Less than ¼ of users have major concern for scenic qualities

The portion of users (one-fourth and three-fourths figures) are provided as a guide only. They indicate the relationship between the types of visitors and their concern for aesthetics on the National Forest. Adjustments in the one-fourth to three-fourths user quantification may be required to meet local situations.

The levels identified are mapped to provide the data base for development of visual quality objectives. An overlay map of seen areas from Level 1 travel routes, use areas, and water bodies is prepared. At this point, distance zones of foreground, middleground and background for seen areas are established for the Level 1 areas just mapped. (Foreground: limited to areas within 1/4 - 1/2 mile of observer; middleground: from foreground to 3-5 miles of observer; background: from middleground to infinity.) All are then labeled with appropriate symbol and sensitivity level number. For example:

fg 1—Foreground Level 1
mg 1—Middleground Level 1
bg 1—Background Level 1

An overlay of seen areas from Level 2 areas are then prepared with appropriate distance zones noted. Level 3 areas are then plotted on a separate overlay with distance zones. When all sets of overlays are put together, the most restrictive sensitivity level is used in areas of conflict.

The most restrictive sensitivity level can be easily determined by use of the chart on the following page. If an area has been identified as both mg 2 and fg 2, these can be compared (mg 2 in the left column vs fg 2 in the top row) to determine that fg 2 is the proper (or most restrictive) term for that area.

	fg1	mg1	bg1	fg2	mg2	bg2
bg2	fg1	mg1	bg1	fg2	mg2	bg2
mg2	fg1	mg1	mg2	fg2	mg2	
fg2	fg1	mg1	fg2	fg2		
bg1	fg1	mg1	bg1			
mg1	fg1	mg1				
fg1	fg1					

The next step in the system involves the development of measurable standards or objectives for the visual management of the lands under consideration. The Visual Quality Objectives are represented by five terms, which can be defined as visual resource management goals. The objectives are:

P	Preservation
R	Retention
PR	Partial Retention
M	Modification
MM	Maximum Modification

Except for preservation, each describes a different degree of "acceptable" allocation of the national landscape based on the importance of aesthetics. Two additional goals may be required. The first is used to upgrade landscapes containing visual impacts which do not meet the quality objectives set for that area. The second is for landscapes having a potential for greater natural-appearing variety. These goals are defined as:

reh	Rehabilitation
e	Enhancement

Once the short-term goal is attained, one of the five quality objectives is then applied. Each of the areas is then "coded" with the appropriate symbol. Detailed guidelines are given in Table 13-12.

Table 13-12. Guidelines for the Visual Management of Lands under Consideration

Visual Quality Parameter	Description
Preservation P	This visual quality objective allows ecological changes only. Management activities, except for very low visual impact recreation facilities, are prohibited.
	This objective applies to wilderness areas, primitive areas, other special classified areas, areas awaiting classification and some unique management units that do not justify special classification.
Retention R	This visual quality objective provides for management activities frequently found in the characteristic landscape. Changes in their qualities of size, amount, intensity, direction, pattern, etc., should not be evident. Retention should be accomplished either during operation or immediately after.
Partial Retention RP	Management activities remain visually subordinate to the characteristic landscape when managed according to the partial retention visual quality objective.
	Activities may repeat form, line, color or texture common to the characteristic landscape but changes in their qualities of size, amount, intensity, direction, pattern, etc., remain visually subordinate to the characteristic landscape.
	Activities may also introduce form, line, color or texture which are found infrequently or not at all in the characteristic landscape, but they should remain subordinate to the visual strength of the characteristic landscape.
	Reduction in form, line, color and texture to meet partial retention should be accomplished as soon after project completion as possible or, at a minimum, within the first year.
Modification M	Under the modification visual quality objective, management activities may visually dominate the original characteristic landscape. However, activities of vegetative and land form alteration must borrow from naturally established form, line, color or texture so completely and at such a scale that its visual characteristics are those of natural occurrences within the surrounding area or character type. Additional parts of these activities such as structures, roads, slash, root wads, etc., must remain visually subordinate to the proposed composition.

Facilities which predominantly introductory, such as buildings, signs, roads etc., should borrow naturally established form, line, color and texture so completely and at such scale that its visual characteristics are compatible with the natural surroundings.

Reduction in form, line, color and texture should be accomplished in the first year or at a minimum should meet existing regional guidelines.

Maximum Modification MM

Management activities of vegetative and land form alterations may dominate the characteristic landscape. However, when viewed as background, the visual characteristics must be those of natural occurrences within the surrounding area or character type. When viewed as foreground or middleground, they may not appear to borrow completely from naturally established form, line, color or texture. Alterations may also be out of scale or contain detail that is incongruent with natural occurrences as seen in foreground or middleground.

Introduction of additional parts of these activities such as structures, roads, slash and root wads must remain visually subordinate to the proposed composition as viewed in background.

Reduction of contrast should be accomplished within five years

Unacceptable Modification

One or more of these characteristics are indicative of unacceptable modification:

• Size of activities is excessive or poorly related to scale of landform and vegetative patterns in characteristic landscape.

• Overall extent of management activities is excessive.

• Activities or facilities that contrast in form, line, color, or texture are excessive. All dominance elements of the management activity are visually unrelated to those in the characteristic landscape.

Unacceptable Modification includes those visual impacts exceeding 10 years duration.

Rehabilitation reh

Landscape rehabilitation is a short-term management alternative used to restore landscape contianing undesirable visual impacts to a desired visual quality. It may not always be possible to immediately achieve the prescribed visual quality objective with rehabilitation, but it should provide a more visually desirable landscape in the interim. Rehabilitation may be achieved through alteration, concealment or removal of obtrusive elements. Such rehabilitation might include:

Table 13-12. Continued

Visual Quality Parameter	Description
	• Vegetative alternatives to eliminate obtrusive edges, shapes, patterns, colors, etc.
	• Terrain alterations to blend better with natural slopes.
	• Alteration, concealment or removal of structures containing obtrusive form, colors or light reflections.
	• Revegetation of cut-and-fill slopes.
	• Alteration, concealment ore removal of slash, root wads or construction debris.
	• Identification of landscapes needing rehabilitation should normally be done at the time quality objectives are applied.
Enhancement e	Enhancement is a short-term management alternative aimed at increasing positive visual variety where little variety now exists. Enhancement may be achieved through addition, subtraction or alteration of vegetation, water, rock earth forms or structures to create additional variety of forms, edges, colors, textures, patterns or spaces. Examples of these might include:
	• Addition of species to plant community to give unique form, color or texture to an area.
	• Manipulation of vegetation to open up vistas or screen out undesirable views.
	• Addition of structures that enhance the natural landscape.

After the Visual Quality Objectives have been identified, they should be mapped by combining Variety Classes and Sensitivity Levels. Using the previously prepared Variety Class and Sensitivity Level overlays, the appropriate visual quality objectives are indicated. These are determined by comparing (on a chart) the Variety Class (A, B or C) with the sensitivity level (fgl, mg2, etc.).

Variety Class	Sensitivity Level						
	fg1	mg1	bg1	fg2	mg2	bg2	3
Class A	R	R	R	PR	PR	PR	PR
Class B	R	PR	PR	PR	M	M	MM
Class C	PR	PR	M	M	M	MM	MM

[a]If 3B area is adjacent to a Retention or Partial Retention visual quality objective, select the Modification visual quality objective. If adjacent to Modification or Maximum Modification objective areas, select Maximum Modification.

By using the "split-circle" concept all findings can be overlayed on the maps. An example of this is given below:

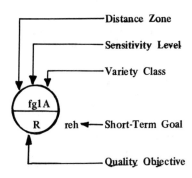

The end product of this procedure is a map of visual quality objectives based upon variety class and sensitivity levels. This system is used for making recommendations for consideration in land use planning. It is recommended that the original reference be reviewed prior to actual use (*e.g.,* Natural Forest Landscape Management, U.S.D.A., Agriculture Handbook No. 462) since detailed mapping examples are given.

REFERENCES

1. The Bechtel Corporation. "Manpower Materials. Equipment and Utilities Required to Operate and Maintain Energy Facilities," San Francisco, CA (1976).
2. Bureau of the Census. "Statistical Abstract of the United States" (1975).
3. Colston, N. V. "Characterization of Urban Land Runoff in Non-Point Sources of Water Pollution," Virginia Water Resources Research Center, Blacksburg, VA (1975).
4. Council on Environmental Quality. "OCS Oils and Gas—An Environmental Assessment," A report to the President, U.S. Government Printing Office (April 1974).
5. Environmental Protection Agency. "Third Report to Congress: Resource Recovery and Waste Reduction," Washington, D.C. (1975).
6. Environmental Protection Agency. "Decision Makers Guide to Solid Waste Management," Washington, D.C. (1976).
7. Federal Bureau of Investigation. "Crime in the United States, 1974," Uniform Crime Reports (1975).
8. Foster, B. J. "Statistics of Public Elementary and Secondary Day Schools," National Center for Education Statistics (1975).
9. Gilmore, J. S., E. F. Jaeckel and M. K. Duff. "Estimate of Local Service Employment and Diversification Potential Related to Development of a Single Oil Shale Plant in Garfield County and an Eight Plant Regional Complex," University of Denver Research Institute (1973).
10. Health, Education, and Welfare, U.S. Department of. "Decennial Census Data for Selected Health Occupations," U.S. HEW Publication Number (HRA) 76-1231, Washington, D.C. (1975).
11. Health, Education and Welfare, U.S. Department of. "Special Analysis K.," *Health Special Anal.* 192-215 (1976).
12. Hindenlang, M. J., E. S. Dunn, A. L. Aumick and L. P. Sutton. Sourcebook of Criminal Justice Statistics Service, Washington, D.C. (1975).
13. Hittman Associates. *Environmental Impact, Efficiency, and Cost of Energy Supply and End Use,* Vol. II. Columbia, Maryland (1975).
14. Hittman Associates. "Coal Conversion Research and Development P Program Study," Prepared for U.S. ERDA by Hittman Associates, Columbia, Maryland (1976).

15. Interior, U.S. Department of, Energy Research and Development Administration. "Synthetic Fuels Commercialization Program," Draft Environmental Statement, ERDA-1547 (December 1975).
16. Interior, U.S. Department of, Bureau of Mines. "Project to Expand Fuel Sources in Western States," Bureau of Mines Circular IC 8719 (1976a).
17. Interior, U.S. Department of, Bureau of Mines. Personal communication (1976b).
18. Interior, U.S. Department of, Energy Research and Development Administration, "Environmental Assessment of a Conceptual Thorium—Uranium Fuel Cycle," Final Environmental Statement, Light Water Breeder Reactor Program, Vol. 4 (1976c).
19. Interior, U.S. Department of, National Park Service. "National Register of Historic Places," *Federal Register* 42FR21:6197-6362 (1977).
20. International Society of Arboriculture. "A Guide to Professional Evaluation of Landscapes, Trees, Specimen Shrubs, and Evergreens" (July 1975).
21. Labor, U.S. Department of. "Bureau of Economic Statistics, Annual Report," Washington, D.C. (1976).
22. Leopold, L. B. "Quantitative Comparisons of Some Aesthetic Factors Among Rivers," *Geol. Surv. Circ.* 620 (1969/1973).
23. LISS. "Illustrated Scenic Value Assessment Criteria," in *Shoreline Appearance and Design Handbook* (1975).
24. Littman, F. E., K. T. Semrua, S. Rubin and W. F. Dabberdt. "A Regional Air Pollution Study (RADA) Preliminary Emission Inventory," EPA, Washington, D.C. (1974).
25. Murray, C. R., and E. B. Reeves. "Estimated Use of Water in the United States in 1970," *Geol. Sur. Cir.* 676, Reston, VA (1975).
26. National Fire Protection Association. *National Fire Protection Guide,* 13th ed., Washington, D.C. (1967).
27. Roy Mann Associates, Inc. Aesthetic Resources of the Coastal Zone (1975).
28. TRW. "Energy Extraction from Coal In-Site: A Five-Year Plan," Contract 27708-6001-TU-01, McLean, VA (1975).
29. Watson, J. W., *et al.* "Infrastructure and Highway Support Needs of Regions Affected by Energy Activity," MITRE Technical Report MS8 (February 1977).

INTRODUCTION

Energy is essential to life. Energy, even more than dollars, is the ultimate common denominator. Therefore, an environmental assessment that does not address energy issues cannot be complete. Energy is a vast and complex subject and cannot be covered in a few pages. Hence, this section will provide an elementary introduction to major issues. We introduce the analyst to dimensions of energy, supply and demand, resources, transportation, international issues and future projections.

Note that no economic information is provided, because the situation is so volatile that the information is rapidly outdated.

DIMENSION OF ENERGY

Table 14-1 and Figure 14-1 provide a context to energy questions by assembling some of the general physical facts on earth characteristics, stored energy reserves and consumption rates. These are first-order estimates.

The unit Bpa or British Thermal Unit per annum is used for reference purposes:

$$1 \text{ Btu} = 2.52 \times 10^{12} \text{ gram carries} = 2.93 \times 10^{-4} \text{ kWh}$$

$$1 \text{ Bpa} = 2.52 \times 10^{12} \text{ gram carries per term} = 3.34 \times 10^{-8} \text{ kW}$$

Figure 14-2 is the U.S. energy metropolism of the pattern of energy known in the year 1970, often considered a base year. Figure 14-3 relates

767

Table 14-1. Earth Characteristics (Gustavson, 1975).

Solar Input	5.3×10^{21} Bpa
Input to Photosynthesis	1.2×10^{18} Bpa
Solar Input per Million Acres	2.1×10^{16} Bpa
Total Geothermal Flux	8.0×10^{17} Bpa
Useful Geothermal Heat Flow	4×10^{15} Bpa
Geothermal Heat to 10-km Depth	4×10^{19} Btu
Tidal Dissipation Energy	9×10^{16} Bpa
Usable Tidal Energy	1.9×10^{15} Bpa
Total Hydrologic Runoff	2.7×10^{17} Bpa
Potential Useful Hydropower	8.6×10^{16} Bpa
Heat Capacity per $^{\circ}$C of Oceans	5.4×10^{21} Btu
Evaporation to the Atmosphere	9.8×10^{20} Bpa
Vaporization Equivalent of Atmospheric Water	3×10^{19} Btu
Heat Capacity per $^{\circ}$C of Atmosphere	5×10^{18} Btu

energy consumption in the U.S. to the gross national product (GNP) and gives the ratio of these two variables over the years. This is a useful indication of the intensity of energy use.

Figure 14-3 shows the historical relationship between U.S. economy growth and energy use. As the economy grew from $468 billion in 1947 to about $1,275 billion in 1976 (1972 constant dollars), gross energy consumption increased from 33 to 74 quadrillion Btus (quads) in the same time period. The ratio of 1000 Btus per GNP dollar declined from 70.5 in 1947 to 60.6 in 1955, indicating a more economically efficient use of energy, and has remained relatively stable since then. The low point of 57.6 for this ratio occurred around 1965. The value of the ratio in 1976 is estimated at 58.1.

SUPPLY AND DEMAND

Figure 14-4 shows gross domestic energy consumption from alternative supply sources. The 1985 values are the Administration's National Energy Plan target goals. Coal use is expected to increase dramatically to provide 28.8% of the 1985 total gross energy input of 97.4 quads. Despite pressures to reduce its use, petroleum consumption will also increase between now and 1985, although its percentage contribution of total energy consumption is projected to drop from 47.1% (1976) to 39.4%.

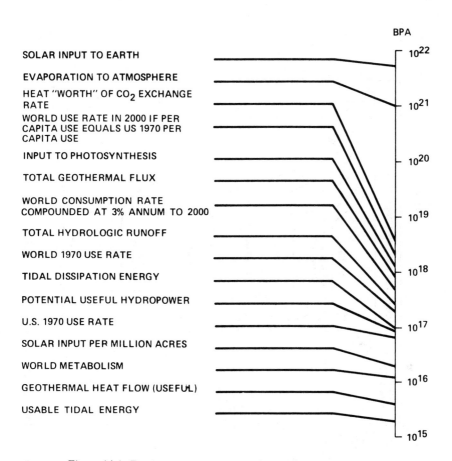

Figure 14-1. Energy rates—some comparisons (Gustavson, 1975).

The historical record and anticipated projection of coal consumption by using sectors is shown in Figure 14-5. The Administration projects use of coal by electrical utilities to follow recent linear growth, and that consumed by industry to sharply reverse a declining trend.

Figure 14-6 gives similar information from petroleum consumption.

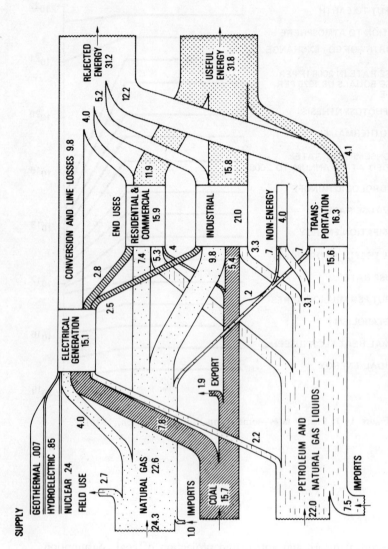

Figure 14-2. Energy flow patterns in the U.S.A.—1970

(NOTE: ALL VALUES ARE x 10^{15} Btu. TOTAL PRODUCTION = 71.6 x 10^{15} Btu.)

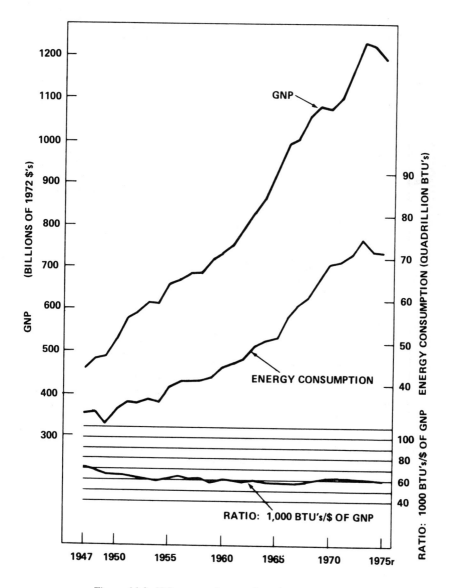

Figure 14-3. U.S. economic growth and energy use.

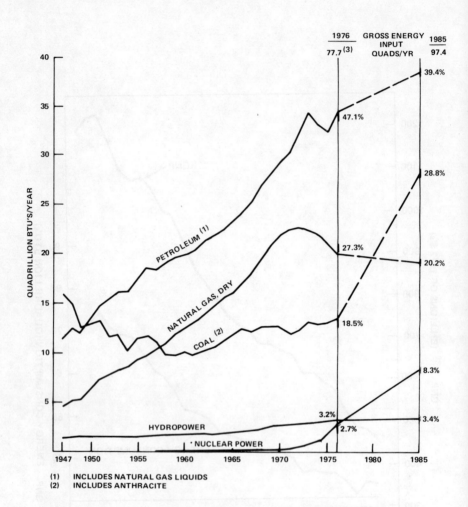

Figure 14-4. U.S. gross consumption of mineral energy resources and electricity from hydropower and nuclear power, 1947-1985.

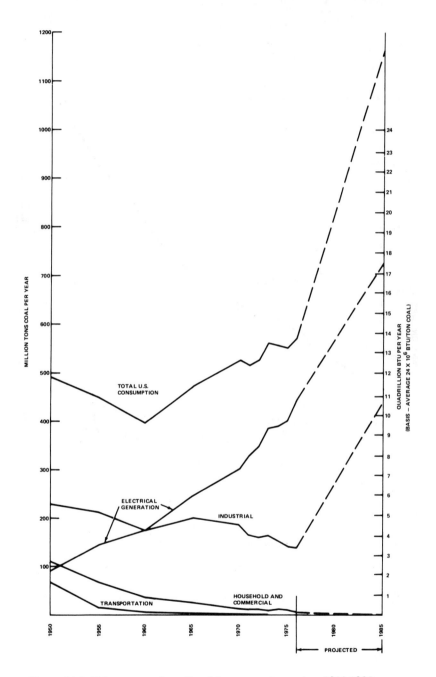

Figure 14-5. U.S. consumption of coal by consuming sector, 1950-1985.

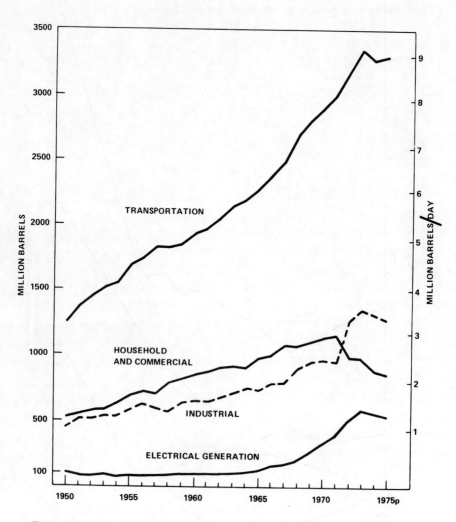

Figure 14-6. U.S. consumption of petroleum by type of customer, 1950-1975.

RESOURCES

Figure 14-7 provides a widely accepted classification scheme for resources and reserves as well as (facts) the specialized terminology currently in use. Table 14-2 provides a glossary of resources terms.

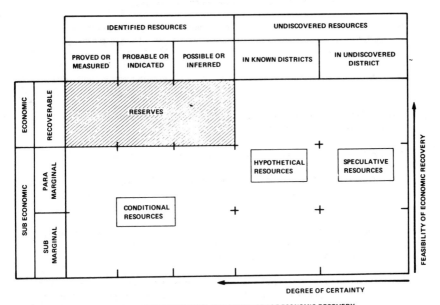

DEGREE OF CERTAINTY INCREASES FROM RIGHT TO LEFT AND FEASIBILITY OF ECONOMIC RECOVERY MEASURES FROM BOTTOM TO TOP.

POTENTIAL RESOURCES = CONDITIONAL & HYPOTHETICAL & SPECULATIVE

Figure 14-7. Classification of mineral resources.

Table 14-2. Glossary of Resource Terms (DOI, 1974a)

Resource—A concentration of naturally occurring solid, liquid, or gaseous materials in or on the earth's crust in such form that economic extraction of a commodity is currently or potentially feasible.

Identified resources—Specific bodies of mineral-bearing material whose location, quality, and quantity are known from geologic evidence supported by engineering measurements with respect to the demonstrated category.

Undiscovered resources—Unspecified bodies of mineral-bearing material surmised to exist on the basis of broad geologic knowledge and theory.

Reserve—That portion of the identified resource from which a usable mineral and energy commodity can be economically and legally extracted at the time of determination. The term ore is also used for reserves of some minerals.

The following definitions for measured, indicated, and inferred are applicable to both the Reserve and Identified-Subeconomic resource components.

Measured—Material for which estimates of the quality and quantity have been computed, within a margin of error of less than 20 percent, from analyses and measurements from closely spaced and geologically well-known sample sites.

Indicated—Material for which estimates of the quality and quantity have been computed partly from sample analyses and measurements and partly from reasonable geologic projections.

Demonstrated—A collective term for the sum of materials in both measured and indicated resources.

Inferred—Material in unexplored but identified deposits for which estimates of the quality and size are based on geologic evidence and projection.

Identified-Subeconomic resources—Known deposits not now economically minable.

Paramarginal—The portion of subeconomic resources that (a) borders on being economically producible or (b) is not commercially available solely because of legal or political circumstances.

Submarginal—The portion of subeconomic resources which would require a substantially higher price (more than 1.5 times the price at the time of determination) or a major cost-reducing advance in technology.

Hypothetical resources—Undiscovered materials that may reasonably be expected to exist in a known mining district under known geologic conditions. Exploration that confirms their existence and reveals quantity and quality will permit their reclassification as a Reserve or identified-subeconomic resource.

Speculative resources—Undiscovered materials that may occur either in known types of deposits in a favorable geologic setting where no discoveries have been made, or in as yet unknown types of deposits that remain to be recognized. Exploration that confirms their existence and reveals quantity and quality will permit their reclassification as reserves or identified-subeconomic resources.

Table 14-3 provides an estimate of the coal resources of the U.S. The total coal resources of the United States remaining in the ground as of 1974, are estimated at 3,968 billion tons. The proportion of coal that can be recovered from an individual deposit varies in a range from 40-90% according to the characteristics of the coal bed, the mining method, legal restraints

Table 14-3. Estimate of U.S. Coal Resources (DOI 1975a)

Category	Billions of Short Tons
Identified Resources	
Reserve base	434[a]
Additional identified resources	1,297
Total identified resources	1,731
Hypothetical Resources	
0-3,000 ft overburden	1,849
3,000-6,000 ft overburden	388
Total hypothetical resources	2,237
Total Remaining Resources	3,968

Identified Coal Resources by Rank and Sulfur Content

Rank	Amount (in billion short tons)	Sulfur Content (% distribution)		
		Low (0-1%)	Medium (1.1-3.0%)	High (over 3%)
Bituminous	747.4	29.8	26.8	43.4
Subbituminous	485.8	99.6	.4	–
Lignite	478.1	90.7	9.3	–
Anthracite	19.7	97.1	2.9	–
All Ranks	1.731.0	65.0	15.0	20.0

[a]Bureau of Mines revision.
Note: Average Btu value per pound:
       Bituminous coal from 11,000 to 15,000 Btu/lb
       Subbituminous coal from 8,000 to 12,000 Btu/lb
       Lignite from 5500 to 8,000 Btu/lb
       Anthracite from 13,000 to 15,000 Btu/lb

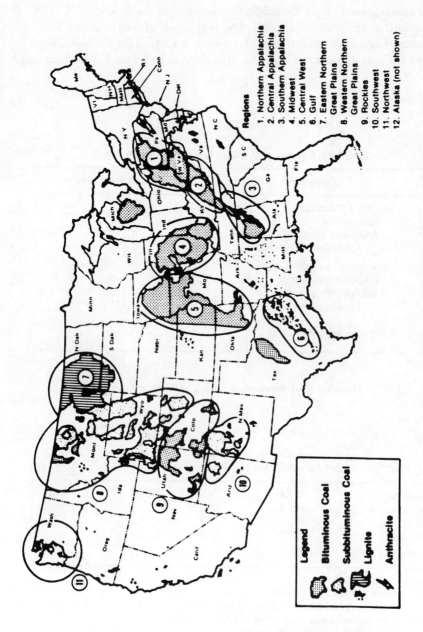

Figure 14-8. U.S. coal supply regions used by FEA-PIES model (FEA, 1976).

and the restrictions placed on mining a deposit because of natural and man-made features. Mining experience in the United States had indicated that on a national basis at least one-half the in-place coals can be recovered. About two-thirds of the identified coal resources have low (0-1%) sulfur content. The major coal supply regions are shown in Figure 14-8.

Tables 14-4 and 14-5 provide, respectively, a picture of the reserve base of coals for western and eastern states. Some facts concerning these reserves are:

1. The reserve base of coals of the Western United States constitutes approximately 22% of the identified coal in the Western United States;

2. The reserve base of low sulfur coal, ≤ 1.0% sulfur, is approximately 167 billion tons (72% of the estimate); medium-sulfur coal, 1.1-3.0% sulfur, is 38 billion tons (16%) and high-sulfur coal, > 3.0% sulfur, is 11 billion tons (4%). The reserve base of coal with an unknown sulfur level is 18 billion tons (8%). The percentages of deep and strippable coal are 56% and 44%, respectively.

Table 14-4. Reserve Base of Western States by Sulfur Content
(DOI, 1975b; 1975e)

State	Sulfur Content				
	≤1.0	1.1-3.0	>3.0	Unknown	Total
Montana	101,647	4,115	503	1,462	107,727
Wyoming	33,912	14,657	1,701	958	51,228
North Dakota	5,389	10,326	269	19	16,003
Colorado	7,476	786	47	6,561	14,870
Alaska	11,458	187	–	–	11,645
Missouri	–	182	5,226	4,080	9,488
New Mexico	3,576	794	1	23	4,394
Utah	1,969	1,547	49	477	4,042
Texas	660	1,885	284	443	3,272
Iowa	2	227	2,106	50	2,885
Washington	604	1,265	39	46	1,954
Kansas	–	309	696	383	1,388
Oklahoma	275	327	241	451	1,294
Arkansas	81	463	46	75	665
South Dakota	103	288	36	1	428
Arizona	173	177	–	–	350
Oregon	1	–	–	–	1
Total	167,326	37,535	11,244	15,529	231,634

Table 14.5. Reserve Base of Eastern States by Sulfur Content
(DOI, 1975a; 1975e)

States	Sulfur Content (million short tons)				
	≤1.0	1.1-3.0	>3.0	Unknown	Total
Alabama	625	1,100	16	1,241	2,982
Georgia	–	–	–	1	1
Illinois	1,095	7,341	42,969	14,260	65,665
Indiana	549	3,306	5,262	1,506	10,623
Kentucky-Eastern	6,558	3,322	299	2,738	12,917
Kentucky-Western	–	564	9,244	2,816	12,624
Maryland	135	691	187	35	1,048
Michigan	5	85	21	8	119
North Carolina	–	–	–	31	31
Ohio	134	6,441	12,634	1,868	21,077
Pennsylvania	1,037	16,731	3,800	9,432	31,000
Tennessee	205	533	157	92	987
Virginia	2,088	1,163	14	385	3,650
West Virginia	14,092	14,006	6,823	4,669	39,590
Total	26,523	55,283	81,426	39,082	202,314

3. The coal reserve base of the Eastern United States totals approximately 202 billion tons. Included in this estimate are 194 billion tons of bituminous coal (96% of the estimate), 7.3 billion tons of anthracite (3.5%), and 1 billion tons of lignite (0.5%).

4. About 13% of the total bituminous coal reserve base, amounting to 26.5 billion tons, contains 1.0% or less sulfur. Twenty-seven percent of the bituminous coal reserve base is in the range of 1.1-3.0% sulfur, and 41% of the coal is of an average sulfur content in excess of 3.0. Nineteen percent, 39 billion tons, is without analytical data.

Table 14-6 A gives the proved and indicated reserves of crude oil, and production by state. Proved reserves of crude oil continued to decline in 1975 from 34.3 billion barrels as of January 1, 1975 to 32.7 billion barrels as of January 1, 1976.

Proved reserves of crude oil and natural gas in various parts of the world are shown in Figures 14-9 to 14-13.

Table 14-6 A. Proven and Indicated Reserves of Crude Oil
and Production by State (API, 1976)
(Million Barrels)

State	Proved Reserves January 1, 1975	Production[a] 1975p	Proved Reserves January 1, 1976	Indicated Added Reserves[b]
Texas	11,001.5	1,176.2	10,080.0	1,867.5
Alaska	10,094.1	69.8	10.037.3	13.0
Louisiana	4,226.5	558.5	3,827.2	209.7
California	3,557.0	322.0	3,647.5	1,863.5
Oklahoma	1,232.4	152.8	1,239.7	227.5
Wyoming	903.4	130.5	877.4	182.1
New Mexico	625.0	90.4	588.1	350.5
Kansas	395.1	58.9	364.4	1.8
Colorado	289.3	37.3	276.1	83.7
Florida	302.7	40.9	262.5	20.9
Mississippi	261.4	45.7	231.2	27.3
Utah	250.6	39.1	208.3	33.2
Montana	207.4	32.3	164.0	58.1
North Dakota	172.8	20.1	158.2	12.7
Illinois	159.8	25.4	161.0	1.4
Ohio	123.9	9.6	121.3	–
Arkansas	106.3	15.6	95.7	21.4
Michigan	82.3	24.5	93.3	5.0
Alabama	68.7	10.0	61.0	4.0
Pennsylvania	50.4	3.2	48.0	22.7
Kentucky	36.6	7.5	39.3	2.4
West Virginia	32.2	2.6	31.4	4.0
Nebraska	26.8	6.1	28.4	4.1
Indiana	24.4	4.6	22.0	2.0
Other States[c]	19.4	2.8	18.8	4.0
Total US	34,250.0	2,886.3	32,682.1	5,022.4

Totals may not add due to independent rounding.
[a]Includes offshore production.
[b]Economically available by fluid injection.
[c]Other states include Arizona, Missouri, Nevada, Virginia, New York, South Dakota and Tennessee.

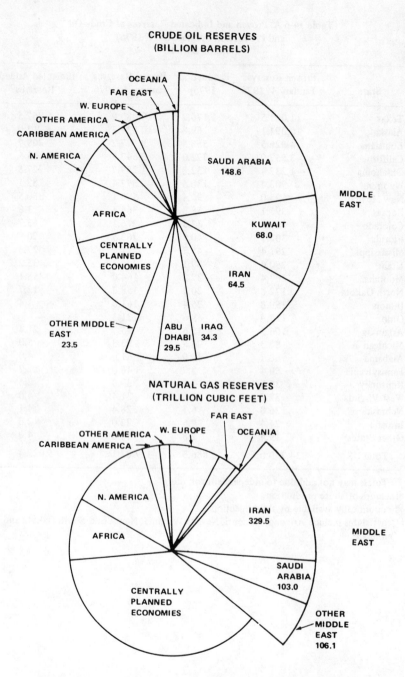

Figure 14-9. Middle East proved reserves of crude oil and natural gas, January 1, 1976.

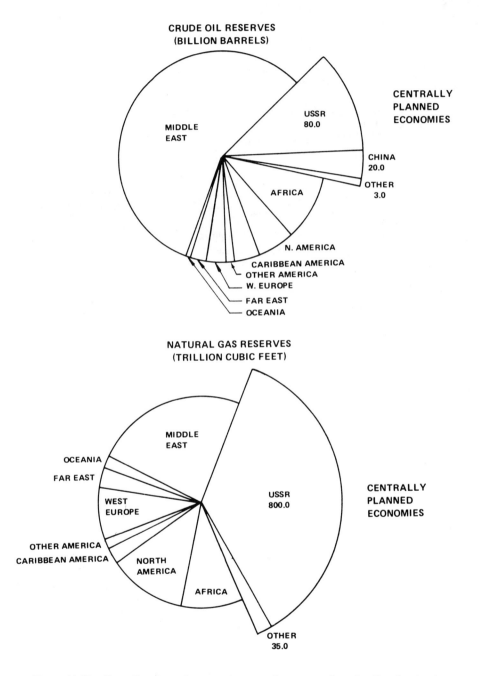

Figure 14-10. Centrally planned economies proved reserves of crude oil and natural gas, January 1, 1976.

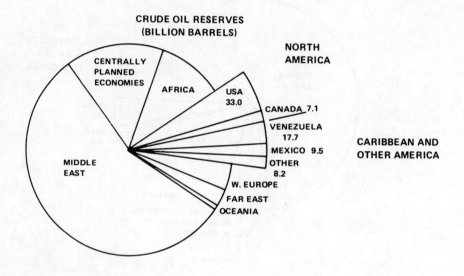

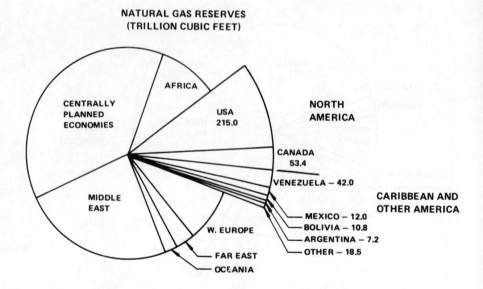

Figure 14-11. North American, Caribbean American and other American nations proved reserves of crude oil and natural gas, January 1, 1976.

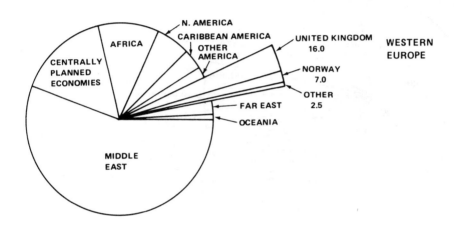

CRUDE OIL RESERVES
(BILLION BARRELS)

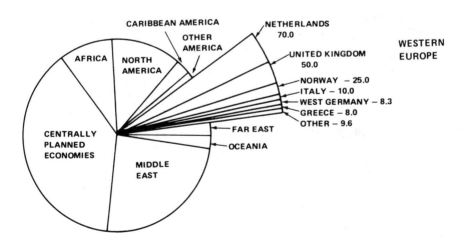

NATURAL GAS RESERVES
(TRILLION CUBIC FEET)

Figure 14-12. Western European proved reserves of crude oil and natural gas, January 1, 1976 (*Oil and Gas J.*, 1975).

CRUDE OIL RESERVES

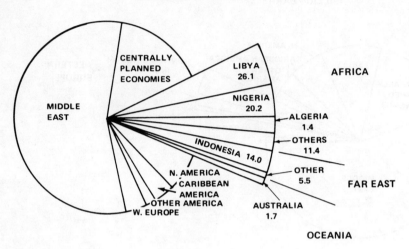

NATURAL GAS RESERVES

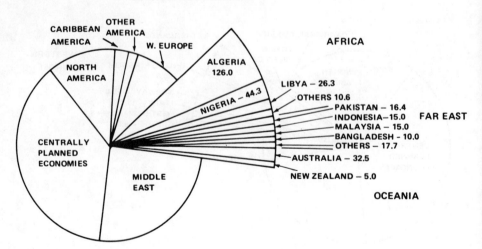

Figure 14-13. Africa, Far East, and Oceania proved reserves of crude oil and natural gas, January 1, 1976.

The natural gas situation in terms of reserve and production is given in Table 14-6 B. Proved reserves of natural gas in 1975 were down 8.9 trillion ft^3 to 228.2 trillion ft^3. Additions to proved reserves amounted to 10.7 trillion ft^3, while production was 19.7 trillion ft^3.

Table 14-7 presents oil shale resources in the U.S., while uranium reserved as a function of price are given in Table 14-8. The total U.S.

Table 14-6 B. Distribution of Proved Reserves of Natural Gas and Production by State as of January 1, 1976 (AGA, 1976a; 1976b)

State	1975 Production (trillion ft^3)	Proved Reserves January 1, 1976 (trillion ft^3)
Texas	7.04	71.0
Louisiana	7.18	61.3
Alaska	0.16	32.1
Oklahoma	1.67	13.1
Kansas	0.85	12.7
New Mexico	1.12	11.8
California	0.33	5.5
Wyoming	0.30	3.7
West Virginia	0.15	2.3
Arkansas	0.12	2.0
Colorado	0.17	1.9
Pennsylvania	0.08	1.7
Michigan	0.11	1.6
Ohio	0.09	1.4
Mississippi	0.08	1.2
Utah	0.06	0.9
Montana	0.05	0.9
Kentucky	0.06	0.8
Alabama	0.02	0.8
North Dakota	0.03	0.4
Illinois	0.001	0.4
Florida	0.04	0.3
New York	0.007	0.2
Other States[a]	0.002	0.4
Total U.S.	19.72	228.2

Totals may not add due to independent rounding.

[a]Other states include Arizona, Missouri, Nevada, Virginia, New York, South Dakota and Tennessee.

Table 14-7. Oil Shale Resources of the U.S. (Billion Barrels) (DOI, 1974b)

Deposits	Identified[a] Currently Exploitable (25-100 gal/ton)[3]	Identified[a] Not Currently Exploitable (10-25 gal/ton)	Hypothetical[b] Currently Exploitable (25-100 gal/ton)[3]	Hypothetical[b] Not Currently Exploitable (10-25 gal/ton)
Green River Foundation— Colorado, Utah and Wyoming	418 (125)[d]	1,400	50 (15)[d]	600
Chattanooga Shale and Equivalent Formations—Central and Eastern U.S.	–	200	–	800
Marine Shale—Alaska	Small	Small	250 (75)[d]	200
Other Shale Deposits	–	Small	Not estimated	Not estimated
Total	418 (125)[d]	1,600	300 (90)[d]	1,600

[a]Identified resources: specific identified mineral deposits that may or may not be evaluated as to extent and grade, and whose contained minerals may or may not be profitably recoverable with existing technology and economic conditions.
[b]Hypothetical resources: undiscovered mineral deposits, whether of recoverable or subeconomic grade, that are geologically predictable as existing in known districts.
[c]The 25-100 gal/ton category is considered virtually equivalent to the category "average of 30 or more gallons per ton."
[d]Figures in parentheses denote the estimates for the amount of oil shale recoverable under present constraints.

Table 14-8. U.S. Uranium Resources by Forward Cost Category[a]
Cumulative Uranium Resources (thousands of tons) DOI, 1976a; 1976c)

Forward Cost Category	Reserves	Potential Probable	Potential Possible	Potential Speculative	Total
≤$10/lb	270	440	420	145	1,275
≤$15/lb	430	655	675	290	2,050
≤$30/lb	640	1,060	1,270	590	3,560
By-product[b]	140	–	–	–	140
Total	780	1,060	1,270	590	3,700

[a]Forward costs are those operating and capital costs yet to be incurred at the time the estimate is made.
[b]By-product of phosphate and copper production.

uranium reserves and potential resources at a maximum forward cost of $30/lb are estimated at approximately 3.5 million tons. Discovered reserve estimates increase about 59% from $10/lb to $15/lb and about 137% from $10/lb to $30/lb. Uranium reserves and resources increase about 61% from $10/lb to $15/lb and about 179% from $10/lb to $30/lb.

Geothermal reserves by reserve category are given in Table 14-9. Geothermal energy is the natural heat contained in the earth's crust. Five types of geothermal resources have been defined:

- Hydrothermal Convection Systems
- Geopressured
- Hot Dry Rock
- Magma
- Normal Gradient

Table 14-9. U.S. Geothermal Resource Base and Estimated Recoverable Heat by Resource Type (Quadrillion Btus) (DOI, 1975c; 1975f)

Resource Type	Resource Base: Heat Content		Resource Base: Recoverable Heat[a]	
	Known[b]	Inferred[c]	Known[b]	Inferred[c]
Hydrothermal Convective ($<$3 km)				
Vapor dominated ($>$150°C)	100	100	2	2
Liquid dominated				
High temperature ($>$150°C)	1,500	4,900	20	110
Low temperature (90-150°C)	1,400	4,100	80	250
Geopressured ($<$10 km)	44,000[d]	132,000[d]		
Methane production			500	1,500
Electricity utilization			100	230
Hot Dry Rock ($<$10 km)	48,000	150,000	80[e]	240[e]
Magma[f] ($<$10 km)	52,000	150,000	80[f]	240[f]
Normal Gradient ($<$10 km)	32×10^6	0	0	0
Total	32.15×10^6	441,100	862	2,572

[a]Amount of heat that may be extracted from resource base with present or near-term technology without regard for cost or type or application.
[b]Identified amount of heat.
[c]Estimate for undiscovered heat content, does not include known heat.
[d]Electrical utilization and methane production.
[e]Assumes low 2% extraction recovery; 8% conversion efficiency.
[f]Magma resources may be renewed by natural resupply from earth's interior making this estimate conservative.

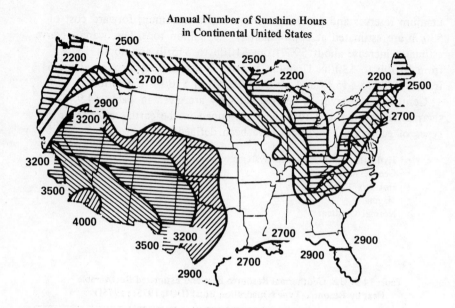

Annual Number of Sunshine Hours in Continental United States

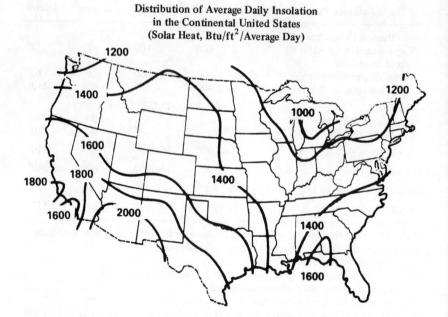

Distribution of Average Daily Insolation in the Continental United States
(Solar Heat, Btu/ft^2/Average Day)

Figure 14-14. Potential of solar energy.

Geothermal energy is useful for electricity generation and nonelectric applications. Nonelectric applications include space heating, industrial process heat, water desalting and agricultural uses.

Figure 14-14 identifies potential solar energy by depicting annual numbers of sunshine hours and average daily insolation for the continental U.S.

TRANSPORTATION

Modes of shipment for several years for coal and petroleum, are given in Tables 14-10, 14-11 and 14-12 indicating trends in modal split and increasing/decreasing volumes moved.

Table 14-10. Shipment of Bituminous Coal from the Mine,
1960-1974 (DOI, 1976b)

Years	Loaded at Mine for Shipment by Rail (%)	Loaded at Mine for Shipment by Water (%)	Trucked to Final Destination (%)	Used at Mine Mouth (%)	Total Production x 10³ Tons
1960	73.13	11.25	12.68	2.92	415,512
1962	72.80	11.39	12.99	2.80	422.149
1964	71.71	12.18	13.45	2.61	486,998
1966	72.48	11.63	12.55	3.33	533,881
1968	72.70	12.26	11.32	3.69	545,245
1970	67.85	13.49	12.26	6.38	602,932
1972	66.17	11.72	11.02	11.06	595,386
1973	67.11	11.59	9.67	11.60	591,738
1974	65.82	11.23	11.00	11.04	603,406

Totals may not equal 100% because small amounts of coal are shipped by slurry pipelines and used for other purposes at the mine.

Table 14-11. Petroleum Transportation, 1938-1974—
Percentage of Total Tonnage Shipped
(Association of Oil Pipelines, 1976)

	Pipelines		Water Carriers		Motor Carriers		Railroad	
Year	Crude	Product[a]	Crude	Product	Crude	Product	Crude	Product
1938	71.01	6.35	25.58	52.65	1.17	10.59	2.24	30.41
1948	68.48	11.36	23.26	44.70	3.86	29.85	4.40	14.09
1958	76.35	20.48	16.90	37.51	6.45	36.76	0.30	5.25
1968	74.08	30.41	18.62	25.60	7.11	41.35	0.19	2.55
1970	74.30	31.12	18.90	26.75	6.65	39.72	0.15	2.41
1972	75.75	32.39	16.10	26.92	7.92	38.55	0.23	2.14
1973	76.89	32.74	14.13	25.78	8.68	39.3	0.30	2.17
1974	74.81	33.54	13.47	25.84	11.29	38.48	0.43	2.17

Petroleum Transportation, 1972-1974—
Percentage of Total Ton-Miles Shipped

	Pipelines		Water Carriers		Motor Carriers		Railroad	
Year	Crude	Product[a]	Crude	Product	Crude	Product	Crude	Product
1972	78.6	40.1	21.0	53.3	0.3	4.6	.5	2.0
1973	83.2	42.9	16.2	49.8	0.4	4.9	.8	2.4
1974	84.4	41.9	14.8	49.8	1.2	5.4	1.6	2.9

[a]Product pipelines move only light petroleum products.

INTERNATIONAL ISSUES

Energy is an international issue, and problems of energy cannot be resolved with national solutions.

Tables 14-13 to 14-17 and Figures 14-11 to 14-14 provide background information on the world reserve of energy. Table 14-18 gives an indication of refining capacity around the world, and Table 14-19 indicates world energy consumption for broad regions and selected countries. The reserves of the world, production and consumption of oil are shown in Figures 14-15 and 14-16.

Table 14-12. Crude Oil and Natural Gas Worldwide Proved Reserves
January 1, 1976 (*Oil and Gas J.*, 1975)

Region	Crude Oil Proved Reserves		Natural Gas Proved Reserves		
	Billion Barrels	Percentage of Distribution	Trillion Cubic Feet	Billion Barrels Crude Oil Equivalent	Percentage of Distribution
Middle East	368.4	55.9	538.6	95.6	24.1
Centrally Planned Economies	103.0	15.6	835.0	148.3	37.4
Africa	65.1	9.9	207.1	36.8	9.3
North America	40.1	6.1	268.4	47.7	12.0
Caribbean America[a]	28.5	4.3	62.0	11.0	2.8
Other America	6.9	1.1	28.5	5.1	1.3
Western Europe	25.5	3.9	180.9	32.1	8.1
Far East	19.4	2.9	74.1	13.1	3.3
Oceania	1.8	0.3	37.5	6.7	1.7
Total	658.7	100.0	2,232.1	396.4	100.0

[a]Includes Colombia, Mexico, Trinidad and Tobago, and Venezuela.

Table 14-13. Middle East Proved Reserves of Crude Oil and Natural Gas
January 1, 1976 (*Oil and Gas J.*, 1975).

Country	Proved Reserves	
	Crude Oil (Billion Barrels)	Natural Gas (Trillion Cubic Feet)
Abu Dhabi	29.5	20.0
Bahrain	0.3	5.5
Dubai	1.4	1.5
Iran	64.5	329.5
Iraq	34.3	27.1
Israel	0.001	0.02
Kuwait	68.0	31.8
Neutral Zone	6.4	7.5
Oman	5.9	2.0
Qatar	5.8	7.5
Saudi Arabia	148.6	103.0
Sharjah	1.4	1.5
Syria	2.2	1.2
Turkey	0.1	0.5
Total	368.4	538.6

Table 14-14. Centrally Planned Economies Proved Reserves of
Crude Oil and Natural Gas, January 1, 1976 (*Oil and Gas J.*, 1975)

Country	Proved Reserves	
	Crude Oil (Billion Barrels)	Natural Gas (Trillion Cubic Feet)
China	20.0	25.0
USSR	80.0	800.0
Others	3.0	10.0
Total	103.0	835.0

Table 14-15. North American, Caribbean American and Other
American Nations Proved Reserves of Crude Oil and Natural Gas
January 1, 1976 (*Oil and Gas J.*, 1975)

Country	Proved Reserves	
	Crude Oil (Billion Barrels)	Natural Gas (Trillion Cubic Feet)
North America		
Canada	7.1	53.4
United States	33.0	215.0
Total	40.1	268.4
Caribbean America		
Colombia	0.6	4.0
Mexico	9.5	12.0
Trinidad and Tobago	0.7	4.0
Venezuela	17.7	42.0
Total	28.5	62.0
Other America		
Argentina	2.5	7.2
Bolivia	0.2	10.8
Brazil	0.8	0.9
Chile	0.2	2.3
Ecuador	2.4	5.0
Peru	0.8	2.3
Total	6.9	28.5

Table 14-16. Western European Proved Reserves of Crude Oil and
Natural Gas, January 1, 1976 (*Oil and Gas J.,* 1975)

Country	Proved Reserves	
	Crude Oil (Billion Barrels)	Natural Gas (Trillion Cubic Feet)
Austria	0.2	0.8
Denmark	0.2	0.5
France	0.1	5.3
Greece	0.04	8.0
Ireland	–	1.0
Italy	0.7	10.0
Netherlands	0.25	70.0
Norway	7.0	25.0
Spain	0.25	0.5
United Kingdom	16.0	50.0
West Germany	0.4	8.3
Yugoslavia	0.4	1.5
Total	25.5	180.9

Coal reserves of the world are given in Figure 14-17, while Tables 14-20 to 14-22 present staticstics on U.S. natural gas and crude oil production, respectively.

World reserves of Uranium and Lithium are given in Figures 14-18 and 14-19, respectively.

U.S. nuclear generation of electricity is presented in Table 14-23.

Table 14-17. Africa, Far East and Oceania Proved Reserves of
Crude Oil and Natural Gas, January 1, 1976 (*Oil and Gas J.*, 1975)

	Proved Reserves	
Country	Crude Oil (Billion Barrels)	Natural Gas (Trillion Cubic Feet)
Africa		
Algeria	7.4	126.0
Angola	1.3	1.5
Congo	2.4	1.0
Egypt	3.9	4.0
Gabon	2.2	2.5
Libya	26.1	26.3
Morocco	–	0.02
Nigeria	20.2	44.3
Tunisia	1.1	1.5
Zaire	0.5	0.05
Total	65.1	207.2
Far East		
Afghanistan	0.1	3.5
Bangladesh	–	10.0
Brunei	2.0	8.7
Burma	–	0.2
India	0.9	2.4
Indonesia	14.0	15.0
Japan	–	1.9
Malaysia	2.5	15.0
Pakistan	–	16.4
Taiwan	–	1.0
Total	19.5	74.1
Oceania		
Australia	1.7	32.5
New Zealand	–	5.0
Total	1.7	37.5

Table 14-18. Worldwide Oil Production and Refining (*Oil and Gas J.*, 1975)

Regions	Oil Production			Refining	
	Producing Wells (7-1-75)	Estimated 1975 Production (1,000 b/d)	% Change in Production From 1974	Number of Refineries (1-1-76)	Crude (b/cd)
Middle East	3,919	20,332.0	- 6.5	33	3,284,951
Centrally Planned Economies	a	11,750.0	9.0	a	a
Africa	3,699	4,863.7	- 9.8	38	1,328,200
North America	512,925	9,820.0	- 6.4	300	17,253,590
Caribbean America	18,493	3,480.0	-10.5	48	5,611,985
Other America	9,467	867.3	- 1.1	42	2,077,518
Western Europe	5,981	540.4	41.1	161	19,972,306
Far East	6,792	1,779.2	- 3.1	96	9,754,394
Oceania	364	418.0	6.4	12	113,950
Total	561,640	53,850.6	- 3.6	730	59,396,894

[a]Data not available

Table 14-19. Worldwide Energy Consumption, 1950-1973 (UN, 1975)

Energy Usage by World Region (quadrillion Btus)

Year	World	North America	Centrally Planned Economies	Western Europe	Far East	Caribbean America[a]	Other America	Africa	Middle East	Oceania
1950	67.8	32.2	13.4	15.7	2.7	0.9	0.9	1.1	0.2	0.7
1955	88.6	38.1	21.2	19.9	3.8	1.3	1.3	1.5	0.4	1.1
1960	115.9	43.1	36.8	22.7	5.9	1.8	1.7	1.9	0.7	1.3
1965	142.5	52.5	42.3	28.9	8.9	2.3	2.2	2.4	1.2	1.8
1970	187.4	66.9	53.6	37.7	15.2	3.6	3.1	3.0	2.3	2.0
1971	194.8	68.3	56.8	38.6	15.8	3.9	3.4	3.3	2.5	2.2
1972	204.5	71.9	59.5	40.0	16.7	4.1	3.6	3.6	2.7	2.4
1973	215.3	74.3	62.1	42.8	18.4	4.4	3.9	3.8	3.0	2.6

[a]Includes Mexico.

Major Energy-Consuming Nations (quadrillion Btus)

Year	US[a]	USSR	Communist China	Japan	Germany	United Kingdom	France	Canada	Total	Percentage of World Consumption
1970	61.7	29.3	10.8	9.4	9.0	8.1	5.5	5.2	139.0	74
1971	62.9	30.9	11.8	9.8	9.1	8.3	5.7	5.3	143.9	74
1972	66.1	32.8	12.2	10.2	9.4	8.2	6.0	5.8	150.7	74
1973	68.3	34.5	12.7	11.6	10.1	8.5	6.4	6.0	158.1	73

[a]US consumed 72.6 Quads in 1974 and 70.9 Quads in 1975. Data for other nations not yet available.

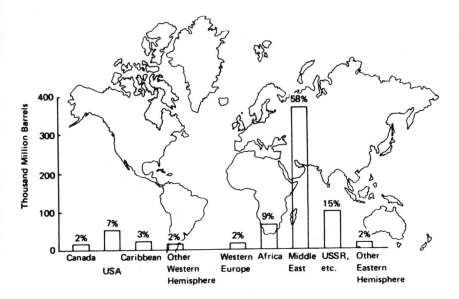

Figure 14-15. World oil reserves–1971.

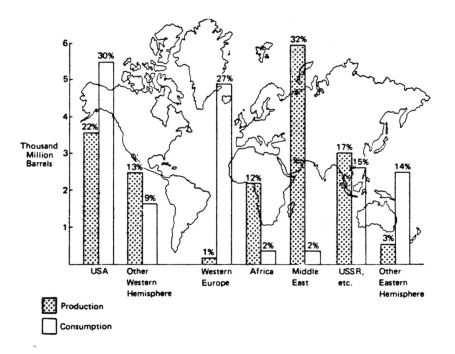

Figure 14-16. World oil production and consumption–1971.

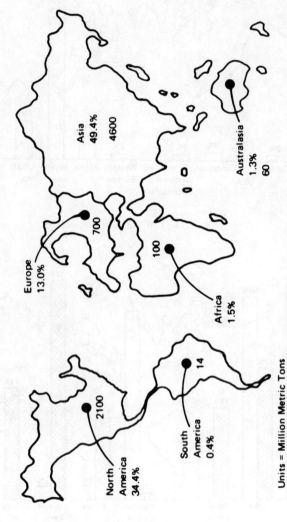

North
America
34.4%
2100

South
America
0.4%
14

Europe
13.0%
700

Africa
1.5%
100

Asia
49.4%
4600

Australasia
1.3%
60

Units = Million Metric Tons

Source: *The MITRE Corporation Report M73-61, June, 1973.*

Figure 14-17. Coal reserves of the world.

Table 14-20. U.S. Coal Production (10^6 tons) Under Selected Scenarios (1985)

Generic Scenario Name	Source					
	$8	$13	$16	Ford Foundation	ERDA	SRI (1986)
Continuation of Historical Trends	890	1040	1090	1170 (domestic oil and gas) 1080 (high nuclear) 880 (high imports)	1010	1500
Conservation	850	930	1020	690 (self-sufficiency) 600 (environ. protection) 600 (ZEG)	880	1060 (nominal) 860 (end-use low variation)
Accelerated Supply	980	1010	1020	–	1070	920 (high oil and gas availability) 1190 (low coal cost)
Accelerated Electrification	1150	1260	1280	–	1010	–
Domestic Oil and Gas Price Regulation ($9/bbl oil)	NA	1000	1020	–	–	–
Nuclear Limitation	–	–	–	–	1000	1430 1120
Supply Limitation	840 NA	920 910	1080 (Regional limit.) 960 (Supply pess.)	–	–	
Coal Limitation	–	–	–	–	–	1020 (coal penalty) 810 (high coal cost)
Import Price Variation	–	–	–	–	–	1070 (high) 940 (low)
Others	–	–	–	–	910 (all technologies)	790 (high nuclear avail.)

Table 14-21. U.S. Natural Gas Production (10^{12} cf) Under Selected Scenarios (1985)

Generic Scenario Name	Source					
	$8	$13	$16	Ford Foundation	ERDA	SRI
Continuation of Historical Trends	20.4	22.3	22.5	28.2 (domestic oil and gas) 28.2 (high nuclear) 25.2 (high imports)	23.5	28.1
Conservation	21.6	22.9	23.5	26.2 (self-sufficiency) 25.2 (environ. protection)	25.7	25.4 (nominal) 26.0 (end-use low variation)
Accelerated Supply	23.2	24.4	24.7	24.3 (ZEG)	25.7	29.3 (high oil and gas avail.) 25.6 (low coal cost)
Accelerated Electrification	20.3	21.3	21.7	—	25.7	—
Domestic Oil and Gas Price Regulation	NA	18.2	18.2	—	—	—
Nuclear Limitation	–	–	–	—	25.7	26.2
Supply Limitation	20.6 NA	22.0 17.9	22.3 (Reg. limit) 17.9 (Supply pess.)	—	—	23.5
Coal Limitation	–	–	–	—	—	26.0 (coal penalty) 25.8 (high coal cost)
Import Price Variation	–	–	–	—	—	25.9 (high) 24.8 (low)
Others	–	–	–	—	25.7 (all technologies)	25.4 (high nuclear avail.)

Table 14-22. U.S. Crude Oil Production (10^6 bbl) Under Selected Scenarios (1985)

Generic Scenario Name				Source		
	$8	$13	$16	Ford Foundation	ERDA	SRI
Continuation of Historical Trends	4150	5060	5460	5490 (domestic oil and gas) 5490 (high nuclear) 4630 (high imports)	3640	4280
Conservation	4060	5110	5510	5150 (self-sufficiency) 4970 (environ. protection) 4800 (ZEG)	4130	4270 (nominal) 4420 (end-use low variation)
Accelerated Supply	4700	5850	6290	—	4130	5220 (high oil and gas avail.) 4360 (low coal cost)
Accelerated Electrification	4090	5050	5450	—	4130	—
Domestic Oil and Gas Price Regulation ($9 bbl oil)	NA	4180	4180	—	—	—
Nuclear Limitation	—	—	5180 (Reg. limit)	—	4130	4300
Supply Limitation	4020	4990	3510	—	—	3610
Coal Limitation	NA	—	—	—	—	4340 (coal penalty) 4310 (high coal cost)
Import Price Variation	—	—	—	—	—	4940 (high) 3260 (low)
Others	—	—	—	—	4130 (all technologies)	4330 (high nuclear avail.)

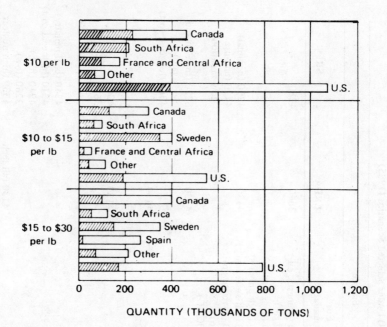

Figure 14-18. Free world reserves of uranium as of 1971. Each horizontal bar is divided into two segments. The left-hand portion shows the reasonably assured reserves, while the right-hand segment shows estimated additional reserves, based on exploration (Hubbert, 1971).

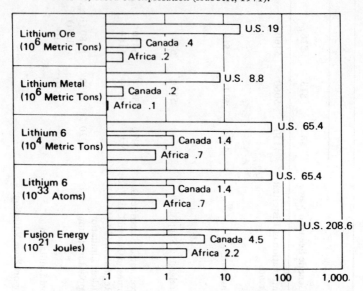

Figure 14-19. World reserves of lithium (Hubbert, 1971).

Table 14-23. U.S. Nuclear Generation of Electricity (10^9 kWh) Under Selected Scenarios (1985)

Generic Scenario Name	Source					
	$8	$13	$16	Ford Foundation	ERDA	SRI
Continuation of Historical Trends	790	870	870	940 (domestic oil and gas) 1130 (high nuclear) 940 (high imports)	1020	1470
Conservation	750	820	810	750 (self-sufficiency) 470 (environ. protection) 470 (ZEG)	1020	1010 (nominal) 730 (end-use low variation)
Accelerated Supply	760	370	870	—	1020	860 (high oil and gas avail) 790 (low coal cost)
Accelerated Electrification	970	990	1000	—	1240	—
Domestic Oil and Gas Price Regulation	NA	870	870	—	—	—
Nuclear Limitation	—	—	—	—	1020	140
Supply Limitation	580	580	580 (Reg. limit) 590 (Supp. pess.)	—	—	1070
Coal Limitation	—	—	—	—	—	Not available (coal penalty) 1420 (high coal cost) 1100 (high) 860 (low)
Import Price Variation	—	—	—	—	—	—
Others	—	—	—	—	1260 (all technologies)	1580 (high nuclear avail.)

FUTURE PROJECTIONS

What will the future look like is a common question. The following tables and figures attempt to provide a broad answer to the question of energy future in terms of alternative scenarios. Figures 14-20 and 14-21 provide boundaries for energy future. Figure 14-22 compares production to marginal cost and Figure 14-23 gives an estimate of future price ranges for imported oil. Tables 14-15 to 14-18 compare a series of scenarios for coal, natural gas crude oil and nuclear generation of electricity.

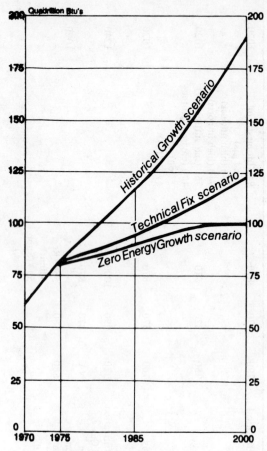

Source: *Energy Policy Project, A Time to Choose: America's Energy Future. Final Report by the Energy Policy Project to the Ford Foundation. Ballinger, 1974.*

Figure 14-20. Total energy consumption in Ford Foundation scenarios.

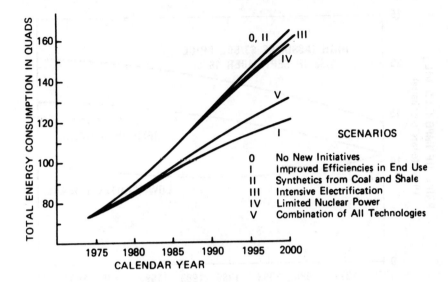

Figure 14-21. Total energy consumption in ERDA scenarios.

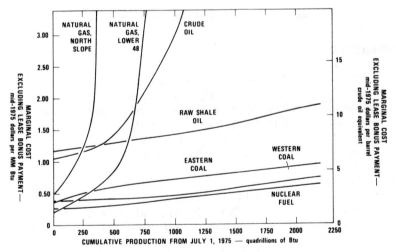

Source: Stanford Research Institute, A Western Region Energy Development Study: Economics Project 4000, SRI, Menlo Park, Ca. 94025. (December 1975).

Figure 14-22. U.S. energy supply curves for SRI "nominal scenario".

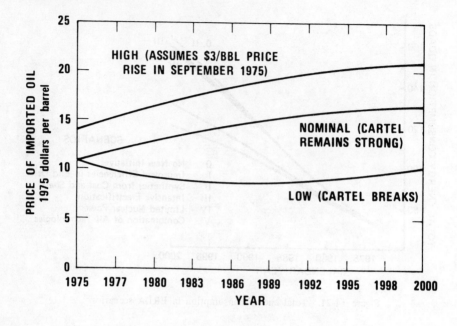

Figure 14-23. Oil import prices (SRI scenarios).

REFERENCES

1. American Gas Association. "News Release" (March 30, 1976a).
2. American Gas Association. *Oil Gas J.* (April 5, 1976b).
3. American Petroleum Institute. "Reserves of Crude Oil; Natural Gas Liquids and Natural Gas in the United States and Canada as of December 31, 1975," *Oil Gas J.* 30 (May 1976).
4. Association of Oil Pipelines. "Press Release." (June 7, 1975; May 26, 1976).
5. Energy Policy Project. *A Time to Choose: America's Energy Future.* Final Report by the Energy Policy Project to the Ford Foundation (Cambridge, MA: Ballinger Publishing Co., 1974).
6. Federal Energy Administration. "1976 National Energy Outlook," FEA-N-75/713, Washington, D.C., (1976).
7. Greeley, R.S. June 1973, *Energy Resources and the Environment— A Set of Presentations,* M73-61 (McLean, VA: The MITRE Corp., 1973).
8. Gustavson, M.R. *Dimensions of World Energy,* M75-4 (McLean, VA: The MITRE Corp., 1975).
9. Hubbert, M. King. " The Energy Resources of the Earth," *Scientific Am.* 224 (3):60 (1971).
10. Interior, U.S. Department of. "News Release," Office of the Secretary (April 1974a).

11. Interior, U.S. Department of, U.S. Geological Survey. "United States Mineral Resources," Professional Paper 820, 1973; Federal Energy Administration Task Force Report, Project Independence Bluepring-Potential Role of Oil Shale: Prospects and Constraints (1974b).

12. Interior, U.S. Department of, Bureau of Mines. The Reserve Base of U.S. Coals by Sulfur Content, The Eastern States, IC 8680 (1975a).

13. Interior, U.S. Department of, Bureau of Mines. The Reserve Base of U.S. Coals by Sulfur Content, The Western States, IC8693 (1975b).

14. Interior, U.S. Department of, Energy Research and Development Administration. "Definition Report—Geothermal Energy Research, Development and Demonstration Program" (1975c).

15. Interior, U.S. Department of, Energy Research and Development Administration. "A National Plan for Energy Research Development and Demonstration," ERDA-48 Vol. 1, Washington, D.C. (1975d).

16. Interior, U.S. Department of, U.S. Geological Survey. "Coal Resources of the U.S.," Bulletin 1412 (1975e).

17. Interior, U.S. Department of, U.S. Geological Survey. "Assessment of Geothermal Resources of the United States" (1975f).

18. Interior, U.S. Department of. "Information from ERDA Weekly Announcements" (April 16, 1976a).

19. Interior, U.S. Department of, Bureau of Mines. The Reserve Base of U.S. Coals by Sulfur Content, The Eastern States, IC 8680 (1975a).

20. Interior, U.S. Department of, Energy Research and Development Administration. "Uranium Supply Developments," Phoenix, Arizona, A.I.F. Fuel Cycle Conference '76 (March 22, 1976c).

21. The *Oil Gas J.* (December 29, 1975).

22. Stanford Research Institute. "A Western Region Energy Development Study," Economics Project 4000, SRI, Menlo Park, CA (December 1975).

23. United Nations. "World Energy Supplies 1970-1973" (1975).

CHAPTER 15

TRANSPORTATION

INTRODUCTION

This section presents historical statistics in the transportation sector of the U.S. economy. These statistics are germane in the environmental assessment level since almost all impact statement incorporate a section on transportation.

The charts and tables presented below provide an historical context, but perhaps more important, they document useful display techniques for aggregating complex data and they refer the analyst to sources who gather such information on a regular basis.

In turn we present data and aggregated information on institutional and economic factors, urban transportation, air transportation, intercity freight, intercity ground passenger transportation, environmental and safety factors, energy considerations and a model assessment.

Many of the charts and figures are taken from U.S. Transportation—A Summary Appraisal (Harris *et al.*, 1975).

INSTITUTIONAL AND ECONOMIC CONSIDERATIONS

Transportation expenditures and revenues of almost $250 billion/yr (Figure 15-2) account for more than 20% of the GNP. The highway systems account for 80% of the transportation sector. Figure 15-2 shows the extent to which highway and air systems have contributed to the growth in national income over the past decade. Tables 15-1 and 15-2 illustrate the importance of transportation to the nation's economy, resources and environment.

Transportation labor represents about 12-13% of the total employed civilian labor force. Figure 15-3 indicates the modal breakdown of the transportation labor force. The motor freight industry is the largest, and grew most during the 1962-1972 decade. The level, however, stabilized during the late 1960's

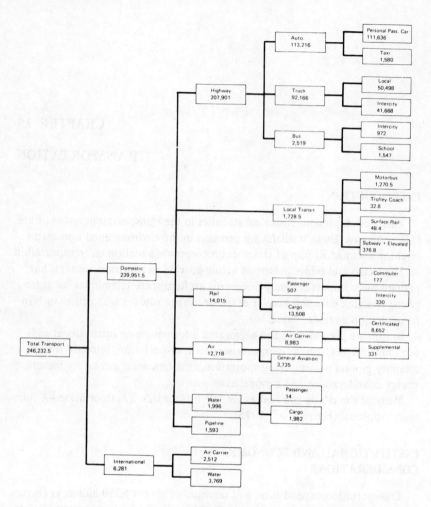

Figure 15-1. Transportation contribution to GNP (1972) (In Millions of Dollars) (DOT, 1974).

and early 1970's as the Interstate Highway System neared completion. The reduction in railroad industry employment complements the trend in that industry to substitute capital for labor. Figure 15-4 shows the transportation sector average annual earnings by mode. No clear trend is descernible, although air system salaries are slightly higher than the other modes.

Transportation is an important item in individuals' personal budgets. Figure 15-5 shows that transportation is outranked only by housing and food as a

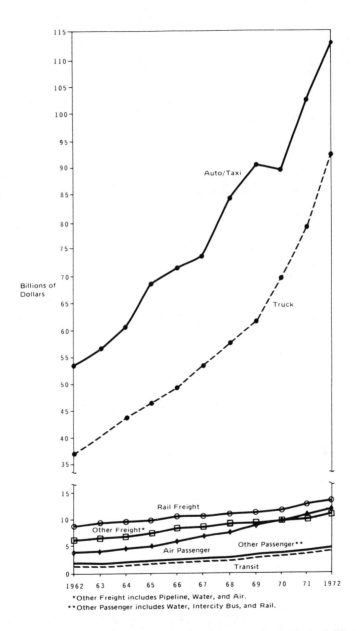

Figure 15-2. Trends of transportation expenditures and revenues (1962-1972) (Harris *et al.*, 1975).

Table 15-1. Comparison of Passenger Transportation Modes in the United States[a] (Harris et al, 1975)

	Urban			Intercity			
	Auto	Transit Bus	Rapid Rail	Auto	Bus	Rail	Air (Certificated)
Usage Patterns (1972)							
Mileage billions							
Vehicle	567.5	1.3	0.4	436.0	1.1	0.4	2.1
Seat	2,270.0	65.0	48.0	1,744.0	46.0	35.1	248.0
Passenger	851.0	23.0	12.0	1,129.0	21.0	13.7	123.0
Passenger trips, billions	109.6	4.6	1.7	39.2	0.4	0.1	0.2
Number of users, millions	210.0	13.0		210.0	21.0	11.0	50.0
% of population using mode (1972 pop. = 210 M)	~100.0	~6.0		~100.0	~10.0	~5.0	24.0
Operating Costs, 1972							
Total annual cost, billions $	75.0	1.5	0.6	46.6	0.9	0.5	7.4
Cost per vehicle mile $	0.13	1.15	1.50	0.11	0.82	1.25	3.52
Cost per seat mile, $	0.033	0.023	0.013	0.027	0.020	0.014	0.030
Labor intensiveness, %	~10	~69		~10	60	69	47
Energy, 1972							
% of total transp. energy	39.3	0.6		14.3	0.3		8.3
Efficiency, pass. mi./gallon	20	50		45	120	50	15
Government Expenditures, 1972							
Federal, millions $	*	491.0		*	*	160.0	1,260.0
State & local, millions $	*	454.0		*	*	0	1,051.0
Total	*	945.0		*	*	160.0	2,311.0
% of total expenditures		45.0				32.0	24.0
Expenditure per user, $		73.00				15.00	46.00
Expenditure per passenger mile		0.027				0.012	0.019
Regulatory Agencies	Emissions-EPA	Fares, level of service, economics, & operational safety-state & local agencies.		Emmissions-EPA	Safety-NTSB	Fare & service -AMTRAK	Safety-FAA & NTSB
	Safety-NHTSA	ICC for economics & safety if inter-state travel. Employee work safety conditions-OSHA.		Safety-NHTSA	Economics-ICC + state & pub. utilities	Economics-ICC Safety-FRA	Economics-CAB & some states
Number of Employees, 1972 (thousands)	2,279.9	138.4		1,719.9	131.6	26.3	314.0

[a] 1972 Government Expenditures for highways were $21.9 billion. $5.9 billion of the funds were contributed by the trucking industry. No attempt has been made to allocate the total to passenger autos and buses, Intercity or Urban.

Note: Figures contained in this table have been aggregated from several sources and, in some cases, different years. Hence, they convey a general understanding rather than an exact comparison.

Table 15-2. Comparison of Major Freight Transportation Modes in the United States[a] (Harris et al., 1975)

	Truck	Rail	Water	Oil Pipeline	Air (Certificated)
Usage Patterns, 1972					
Tonnage, millions	1,934[b]	1,531	660	876	3
Ton miles, millions	992,000	784,000	339,000	476,000	3700
Operating Costs, 1972					
Total annual cost, billions $	86.7	13.0	1.7	0.9	0.7
Cost per ton mile, $	0.087	0.017	0.005	0.002	0.189
Labor intensiveness, %	60	69	59	27	47
Number of employees, thousands	9,050	479	78	18	32
Energy, 1972					
Percent of total transportation energy	8.9	3.3	3.5	0.5	1.2
Efficiency (ton mi/gal)	45	213	193	342	3
Government Expenditures, 1972					
Federal, millions $	1,900	—	153	—	126
State & local, millions $	4,000	—	190	—	105
Total	5,900	—	343	—	231
Percent of total expenditures	6	—	17	—	25
Expenditure per ton mile, $	0.0006	—	0.001	—	0.062
Regulatory Agencies, % for 1972	ICC-42% (some state + local for other 58%) EPA-Emissions Bureau of Motor Carrier Safety-DOT	ICC-100% FRA-safety	ICC-small percentage Coast Guard, navigation & safety Corps of Engineers, maintenance	ICC-85% DOT-Office of Pipeline Safety	CAB-100% FAA-safety, airports, airways

[a] The main freight transportation modes by weight of cargo are shown in this table. Other carriers—such as REA and United Parcel—account for a small percentage, by weight, of freight.

[b] Intercity tonnage only.

Note: Figures contained in this table have been aggregated from several sources and, in some cases, different years. Hence, they convey a general understanding rather than an exact comparison.

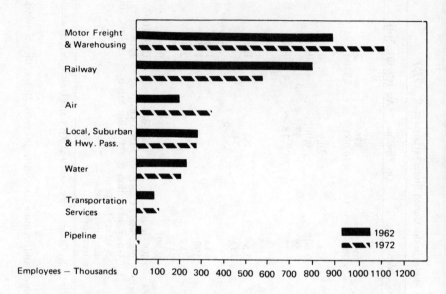

Figure 15-3. Average number of full-time and part-time employees by transportation sector (1962-1972) (DOT, 1974).

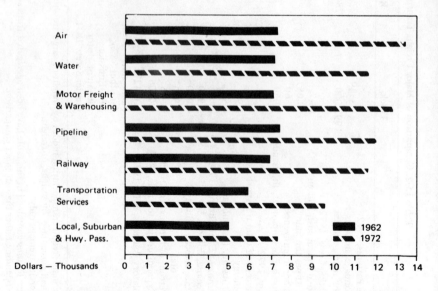

Figure 15-4. Average annual earnings per full-time employee by transportation sector (1962-1972) (DOT, 1974).

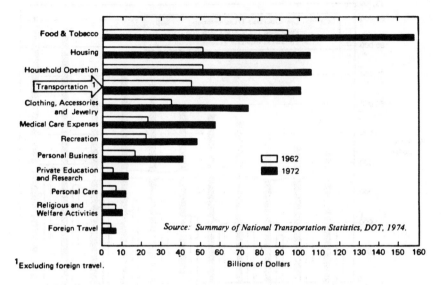

Figure 15-5. Personal consumption expenditures, by type of product (1962-1972) (DOT, 1974).

personal expense. While its rank in the household budget has remained fairly constant during the 1962-1972 time period, a larger portion went to automobile expenses than previously when public transit was more popular. Figure 15-6 shows clearly how the automobile dominates personal transportation expenditures, and that auto expenses are growing. This trend accelerated during the 1973-1974 period as costs of gasoline and cars rose drastically.

URBAN TRANSPORTATION

Eighty-three million Americans currently live in 34 metropolitan areas, each with a population of 1 million or more people; 24 million more people live in 35 urban areas with populations between 500,000 and 1 million people. At the same time, 70% of the 100 million automobiles in the U.S. are registered in urban areas, up from 55% a decade earlier (Table 15-3). With more than 90% of all urban area trips by autos, buses and trucks, the street capacity of our cities has been severely overloaded, and vehicular congestion is the familiar, frustrating result. Expansion of the city highways seemed to be one way to resolve the congestion. However, urban auto mileage has increased by more than 70% in 10 years, one-third of the journeys being to and from work, and truck urban mileage increased by 80% over the same period (Figure 15-7). Continued expansion of the urban highway network is now recognized as impracticable, in such an environment of growth, rising costs and limited available right-of-way.

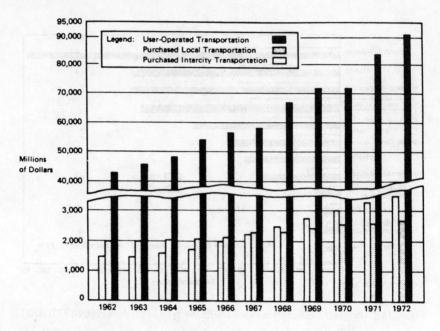

Figure 15-6. Personal consumption expenditures by transportation sector (1962-1972) (DOT, 1974).

Passenger cars, as operated in urban areas to transport people, include taxis, rental cars and fleet cars, as well as the private automobile. Most of these cars use gasoline fuel. *Highway statistics*, published by the U.S. Department of Transportation, presents the following vehicle mileage data for all personal passenger vehicles (in millions of vehicle-miles) in 1972.

	Passenger Cars	Motorcycles	All Personal Passenger Vehicles	Percentage of Total
Rural Roads	–	–	428,943	45%
Urban Streets	–	–	525,212	55%
TOTAL	939,102	15,053	954,155	100%

At the same time that city streets were reaching their limits of vehicle capacity public transit was rapidly declining in patronage. Figure 15-8 shows the steady deterioration of transit ridership. Today, about 50,000 urban transit buses operated by about 1,000 transit companies are in use in the U.S. About 80% of these bus companies operate fewer than 50 buses. Falling patronage, inflexible pricing and operating policies, and increasing costs have led to operating deficits.

Table 15-3. Cars and Population

Year	Estimated Population Residing in U.S. (Millions)	Estimated Passenger Cars Registered at End of Year (Millions)	Persons per Car
1910	92.4	0.5	202
1920	106.5	8.1	13
1930	123.1	23.0	5.4
1940	132.5	27.5	4.8
1950	153.0	40.3	3.80
1955	166.7	52.1	3.10
1960	181.7	61.7	2.94
1961	184.6	63.4	2.91
1962	187.2	66.1	2.83
1963	189.9	69.1	2.75
1964	192.5	72.0	2.67
1965	194.6	75.3	2.58
1966	196.5	78.1	2.52
1967	198.5	80.4	2.47
1968	200.4	83.7	2.39
1969	202.6	86.9	2.33
1970	205.1	89.3	2.30
1971	207.0	92.8	2.23
1972	208.8	96.9	2.15
1973	210.4	101.2	2.08
1975	213.9	109.2	1.96
1980	224.1	126.7	1.77

Looking to the future, urban population growth is expected to continue, but with a moderating trend to lower urban densities (Figure 15-9). This type of lower density growth implies that fixed-route systems (*e.g.*, rapid rail) will not provide the dispersed service required. Conversely, automobile use must be expected to increase to meet this dispersed service requirement.

AIR TRANSPORTATION

The United States civil aviation industry has developed over the past 70 years of manned flight into the largest and most diversified system of air transportation in the world. The U.S. has over three-quarters of a million licensed fliers, a civil aviation fleet of 135,000 aircraft (of which over 3,000 are engaged in common carriage), and a system of 12,000 airports and airfields. The federal government operates an extensive network of air traffic control and navigation/communication facilities. Civil aviation direct employment accounts for about

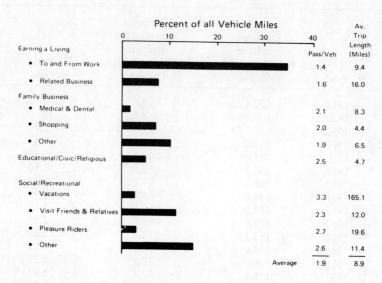

Figure 15-7. Current use of automobile (Motor Vehicle Manufacturers Association, 1972).

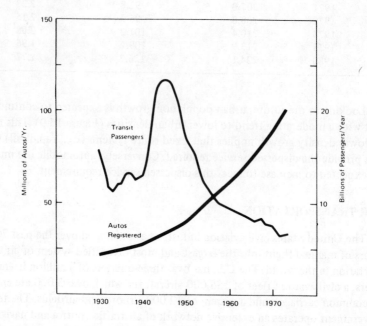

Figure 15-8. Auto ownership vs transit patronage (1930-1973) (Harris *et al.*, 1975).

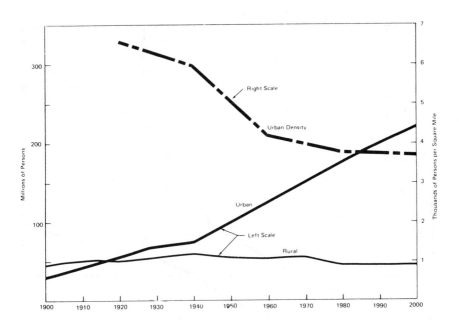

Figure 15-9. U.S. urban/rural population (1900-2000) (Harris *et al.*, 1975).

1% of the U.S. work force, and the industry's contribution to the GNP is 1.3%. In international trade, the manufacture of commercial airliners alone contributes $3 billion per year to exports—the Free World airline fleet is over 90% U.S.-made.

Demand for domestic air service has grown to its present high level in a climate of strong federal regulation provided by the Civil Aeronautics Board. The U.S.-certificated air carriers move over 200 million passengers per year. As shown in Figure 15-10, demand grew sharply in the mid-1960s with the advent of the jet transport and markedly lower air fares. This growth has tapered since 1969.

The growth in airline capacity has not matched well with the growth in demand (Figure 15-10). A combination of overoptimistic traffic forecasts and the long lead time on orders for high-capacity, wide-body aircraft in the late 1960s brought about the present overcapacity of the airlines. Only by cutting capacity (*i.e.,* reducing the amount and frequency of service provided) through 1974 were the carriers able to achieve profitable load factors on their aircraft (Figure 15-11). To meet rising costs, substantial fare increases were requested that have maintained a moderate growth in current dollar revenues, but, as shown in Figure 15-12, constant dollar revenues have remained stagnant since 1969.

Costs have risen sharply in the airline industry. Operating costs (in particular

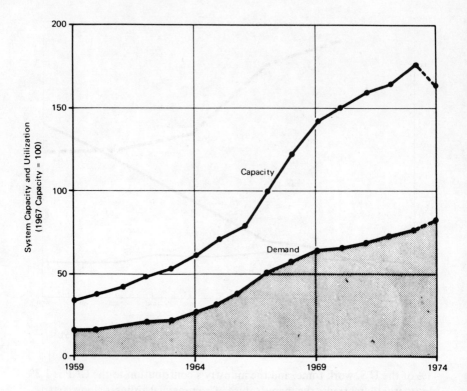

Figure 15-10. Fifteen-year growth in airline capacity and utilization (Harris *et al.,* 1975).

fuel and labor) and the costs of new capital have grown at a rate higher than those of the general economy and have pushed up the relative cost of air travel. Figure 15-13 shows the cost trend in which inflation has canceled out the economies achieved by the jet transport. The continued impact into 1975 of rising fuel costs has not been completely shown in these data. The response of the industry to rising costs has been to resort to higher fares and lower service (capacity cutbacks) to maintain revenues, generate profits, and maintain a rate of return on investment (ROI) that is competitive with other industrial groups.

In addition to the short-haul air service provided by many of the 20 major trunk and local airlines, there exists a third level of air service provided by the scheduled computer and intrastate carriers as well as licensed air taxi operators. These third-level carriers range from the large operations such as Pacific Southwest Airlines and the Allegheny Commuter system to small charter operators. Third-level, short-haul carriers have become a substantial segment of the air transport industry. Commuter carriers carry over 5 million passengers per year. Growth in this segment has been high when compared to that of the certified carriers, and nearly half of all air passenger trips can be classified as short-haul (Figure 15-14).

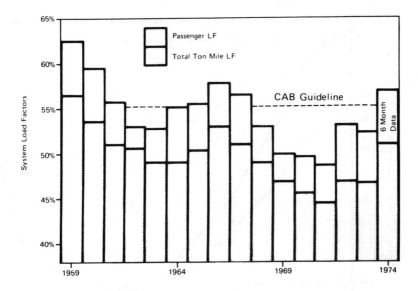

Figure 15-11. Airline passenger and ton mile load factors (1959-1974) (Harris *et al.,* 1975).

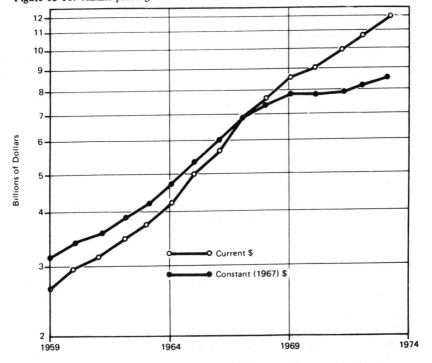

Figure 15-12. Fifteen-year growth of airline revenues (Harris *et al.,* 1975).

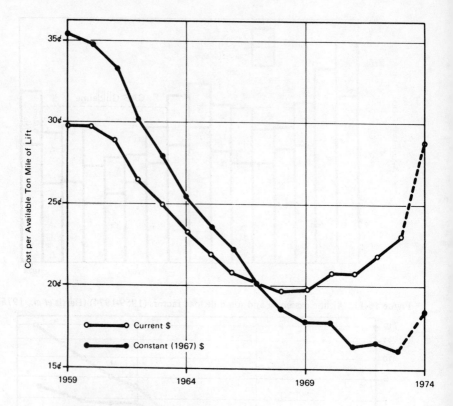

Figure 15-13. Cost trends in airline lift (1959-1974) (Harris *et al.*, 1975).

INTERCITY FREIGHT

The U.S. Intercity Freight System moves over 2 trillion ton mi/yr and contributes over $61 billion to our economy (about 5% in terms of GNP). Table
15-4 breaks down the U.S. estimated freight bill by mode. Note the dominance
of trucking in terms of freight revenues. Although large portions of this system
work reasonably well, substantial problems exist and must be rectified.

The railroad share of the intercity freight market (in total ton miles) has
declined from 67% in 1946 to 39% by 1973, even though the amount moved
by the railroads increased from 602 billion ton miles to 854 billion ton miles
during the same period. This decrease in the railroad share was accompanied by
a steady increase in the trucking and oil pipeline share during the same period
(Figure 15-15). The shift in relative distribution of total revenues over time also
illustrates the decline of the railroads (Figure 15-16). Of particular importance
is the trucking competition; the U.S. economy is expanding and diversifying
into market areas that are not well suited to conventional rail transport (*i.e.*,

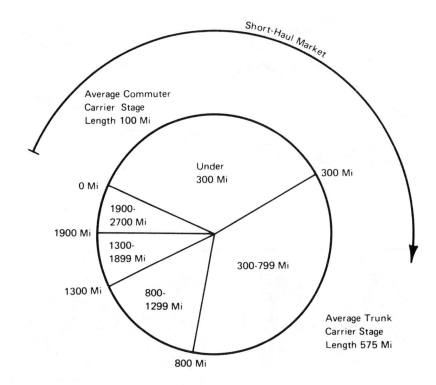

Figure 15-14. 1972 domestic air travel market (Boeing, 1974).

Table 15-4. U.S. Estimated Freight Bill (1972) (Billions of Dollars)

● Highways, Trucks	92.3 (41.8 intercity)
● Rail	13.5
● Pipeline, oil	1.6
● Domestic waterways	2.0
● International Waterways	3.5
● Air	1.5
● Other (*e.g.*, cost of loading and unloading)	1.9
TOTAL	116.3 (61.7 intercity)

high unit value, low-weight manufactured goods that have diverse origins and destinations). The rate of growth of bulk commodities that form the railroad's basic markets has been slower than that for GNP and other sectors of the economy.

Trucks represent a major use of highway and fuel (Table 15-5).

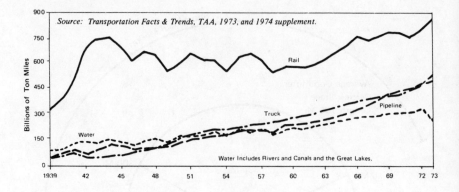

Figure 15-15. Freight handled by mode.

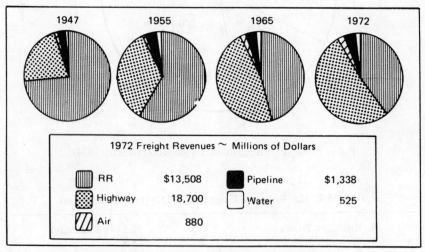

Source: Transportation Facts & Trends, TAA, 1973 and 1974 supplement.

Figure 15-16. Relative distribution of freight revenues (1947-1972) and 1972 revenues of regulated carriers.

INTERCITY GROUND PASSENGER TRANSPORTATION

Intercity passenger travel by all modes amounted to 1.4 trillion passenger miles in 1973, with 1.2 trillion in private autos and aircraft and the remainder in public carrier vehicles. As shown in Figure 15-17, the most important public carriers were the airlines, with 130 billion passenger miles (77%), followed by the bus lines (16%) and the rail lines (5%). Water transport on the Great Lakes and to Hawaii and Alaska accounted for the remaining 2%.

Table 15-5. Estimated Truck Travel Data for the United States (1973) (Bisselle, 1976)

Item	Single-Unit Trucks	Combination Units	All Trucks
Truck Miles, Millions			
Main rural roads	86,764	32,772	119,536
Local rural roads	33,292	1,165	34,457
Urban streets	99,072	14,082	113,154
TOTAL	219,128	48,019	267,147
Trucks Registered	22,205,000	1,027,900	23,232,900
Average Miles per Truck	9,868	46,716	11,538
Fuel Consumed, million gallons	22,755	8,860	31,615
Average Fuel Consumption per Truck, gallons	1,025	8,620	1,361
Average Miles per gallon	1, 9.63	5.42	8.45

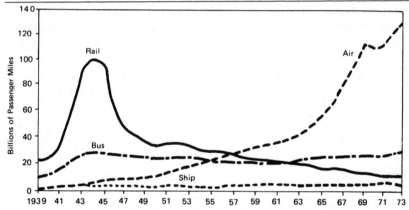

Source: Transportation Facts & Trends, TAA, 1973.

Figure 15-17. Travel by public carrier.

The estimated contribution of all intercity passenger travel to the GNP totals $69 billion, or 6%. By contrast, the contribution for all automobile travel is $111.6 billion.

The intercity bus system of this country is a mature, stable and generally healthy industry. Greyhound and Trailways account for 85% of intercity bus passengers. The remaining 15% is distributed among a large number of small operations. As indicated in Table 15-6, intercity buses go almost everywhere and perform the service more cheaply than either auto or railroad, with approximately the same highway speed (but not door-to-door time) as auto; also, the bus lines are generally profitable. In 1972, 270,000 miles of highway were

Table 15-6. 1972 Comparative Statistics: Bus, Rail, Auto (DOT, 1974)

	Intercity Bus	Noncommuter Railroad	Private Auto
Average Speed, Main Rural Roads			
Roads	60 mph	49 mph	62 mph
Miles of Road Served	270,000	30,000	300,000
Passenger Mile Costs	3.9¢	6.6¢	6.5¢ [a]
Financial State, Generally	Profitable	45% subsidized	Privately owned
Passenger Miles per Year,			
Millions	25,500	1,234	750,000

[a]Calculated on the basis of nationwide average 2.1 passengers/auto for intercity traffic.

served by intercity buses. To appreciate the magnitude of this number, the interstate highway network is only 42,500 miles at present—and all of AMTRAK's mileage is only 30,000 miles. For many communities, intercity bus is the only mode of public transportation available, and the advantage of bus service to lower income passengers is significant.

The completion of a major part of the interstate highway system had increased the average speed of buses for that portion of bus travel, and this may account for the average speed rise from 57 mph in 1962 to 60.5 mph in 1972. Utilization has risen modestly—20% in the last decade, roughly in tune with population growth (Figure 15-18). Still, public subsidy has been needed in many states to continue bus service to small rural communities not on main highways.

ENVIRONMENT

The contribution of the separate transportation modes to that portion of the atmospheric pollution load which is chargeable to transportation may be estimated through the use of Figure 15-19 and Table 15-7. The table shows that highway vehicles (auto, truck, bus) produce nearly all the atmospheric pollutants chargeable to transportation: 95% of UHC from transportation is due to highway vehicles; similarly, 96% of CO and 89% of NO_x come from the highway sector of U.S. transportation. The contribution of freight trucking is by no means negligible (16% for CO to 23% for NO_x) with the gasoline-fueled truck polluting considerably more on an aggregate basis than the diesel truck. The diesel truck is a significant polluter only with respect to NO_x emissions.

Emissions per seat mile at cruise speed for several passenger modes are given in Figure 15-20. Emissions for the auto are based on a vehicle meeting the

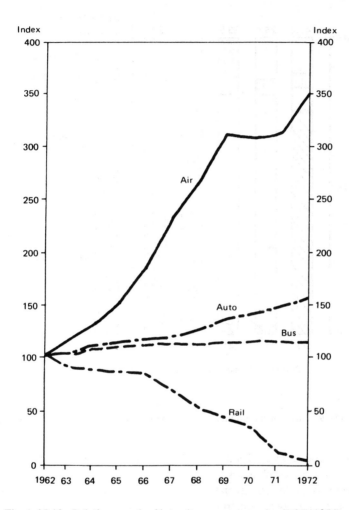

Figure 15-18. Relative growth of intercity passenger service (DOT, 1974).

original 1976 federal standards (before relaxation of the time frame). The electrically driven Metroliner has an emissions spectrum which depends on the level of emissions control applied at the generating station. Three levels of control are indicated, and they show that for today's situation (emission level "A"), electric rail systems are by no means nonpolluting. The AMTRAK Turbotrain (gas turbine-powered) is the "cleanest" of the systems shown. The diesel bus, while efficient from an energy standpoint, exhibits a relatively high level of CO and NO_x emissions. The intermediate-sized aircraft, to which only the emissions due to the landing and takeoff (LTO) cycle (below 3000 ft) are

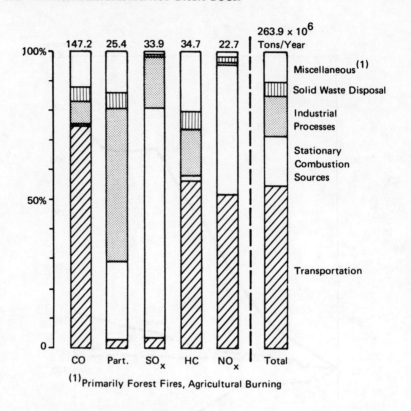

Figure 15-19. Atmospheric pollutants on a weight basis in the U.S. (1970) (CEQ, 1972).

assigned, produces significant CO, NO_x and particulate emissions, even with the "smokeless" combustors.

The major pollution associated with transportation is the storm runoff associated with highway construction (Table 15-8). Highway storm runoff is about half of the same stream loading from industrial areas. An important form of environmental effect is land pollution or the dedication of increasing acreage or the transportation network (Table 15-9).

Our highways are not safe, as is evident from the total number of yearly accidents and fatalities (Tables 15-10 and 15-11). The situation has improved (Table 15-12) with the passing of the 55-mph speed limit on highways.

One measure of the serious degradation of the railroad system is the number of accidents due to maintenance of way deficiencies. The percentage of accidents due to poor maintenance of ways has markedly increased from 11% in 1957 to 37% in 1973 (Figure 15-21).

Table 15-7. Atmospheric Pollutants from U.S. Transportation,
1970–% Breakdown by Mode (Fraize, 1974)

	UHC	CO	NO_x
Passenger Mode			
Auto: Urban	45.0	48.0	33.4
Rural Rural	28.0	25.6	27.8
Total	(73.0)	(73.6)	(61.2)
Light Truck, Urban	5.3	5.6	3.7
Bus: Diesel	0.1	0.1	0.9
Gasoline (school)	0.4	0.4	0.3
Total	(0.5)	(0.5)	(1.2)
Rail: Urban (electric)	–	–	0.3
Intercity	–	–	0.1
Total	–	–	(0.4)
Air (LTO & Cruise)	0.7	0.3	1.1
Total Passenger	(79.5)	(80.0)	(67.6)
Freight Modes			
Truck: Gasoline	15.8	15.4	13.9
Diesel	0.5	0.6	9.3
Total	(16.3)	(16.0)	(23.2)
Rail	0.5	0.1	1.2
Pipelines & Waterways	0.6	0.1	1.5
Air	0.1	–	0.2
Total Freight	(17.5)	(16.2)	(26.1)
Other			
General Aviation	0.1	0.5	0.2
Recreation Vehicles	0.8	0.9	0.1
Military	2.1	2.4	6.0
Total	100.0	100.0	100.0

One visible impact of transportation on ecosystems is the number of animals killed by fast-moving vehicles (Table 15-13).

ENERGY

Transportation depends on expensive liquid petroleum. Long lines at the gas station during the fuel embargo have, more than anything, driven home the facts of the energy crisis.

Transportation, according to Figures 15-22 and 15-23, consumes 25% of the nation's energy budget, is nearly 100% dependent on petroleum as a fuel,

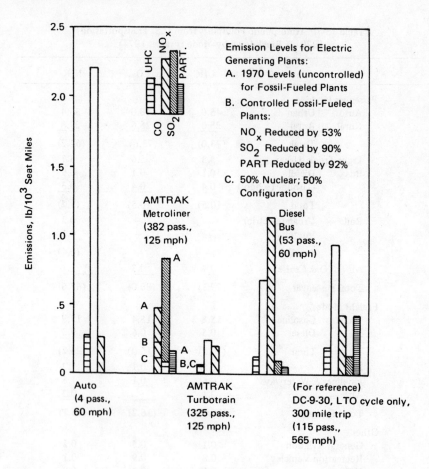

Figure 15-20. Emissions for Various Transportation Modes at Cruise Speed (Fraize *et al.*, 1974).

and consumes more than half of all petroleum used in the United States. These figures represent direct fuel use only; they do not include the energy input to that portion of the industrial sector which is transportation-related.

A more detailed look at transportation energy, according to mode and type of service, is given in Figure 15-24. The largest category, by far, for transportation energy use is urban passenger service, which is overwhelmingly dominated by the automobile. In total, the automobile accounts for 54% of the transportation energy budget. The air mode plays a major role in intercity passenger service. The mass modes, except for air, contribute only fractions of a percent to the total.

Among the freight modes, truck is the largest energy consumer. A large

Table 15-8. Water Pollutant Characteristics of Storm Runoff
(Highways, Urban and Industrial Areas) (Guy, 1975)

Contaminant	Residential Area (lb/mi/day)	Industrial Area (lb/mi/day)	Average (mg/l)
Total Solids	590.0	1400.0	1440
Volatile Solids	44.0	77.0	205
BOD	3.6	7.2	–
COD	20.6	81.0	170
Kjeldahl Nitrogen	0.60	1.2	0.96
Nitrates	0.019	0.055	–
Phosphates	0.37	1.1	0.82
Heavy Metals	1.2	1.6	0.15 - 16.0
Street Sweepings[a]	1.05 Ton/ac/yr	–	–

[a]4% rags and paper; 64% dust and dirt; 22% vegetation; and 10% organic matter.

Table 15-9. Typical Widths for Highway Rights-of-Way Transportation
(American Association of State Highway Officials, 1965).

	Minimum (ft)	Desirable (ft)	Paved Width (ft)	Maximum Acres per Mile
Two-Lane Road				
Low type[a]	66	80	18-20	9.6
Intermediate	80	100	20-24	12.1
High type	100	120	24	14.5
Four-Lane Road				
Restricted[b]	90	110	48	13.3
Intermediate	140	180	48	21.7
Desirable[c]	210	310	48	37.5
Railroad	118	200	26	24.2

[a]Rural dirt road or construction road.
[b]In Mountainous areas.
[c]Approaching Interstate standards.

Table 15-10. Motor Vehicle Accidents, Deaths and Injuries According to Urban and Rural Places, (1973)

Place	Fatal Accidents	Injury Accidnets	Property Damage Accidents	Injuries	Deaths No.	Deaths Rate
Total	48,100	1,300,000	15,000,000	2,000,000	55,800	26.6
Urban	16,800	870,000	10,900,000	1,240,000	18,200	13.1
Over 1,000,000	2,000	150,000	2,200,000	200,000	2,200	11.7
250,000 - 1,000,000	3,100	200,000	2,400,000	300,000	3,300	13.7
100,000 - 250,000	2,100	110,000	1,500,000	160,000	2,200	14.6
50,000 - 100,000	2,100	110,000	1,500,000	160,000	2,300	13.1
10,000 - 50,000	4,300	200,000	2,150,000	270,000	4,700	11.4
Under 10,000	3,200	100,000	1,150,000	150,000	3,400	15.5
Rural	31,300	430,000	4,100,000	760,000	37,600	—
State Roads	19,300	230,000	2,240,000	420,000	23,300	—
County Roads	7,400	120,000	1,230,000	200,000	8,600	—
Controlled Access Roads	2,800	42,000	230,000	80,000	3,500	—
Other	1,800	38,000	400,000	60,000	2,200	—

[a]Deaths per 100,000 population.

Table 15-11. Age of Drivers - Total Number and Number in Accidents (1973)

Age Group	All Drivers		Drivers in Accidents						
			Fatal		All		Per No. of Drivers		
	Number	%	Number	%	Number	%	Fatal[a]	All[b]
Total	122,400,000	100%	67,300	100.0%	27,700,00	100.0%	55	23
Under 20	12,600,000	10.3	11,300	16.8	5,700,00	20.6	90	45
20-24	13,900,000	11.4	13,100	19.5	5,200,000	18.8	94	37
25-29	13,400,000	11.0	7,900	11.7	3,300,000	11.9	59	25
30-34	12,500,000	10.2	6,900	10.2	2,600,000	9.4	55	21
35-39	1,400,000	9.3	4,700	7.0	2,100,000	7.6	41	18
40-44	1,400,000	9.3	4,700	7.0	1,800,000	6.5	41	16
45-49	1,500,000	9.4	4,600	6.8	1,800,000	6.5	40	16
50-54	10,700,000	8.7	3,500	5.2	1,500,000	5.4	33	14
55-59	8,100,000	6.6	2,900	4.3	1,300,000	4.7	36	16
60-64	8,400,000	5.2	2,500	3.7	900,000	3.2	39	14
65-69	4,900,000	4.0	2,000	3.0	800,000	2.9	41	16
70-74	3,300,000	2.7	1,400	2.1	300,000	1.1	42	9
75 and Over	2,300,000	1.9	1,800	2.7	400,000	1.4	78	17

[a]Drivers in fatal accidents per 100,000 drivers in each age group.
[b]Drivers in all accidents per 100 drivers in each age group.

Table 15-12. Report of Traffic Fatalities Based on Early Reports
(National Highway Safety Administration, 1974)
Month of December, 1974
Data as of January 31, 1975
Adjusted Traffic Fatalities

State	Dec. 1974	Dec. 1973	% Change	Comparison of 12 Months 1974	1973[a]	% Change
Alabama	75	102	- 26.5	978	1235	- 20.8
Alaska	7	4[b]	+75.0	85	74	+14.9
Arizona	61	58[b]	+ 5.2	714	958	- 25.5
Arkansas	40	60	- 33.3	526	671	- 21.6
California	378	316[b]	+19.6	3983	4905	- 18.8
Colorado	53	47[b]	+12.8	614	675	- 9.0
Connecticut	41	37	+19.8	400	517	- 22.6
Delaware	10	6[b]	+66.7	112	127	- 11.8
Florida	212	199	+ 6.5	2263	2662	- 15.0
Georgia	145	170	- 14.7	1534	1924	- 20.3
Hawaii	9	12	- 25.0	127	136	- 6.6
Idaho	24	16	+15.0	329	349	- 5.7
Illinois	146	179[b]	- 18.4	1973	2369	- 16.7
Indiana	101	92[b]	+99.8	1164	1605	- 27.5
Iowa	62	49	+26.5	687	813	- 15.5
Kansas	56	48	+16.7	512	623	- 17.8
Kentucky	64	51	+25.5	790	1117	- 29.3
Louisiana	79	89	- 11.2	841	1156	- 27.2
Maine	19	19[b]	0	214	247	- 13.4
Maryland	91	55[b]	+65.5	734	819	- 10.4
Massachusetts	104	67[b]	+55.5	964	1010	- 4.6
Michigan	124	137[b]	- 9.7	1847	2213	- 16.5
Minnesota	49	70[b]	- 30.0	836	1024	- 18.4
Mississippi	43	74[b]	- 41.9	644	883	- 27.1
Missouri	81	78[b]	+ 3.8	1027	1452	- 29.3
Montana	30	30[b]	0	298	323	- 7.7
Nebraska	28	28	0	388	433	- 10.4
Nevada	18	23	- 21.7	215	266	- 19.2
New Hampshire	10	13[b]	- 23.1	166	145	+14.5
New Jersey	128	100[b]	+28.0	1110	1355	- 18.1
New mexico	54	50	+ 8.0	540	638	- 15.4
New York	245	200[b]	+22.5	2534	3082	- 17.8
North Carolina	135	147	- 8.2	1566	1892	- 17.2
North Dakota	14	5	+180.0	161	208	- 22.6
Ohio	130	167[b]	+22.2	1965	2385	- 17.6
Oklahoma	70	57	+22.8	751	797	- 5.8
Oregon	67	37[b]	+81.1	674	635	+ 6.1
Pennsylvania	188	208[b]	- 9.6	2154	2444	- 11.9
Rhode Island	6	6[b]	0	96	131	- 26.7
South Carolina	64	93	- 31.2	865	967	- 10.5
South Dakota	22	23	- 4.3	229	286	- 19.9
Tennessee	103	107	- 3.7	127	1427	- 14.8

Table 15-12, continued

State	Dec. 1974	Dec. 1973	% Change	Comparison of 12 Months		
				1974	1973[a]	% Change
Texas	185	278[b]	- 33.5	2934	3692	- 20.5
Utah	13	23	- 43.5	229	361	- 36.6
Vermont	17	10	+70.0	127	155	- 18.1
Virginia	91	90[b]	+ 1.1	1045	1220	- 14.3
Washington	60	53	+13.2	752	776	- 3.1
West Virginia	26	24[b]	+ 8.3	440	477	- 7.8
Wisconsin	80	83	- 3.6	908	1156	- 21.5
Syoming	5	18	- 72.2	195	192	+ 1.6
District of Columbia	5	7	- 28.6	78	76	+ 2.6
Puerto Rico	57	78	- 26.9	544	575	- 5.4
Total	3925	3993	- 1.7	46,078	55,658	- 17.2

[a]All 1973 totals are updated, but may not reflect final state figures.
[b]Officially updated by state.
Note: The Virgin Islands report one Rural Motor Vehicle fatality for the first eight months of 1974.

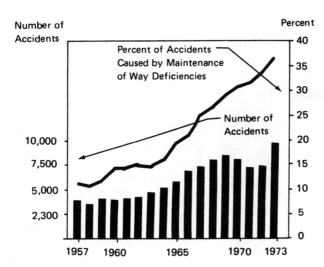

Figure 15-21. Number of train accidents and percentage caused by maintenance of way deficiencies.

Table 15-13. Animals Killed per Mile of Highway
(Oxley *et al.*, 1974; Bellis and Graves, 1971)

| Biota | Meters | Number Dead per Mile per Right-of-Way Width | | | | |
		<10.0	14.5-20.0	30.0-36.0	>93.0	Interstate
Amphibians[a]		0.07	0.86	1.46	0.91	–
Reptiles[a]		0.41	1.43	1.92	1.97	–
Birds[a]		0.14	1.31	1.84	2.00	–
Mammals						
Woodchuck[a]		0.07	0.59	0.93	0.91	–
Skunk[a]		0.0	0.21	0.35	0.41	–
Raccoon[a]		0.07	0.07	0.30	0.41	–
Rabbit[a]		0.0	0.03	0.17	0.26	–
Squirrel[a]		0.07	0.27	0.21	0.03	–
Deer[b]		–	–	–	–	7.6

[a]Canadian data: only 116 days available (June-September).
[b]Pennsylvania data: kill records higher for spring and fall months.

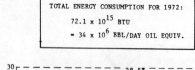

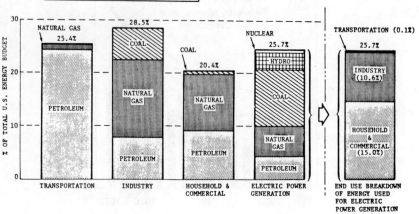

Source: Project Independence Summary, FEA, W. E. Fraize, A Program Plan of Policy-Oriented Research for Transportation Energy Conservation, The MITRE Corporation, MTR-6843, January 1975.

Figure 15-22. U.S. total energy budget, by sector and energy resource for 1972.

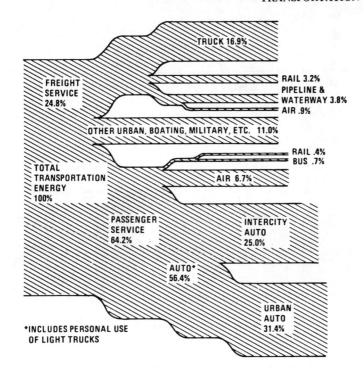

TRUCK 16.9%

FREIGHT
SERVICE
24.8%

RAIL 3.2%
PIPELINE &
WATERWAY 3.8%
AIR .9%

OTHER URBAN, BOATING, MILITARY, ETC. 11.0%

RAIL .4%
BUS .7%

TOTAL
TRANSPORTATION
ENERGY
100%

AIR 6.7%

PASSENGER
SERVICE
64.2%

INTERCITY
AUTO
25.0%

AUTO*
56.4%

URBAN
AUTO
31.4%

*INCLUDES PERSONAL USE
OF LIGHT TRUCKS

Source: Fraize, W. E. et al, Energy and Environmental Aspects of U.S. Transportation,
The MITRE Corporation, MTP-391, February 1974.

Figure 15-23. U.S. transportation energy distribution by mode (1970).

portion (8.1%) of energy use due to trucking is for nonfreight trucking service, and is, therefore, subject to different policy and control measures than
would apply for the truck freight industry.

Not only has energy intensiveness changed in the past few decades,
but so has the distribution of energy use among the several modes.
Figure 15-25 illustrates that while the energy consumed by railroads was
declining, partly from improvements in energy use efficiency and partly
from a decrease in traffic, the energy consumed by the more energy-
intensive modes increased steadily. The air mode has shown the greatest
percentage growth.

Total transportation energy use increased for the same period, as
shown in Figure 15-25. This growth is due principally to increases in
per-capita transportation use, while increases in population and changes

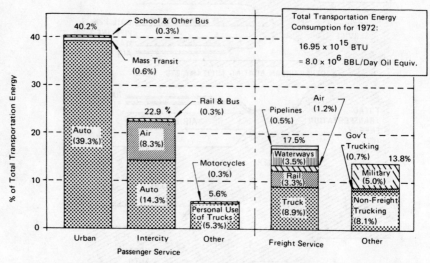

Source: W. E. Fraize, A Program Plan of Policy-Oriented Research for Transportation Energy Conservation, The MITRE Corporation, MTR-6843, January 1975. Data Source—Jack Faucett Assoc., Inc.

Figure 15-24. U.S. transportation energy consumption by mode (1972).

in energy intensiveness, including the effect of mode shifts, had important, but secondary, influences on energy growth.

The trend toward shorter weeks and more leisure time will result in diminished use of the auto in its most energy-intensive (Btu/pass. mi) function and increased use in its least energy-intensive function. Figure 15-26 shows current automobile usage according to trip purpose. Work-related trips currently consume more than 40% of all auto vehicle miles at relatively low load factors (1.4 pass/vehicle). However, more leisure is apt to encourage greater overall usage of the automobile so that the efficiency improvement noted above may well be overshadowed by potential increases in vehicle usage; hence, energy consumption for automobiles may continue rising in spite of increased energy costs.

Figure 15-27 shows the trend of U.S. automobile ownership, and indicates that car ownership is approaching the saturation level at a little over 80% of all households. The remaining, no-car group includes the infirm, certain poor and other persons for whom a car is a net inconvenience. The proportion of multicar households is seen to be rising rapidly, emphasizing the trend to more specialized vehicles.

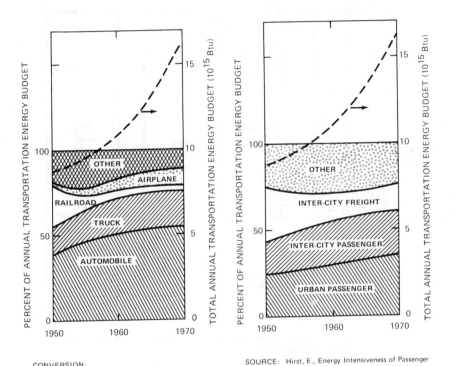

SOURCE: Hirst, E., Energy Intensiveness of Passenger
and Freight Transport Modes, 1950-1970,
Oak Ridge National Laboratory, Report
ORNL-NSF-EP-44, April 1973.

CONVERSION:

1 BTU = 1055 HOULE

Figure 15-25. Distribution of transportation energy by mode.

Figure 15-26. Distribution of transportation energy by purpose.

As suggested by Figure 15-28, the energy consumption rate of the vehicle appears to be closely correlated to vehicle weight: the larger the vehicle, the greater the rate. This relationship is more clearly illustrated in Figure 15-29. However, fuel consumption is not directly proportional to vehicle weight alone: a rapid-rail vehicle weighs 20 times more than a standard auto but only consumes 6 times more energy. Also, the weight ratio of a bus and auto are 5 to 1 but the fuel consumption ratio is 3 to 1. Fuel consumption is also a function of design characteristics, such as wheel type (rubber vs steel) or aerodynamic drag qualities, and is very much a function of duty cycle. A rapid-rail vehicle averages

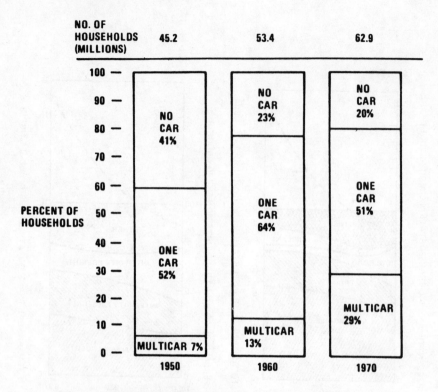

Source: W. E. Fraize et al., Energy and Environments Aspects of U.S. Transportation, MTP-391, February 1974.

Figure 15-27.   Automobile ownership by U.S. households.

one stop per mile, whereas a transit bus averages more than four stops per mile. An automobile stops an average 2.4 times per mile, as suggested by the Federal Urban Driving Cycle. Barring bad data or improper interpretation of existing data, the difference in duty cycles is probably responsible for the difference in energy consumption of the transit bus and trolley bus, which are of equal weight.

As discussed previously, energy consumption per vehicle mile and the number of passengers per vehicle are important when determining the efficiency of the various urban ground transportation modes. Figure 15-30 graphically portrays the relationship between the energy rate and passenger load. Lines of constant energy rate per vehicle mile and of constant passenger load are superimposed on lines of energy required per passenger load. The energy rates of the various modes are shown on bars along lines on constant energy rate per vehicle mile. The bars for each mode

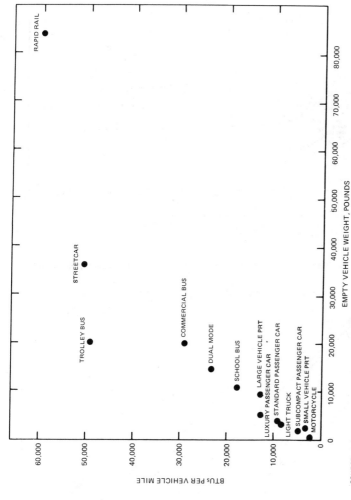

SOURCE: J. G. Lieb, A Comparative Analysis of the Energy Consumption
for Several Urban Passenger Ground Transportation Systems,
The MITRE Corporation, MTR-6606, February 1974.

Figure 15-28. Energy consumption and vehicle weight (vehicle-mile basis).

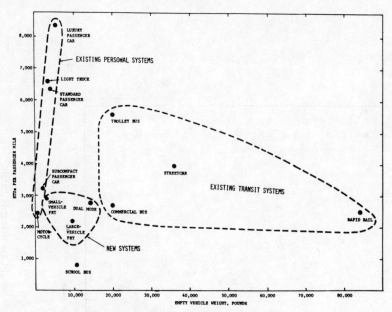

Source: J. G. Lieb; A Comparative Analysis of the Energy Consumption for Several
Urban Passenger Ground Transportation Systems, The MITRE Corporation,
MTR-6606, February 1974.

Figure 15-29. Energy consumption and vehicle weight (passenger mile basis).

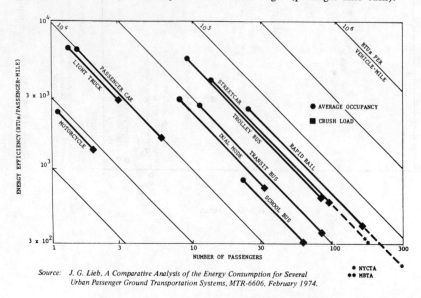

Source: J. G. Lieb, A Comparative Analysis of the Energy Consumption for Several
Urban Passenger Ground Transportation Systems, MTR-6606, February 1974.

Figure 15-30. Composite energy consumption rates.

extend from the energy rate with an average occupancy to the energy rate with a crush load. The chart illustrates that mass transit vehicles with crush load occupancy rates are significantly more efficient than existing personal modes, such as the passenger car; with low occupancy rates, mass transit is significantly less efficient.

A detailed analysis of transporation energy consumption, again for 1970, is given by Table 15-14, which presents not only the energy consumption for each mode, but the useful transport work (passenger miles), the load factor and the energy intensiveness (Btu/pass. mi, or Btu/ton mi). Energy intensiveness is the energy consumed per unit of useful transport work (passenger miles or ton miles), and is, therefore, inversely related to a transport mode's efficiency. The values in the table represent the exercising of the authors' judgment on the range of values presented by the data sources listed on the table.

Table 15-15 looks in more detail at the automobile, presenting energy intensiveness and the breakdowns of fuel consumption and travel (number of trips, vehicle miles and passenger miles) according to trip purpose. The energy intensiveness and % fuel consumed are based on the fuel economies assumed for each trip purpose.

The energy intensiveness for the various automobile-type purposes is displayed graphically in Figure 15-31. The least efficient (most energy-intensive) use of the automobile is in commuting, primarily because of the low load factor (1.4 occupants per car, as noted in parentheses on the figure).

On the other hand, social and recreational trips, with nearly double the load factor of commuting trips, constitute the more efficient use of the automobile. In fact, for long distance intercity vacation trips at an average occupancy of 3.3 persons per car, the automobile is less energy-intensive than intercity rail; however, intercity bus still offers an energy savings of a factor of two over automobile vacation trips. Of course, those who travel by automobile at a full loading of six occupants per standard-sized car can nearly match the energy performance of intercity buses which, as noted in Table 10, travel with an average load of only 22 passengers per vehicle (approximately half full).

To compare the energy consumption rate and efficiency of various transportation modes, quantitative measures must be defined and evaluated. Five measures appear to be useful, and energy is measured in Btus in each measure. The measures are:

1. Btus per vehicle mile (Btu/vm),
2. Btus per seat mile (Btus/sm),
3. Btus per full-load mile (Btus/flm),
4. Btus per crush-load mile (Btus/clm), and
5. Btus per passenger-mile (Btus/pm).

Table 15-14. U.S. Transportation Energy (1970) (Fraize et al., 1974)

Mode		Transport Work (pass. mi or ton mi)	Load Factor	Energy Intensiveness (Btu/pass. mi or Btu/ton mi) (At current load factor)	Energy Consumption (10^{15} Btu) Subtotals	Energy Consumption (10^{15} Btu) Additive Totals
Passenger Service						
Auto: Urban		0.69×10^{12}	1.4 pass./veh.	7,550 (12.1 mpg)	5.2	
Intercity		1.04	2.5	3,250 (16.0 mpg)	3.4	
(Small cars)	Alternate	(0.27	1.9	3,220 (21.2 mpg)	(0.87)	
(Standard & compact cars)	Breakdown	1.46)	1.9	5,300 (12.9 mpg)	(7.73)	
Auto Mode		1.73	1.9	4,980 (13.6 mpg)	8.6	8.6
Light Truck		0.08	1.4	9,000 (10.1 mpg)		0.72
Air: Short haul (<500 mi)		0.018		12,200	0.22	
Long haul (>500 mi)		0.101		8,720	0.88	
Air Mode		0.119	49%	9,300	1.10	1.10
Bus: Urban		0.017	10 pass./veh.	2,940 (4.4 mpg)	0.05	
Intercity		0.028	22	1,070 (5.5 mpg)	0.03	
School		0.052	25	770 (6.75 mpg)	0.04	
Bus Mode		0.097	19.2	1,240 (5.5 mpg)	0.12	0.12
Rail: Urban		0.007	25%	4,300	0.03	
Intercity		0.011	37%	2,730	0.03	
Rail Mode		0.018		3,330	0.06	0.06
All Passenger Service		2.044×10^{12} pass mi		5,250 Btu/pass mi		10.6

Freight Service		Alternate Breakdown	1.09 ton mi/veh. mi	10,650 Btu/ton mi	
Truck: Single units	0.15		1.09 ton mi/veh. mi	10,650 Btu/ton mi	1.6
Combinations (Motor Carrier	0.35	(0.39)	9.21	3,440	1.2
Private Truck)		0.11			
					2.8
Truck Mode	0.50		2.63	5,600	2.8
Rail	0.77			675	0.52
Air	0.004			37,500	0.15
Pipeline	0.43			420	0.18
Waterway	0.60			750	0.45
All Freight Service	2.304×10^{12} ton mi			1,780 Btu/ton mi	4.1
Other					
General Aviation					0.10
Recreational Vehicles					0.20
Military					1.5
Total Transportation					16.5

Conversion: 1 Btu = 1,055 Joule; 1 ton = 907.2 kg; 1 mile = 1.62 km; 1 ton mile = 1,470 mg km; 1 Btu/pass mi = 650 joule/pass km; 1 Btu/ton mi = .717 joule/kg km.

Table 15-15. Automobile Usage and Efficiency—by Trip Purpose (1970)
(Fraize et al., 1974; Motor Vehicle Manufacturers' Association, 1972)

Trip Purpose	Average Trip Length (One Way)	Average Occupancy	Assumed Fuel Consumption	% Trip	% Vehicle Miles	Passenger Miles	% Fuel Consumed	Energy Intensiveness (Btu/Pass. mi)
Earning a Living								
To & from work	9.4 ml	1.4 pass/veh	13.0 mpg	32.3	34.1	24.0	35.6%	7400
Related business	16.0	1.6	16.0	4.4	8.0	6.4	6.9	5370
	10.2	1.4	13.4	36.7	42.1	30.4	42.5	6970
Family Business								
Medical & dental	8.3	2.1	13.5	1.8	1.6	1.8	1.6	4430
Shopping	4.4	2.0	11.5	15.4	7.6	8.0	9.0	5600
Other	6.5	1.9	12.5	14.2	10.4	10.4	11.3	5400
	5.5	2.0	12.1	31.4	19.6	20.2	21.9	5390
Educational/Civic/Religious	4.7	2.5	11.5	9.4	5.0	6.6	6.0	4530
Social/Recreational								
Vacations	165.1	3.3	18.0	0.1	2.5	4.1	1.9	2310
Visits to friends & relatives	12.0	2.3	15.0	9.0	12.2	14.2	11.0	3860
Pleasure rides	19.6	2.7	16.0	1.4	3.1	4.2	2.7	3200
Other	11.4	2.6	15.0	12.0	15.5	20.3	14.0	3440
	13.1	2.5	15.3	22.5	33.3	42.8	29.6	3450
All Trips	8.9	1.9	13.6	100.0	100.0	100.0	100.0	4980

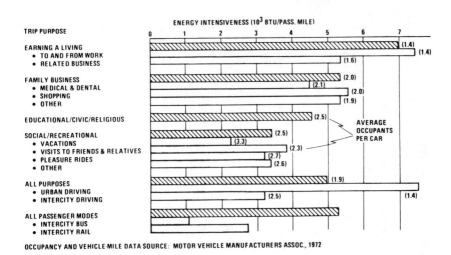

OCCUPANCY AND VEHICLE-MILE DATA SOURCE: MOTOR VEHICLE MANUFACTURERS ASSOC., 1972

Figure 15-31. Automobile energy intensiveness—by trip purpose.

"Btus per vehicle mile" is the average fuel consumption rate required to propel the vehicle through its daily duty cycle and power its accessories. The other four measures are indications of the efficiency of the modes while performing the desired function—transport of people.

Btus per passenger mile is a measure of the efficiency of the transportation mode with an average passenger occupancy that represents either actual experience or, in the case of the new systems, the expected average occupancy. Average occupancy is defined as the total annual passenger miles divided by the total annual vehicle miles. This measure is the best indication of the efficiency of existing transportation modes as they are currently performing. But many of the proposed energy conservation options are directed toward increasing the average occupancy (*e.g.*, car-pooling). Hence, the other measures that reflect potential efficiency are useful. The three measures of the potential efficiency of the modes were calculated by assuming that the occupancy of the vehicle is the maximum possible within three comfort categories: all passengers seated, all seats occupied and comfortable standees, and all seats occupied and a crush load of standees. The results are shown in Tables 15-16 and 15-17 and Figure 15-32.

The last charts (Figure 15-33 and 15-34, and Table 15-18) are proposed as a model on how to appropriate transportation environmental assessment. They are taken from a study on the 55-mph limit (Doherty, 1975).

Table 15-16. 1971 Urban Passenger Ground Transportation Energy Consumption (Lieb, 1974)

	Passenger Car	Light Truck	Motorcycle	Commercial Bus	Rapid Rail	Streetcar	Trolley Bus	School Bus	Total
Vehicle Mileage, miles x 10^6 (% of total)	516,506.0 (94.662)	18,179.0 (3.332)	8,279.0 (1.517)	1,767.0 (0.324)	407.4 (0.075)	32.7 (0.006)	30.8 (0.006)	429.0 (0.079)	545,630.9 (100%)
Energy Source	Gasoline	Gasoline	Gasoline	Diesel Oil	Electricity	Electricity	Electricity	Gasoline	
Fuel Consumption, gallons, 10^6	42,686.0 (95.453)	1,377.0 (3.078)	186.0 (0.416)	401.6 (0.898)	NA	NA	NA	69.2 (0.155)	44,719.0 (100%)
Electricity Consumption, kWh 10^6	NA	NA	NA	NA	2,262 88.498	153 5,986	141 5.516	NA	2,556 (100%)
Total Energy Consumption, Btus, 10^12	4,972.92 (94.935)	155.76 (2.973)	21.67 (0.414)	52.13 (0.995)	24.51 (0.468)	1.66 (0.032)	1.53 (0.029)	8.06 (0.154)	5,238.24 (100%)
Petroleum-Based Energy Consumption, Btus, 10^12	4,972.92 (95.369)	155.76 (2.987)	21.67 (0.415)	52.13 (1.000)	3.43[a] (0.066)	0.23[a] (0.004)	0.21[a] (0.004)	8.06 (0.155)	5,241.41 (100%)

[a]Assuming 14% of fuel used to generate electricity is petroleum based.

Table 15-17. Urban Passenger Ground Transportation Energy Consumption Rates (Lieb, 1974)

	Existing Modes								New Systems		
	Passenger Car	Light Truck	Motor-cycle	Commercial Bus	Rapid Rail	Street Car	Trolley Bus	School Bus	Large-Vehicle PRT	Small-Vehicle PRT	Dual Mode
Btus/vm	9,600	8,600	2,600	29,400	60,200	50,800	49,700	18,800	13,200	3,500	23,500
Btus/sm	1,600	2,900	1,300	600	1,000	1,400	1,000	300	1,100	900	1,200
Btus/flm	1,600	2,900	1,300	400	500	700	700	300	700	900	800
Btus/clm	1,600	2,900	1,300	400	400	600	600	300	500	900	700
Btus/pm	6,400	6,600	2,400	2,700	2,500	3,900	5,520	800	2,200	2,900	2,800

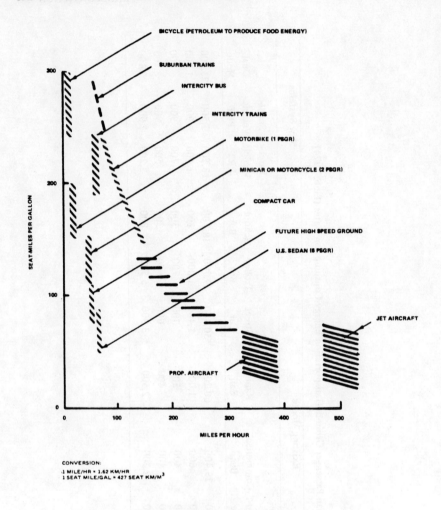

Source: Nutter, R. D., A Perspective of Transportation Fuel Economy, The MITRE Corporation, MTP-396, March 1974.

Figure 15-32. Modal comparison of fuel economy.

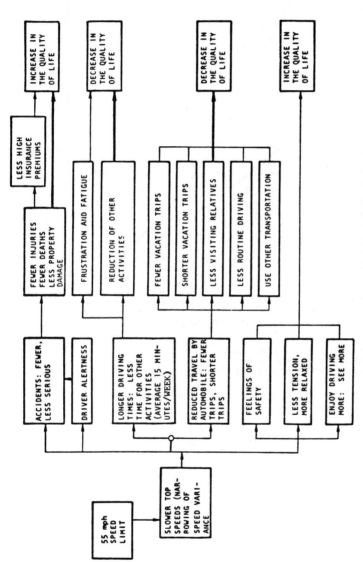

Source: M. G. Doherty et al., Policy Assessment of the 55 Miles Per Hour Speed Limit, The MITRE Corporation, MTR-6966, July 1975.

Figure 15-33. Causal path flow diagram of the direct and significant impacts on individuals.

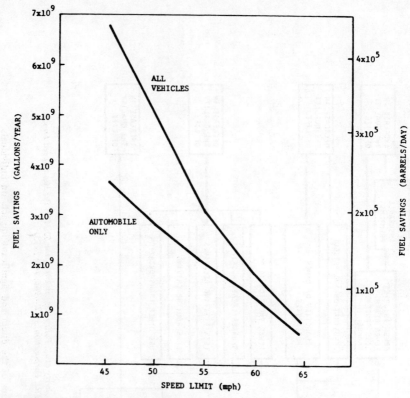

Source: *M. G. Doherty et al., Policy Assessment of the 55 Miles Per Hour Speed Limit, The MITRE Corporation, MTR-6966, July 1975.*

Figure 15-34. Theoretical motor vehicle fuel savings.

Table 15-18. Summary Table of Social Impact Analysis (Doherty et al., 1975)[a]

Event	First-Order Consequences A	Second-Order Consequences B	Third-Order Consequences C	Fourth-Order Consequences D	Fifth-Order Consequences E
1		Fewer injuries	Reevaluation of Car Insurance premium rates	Savings to consumers	
2 Fewer accidents		Fewer deaths 1C	Lower life insurance Premiums	Savings to consumers	
3		Less property damage	Less business for body shops	Savings to consumers	
4 Reduced Travel by automobile	Fewer vacation trips	Resort and tourist industry decline	Slowed development in resort areas	Better planning of Resort area developments	
5 55-mph Speed Limit and Lower Top Speeds	Shorter distance vacation trips	Expansion of close-by tourism	Possible increase or initiation of mass transit to close-by tourist attractions	Reduced attractiveness of close-by tourist	Development of additional close-by tourist attraction
6	Less visiting of relatives	Weakening of family ties	Increase isolation of the elderly		
7	Less routine driving	Slight decline in entertainment and sales	Fewer shopping centers located near speedways	Increased sense of community	
8	Shift to airplane or train	Greater profits for airlines and railroads	Smaller increases in fares	Savings to consumers	
9 Longer Driving Times	Reduced 10B time for other activities	Reduced leisure activities	Increased family tensions 10B		
10	Frustration and fatigue 8A	Increased family tensions	Greater hostility expressed in other relationships		
11 Psychological Impacts	Less tension, more relaxed	Less hurried lifestyle 25A			
12	Feelings of safety	Driving used less for agressive tension release	Fewer accidents 2A		

Table 15-18, continued

Event	First-Order Consequences A	Second-Order Consequences B	Third-Order Consequences C	Fourth-Order Consequences D	Fifth-Order Consequences E
13	Enjoy driving more because sees more 25A	Increases leisurely pleasure driving	Reeuced gasoline savings 15A		
14	Driver alertness	Fewer accidents 2A			
15	Gasoline savings	Shorter gas lines More heating fuel	Less-severe energy shortages	More driving, higher driving speeds	Accidents increase 2A
16	Impact on Trucking Industry	Longer delivery times, *i.e.,* reduced productivity 17B	Longer separation from family - interrupts drivers' rest stop patterns	Truckers complain and strike	Economic losses to food industries/food shortages and higher food prices	Losses to consumers
17	Regearing Trucks	Increased trucking costs 16C	Higher trucking rates	Higher prices	
18	Clustering	Slows highway traffic	Frustration and fatigue 10A		
19	Impact on Bus Companies	Schedule changes			
20		Reduced productivity	Higher fares	Losses to consumers	
21	Impact on Automobile Industry	Increases demand for smaller cars	Steel, energy, etc. savings 23B	Gasoline savings 15A	
22		Engine redesign to be efficient at lower cruising s speed	Longer-lasting engines	Fewer new cars sold 23B	
23		Reduced production	Reduced profits and employment	Economic decline in Detroit	

55-mph Speed Lmit and Lower Top Speeds

55-mph Speed Limit and the Same Top Speeds	24	Value Changes	Increase conservation values 25A	Drive slower and save Gas and many other effects
	25		Less hurried lifestyle 24A	Save energy, greater emphasis on personal relationships	Improved family relationships 10B
	26	Increased workload for enforcement personnel	More citations given	Increased workload for courts
	27		Increased employment for highway patrols	More police cars and radar units
	28	Less respect for the law	Lower status for patrolman	

LEGEND: Alpha numerics in the table refer the reader to other cells of the matrix for additional impacts. Not all orders of impacts have been explicitly covered in the analysis.

REFERENCES

Federal Railroad Administration. "Accident Bulletin," in *A United States Railroad Trust Fund* (1974).

American Association of State Highway Officials. "A Policy on Geometric Design of Rural Highways," Washington, D.C. (1965).

Bellis, E.D., and H. B. Graves. "Der   Mortality on a Pennsylvania Interstate Highway," *J. Wildlife Managem.* 35 (2):232-237 (1971).

Bisselle, C. A. *Preliminary Assessment of Empty Miles Traveled by Selected Regulated Motor Carriers* MTR-7081 (McLean, VA: The MITRE Corp., 1976).

Boeing Commercial Airplane Co. "Passenger Origin–Destination Data," *Aviation Week* (October 28, 1974), p. 119.

Doherty, M. G., J. L. Pfeffer, B. B. Stokes and H. W. Williams. *Policy Assessment of the 55 Miles per Hour Spped Limit,* MTR 6966 (McLean, VA: The MITRE Corp., 1975).

Council on Environmental Quality. "Environmental Quality," (August 1972).

Fraize, W. E., P. Dyson and S. W. Gouse. *Energy and Environmental Aspects of U.S. Transportation,* MTP-391 (McLean, VA: The MITRE Corporation, 1974).

Fraize, W. E. *A Program Plan of Policy-Oriented Research for Transportation Energy Conservation,* MTR-6843 (McLean, VA: The MITRE Corp., 1975).

Guy, H. P. "An Overview of Non-Point Water Pollution from the Urban Suburban Area," in *Non-Point Sources of Resources Research Center,* Blacksburg, VA (1975).

Harris, R. M., J. W. F. Mason, W. L. McCade, R. H. Winslow and C. A. Zraket. *U.S. Transportation–A Summary Appraisal,* M75-22, (McLean, VA: The MITRE Corp., 1975).

Hirst, E. "Energy Intensiveness of Passenger and Freight Transport Modes, 1950-1970," Oak Ridge National Laboratory, Report ORNL-NSF-EP-44 (April 1973).

Lieb, J. G. *A Comparative Analysis of the Eer   Consumption for Several Urban Passenger Ground Transportation Systems,* MTR-6606 (McLean, VA: The MITRE Corp., 1974).

Motor Vehicle Manufacturers Association of the U.S., Inc. "1972 Automobile Facts and Figures" (1972).

National Highway Traffic Safety Administration. "Highway Fatality Statistics" (December 1974).

Nutter, R. D. *A Perspective of Transportation Fuel Economy,* MTP-396 (McLean, VA: The MITRE Corp. 1974).

Oxley, D. J., M. B. Fenton and G. R. Carmondy. "The Effects of Roads on Populations of Small Mammals," *J. Appl. Ecol.* II(a):51-59 (1974).

Transportation, U.S. Department of. "Summary of National Transportation Statistics" (1974).

INDEX

acid-base characteristics   705
agricultural materials, open burning
    of   291
agricultural systems   610-612
air quality   258,277
    control regions   294,308
    Also see ambient air quality
air transportation   819-824
aircraft   254,256
    disturbances to wildlife   517
    landing-takeoff cycle   286
    noise   156,255,257,509
    noise levels   518,519
    supersonic   256
Alaska   670
ambient air quality   171
    modeling   171,174
    monitoring   78
animal unit equivalent   611,612
aquatic ecosystem   613,614
aquatic life
    freshwater   447
    marine   251,446
    Also see fish
atmospheric diffusion particle in
    cell   188
autooxidation   705

backdune   669
Batelle Environmental Evaluation
    System   39
Batelle Hierarchical System   39

beach and dune succession
    665-669
    primary dune   665
    colonization   667
    trough   668
Bibliographic Computerized
    Systems   133
bioaccumulation   706
bioconcentration   701,706
biomagnification   706
biomes   602
    eastern   682-688
    forest   670,687
    grassland   689,692
    northern   670,687,688
    representatives   678-680
    sagebrush   696
    southern   682
    steppe   696
    tropical   676-681
    tundra   673
    western   688-697
birds   629
black spruce forest   672
brush regrowth   671
bulk effect   718
butterflies   627

C values   567
California   636
chemicals
    control   700

effects of 717-729
entry into environment   701,
    702
movement   703,704
process industry   279
risk to marine biota   482
stability   704-708
toxicity   708-716
coal
    anthracite combustion   280
    resources, U.S.   777,779,780,
        791,801
coastal
    resources   250,251
    salt meadow   671
    shallow fresh marsh   676
Coastal Zone Management Act
    252,270
Colorado   637
combustion sources   278
Committee Prints   250
Commonwealth Environmental
    Analysis System   40
community development   737,739
    cost analysis   739
    expanding population factors
        740
    recreational needs and   741
condenser cooling   496
Connecticut   637
construction equipment   281
    noise   507,508
cooling tower plume models   159,
    162
Council on Environmental Quality
    (CEQ) Guidelines   4,11,12
Cross Impact Matrix   48
crude oil
    See oil

data
    collection   16
    retrieval and information services,
        federal   81,84,88-92
    sources on water resources   434

systems, energy   97,99,104,
    115,118-126
data banks
    specimen   130-143
    toxic chemical   96-130
data bases
    environmental   78ff
    environmental radiation ambient
        monitoring system and
        78,96
Delphi technique   34,35
dune
    back-   699
    building   667
    primary   665
    stabilization   668
    Also see beach and dune
        succession

earthquake   580,584,586,588
    risk   584,585
    shaking hazards   586
    water requirements   496
eastern biomes   682
ecosystem productivity rates
    603-608
effluent guidelines   451
emission factors   277,278,280-
    291
endangered species   618,619,632,
    636
ENDEX   145
energy
    consumption, worldwide   798
    international issues   792-808
    models   147
    nuclear   805
    resources   775-791
    solar   791
    supply and demand   768-774
    transportation and   791,792,
        831-857
environmental assessment   12-57
    cost/benefit analysis   31-33
    method selection   26-28
    techniques   28-57

environmental data services   74
environmental impact statement
    (EIS)   241,249,250
Environmental Protection Agency
    Environmental Radiation Ambient
        Monitoring System   95
    National Emission Report   317-
        439
    Numerical Water Quality Criteria
        445-447
    regulations under consideration
        258
    Water Quality Data (STORET)
        432
evaporation loss sources   279
everglade hammock   680
explosion, underwater—effects   483,
    484,487,488,492

FAA   255-257
factor analysis   37
federal regulations   243,250,253
    Also see Environmental Protec-
        tion Agency
FHWA   253
fires   568,578,579,581,671
    forest, succession   670-677
First National Bank v Richardson
    11
fish   616,619,627,628
    effect of pollution on   710,713
    spawning requirements of   489
fish production   617
    and wildlife   251,252
fishery and stream habitat flow
    438
Florida   638
food and agricultural industry   279
    chains   603-605
forest biome   687
    fire succession   670
FRA   254
Froude Number   216

generic assessment   15
geochemical cycles   718
geological maps   550
Georgia   639
goal matrix   48
goal structuring   38
grassland biome   689,692

hardwood forest   679
hearing loss   145,156,158
Hirst's Model   224
historic preservation offices   749-
    754
historic sites   745-749
HUD   255
hydrolysis   706

Illinois   643
impact
    allocation   25
    analysis   156
    determination   24
    integration   25
    measurement   25
    on wildlife   608
    quotient   39
    value function   54

jet models   218

K values   565
Kentucky   645

landmarks   145
Lattice Theory   41
LD_{50} 709
lead   258
Lexicographic ranking   41
lightning   583

lithium   804
Livermore Regional Air Quality
    Model   189
Louisiana   647

mangrove forest   681
Maryland   647
mesophytic forest   686
metallurgical industry   279
meteorological effects   717
Michigan   647
mine, surface—reclamation   569
minerals   589,594
    production   279,592,596,598
    resources   594
    supply   596
Minnesota   648
Missouri   648
models
    air quality   171-190
    compartment   213
    complete field   222
    cooling tower plume   159-169
    elements   24
    far field   220
    jet   218
    Modified Prichard-Carpenter   217
    noise   153-159
    pollutants transport   191-214
    selection   215-217
    transportation   169-171
    water   189,192,196-198,200,202,
        208
    water thermal discharge   214-226
Montana   652
moot courts   48
Morningstar Renewal Council v AED
    19
morphological analysis   49
municipal waste, pollutant yield
    442
mutagenesis   709

National Ambient Air Quality
    Standards   278
National Environmental Policy
    Act   1,251
National Inventory of Recreational
    Facilities   143
national parks   145
natural gas   775-796,802
Negative Determination   10,15
NEPA Procedures   5
    Statutory Requirements   4-12
NESB survey   130-132
New Jersey   653
New York   654
nitrogen stream concentration
    444
NOAA   145,251
noise
    abatement   255,256
    aircraft   156,255,257,509,517-
        519
    audibility   487
    construction   505,507
    effects   158,510,512,516
    emission standards   254
    levels   506,512
    limits   518,519
    modeling   153
    railroad   254
    regulations   252,255
    sources   507
    standards   253,256,257
    state restrictions   520,522
    vehicular   508,520
    weapons   509
noise impact for various land uses
    514
    analysis   513,515
    index   154
North Carolina   655
North Dakota   655
northern biome   688
northern coniferous biome   687
northern spruce forest fire   670
nuclear energy   805
    fast breeder reactor   13

Ohio   655
oil
   and gas   252
   in the oceans   445
   international issues   792-808
   resources   775-797
Oklahoma   656
Oregon   657
Orlook Program   73
OSHA   257,258

palmetto prairie   683
partition coefficient   705,706
Pennsylvania   657
photolysis   704-706
pine scrub   683
pollutant material balance for water
   212
   model   189,191
   transport in soils   191

radiation   78
railroads
   See transportation
redox potential   705
relevance numbers   54
resource term glossary   776
Rhode Island   658
Richter Scale   589
river basin planning   251
   and harbors   250
RUSTIC   73

sagebrush biome   696
Scientists' Institute v The Atomic
   Energy Commission   13,
   21
sediment control systems   566,567
soil
   capability   555
   classification   556
   data   565
   erodibility factor   566

loss prediction method   568,
   578
orders   552
properties   559
surveys   557
types   560
Also see erosion
solar energy   791
sound level   512,514
   weighted population   154-157
   Also see noise
South Dakota   658
southern floodplain forest   682
   mixed forest biome   682
speech
   intelligibility   505
   interference   511
standard metropolitan statistical
   areas   (SMSA)   144
state codes   268,270,271,433
state mineral production   592
state noise restrictions   520,522
state numerical water quality
   standards   462
steam generators   258
   steppe biome   696
stream analysis   436,493
structural value analysis   52
sulfur dioxide   258
surface-mined area reclamation
   569
surface stabilizing treatment   567
surface water temperature
   isotherms   491

technology assessment   41
teratogenesis   709
terrestrial ecosystem   606
Texas   658
threshold limit value   709
   testing   56
topographical maps   549,550
toxicity   701,708,709,717
transportation
   affect on environment   828-831

air   819-824
automobiles   819,848
comparison: bus, rail, auto   828
energy and   791,792,831-857
equipment   253,258
intercity freight   815,824-826
intercity ground passenger   826-828,850,851
passenger   814,816-828
pollutants from   831,833
truck   827
urban   817-819
treaties   241,250
trend extrapolation   56
tropical biome   676-681
tundra biome   673

universal soil loss equation   597
uranium   787,788,804
urban runoff, pollutant yield   442
USDA Soil Conservation Service   555
U.S. Environmental Protection Agency
See Environmental Protection Agency
utility assessment   57
matrix   48

vehicular noise   508,520
Virginia   660
visual management system   754-764
volcanic activity   587,590,591

Washington   660
water
assessment process   431
coastal, biocides in   481
consumption requirements   495-499,502
models   189,192,196-198,200,202,208
navigable   250,252
resources   251,431,434
supply   445,448,450
thermal discharge   214
Water Bank Act   251
water quality   432,445,462
Water Resources Council   251
weapons noise   509
western biome   688
wetland   250,252
ecosystem   674
laws   270
wildlife
densitites   609
effects of noise on   517,520
Wisconsin   661
Wyoming   661